# Human Diseases

*SECOND EDITION*

# Human Diseases

DELMAR
CENGAGE Learning    Australia    Canada    Mexico    Singapore    Spain    United Kingdom    United States

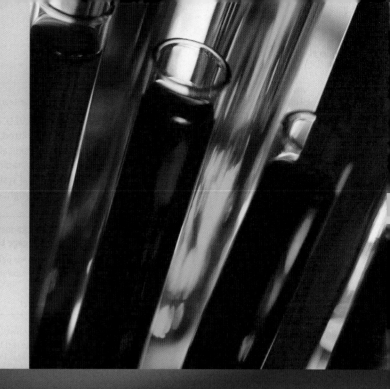

# MARIANNE NEIGHBORS, EdD, RN

**Professor**
**University of Arkansas**
**Eleanor Mann School of Nursing**
**Fayetteville, Arkansas**

# RUTH TANNEHILL-JONES, MS, RN

**Vice President-Patient Care Services**
**Chief Nurse Executive**
**St. Mary's—Mercy Health System NW Arkansas**

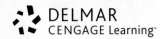

**DELMAR**
CENGAGE Learning™

**Human Diseases,**
**Second Edition**
**By Marianne Neighbors and**
**Ruth Tannehill-Jones**

Vice President,
Health Care Business Unit:
**William Brottmiller**

Editorial Director:
**Matthew Kane**

Acquisitions Editor:
**Marah Bellegarde**

Developmental Editor:
**Deb Flis**

Editorial Assistant:
**Jadin Babin-Kavanaugh**

Marketing Director:
**Jennifer McAvey**

Marketing Channel Manager:
**Tamara Caruso**

Marketing Coordinator:
**Michele Gleason**

Technology Director:
**Laurie Davis**

Technology Project Manager:
**Mary Colleen Liburdi**

Production Director:
**Carolyn Miller**

Production Manager:
**Barbara A. Bullock**

Art and Design Coordinator:
**Alexandros Vasilakos**

Production Coordinators:
**Jessica McNavich**
**Thomas Heffernan**

Project Editor:
**Ruth Fisher**

For product information and technology assistance, contact us at
**Cengage Learning Customer & Sales Support, 1-800-354-9706**

For permission to use material from this text or product,
submit all requests online at **cengage.com/permissions**
Further permissions questions can be emailed to
**permissionrequest@cengage.com**

ExamView® and ExamView Pro® are registered trademarks of FSCreations, Inc. Windows is a registered trademark of the Microsoft Corporation used herein under license. Macintosh and Power Macintosh are registered trademarks of Apple Computer, Inc. Used herein under license.

© 2007 Cengage Learning. All Rights Reserved. Cengage Learning WebTutor™ is a trademark of Cengage Learning.

Library of Congress Control Number: 2005049726

ISBN-13: 978-1-4018-7088-1

ISBN-10: 1-4018-7088-0

**Delmar Cengage Learning**
5 Maxwell Drive
Clifton Park, NY 12065-2919
USA

Cengage Learning products are represented in Canada by Nelson Education, Ltd.

For your lifelong learning solutions, visit **delmar.cengage.com**

Visit our corporate website at **www.cengage.com**

**Notice to the Reader**
Publisher does not warrant or guarantee any of the products described herein or perform any independent analysis in connection with any of the product information contained herein. Publisher does not assume, and expressly disclaims, any obligation to obtain and include information other than that provided to it by the manufacturer. The reader is expressly warned to consider and adopt all safety precautions that might be indicated by the activities described herein and to avoid all potential hazards. By following the instructions contained herein, the reader willingly assumes all risks in connection with such instructions. The publisher makes no representations or warranties of any kind, including but not limited to, the warranties of fitness for particular purpose or merchantability, nor are any such representations implied with respect to the material set forth herein, and the publisher takes no responsibility with respect to such material. The publisher shall not be liable for any special, consequential, or exemplary damages resulting, in whole or part, from the readers' use of, or reliance upon, this material.

Printed in China
7 8 9 10 11 12 11 10 09 08

***To my husband, Larry Butler,*** *my son Jeremy, my parents Louis and Lillian Zadra, and my super supportive sister, Marji Schwickrath. They are always there when I need inspiration and encouragement. I love you and thank you. Marianne*

***To my husband, Jim,*** *the quite solid, love of my life for over 30 years, and to the other man in my life, my brother Bob Tannehill, who has always loved and supported me "his younger, little sister." Ruth*

# Contents

## UNIT I
## Concepts of Human Disease                        1

### CHAPTER 1
### Introduction to Human Diseases                  2

### CHAPTER 2
### Mechanisms of Disease                           12

### CHAPTER 3
### Neoplasms                                       24

**UNIT II**
# Common Diseases and Disorders of Body Systems   61

**CHAPTER 5**
# Immune System Diseases and Disorders   62

**CHAPTER 6**
# Musculoskeletal System Diseases and Disorders   84

## UNIT III
# Genetic/Developmental, Childhood, and Mental Health Diseases and Disorders    363

## CHAPTER 19
## Genetic and Developmental Diseases and Disorders    364

## CHAPTER 20
## Childhood Diseases and Disorders    386

**CHAPTER 21**

# Mental Health Diseases and Disorders   406

**APPENDIX A:**

**APPENDIX B:**

**APPENDIX C:**

**APPENDIX D:**

**APPENDIX E:**

# List of Tables

As the medical field has undergone an explosion in new techniques and therapies, there has been a matched explosion in the need for technicians, patient care providers, and general health care professionals to support this growth. These new and developing careers assist and support physicians in a variety of health care settings. These health professionals include nurses, medical assistants, nursing assistants, surgical technologists, respiratory therapy assistants, physical therapy assistants, radiographic technologists, medical transcriptionists, medical office assistants, and emergency medical technicians, to name only a few.

## APPROACH

Many pathophysiology books have been written to address the informational needs of the medical community, but few basic disease textbooks exist for the benefit of the health care professional. This book has been designed and written specifically for this group. It is intended to meet the needs of the student in the classroom as well as serve as a valuable resource for health care professionals on the job. In addition, this text may be used as a resource on basic diseases by anyone within the medical arena or lay community. Current information for this book was based on the authors' own experiences, and research sought from current literature, books, Internet resources, and physician consultations. Students will best understand this text if a basic medical terminology or anatomy and physiology course has been completed before this course of study.

Several dilemmas immediately emerge when one considers writing a textbook for such a large and diverse audience as the health care field. Questions arise as to how much content to include, what to exclude, how detailed the content should be, and how to organize the content in the most understandable manner. Another common concern is the question of the appropriate reading level.

In an attempt to resolve these dilemmas, it was decided to organize the book in such a way that blocks of material or even entire chapters could be omitted or covered in detail, depending on the format of the class and needs of the student. At the same time, information on each disease is written in such a way that it can "stand alone" or be viewed as all-inclusive. This concept allows the instructor, student, or individual to select and study only those specific diseases or individual disease of interest. Our intention also was to keep the reading level of the text at an easy-to-read basic level to promote understanding. We did not want to write beneath the level of the student but, at the same time, felt that a difficult reading level would only increase the complexity of the material and thus fail to promote understanding of the subject matter.

## ORGANIZATION OF THE TEXT

*Human Diseases*, Second Edition, consists of 21 chapters organized into three units. **Unit I**, Chapters 1 through 4, lays the foundation for some basic disease concepts, including mechanisms of disease, neoplasms, inflammation, and infection. **Unit II**, Chapters 5 through 18, is organized by body systems, and opens with a basic *Anatomy and Physiology* review of the system before discussion of the *Common System Diseases and Disorders*. Included with this discussion, where appropriate, are *Common Signs and Symptoms, Diagnostic Tests, Trauma,* and *Rare Diseases.* In addition, a unique section toward the end of each chapter discusses the *Effects of Aging* to help learners understand the natural aging process of the human body. **Unit III**, Chapters 19 through 21, includes specialty areas covering genetics, childhood diseases, and mental health disorders.

Several features were especially developed to promote learning and accessibility of information. Review the "How to Use This Book" on page xxiii for a detailed description and benefit of each feature.

## CHANGES TO THE SECOND EDITION

Major changes to the second edition include:

- Reorganization and delineation of Etiology, Symptoms, and Treatment headings and content so that each disease and disorder follows the same presentation

- **New** feature entitled "Glimpse of the Future" that details cutting-edge information or treatments

- **New** feature entitled "Complementary and Alternative Therapy" that discusses herbal and other nontraditional treatments

- Content on bio- and medical ethics was added

- Color photographs replaced many of the line drawings to enhance understanding of the diseases and disorders presented in the text

- Disease statistics were updated to reflect the latest statistics available

- The breast self-exam content and images in Chapter 5 were updated to reflect the American Cancer Society's most current recommendations. New figures were also added to display cancer data.

- Details about the emerging infection SARS was added to Chapter 9

- An additional Healthy Highlight on vitamins and vision was added to Chapter 16

- Updates on female hormone replacement therapy were added to Chapter 17

- Bibliographies for each chapter and the reference list were updated

- Quizzes and activities on the StudyWARE™ CD-ROM in the back of the book

- **New** accompanying workbook is available that offers learners additional practice with exercises corresponding to each chapter in the book.

## LEARNING SUPPLEMENTS

### *Human Diseases*, Second Edition, StudyWARE™

The StudyWARE™ CD-ROM offers an exciting way to enhance your learning of human diseases. The quizzes and activities are an interactive and engaging way to reinforce the content in the book. Review the "How to Use StudyWARE™ on page xxv for a detailed description of this component.

### Workbook

The workbook offers additional practice with exercises corresponding to each chapter in the book, including multiple choice, fill-in-the-blank, true/false, short answer, and matching questions.

## INSTRUCTOR TOOLS

A comprehensive package of instructor tools was designed to assist you in teaching the content.

### The Electronic Classroom Manager

The Electronic Classroom Manager is a robust CD-ROM that includes the following.

- **The Instructor's Manual** includes a sample course syllabus and outline as a guide for setting up a course. Additional materials for each chapter include detailed content outlines, learning objectives, expanded chapter summaries, discussion topics, learning activities, answers to the text review questions, answers to the workbook activities, and chapter tests with answer keys.

- **Correlation Guides** help you change previously developed curriculum to this text.

- **ExamView® Computerized Testbank** contains 1,000 questions. You can use these questions to create your own tests.

- **PowerPoint® Presentations** are designed to help you plan your class presentations. If a learner misses a class, a printout of the slides for a lecture makes a helpful review page.

## WebTUTOR™

Designed to complement the book, WebTUTOR™ is a content-rich, Web-based teaching and learning aid that reinforces and clarifies complex concepts. The WebCT™ and Blackboard™ platforms provide rich communication tools to instructors and learners, including a course calendar, chat, e-mail, and threaded discussions.

*Human Diseases*, 1e WebTUTOR™ on WebCT™, ISBN 0-7668-3946-X

Text Bundled with WebTUTOR™ on WebCT™, ISBN 1-4180-2479-1

*Human Diseases*, 1e WebTUTOR™ on Blackboard™, ISBN 0-7668-3948-6

Text Bundled with WebTUTOR™ on Blackboard™, ISBN 1-4180-2480-5

## ABOUT THE AUTHORS

Ruth Tannehill-Jones has been a Registered Nurse for over 20 years. She began her nursing education at the University of Arkansas, Fayetteville, with completion of an associate degree in nursing. Ms. Tannehill-Jones was not a newcomer to this campus, as she had previously completed a bachelor's degree in home economics some years earlier. On receiving her RN license, she worked at St. Mary-Rogers Memorial Hospital in the capacities of staff nurse, head nurse, and nursing supervisor. Other nursing experience includes assisting orthopedic surgeons while employed by Ozark Orthopedic and Sports Medicine Clinic located in the Northwest Arkansas area. Ms. Tannehill-Jones gained experience in education by working as an instructor of surgical technology while serving as the Divisional Chair of Nursing and Allied Health Programs at Northwest Technical Institute in Springdale, Arkansas. She obtained her bachelor's degree in nursing from Missouri Southern State College in Joplin and her master's degree in health service administration at Southwest Baptist University at Bolivar, Missouri. She is currently the Vice President of Patient Care Services, Chief Nurse Executive for St. Mary's–Mercy Health System of Northwest Arkansas.

Dr. Marianne Neighbors has been in nursing practice and nursing education for over 30 years. She received her bachelor's degree in nursing at Mankato State, a master's degree in health education at the University of Arkansas, a master's degree in nursing at the University of Oklahoma, and a doctoral degree in education with a focus on health science at the University of Arkansas. Dr. Neighbors has taught in associate degree nursing education for 18 years, focusing on medical/surgical nursing, and in baccalaureate nursing education for 9 years, focusing on health promotion and community health. She has coauthored several research articles, four medical/surgical nursing texts, along with two medical/surgical handbooks, a health assessment handbook, and a home health handbook. She is currently a Professor in the Eleanor Mann School of Nursing at the University of Arkansas, Fayetteville, Arkansas.

## ACKNOWLEDGMENTS

A special thanks goes out to all our colleagues, friends, and family members who have supported us throughout this project.

## Feedback from the User(s)

The authors would like to hear from instructors, learners, or anyone using the textbook about its strengths and/or suggestions for revisions. They are truly interested in making the textbook user-friendly and comprehensive but not too detailed or too in-depth for the reader. The authors want to know how the text is being used and what features are most helpful. Please feel free to forward comments to the authors via Delmar, Cengage Learning or directly by e-mail to Dr. Neighbors at *neighbo@uark .edu* and Ms. Tannehill-Jones at *rjonesnwark@ hotmail.com*.

*Marianne Neighbors, EdD, RN*
*Ruth Tannehill-Jones, MS, RN*

We would like to thank all of the reviewers who have been an invaluable resource in guiding this book as it has evolved. Their insights, comments, suggestions, and attention to detail were extremely important in developing this textbook.

**Kathrine Ivester, CMA, CLS (NCA), MPA**
Director/Instructor, Medical Assisting Program
North Georgia Technical College
Clarkesville, Georgia

**Rosemary C. Johnson, RN (retired), MSPA, FHFMA**
Instructor, Medical Assisting Department
Goodwin College
East Hartford, Connecticut

**Jacqueline J. Jones, RHIA**
Instructor, Health Information Technology
Delgado Community College
New Orleans, Louisiana

**Pamela S. McLaughlin**
Instructor, Life Science & Health Science Division
Harper College
Palatine, Illinois

**Bess Porter, BS, RHIA**
Instructor, Health Information Systems
St. Phillip's College
San Antonio, Texas

**Linda Scarborough, RN, CMA, CPC, BSM**
Director, Health Care Management Technology Program
Lanier Technical College
Gainesville, Georgia

**Pamela K. Terry, PhD, CHES, CADP**
Associate Professor, Community Health & Health Services Management
Western Illinois University
Macomb, Illinois

*Human Diseases,* Second Edition, helps you learn basic disease information. The following features are integrated throughout the book to assist you in learning and mastering human disease core concepts and terms.

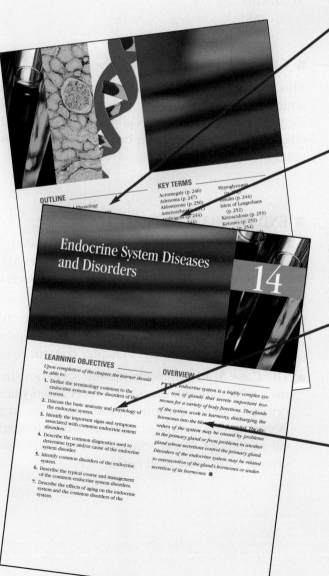

### ■ OUTLINE

The content outline provides you with an overview of concepts you will learn by presenting the major topics in the chapter.

### ■ KEY TERMS

A list of key terms at the beginning of each chapter references the page number where each term can be found within the text. Turn to the page to understand the term used in context; turn to the glossary for the term definition. Within the text, the term is highlighted in color for easy identification.

### ■ LEARNING OBJECTIVES

The learning objectives alert you to concepts you should understand after reading the chapter and completing the review questions.

### ■ OVERVIEW

The overview provides a snapshot of the core concepts you will learn about in the chapter.

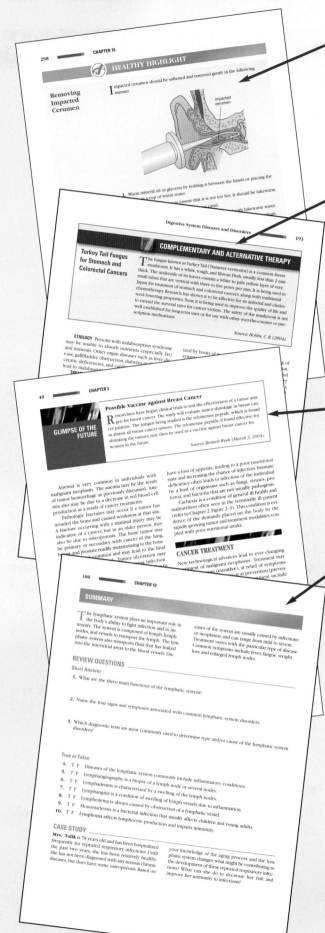

### ■ HEALTHY HIGHLIGHT

Healthy Highlights include tips for health promotion and disease prevention. They are presented to help learners more fully understand how they, as health professionals, can help promote healthy living for themselves and their patients.

### ■ COMPLEMENTARY AND ALTERNATIVE THERAPY

This **new** feature highlights information about treatments or special therapies that have research-based evidence of success. These therapies are being used by consumers of health care and health care practitioners, either in combination with traditional therapy and medicines or as an alternative to traditional treatments.

### ■ GLIMPSE OF THE FUTURE

This **new** feature focuses on new procedures, medicines, or therapies that are presently being tested for usefulness in medical regimens. These cutting-edge treatments might soon be commonplace therapies.

### ■ END OF CHAPTER FEATURES

■ The **Summary** is a succinct textual conclusion of basic chapter concepts. This differs from the overview because it consolidates the material rather than highlighting basic ideas.

■ **Review Questions** reinforce material learned by testing comprehension through structured questions that directly relate to chapter content.

■ The **Case Study** presents real-life scenarios that may occur in health care situations. Learners think critically about questions posed to arrive at a deeper understanding of the effects of pathological conditions. These scenarios often delve into critical ethical and legal issues.

# How to Use StudyWARE™

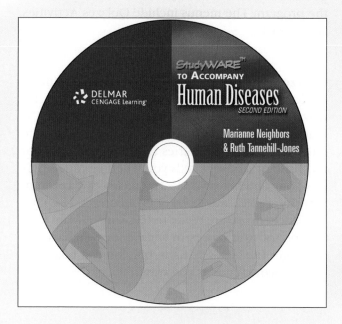

## ■ MINIMUM SYSTEM REQUIREMENTS

- Operating System: Microsoft Windows 98 SE, Windows 2000, or Windows XP
- Processor: Pentium PC 500 MHz or higher (750 Mhz recommended)
- RAM: 64 MB of RAM (128 MB recommended)
- Screen Resolution: 800 x 600 pixels
- Color Depth: 16-bit color (thousands of colors)
- Macromedia Flash Player V7.x. (The Macromedia Flash Player is free and can be downloaded from http://www.macromedia.com.)

## ■ INSTALLATION INSTRUCTIONS

1. Insert disk into CD-ROM player. The *Human Diseases*, Second Edition, StudyWARE™ installation program should start up automatically. If it does not, go to step 2.
2. From My Computer, double-click the icon for the CD drive.
3. Double-click the *setup.exe* file to start the program.

## ■ TECHNICAL SUPPORT

Telephone: 1-800-648-7450, 8:30 A.M.–5:30 P.M. Eastern Time

Fax: 1-518-881-1247

E-mail: delmar.help@cengage.com

StudyWARE™ is a trademark used herein under license. Refer to the license agreement in the back of the book following the index.

## ■ GETTING STARTED

The StudyWARE™ software will help you learn core concepts and terms in *Human Diseases*, Second Edition. As you study each chapter in the text, be sure to explore the activities in the corresponding chapter in the software. Use StudyWARE™ as your own private tutor to help you learn the material in the text.

Getting started is easy. Install the software by inserting the CD-ROM into your computer's CD-ROM drive and following the on-screen instructions. When you open the software, enter your first and last name so that the software can store your quiz results. Then choose a chapter from the menu to take a quiz or explore one of the activities.

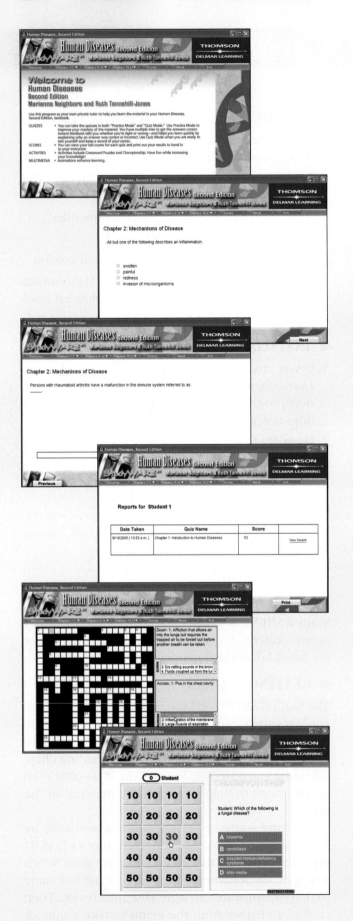

## ■ MENUS

You can access the menus from wherever you are in the program. The menus include Quizzes, Activities, and Scores.

**Quizzes.** Quizzes include fill-in-the-blank, multiple choice, and true/false questions. You can take the quizzes in both Practice Mode and Quiz Mode. Use Practice Mode to improve your mastery of the material. You have multiple tries to get the answers correct. Instant feedback tells you whether you're right or wrong and helps you learn quickly by explaining why an answer was correct or incorrect. Use Quiz Mode when you are ready to test yourself and keep a record of your scores. In Quiz Mode, you have one try to get the answers right, but you can take each quiz as many times as you want.

**Scores.** You can view your last scores for each quiz and print your results to hand in to your instructor.

**Activities.** Activities include crossword puzzles and a Jeopardy!-style Championship Game. Have fun while increasing your knowledge!

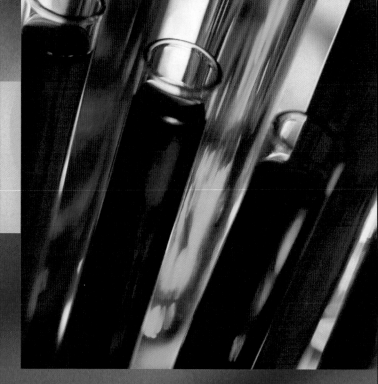

# Concepts of Human Disease

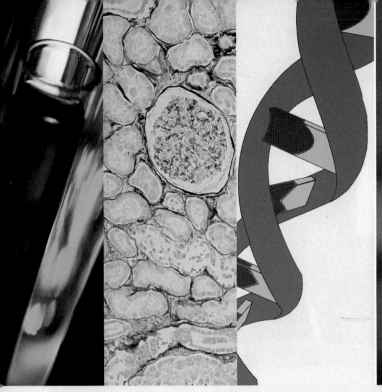
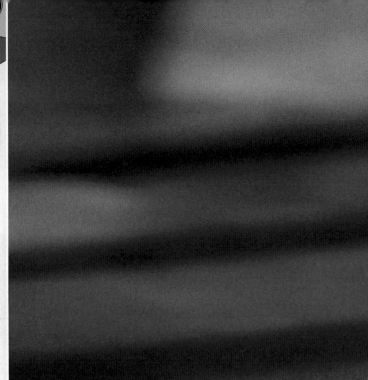

# OUTLINE

# KEY TERMS

# Introduction to Human Diseases

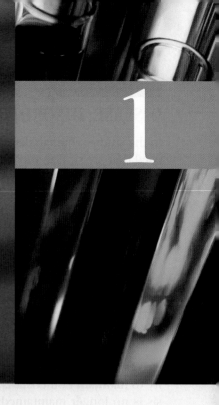

**1**

## LEARNING OBJECTIVES

*Upon completion of the chapter, the learner should be able to:*

1. Define basic terminology used in the study of human diseases.

2. Discuss the pathogenesis of disease.

3. Describe the Standard Precaution guidelines for disease prevention.

4. Identify the predisposing factors to human diseases.

5. Explain the difference between the diagnosis and prognosis of a disease.

6. Describe some common tests used to diagnose disease states.

## OVERVIEW

*The study of human diseases is important to understanding a variety of other topics in the health care field. Diseases that affect humans can range from mild to severe, and may be acute (short term) or chronic (long term). Some diseases affect only one part of the body or a particular body system, whereas others affect several parts of the body or body systems at the same time. There are many factors that influence the body's ability to stay healthy or predispose the body to a disease process. Some of these factors are controllable, but some are strictly related to heredity. Diseases can be diagnosed by professional health care providers using a variety of techniques and tests.* ∎

## DISEASE, DISORDER, AND SYNDROME

In the study of human disease, there are several terms used that are similar and often used interchangeably, but may not have the exact same definition. **Disease** may be defined in several ways. It may be called a change in structure or function within the body, which is considered to be abnormal, or it may be defined as any change from normal. It usually refers to a condition in which abnormal symptoms occur and a pathological state is present such as in pneumonia or leukemia. Both of these definitions have one underlying concept. That concept is the alteration of **homeostasis** (HOME-ee-oh-**STAY**-sis). Homeostasis is the state of sameness or normalcy that the body strives to maintain. The body is remarkable in its ability to maintain homeostasis, but once this homeostasis is no longer maintained, the body is diseased or "not at ease."

**Disorder** is defined as a derangement or abnormality of function. The term disorder can also refer to a pathological condition of the body or mind, but more commonly, is used to refer to a problem such as a vitamin deficiency (nutritional disorder). It is also used to refer to structural problems such as a malformation of a joint (bone disorder) or a condition where the term disease does not seem to apply such as dysphagia (swallowing disorder). Because disease and disorder are so closely related, they are often used synonymously.

The term **syndrome** (SIN-drome) refers to a group of symptoms, which may be caused by a specific disease but may also be caused by several interrelated problems. Examples include Tourette's syndrome, Down syndrome, and acquired immunodeficiency syndrome (AIDS), which are discussed later in the text.

## PATHOLOGY

**Pathology** (pah-THOL-oh-jee) can be broadly defined as the study of disease (patho = disease, ology = study). A **pathologist** (pah-THOL-oh-jist) is one who studies disease. Even a student studying diseases might be considered a pathologist using the strict definition of the word. There are many types of pathologists because there are numerous ways to study disease. One of the more commonly known pathologists is the surgical pathologist, who inspects

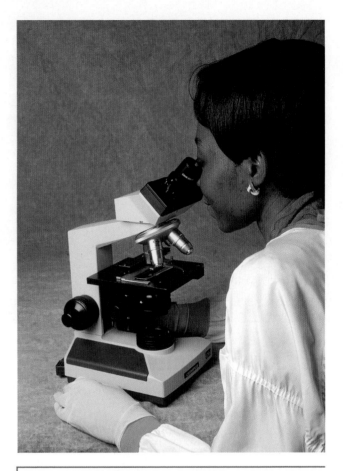

**FIGURE 1–1**  Pathologist looking through a microscope.

surgical tissue or biopsies for evidence of disease (Figure 1–1). The medical examiner or coroner may be a pathologist who studies human tissue to determine the cause of death and to provide evidence of criminal involvement in a death. Other types of pathologists are outlined in Table 1–1.

The prefix "patho" can be used in a variety of ways to describe disease processes or the disease itself. Microorganisms or agents that cause disease

**TABLE 1–1**  Types of Pathologists

| Pathologist | Role or Subject |
| --- | --- |
| Experimental | Research |
| Academic | Teaching |
| Anatomic | Clinical Examinations |
| Autopsy | Postmortem |
| Surgical | Biopsies |
| Clinical | Laboratory Examinations |
| Hematology | Blood |
| Immunology | Antigen/Antibodies |
| Microbiology | Microorganisms |

are called **pathogens** (PATH-oh-jens). These include bacteria, viruses, fungi, protozoans, and helminths (worms). All are pathogens that cause a pathogenic reaction. Fractures that are caused by a disease process that weakens the bone such as osteoporosis would be called **pathologic** (path-oh-LODGE-ick) fractures.

## PATHOGENESIS

The **pathogenesis** (PATH-oh-**JEN**-ah-sis; patho = disease, genesis = arising) is a description of how a particular disease progresses. Many of us are familiar with the pathogenesis of the common cold. A cold begins with an inoculation of the cold virus. This may occur following a simple handshake with someone who has a cold. Afterward, the target person may rub his or her eyes or nose, allowing entry of the virus into the body. After the inoculation period comes incubation time. During this period, the virus multiplies and the target person begins to have symptoms such as a runny nose and itchy eyes. The pathogenesis of the cold then moves into full-blown illness, usually followed by recovery and return to the previous state of health.

| TABLE 1–2 | Examples of Acute and Chronic Diseases |
|---|---|
| **Acute** | **Chronic** |
| Upper Respiratory Infections | Arthritis |
| Lacerations | Hypertension |
| Middle Ear Infections | Diabetes Mellitus |
| Gastroenteritis | Low Back Pain |
| Pneumonia | Heart Disease |
| Fractures | Asthma |

The pathogenesis of a disease may be explained in terms of time. An **acute** (a-CUTE) disease is short term and usually has a sudden onset. If the disease lasts for an extended period of time or the healing process is progressing slowly, it is classified as a **chronic** (KRON-ick) condition. See Table 1–2 for examples of acute and chronic diseases.

## ETIOLOGY

The **etiology** (EE-tee-OL-oh-jee) of a disease means the study of cause. The term etiology is commonly used to simply mean "the cause." One may say that

## HEALTHY HIGHLIGHT

**Hand Washing Technique**

To prevent the spread of disease between oneself and others, good and frequent hand washing is the best prevention. Follow the good hand washing steps listed below.

- Use an antimicrobial soap when possible. Have paper towels available to dry hands and to turn off the water.

- Adjust water temperature and force. Wet hands and wrists, and use a fingernail cleaner (if available) to gently clean under the nails on both hands, while holding hands under the running water.

- Apply a small amount of liquid soap. Work into a lather on wrists and hands. Briskly rub hands together, being sure to wash areas between fingers and around each wrist.

- Rinse well from fingertips to wrists. Be careful not to touch the sides of the basin.

- Dry each hand from fingertips to wrist using a paper towel. When finished, turn off the water using a paper towel as a barrier between the hands and the faucet.

- Discard soiled towels into the trash basket.

the cause is unknown or of "unknown etiology." The cause or etiology of pneumonia may be a virus or a bacterium. The etiology of athlete's foot is a fungus named *tinea pedis.* Another term used to mean the cause is unknown is **idiopathic** (ID-ee-oh-**PATH**-ick). If an individual is diagnosed as having idiopathic gastric pain, it means the cause of the pain in the stomach is unknown.

Other terms related to cause of disease are **iatrogenic** (eye-AT-roh-**JEN**-ick) and **nosocomial** (NOS-oh-**KOH**-me-al). Iatrogenic (iatro = medicine, physician, genic = arising from) means that the problem arose from a prescribed treatment. An example of an iatrogenic problem is the development of anemia in a patient undergoing chemotherapy treatments for cancer. Nosocomial is a closely related term. Nosocomial implies that the disease was acquired from a hospital environment. An example would be a postoperative patient developing an incisional staphylococcal infection. The best way to prevent nosocomial infections is through the practice of good hand washing. A good hand washing technique is described in the Healthy Highlight on the previous page.

## PREDISPOSING FACTORS

**Predisposing factors**, also known as risk factors, make a person more susceptible to disease. Predisposing factors are not the cause of the disease, and people with predisposing factors do not always develop the disease. These factors include age, sex, environment, lifestyle, and heredity. Some risk factors are controllable, such as lifestyle behaviors, whereas others, such as age, are not.

 **HEALTHY HIGHLIGHT**

**Standard Precautions**

The use of Standard Precautions is recommended by the Centers for Disease Control and Prevention for the care of all patients or when administering first aid to anyone.

- Hand washing—after touching blood and/or body fluids, even if gloves are worn; use an antimicrobial soap.

- Gloves—wear gloves when touching blood, body fluids, and contaminated items; change gloves after patient contact or contact with contaminated items; wash hands before and after.

- Eye wear, mask, and face shield—wear protection for the eyes, mouth, and face when doing procedures where there is a risk of splashing or spraying of blood or body secretions.

- Gown—wear a waterproof gown to protect the clothing from splashing or spraying of blood or body fluids.

- Equipment—wear gloves when handling equipment contaminated with blood or body fluids; clean equipment appropriately after use; discard disposable equipment in proper containers.

- Environment control—follow proper procedures for cleaning and disinfecting the patient's environment after completion of a procedure.

- Linen—use proper procedure for disposing of linen contaminated with blood or body fluids.

- Bloodborne pathogens—do not recap needles; dispose of used needles and other sharp instruments in proper containers; use a mouthpiece for resuscitation; keep one available in areas where there is likelihood of need.

## Age

From the beginning of life until death, our risk of disease follows our age. Newborns are at risk of disease because their immune systems are not fully developed. On the other hand, older persons are at risk because their immune systems are degenerating or wearing out. Girls in their early teens are at high risk for a difficult or problem pregnancy; women over the age of thirty are also considered high risk. The older we become, the higher the risk for diseases such as cancer, heart disease, stroke, senile dementia, and Alzheimer's.

## Sex

Some diseases are more **prevalent** (occurring more often) in one gender or the other. Men are more at risk for diseases such as lung cancer, gout, and parkinsonism. Other disorders or diseases occur more often in women including osteoporosis, rheumatoid arthritis, and breast cancer.

## Environment

Air and water pollution may lead to respiratory and gastrointestinal disease. Poor sanitation, excessive noise, and stress are also environmental risk factors. Occupational diseases such as lung disease are high among miners and persons working in areas where there are increased amounts of dust or other particles in the air. Farmers are considered to be at higher risk for diseases because of their increased exposure to dust, pesticides, and other pollutants. Farmers are also at higher risk for trauma injuries due to safety problems around farm machinery. People living in remote, rural areas do not have health care availability comparable to those living in urban areas. This increases their risk for chronic illnesses.

## Lifestyle

Lifestyle factors fall into a category over which the individual has some control. Choosing to improve health behaviors in these areas could lead to a reduction in risk and thus a possibility of avoiding the occurrence of the disease. Such factors include smoking, drinking alcohol, poor nutrition (excessive fat, salt, and sugar, and not enough fruits, vegetables, and fiber), lack of exercise, and stress.

Practicing health behaviors to prevent contamination, and thus disease, is also an important lifestyle behavior. The Centers for Disease Control and Prevention recommend the use of Standard Precautions when caring for any individual where there is a chance of being contaminated with blood or body fluids (see Healthy Highlight page 6). This is an important measure to prevent transmission of any disease that can be passed between humans in blood or body fluids such as hepatitis, *E. coli* infections, and AIDS.

## Heredity

Although one cannot change genetic makeup, being aware of hereditary risk factors may encourage the individual to change lifestyle behaviors to reduce the risk of disease. For example, coronary heart disease has been shown to have a high familial tendency. Persons with this family inheritance are compounding their chances if they smoke, have poor nutritional intake, and do not exercise routinely. Breast cancer and cervical cancer also have familial tendencies. Women with family members who have been diagnosed with breast cancer or cervical cancer are at a higher risk for developing these diseases. These women should be screened routinely for evidence of cancer and should complete monthly breast self-exams. With this knowledge about hereditary factors, individuals may choose to decrease their overall risk by improving their lifestyle health behaviors.

## DIAGNOSIS

**Diagnosis** (DIE-ag-**KNOW**-sis) is the identification or naming of a disease. When an individual seeks medical attention, it is the duty of the physician to determine a diagnosis of the problem. A diagnosis is made after a methodical study by the physician utilizing data collected from a medical history, physical examination, and diagnostic tests (Figure 1–2).

A medical history is a systems review that may include such information as previous illnesses, family illness, predisposing factors, medication allergies, current illnesses, and current **symptoms** (SIMP-tums; what patients report as their problem or problems). Examples of symptoms may include stomach pain, headache, and nausea.

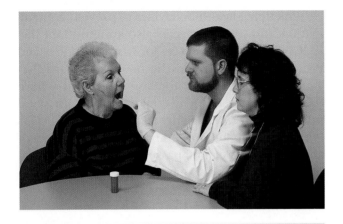

**FIGURE 1–2** Physician checking a patient.

The physician proceeds with a head-to-toe physical examination of the patient looking for **signs** of the disease. Signs differ from symptoms in that signs are observable or measurable. Signs are what the physician sees or measures. Examples of signs could include vomiting, elevated blood pressure, and elevated temperature. In some cases a patient's concern may be considered as both a symptom and a sign. Some references call this an objective or observable symptom, while others state that it is also a sign. An example would be a patient complaining of a runny nose. The runny nose is the patient's symptom and because it is observable to the physician it is also a sign.

During the physical examination, the physician may utilize other skills such as **auscultation** (AWS-kul-**TAY**-shun; using a stethoscope to listen to body cavities), **palpation** (pal-PAY-shun; feeling lightly or pressing firmly on internal organs or structures), and **percussion** (per-KUSH-un; tapping over various body areas to produce a vibrating sound). All of the results are compared to a normal standard to identify problems.

Diagnostic tests and procedures to assist in determining a diagnosis are numerable. The routine or most common include urinalysis, complete blood count (CBC), chest X-ray (CXR), and electrocardiography (EKG or ECG). See Table 1–3 for examples of common diagnostic tests and procedures.

## PROGNOSIS

**Prognosis** (prawg-KNOW-sis) is the predicted or expected outcome of the disease. For example, the prognosis of the common cold would be that the individual should feel better in seven to ten days.

The duration of the disease may be described as acute in nature. An acute disease is one that usually has a sudden onset and lasts a short amount of time (days or weeks). Most acute diseases are related to the respiratory system. Again, the common cold would be a good example.

If the disease persists for a long time, it is considered to be chronic. Chronic diseases may begin insidiously (slowly and without symptoms) and may last for the entire life of the individual. As one ages, the occurrence of chronic disease increases. One of the most common chronic diseases is hypertension or high blood pressure.

Chronic diseases often go through periods of **remission** and **exacerbation** (x-AS-er-**BAY**-shun). Remission refers to a time when symptoms are diminished or temporarily resolved. Exacerbation refers to a time when symptoms flare up or become

**TABLE 1–3** Examples of Common Diagnostic Tests and Procedures

| Test | Description |
| --- | --- |
| Complete Blood Count (CBC) | An examination of blood for cell counts and abnormalities |
| Urinalysis (UA) | An examination of urine for abnormalities |
| Chest X-ray (CXR) | X-ray examination of the chest cavity |
| Electrocardiography (ECG or EKG) | A procedure for recording the electrical activity of the heart |
| Blood Glucose | A test of the blood to determine its glucose or sugar levels |
| Computerized Axial Tomography (CT or CAT) | A special X-ray examination showing detailed images of body structures and organs |
| Serum Electrolytes | An examination of blood serum to determine the levels of the common electrolytes (sodium, potassium, and chloride) |

worse. Leukemia is a disease that progresses through periods of remission and exacerbation. Both acute and chronic diseases may range from mild to life threatening.

The prognosis may be altered or changed at times if the individual develops a **complication**. A complication is the onset of a second disease or disorder in an individual who is already affected with a disease. An individual with a fractured arm may have a prognosis of the arm healing in six to eight weeks. If the individual suffers the complication of bone infection, the prognosis may change drastically.

Diseases commonly leading to the death of an individual have a high **mortality** rate. Mortality is defined as the quality of being mortal or destined to die. The mortality rate of a disease is related to the number of people who die with the disease in a certain amount of time. Other terms the medical community uses to refer to a deadly disease include **fatal** and **lethal**.

A physician's prognosis may also consider survival rate. Survival rate is the percentage of people with a particular disease who live for a set period of time. For example, the two-year survival rate of individuals with lung cancer would be the percentage of people alive two years after diagnosis.

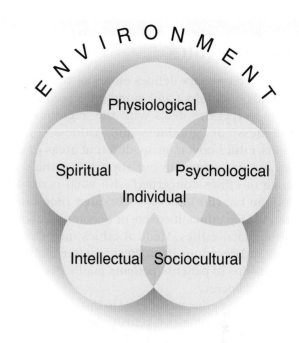

**FIGURE 1–3**  Holistic medicine.

# TREATMENT

After the diagnosis is established, the physician will work with the individual to explain or outline a plan of care. The physician may offer treatment options to the individual with expected outcomes or prognoses. The individual's entire being should be taken into consideration. The concept of considering the whole person rather than just the physical being is called **holistic medicine**. From a holistic viewpoint, there is interaction between the spiritual, cognitive, social, physical, and emotional being. These areas do not work independently, but have a dynamic interaction (Figure 1–3).

Treatment interventions may include (1) medications, (2) surgery, (3) exercise, (4) nutritional modifications, (5) physical therapy, and (6) education. Individuals and family members should be educated and involved in the treatment plan. Failure to involve the individual and family may decrease compliance and lead to failure of the plan.

After the treatment plan is implemented, the physician will follow up with the individual to determine effectiveness. The individual and physician should work together to modify the plan if it is found to be ineffective. Implementation of the plan usually requires an entire health care team. The team may include nurses, a physical therapist, a social worker, clergy, and other health care professionals as needed.

The best treatment option is a **preventive** plan. In preventive treatment, care is given to prevent disease. Examples of preventive care are breast mammograms to screen for breast cancer, blood pressure screening for hypertension, routine dental care to prevent dental caries, and Hemoccult stool test to screen for colon cancer.

Other treatment plans may include **palliative** (**PAL**-ee-AY-tiv) treatment. Palliative treatment is aimed at preventing pain and discomfort, but does not seek to cure the disease. Treatment for end-term cancer and other serious chronic conditions may be palliative.

Decisions concerning treatment plans may be very difficult for the patient, the patient's family, and the health care team. This is especially true when those decisions involve palliative treatment and end-of-life issues. During these times, professionals often seek assistance in decision making by utilizing their knowledge of medical ethics.

## MEDICAL ETHICS

Webster's dictionary defines ethics as "the study of standards of conduct and moral judgement." More simply put, ethics deals with the "rightness and wrongness" or "goodness and badness" of our actions. Ethics covers many different areas of conduct and judgement in our society. Bioethics is a branch of ethics concerned with what is right or wrong in bio (life) decisions. Because bioethics is a study of life ethics, it covers or becomes entwined with medical ethics. Medical ethics includes the values and decisions in medical practice including relationships to patients, patients' family, peer physicians, and society.

Part of our ethical challenge in this age of rapidly advancing technologies is actually determining what is right, wrong, good, or bad. New scientific discoveries are challenging our familiar or usual human behaviors, and are leading us to reconsider the way we feel, think, and act. Ethical dilemmas, once rare, are now common, and often happen so quickly that we are unable to understand how these decisions will affect our future.

Bioethical decisions are often very difficult because they touch the core of our humanity as we deal with issues of birth, death, sickness, health, and dignity. This generation and generations to come will be faced with ethical decisions formerly unknown to man. Many of these decisions will have great impact on medical ethics and will actually shape the future of mankind.

When challenges concerning medical ethics arise in a health care facility, an ethics committee may be called on to make a decision. This committee may involve one or more persons at each of these levels: physician, nurse, ethicist, social worker, case manager, chaplain, legal representative, and administrator and/or director.

Groups or committees involved in decision making may need to consider previous works of philosophy, history, law, and religion to assist them in reaching a conclusion. Participation in ethical decision making requires that members follow some basic rules, which may include:

■ keeping the discussion focused and civil

■ listening with an open mind to all opinions

■ entertaining diverse ideas

■ weighing out the pros and cons of each idea

■ considering the impact of the decision on all persons involved

Every individual at some time or another will encounter or be called on to make a decision that is bioethical in nature. Examples of these may include one or more of the following:

■ In the case of infertility, am I willing to use a surrogate mother or father in order to have a biological child?

■ Will I control the sex of my children through chromosome selection?

■ Do I support the use of fetal stem cells to grow new organs and tissues?

■ Is it right to use prescription stimulants in children?

■ Am I for or against abortion?

■ What do I think about the use of mood-altering drugs for older persons?

■ Should we clone humans?

■ Should we treat disease by replacing damaged or abnormal genes with normal genes?

■ How do I feel about xenotransplants (using animal organs/tissues in humans)?

■ Do I support euthanasia?

■ Should we allow physician-assisted suicide?

Each of the above issues can be overwhelming. And even so, there is yet another concern that must be addressed. That concern involves the economics of our choices: in other words, the "how do we pay for this?" decision.

Let us consider, for example, the economics of human cloning. If we choose to clone humans, who will pay for the research, technology, and intervention? If costs are funded by individuals, only the wealthy would be able to afford clones. Is that fair and/or right? If costs are funded by the government, what criteria will be used for selection? Will selection be based on intelligence, physical ability, or artistic skills? Who decides?

Medical ethics includes some very complicated life issues. Bioethical decision making, or determining the rightness or wrongness of such issues, will continue to be a challenge for society well into the future.

## SUMMARY

The study of human diseases is important to any health care or allied health professional. Disease can affect any body system or organ, and can range from mild to severe, depending on many factors. There are several risk factors for disease that can be controlled to some extent by one's lifestyle. Other diseases may not be prevented or controlled, but need medical intervention for treatment or cure. Diagnosis and treatment of a disease is usually accomplished by a team of health care professionals led by the physician. Ethical decision-making has become a challenge in health care today. As technology continues to grow and develop, medical ethics will become a more difficult issue than ever before.

## REVIEW QUESTIONS

### Short Answer

1. Identify why it is important to study human diseases.

2. Describe the types of pathologists and their roles in the study of disease.

3. List the five predisposing factors for disease and one disease related to each factor.

### Matching

4. Match the terms in the left column with the correct definition in the right column.

| | |
|---|---|
| _____ Pathogenesis | **a.** the cause of a disease |
| _____ Etiology | **b.** interventions to cure or control a disease |
| _____ Diagnosis | **c.** the development of a disease |
| _____ Prognosis | **d.** the identification or naming of a disease |
| _____ Treatment | **e.** the predicted or expected outcome of a disease |

## CASE STUDY

**Stan Cotton** was injured at a soccer game you were coaching. He was accidentally tripped by another player while running down the field. He is able to walk to the sideline with assistance, but has obvious bleeding on his legs and one arm. You grab the first aid box and go to his side. What do you do next? What equipment might you use to give aid to Stan? What Standard Precautions should apply to this case?

## BIBLIOGRAPHY

Ames, B. N. (2004). A role for supplements in optimizing health: The metabolic tune-up. *Archives of Biochemistry & Biophysics 29*(3), 152–159.

Brody, J. E. (2001, February 4). Herbal and natural don't always mean safe. *New York Times 152*(52348), 7.

Childs, S. G. (2002). Pathogenesis of anterior cruciate ligament injury. *Orthopaedic Nursing 21*(4), 35–40.

Reasons to be wary of herbal treatments. (2001). *NCAHF Newsletter 24*(2), 3.

Stuart-Shor, E. M., Buselli, E. F., & Carroll, D. L. (2003). Are psychological factors associated with the pathogenesis and consequences of cardiovascular disease in the elderly? *Journal of Cardiovascular Nursing 18*(3), 169–183.

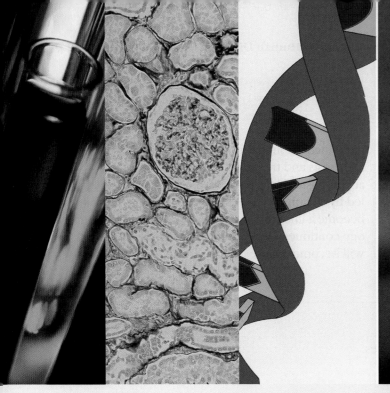
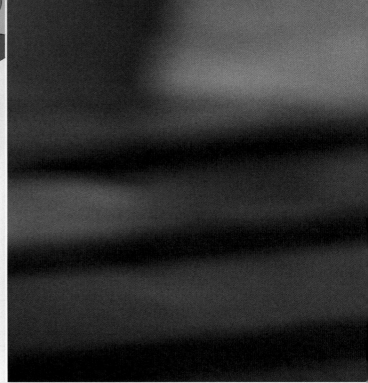

## OUTLINE

## KEY TERMS

# Mechanisms of Disease

## LEARNING OBJECTIVES

*Upon completion of the chapter, the learner should be able to:*

1. Identify important terminology related to the mechanisms of human disease.

2. Describe the causes of disease.

3. Identify disorders in each category of the causes of disease.

4. Describe behaviors important to a healthy lifestyle.

5. Compare the various types of impaired immunity.

6. Identify the basic changes in the body occurring in the aging process.

7. Describe the process of cell/tissue injury, adaptation, and death.

## OVERVIEW

The human body is a complex machine that normally runs in an efficient, balanced manner. When changes occur in the body due to lifestyle behaviors, abnormal growths, nutritional problems, bacterial invasion, or any other factor that upsets the balance, the result may be a disease process. Human disease may be very minor or life threatening. Diseases are caused by a variety of factors; some are controllable and some are not. Even normal changes in the body can make an individual more susceptible to disease. As the body ages, some changes put the individual at higher risk for developing disease. Many changes or alterations in cell and tissue structure may occur. Some of these changes are reversible, but some may cause cellular, tissue, organ, or system death. ■

## CAUSES OF DISEASE

To gain a better understanding of the different causes of diseases, it is usually helpful to classify or divide them into smaller groups. This classification may be approached in several different yet logical ways. One commonly used approach is to divide the causes of disease into the following six categories:

1. Heredity
2. Trauma
3. Inflammation/Infection
4. Hyperplasias/Neoplasms
5. Nutritional Imbalance
6. Immunity

### Heredity

Hereditary diseases are caused by an abnormality in the individual's genetic or chromosomal makeup. These diseases may or may not be apparent at birth. Hereditary diseases that are present at birth, even if not apparent, are called **congenital** (kon-JEN-ih-tahl) disorders. However, not all congenital disorders are inherited. Some other causes of congenital disorders include disease during pregnancy (fetal alcohol syndrome) or difficulty with delivery (cerebral palsy) to name only a few.

Hereditary diseases are classified in three basic ways. They are described as (1) a single gene abnormality, (2) an abnormality of several genes (polygenic), or (3) an abnormality of a chromosome (either entire absence of a chromosome or the presence of an additional chromosome). See Table 2–1 for the classification of hereditary diseases and examples.

Chromosomal and genetic abnormalities may or may not be compatible with life. Some abnormalities may be present but cause no effect on the individual, whereas others may lead to the death and spontaneous abortion of the unborn child.

More information related to hereditary diseases can be found in Chapter 19.

### Trauma

Traumatic diseases are caused by a physical injury from an external force. Trauma is the leading cause of death in children and young adults. The type of **trauma** (TRAW-mah) or traumatic disease most commonly affecting individuals varies with age, race, and residence. For example, accidents, especially falls, are a common cause of traumatic disorders in older adults, whereas gunshot wounds are the most common cause of traumatic disease and even death in young adult black males living in urban areas. However, motor vehicle accidents (**MVAs**) are the most frequent cause of serious injury overall.

In general, classification of trauma in order of prevalence (or occurrence) includes:

- motor vehicle accidents
- falls
- drowning
- burns
- ingested or inhaled objects
- poisoning
- penetrating injuries (such as a stab or gunshot wound)
- physical abuse

Emergency management of trauma is often necessary to prevent the complications of shock, hemorrhage, and infection. On arrival at an emergency department, patients are assessed according to signs/symptoms, age, and previous medical history. Needs are then prioritized and care is given in order of severity of injury. This prioritizing of care is called **triage** (tree-AUZH). Triage incorporates an ABC prioritizing method with A = Airway, B = Breathing, C = Cardiac function. After these areas are assessed, attention is turned to other areas of trauma such as

**TABLE 2–1**　Classification of Hereditary Disease with Examples

| Single Gene | Polygenic | Chromosomal |
|---|---|---|
| Cystic Fibrosis | Gout | Klinefelter's Syndrome |
| Phenylketonuria | Hypertension | Turner's Syndrome |
| Sickle Cell Anemia | Congenital Heart Anomalies | Down Syndrome |

bleeding and fractures. An example of triage, in general, would be giving priority care to a patient who is not breathing before assisting a patient who has a bleeding leg wound.

Types of trauma commonly occurring in each body system are discussed in the specific system chapters.

## Inflammation/Infection

**Inflammation** (IN-flah-**MAY**-shun) is a protective immune response that is triggered by any type of injury or irritant. Even the slightest trauma can initiate the inflammatory response. Signs of inflammation are redness, heat, swelling, pain, and loss of motion.

**Infection** (in-FECT-shun) refers to the invasion of microorganisms into tissue that causes cell or tissue injury. Inflammation and infection are often used synonymously even though they are quite different. A tissue may be inflamed but not infected, but usually, tissue that is infected will also be inflamed. An example of inflammation is a sunburn. The tissue is red, warm to the touch, swollen, painful, and uncomfortable when moving. Although this area is inflamed, it is usually not infected.

For tissue to be infected or for infection to occur, there has to be an invasion of microorganisms. Usually, inflammation and infection go hand in hand. For example, when the skin is cut, the tissue around the cut will undergo a mild inflammation. As skin bacteria invade the cut tissue, the area becomes infected and usually becomes even more inflamed due to the irritation to the tissue caused by the bacteria (Figure 2–1).

Diseases that are related to inflammation are identified with the suffix "itis." Examples include appendicitis (inflammation of the appendix), gastritis (inflammation of the stomach), colitis (inflammation of the colon), and encephalitis (inflammation of the brain). In many cases, the inflammation will progress to an infection due to the presence of bacteria in the region. For example, appendicitis may be caused by an obstruction of the appendix. Because the bacteria *Escherichia coli* (*E. coli*) are commonly found in the colon, the appendix becomes infected.

## Hyperplasias/Neoplasms

**Hyperplasias** (HIGH-per-**PLAY**-zee-ahs; hyper = excessive, plasia = growth) and **neoplasms** (NEE-oh-plazms; neo = new, plasm = growth) are similar

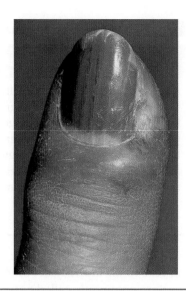

**FIGURE 2–1** Inflammation of a finger.

because in both there is an increase in cell number leading to an increase in tissue size. Hyperplasias differ from neoplasms, however, in terms of cause and growth limits. Hyperplasias are an overgrowth in response to some type of stimulus. An example of a hyperplasia would be enlargement of the thyroid gland (goiter) in response to a hormone deficiency.

Neoplasms (new growths) are commonly called **tumors**. The Latin word tumor means "swelling" and originally was used in the description of the swelling related to inflammation. The Greek term for swelling is *onkos*, which has been used to construct the word **oncology** (ong-KOL-oh-jee; onco = tumor, logy = study of, or the study of cancer). Although all tumors are not neoplasms, the words are often used synonymously.

Diseases with tumor involvement usually end with the suffix "oma." Examples include lipoma, carcinoma, melanoma, and sarcoma (Table 2–2). An exception to this is the word hematoma, which is a clot of blood in an area. A hematoma on the head due to a blunt blow would be an example.

Neoplasms or tumors (omas) may be classified as **benign** (beh-NINE) or **malignant** (mah-LIG-nant). Generally speaking, benign tumors have a limited growth, are **encapsulated** (enclosed in a capsule), and thus easily removed, and are not deadly. Malignant tumors are just the opposite. These tumors usually grow uncontrollably, have finger-like projections into surrounding tissue making removal very difficult, and are usually deadly. Malignant means deadly or progressing to death. With these definitions, it is understandable why the terms tumor, malignancy, and

**TABLE 2–2** Examples of Neoplasms or Tumors

| Neoplasms/Tumors | Description |
|---|---|
| Adenoma | Usually benign tumor arising from glandular epithelial tissue |
| Carcinoma | Malignant tumor of epithelial tissue |
| Fibroma | Benign encapsulated tumor of connective tissue |
| Glioma | Malignant tumor of neurological cells |
| Lipoma | Benign fatty tumor |
| Melanoma | Malignant tumor of the skin |
| Sarcoma | Malignant tumor arising from connective tissue like muscle or bone |

cancer bring fear to an individual. Some "omas" or tumor diseases are commonly called **cancer**. Cancer is defined as any malignant tumor.

Malignant tumors invade surrounding tissue with finger-like or "crab-like" projections. This explains why cancer comes from the Greek word *karkinos*, meaning crab. This characteristic makes surgical removal of cancer quite difficult (Figure 2–2). Another characteristic of malignant neoplasms is that they **metastasize** (meh-TAS-tah-sighz). Metastasize means to move. **Metastatic** (MET-ah-STAT-ic) cancers move from a site of origin to another secondary site in the body. For example, lung cancer commonly metastasizes to the bone. More detailed information on hyperplasias and neoplasms is found in Chapter 3.

## Nutritional Imbalance

Good nutrition is important in maintaining good health and reducing the chance of disease. Nutritional disorders may cause problems with physical growth, mental and intellectual retardation, and even death in extreme cases. Most nutritional diseases are related to overconsumption or underconsumption of nutrients. Specific problems are malnutrition, obesity, and excessive or deficient vitamins and/or minerals.

Malnutrition may be due to inadequate nutrient intake or an intake of an adequate amount with poor nutritive value. Diseases that cause a problem with absorption of nutrients may also lead to malnutrition. Children and older persons are the age groups most affected by malnutrition. Persons suffering with cancer often experience problems with malnutrition and develop cachexia. **Cachexia** (ca-KECK-see-ah) is a term used to describe any individual who has an ill, thin, wasted appearance (Figure 2–3).

Persons who are unable to eat enough to maintain their body weight may have nutritional supplements provided in a liquid drink. Another way to supplement or provide for total nutritional intake is not through the alimentary canal or digestive system, but through a **parenteral** (pah-REN-ter-al; to administer by injection) route. Parenteral routes may include subcutaneous (sub = under, cutaneous =

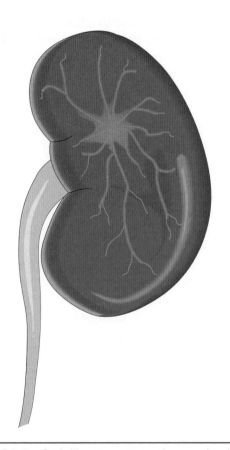

**FIGURE 2–2**   Crab-like appearance of cancer in a kidney.

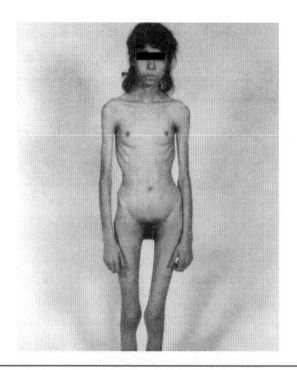

**FIGURE 2–3** Cachexia. (*Reproduced by permission from R. P. Rowlings, S. R. Williams, & C. K. Beck.* Mental health—Psychiatry nursing *(3rd ed.), St. Louis, MO: Mosby-Year Book, 1992.*)

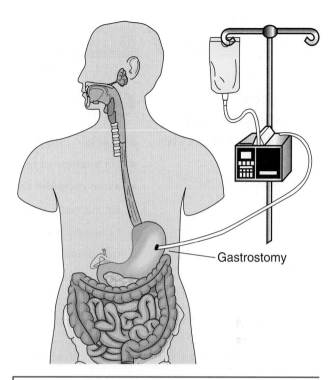

**FIGURE 2–4** Gastrostomy feeding.

skin) or under the skin, intramuscular (intra = within, muscular = muscle) or in the muscle, or intravenous (intra = within, venous = vein) or in the vein administration. The intravenous route is the most common parenteral route utilized. Providing the total nutrition needed by giving nutritive liquid through a venous (vein) route is called total parenteral nutrition (**TPN**).

Nutrition may also be provided through an **enteral** (small intestine) route. A nasogastric (naso = nose, gastric = stomach) tube or a tube running through the nose and into the stomach may be utilized for feedings if the supplement is planned short term. For longer term enteral feeding, a gastrostomy (gastro = stomach, ostomy = opening; opening into the stomach) procedure is performed to place a tube through the abdominal and stomach wall. Enteral feeding, commonly called "tube feeding," is accomplished utilizing this method (Figure 2–4).

Although there are many individuals in the United States who have a nutritional deficiency, the most common problem is obesity. Obesity is primarily due to overconsumption of nutrients and lack of exercise. Although obesity is difficult to define specifically for each individual, it is obvious that it is a major nutritional problem. Obesity shortens the life span of the individual by increasing the chance for arteriosclerosis, leading to cardiovascular diseases. It also affects the individual's risk for developing bone/joint problems due to the increased pressure on the skeletal system.

Vitamin and mineral excesses and deficiencies are usually related to diet, metabolic disorders, and some medications. Hypervitaminosis may occur in individuals who consume large amounts of vitamins for an extended period of time.

Nutritional guidelines for a healthy lifestyle are difficult to determine because they must cover a variety of ages and nutritional needs. Children, teens, and pregnant women have very specific nutritional needs. General guidelines for a healthy lifestyle are found in the Healthy Highlight on the following page.

## Impaired Immunity

The immune system of the body is a specialized group of cells, tissues, and organs that are designed to defend the body against pathogenic attacks. The body's first line of defense against pathogens is its normal structure and function including an intact skin, mucous membranes, tears, and secretions. The

## HEALTHY HIGHLIGHT

**General Guidelines for a Healthy Lifestyle**

General guidelines for a healthy lifestyle include the following tips:

- Maintain proper body weight
- Eat a variety of foods
- Avoid excessive fat, salt, and sugar
- Eat adequate amounts of fiber
- Consume alcohol in moderation
- Get enough rest and sleep
- Always eat breakfast
- Maintain a moderate exercise schedule

---

immune system protects the body in basically two other ways through:

1. The inflammatory response in which leukocytes play a vital part in the killing of foreign invaders.
2. The specific antigen–antibody reaction in which the body responds to **antigens** (AN-tih-jens) by producing **antibodies**. Antigens are substances that cause the body some type of harm, thus setting off this specific reaction. Antibodies, also called immune bodies, are proteins that the body produces to react to and render the antigen harmless.

Impaired immunity occurs when some part of this system malfunctions. Common ways the system malfunctions are as follows:

1. **Allergy**—the immune response is too intense or hypersensitive to an environmental substance. The **allergen** (environmental substance that causes a reaction) in an allergy may be such things as house dust, grass, pets, perfumes, or insect bites to name a few. The allergens do not usually cause this type of reaction in most persons, but cause an allergic reaction in affected persons.
2. **Autoimmunity**—the immune response attacks itself. In autoimmunity (auto = self), the body's lymphocytes (a white blood cell that produces antibodies) cannot identify the body's own self-antigens, which are harmless. In response, the lymphocytes form antibodies that then attack the body's own cells. Examples of autoimmune dis-

eases include rheumatoid arthritis and rheumatic fever.

3. **Immunodeficiency**—the immune response is unable to defend the body due to a decrease or absence of leukocytes, primarily lymphocytes. Persons with immunodeficiency are usually asymptomatic (without symptoms) except for recurrent infections. It is these recurrent infections that often lead to death. An example of an immunodeficiency disease is **AIDS** (Acquired Immunodeficiency Syndrome). Immunodeficiency may be caused by medications, chemotherapy, or radiation. Organ recipients are intentionally immunosuppressed or immunodeficient to save their transplanted organ. Without immunosuppressant medications, the body's immune system would recognize the organ as foreign and attack it, leading to organ death. This process is called **organ rejection**. Cancer patients often undergo chemotherapy and radiation treatments that may cause immunodeficiency. Some medications also affect the system by depressing its ability to function properly. Chapter 5 discusses the immune system and related diseases in more detail.

## AGING

There is no definite age in years when an individual becomes "aged." However, some statisticians consider the retirement age or age 65 as aged. An individual's body actually begins to age at physical maturity around age 18. The aging process is complicated and not completely understood, but it is progressive and is not reversible. Diseases related to aging are often called **degenerative** diseases. Tissue degeneration is a change in functional activity to a lower or lesser level. Examples of degenerative diseases are degenerative joint disease and degenerative disk disease.

The mechanisms of aging are complex and thought to include such factors as heredity, lifestyle, stress, diet, and environment. One may slow the process of aging to some degree by living a healthy lifestyle, and controlling stress and environmental factors.

Hereditary factors may include increased life span related to an inherited ability to resist disease. Just as families have a history of disease patterns, they also appear to have a pattern of longevity. Thus, individuals who have relatives who live to be in their 90s may themselves live to that age. Individuals with a family history of members who have died of heart disease in their early years may also suffer the same problem. Although hereditary patterns cannot be controlled, longevity can be increased and disease decreased by controlling lifestyle behaviors that increase risk of chronic disease as previously mentioned.

The body replaces and repairs itself throughout its lifetime, but with aging, this process slows. As early as age 40, there are changes in skin, endocrine function, vision, and muscle strength. Other changes in the aging process may include bone loss leading to osteoporosis, decreased melanin pigment production leading to graying of the hair, decreased immunity leading to an increase in infections, possible development of cancer, loss of brain and nerve cells that may lead to senile dementia, and decrease in intestinal motility leading to constipation and possible diverticulosis.

## DEATH

Humans are mortal, so eventually, everyone will die. Even though we are unable to fully understand the aging process, cellular, tissue, and organ death can be reviewed in an effort to understand the death of the organism as a whole.

### Cellular Injury

Cellular injury and death may be due to some type of trauma, **hypoxia** (HIGH-**POCK**-see-ah; not enough oxygen), **anoxia** (ah-NOCK-see-ah; no oxygen), drug or bacterial toxins, or viruses. Cells may undergo near-death experiences and actually recuperate. This is considered to be reversible cell injury.

The ability of the cell to survive depends on several factors including the amount of time the cell suffers and the type of cell injury that occurred. If the cause of the injury is short term, the cell has a greater chance of survival.

The type of cell also plays a part in its ability to recuperate. The heart, brain, and nerve cells are easily injured and often suffer death. This is particularly important because these cells do not replace themselves. Even short-term injury may readily lead to death in these cells. Other cells are not as easily damaged. Connective and epithelial

## COMPLEMENTARY AND ALTERNATIVE THERAPY

**Herbal Therapies for Older Persons**

The use of herbal remedies by older persons is on the rise. Some of the most common herbal therapies have been well researched and are effective for some problems common to older adults. St. John's Wort (*Hypericum perforatum*) has been shown to help mild depression and Valerian (*Valerina officinalis*) is known to be effective for insomnia. There is research showing that ginkgo (*Ginkgo biloba*) delays dementia in some cases and that Saw palmetto (*Serenoa repens*) helps reduce the symptoms of benign prostatic hypertrophy. However, these are only a few of the herbal products on the market. Consumers should be careful when using herbal preparations. Some are ineffective or untested, and others may interact with prescription medications the individual is already taking (Ernst, 1999).

cells often recuperate, and even readily replace themselves by mitosis (cell division).

## Cellular Adaptation

Cells that are exposed to adverse conditions often go through a process of adaptation. Once the condition is changed, these cells may have the ability to change back to their normal structure and function. However, some adaptations are permanent, so even if the condition improves, the cells are not able to return to normal. Types of adaptation include **atrophy** (AT-tro-fee), **hypertrophy** (HIGH-**PER**-tro-fee), hyperplasia, **metaplasia** (MET-ah-**PLAY**-zee-ah), **dysplasia** (dis-PLAY-zee-ah), and **neoplasia** (nee-oh-PLAY-zee-ah).

Atrophy (a = without, trophy = growth) is a decrease in cell size, which leads to a decrease in the size of the tissue and organ (Figure 2–5). Atrophy is often due to the aging process itself or to disease. An example of atrophy related to aging would be the smaller size of the muscles and bones of older people. As the female ages, the breasts and female reproductive organs atrophy, especially after menopause. Examples of disease or pathologic atrophy are usually related to decreased use of the organ, especially muscles. Spinal cord injuries lead to an inability to move muscles. Without use, muscle cells decrease in size and the muscle atrophies.

Hypertrophy (hyper = excessive, trophy = growth) is an increase in the size of the cell leading to an increase in tissue and organ size (Figure 2-6). Skeletal muscle and heart muscle cells do not increase in number by mitosis. Literally, what an individual has at birth is what the individual gets. This

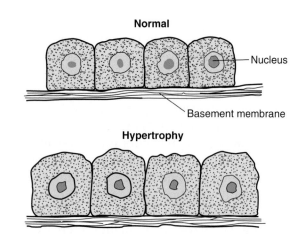

**FIGURE 2–6**  Normal cell versus hypertrophied cell.

helps explain why some athletes bulk up with exercise while others do not. The inherited number of muscle cells does not change with exercise, just the size of each cell. To adapt to an increased workload, muscle cells increase in size. Increased workload on the skeletal muscles causes cellular hypertrophy and an increase in muscle size. Heart muscle hypertrophy is usually seen in the left ventricle of the heart (left ventricular hypertrophy). The left ventricle must work harder to pump blood through diseased valves and arteries. To adapt to this need, the cells increase in size and the left side of the heart enlarges.

Hyperplasia (hyper = increased, plasia = growth) is an increase in cell number that is commonly due to hormonal stimulation (Figure 2-7). Hyperplasia is discussed in more detail in Chapter 3.

Dysplasia (dys = bad or difficult, plasia = growth) usually follows hyperplasia. It is an alteration in size, shape, and organization of cells (Figure 2-8). Dys-

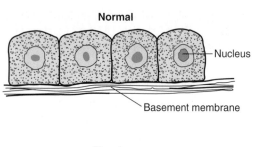

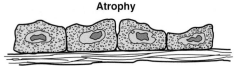

**FIGURE 2–5**  Normal cell versus atrophied cell.

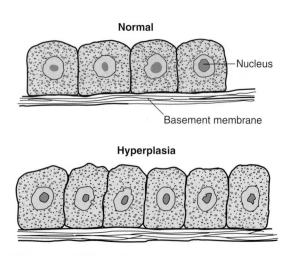

**FIGURE 2–7**  Normal tissue versus hyperplasia.

**Normal**

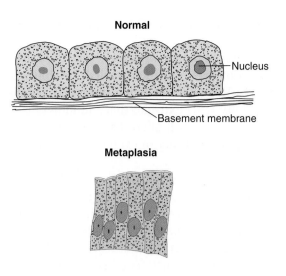

Nucleus

Basement membrane

**Metaplasia**

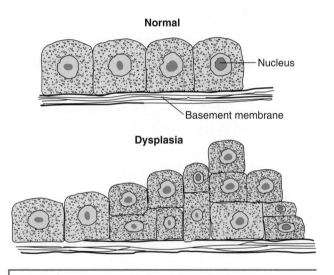

FIGURE 2–8   Normal tissue versus metaplasia.

**Normal**

Nucleus

Basement membrane

**Dysplasia**

FIGURE 2–9   Normal tissue versus dysplasia.

plastic cells may change back to the normal cell structure if the irritant or stimulus is removed, but usually these cells progress to neoplasia.

Metaplasia (meta = changed, plasia = growth) is a cellular adaptation in which the cell changes to another type of cell (Figure 2-9). An example is the columnar epithelial cells of the respiratory tree, which often change to stratified squamous epithelial cells when exposed to the irritants of cigarette smoking. This protective adaptation may be reversible if the individual quits smoking.

Neoplasia (neo = new, plasia = growth) is the development of a new type of cell with an uncontrolled growth pattern (Figure 2-10). Neoplasia is discussed in more detail in Chapter 3.

**Normal**

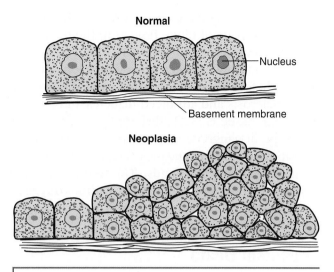

Nucleus

Basement membrane

**Neoplasia**

FIGURE 2–10   Normal tissue versus neoplasia.

## Cell and Tissue Death

**Necrosis** (nee-CROW-sis) is defined as cellular death. This cell death may involve a group of cells, and thus tissue. When referring to dead cells or tissue, one would describe the area as necrotic. Cell death, as previously mentioned, may be caused by trauma, hypoxia, anoxia, drug or bacterial toxins, or viruses. The most common causes of cell death are anoxia and hypoxia. Hypoxia caused by decreased blood flow is called **ischemia** (iss-KEE-me-ah; isch = hold back, emia = blood). When necrosis occurs due to ischemia, the area of dead cells (ischemic necrosis) is called an **infarct** (in-FARKT). Infarcts are commonly due to obstruction of arteries.

Cells that are injured and not able to recover eventually die. The cause of cell death can be determined by a pathologist because the gross and microscopic appearance of the tissue differs with the type of death. There are several types of necrosis primarily named by the microscopic appearance of the dead cells. The most common type of necrosis is called coagulation necrosis and is due to cellular anoxia. A cell without oxygen cannot produce needed energy and eventually dies. Coagulation necrosis is the type of cell death experienced with myocardial infarction.

A common alteration in necrosis occurs when saprophytic (dead tissue-loving) bacteria become involved in the necrotic tissue. With this occurrence, the necrotic tissue is now described as gangrenous or having **gangrene** (GANG-green). The type of gangrene may be wet, dry, or gas, depending on the appearance of the necrotic tissue. Wet gangrene usually occurs when the necrosis was caused by the sudden stoppage of blood flow as in the trauma of burning, freezing, or embolism. Dry gangrene occurs when blood flow has been slowed for a long period of time before necrosis occurred as in the case of arteriosclerosis and advanced diabetes. In dry gangrene, the tissue is black, shriveled, or mummified. This type of gangrene only occurs on the extremities, primarily the feet and toes. Gas gangrene occurs with dirty, infected wounds. The tissue becomes infected with anaerobic (growing without oxygen) bacteria that produce a toxic gas. This is an acute, painful, and often fatal type of gangrene.

## Organism Death

Human death may be related to any of the aforementioned causes of disease. The aging process as we have discussed leads to death due to a decrease in the ability to fight disease. Diseases that would not be lethal in our younger years, like respiratory infections, will be the cause of death in an older individual. The most common cause of death in the United States is heart disease, followed by cancer and strokes (cerebrovascular accident). Heart disease is such a major cause of death that finding the cure for cancer would not produce as great an effect in human lives

as decreasing heart disease. (See Chapter 8 for more information.)

Many times, the human organism—like the cell—is not killed but may become disabled. Disability is called **morbidity** (state of being diseased). Oftentimes, morbidity is so extreme that the individual's quality of life is severely limited. This is often seen in cases of severe brain injury or even some congenital disorders.

Prior to death, major organs such as the heart, lungs, and brain stop functioning. Once the brain ceases to function, the individual is considered brain dead. Although death is difficult to define and difficult to determine in some cases, one guideline used is that of brain death. The criteria for determining brain death include:

- a lack of response to stimuli
- loss of all reflexes
- absence of respirations or breathing effort
- lack of brain activity as shown by an electroencephalogram (EEG)

This issue of "death" and when an individual is actually dead is still controversial in the medical profession.

## SUMMARY

Human diseases are caused by heredity, trauma, inflammation/infection, hyperplasias/neoplasms, nutritional imbalances, and/or impaired immunity. Lifestyle behaviors can also be contributing factors to disease development as can the aging process. Eventually, all organisms die, and the process of death can occur at the cellular, tissue, or whole organism level.

## REVIEW QUESTIONS

### Matching

1. Match the cause of diseases in the left column with the example of a disease for that category in the right column.

| | |
|---|---|
| _____ Heredity | **a.** pneumonia |
| _____ Trauma | **b.** motor vehicle accident |
| _____ Inflammation/Infection | **c.** cancer |
| _____ Hyperplasias/Neoplasms | **d.** obesity |
| _____ Nutritional Imbalance | **e.** allergies |
| _____ Impaired Immunity | **f.** cystic fibrosis |

## True or False

**2.**   T   F    In autoimmunity, the body's immune system attacks itself.

**3.**   T   F    Some medications used to prevent or cure some diseases can cause immunodeficiency.

**4.**   T   F    Diseases related to the aging process are called regenerative disorders.

**5.**   T   F    Congenital disorders are easily recognized at birth.

**6.**   T   F    Heart and brain cells are easily injured by hypoxia.

**7.**   T   F    Heredity does not affect the aging process.

**8.**   T   F    Cellular death occurs only in the event of hypoxia (lack of oxygen).

## Short Answer

**9.** List the factors that affect a cell's ability to survive after injury.

**10.** How do cells adapt when exposed to adverse conditions?

## CASE STUDY

**Cann Ragland**, age 29, was seriously injured in a motorcycle accident. He is comatose and on life support equipment to maintain his breathing. He has not improved in two weeks with aggressive medical treatment. The family is questioning whether he is alive or dead at this time. What criteria can be used to determine this? What are the issues surrounding this determination?

## BIBLIOGRAPHY

Ahijevych, K., & Wewers, M. E. (2003). Passive smoking and vascular disease. *Journal of Cardiovascular Nursing 18*(1), 69-74.

Bloedon, L. T., & Szapary, P. O. (2004). Flaxseed and cardiovascular risk. *Nutrition Reviews 62*(1), 18-27.

Castle, N. (2003). Effective relief of acute coronary syndrome. *Emergency Nurse 10*(9), 15-19.

Coviello, J. S., & Nystrom, K. V. (2003). Obesity and heart failure. *Journal of Cardiovascular Nursing 18*(5), 360-366.

Davis, S. L. (2002). How the heart failure picture has changed. *Nursing 32*(11), 36-47.

Ernst, E. (1999). Herbal medications for common ailments in the elderly. *Drugs and Aging 15*(6), 423-428.

King, K. M., & Arthur, H. M. (2003). Coronary heart disease prevention. *Journal of Cardiovascular Nursing 18*(4), 274-281.

Quinn, L. (2002). Mechanisms in the development of type 2 diabetes mellitus. *Journal of Cardiovascular Nursing 16*(2), 1-16.

Ship, J. A. (2002). Improving oral health in older people. *Journal of the American Geriatrics Society 50*(8), 1454-1455.

Storry, J. R. (2003). Human blood groups: Inheritance and importance in transfusion. *Journal of Infusion Nursing 26*(6), 367-372.

Whitehead, D. (2003). Beyond metaphysical: Health-promoting existential mechanisms and their impact on the health status of clients. *Journal of Clinical Nursing 12*(5), 678-688.

Zinkernagel, R. M. (2003). On natural and artificial vaccinations. *Annual Review of Immunology 21*(1), 515-546.

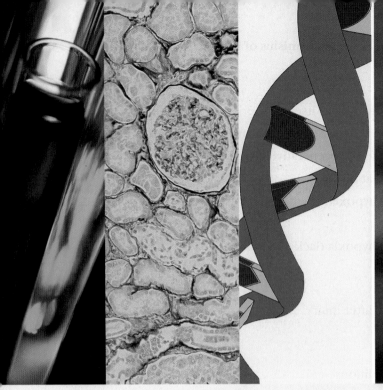
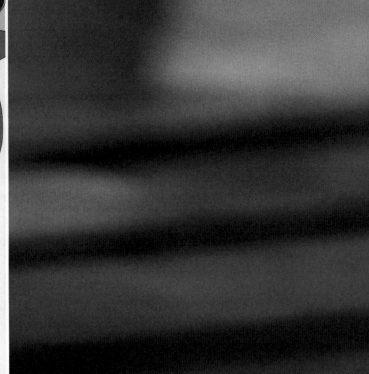

## OUTLINE

## KEY TERMS

# Neoplasms

## LEARNING OBJECTIVES

*Upon completion of the chapter, the learner should be able to:*

1. Define basic terminology used in the study of neoplasms.

2. Explain the system used to classify neoplasms.

3. Compare hyperplasias to neoplasms.

4. Identify the progression of cancer development.

5. State the signs and symptoms of cancer.

6. Identify some common carcinogenic substances.

7. Identify high-risk behaviors for cancer development.

8. State the frequency of cancer development in the population.

9. Describe the curative, palliative, and preventive methods used in cancer treatment.

## OVERVIEW

Thousands of individuals are diagnosed with neoplasms each year. The diagnostic statement "you have a tumor" often causes instant fear, dread, and tears for the individuals and families involved. Few statements in our society carry the emotional impact this one does. To most people, this diagnosis is equivalent to a pronouncement of death. But not all tumors are malignant and not all are deadly. However, there are more than 1.3 million individuals diagnosed with malignant neoplasms each year (American Cancer Society, 2004). This includes all types of cancers. Cancer can be diagnosed using a variety of diagnostic tests. Treatment of cancer is most successful when the cancer has been diagnosed early. Individuals can reduce their risk of developing some types of cancer by following preventive measures recommended by the American Cancer Society. ■

## TERMINOLOGY RELATED TO NEOPLASMS AND TUMORS

The term **neoplasm** (NEE-oh-plazm; neo = new, plasm = growth) means a new growth. The term **tumor** may be defined simply as a swelling or as a neoplasm. Tumor is used as a sign of inflammation, and in this instance, describes swelling. The term tumor as related to neoplasm means a new growth. Even though the terms tumor and neoplasm are used synonymously, not all neoplasms form tumors. **Leukemia** (loo-KEE-me-ah; leuk = white, emia = blood) is a malignant disease of the bone marrow that causes an increase in white blood cell production and may not form distinctive tumors. Likewise, not all tumors are neoplasms. A **hematoma** (HEM-ah-**TOH**-mah; hemat = blood, oma = tumor) is a large tumor or swelling filled with blood commonly called a bruise or contusion (Figure 3–1).

## CLASSIFICATION OF NEOPLASMS

Neoplasms may be classified in a variety of ways. Two of the most common ways are according to the

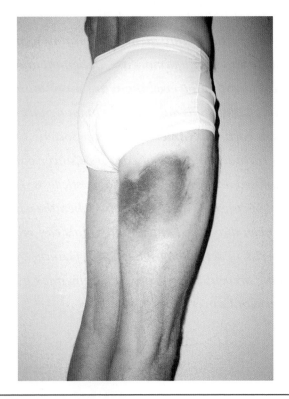

**FIGURE 3–1** Hematoma.

1) appearance and growth pattern, and 2) type of body tissue from which they arise.

Classification by appearance and growth pattern identifies neoplasms (tumors) as **benign** (beh-NINE) or **malignant** (mah-LIG-nant). Tumors that are confined to a local area and do not spread are called benign. If the tumor spreads into local tissue (**invasion**) or to distant sites (**metastasis**; meh-TAS-tah-sis), it is called a malignant (deadly) tumor or neoplasm. The general term for any malignant neoplasm or tumor is cancer.

Benign tumors are generally harmless whereas malignant neoplasms are considered deadly because they exhibit characteristics of invasion and metastasis. Invasion refers to the spreading of the neoplasm into surrounding tissue. Metastasis is the spread of the neoplasm to distant sites.

Tumors are classified or named according to the tissue they resemble along with the suffix "oma" for tumor. A benign tumor will have the suffix "oma" added after the name of the tissue. An example would be lipoma, a benign tumor of fatty tissue. A malignant neoplasm will have the term **carcinoma** (KAR-sih-**NO**-mah) or **sarcoma** (sar-KOH-mah) added to the name of the tissue type.

Carcinoma is the largest group of malignant neoplasms, and indicates a tumor of epithelial tissue found on external or internal body surfaces. A benign tumor of epithelial tissue such as a gland would be adenoma; if it is a malignant neoplasm, the name becomes adenocarcinoma.

Sarcoma is used if the neoplasm is from connective tissue such as muscle, fat, and bone. Sarcomas are less common than carcinomas, but spread more rapidly and are highly malignant. A benign tumor of connective tissue such as bone would be an osteoma; if it is a malignant neoplasm, the name is osteosarcoma.

Leukemias and **lymphomas** (lim-FOH-mas) are malignant neoplasms of blood-forming organs and lymphatic tissues, respectively. These malignant neoplasms do not have benign counterparts. All leukemias and lymphomas are malignant although their prognoses may vary considerably (Figure 3–2).

There are, of course, some tumors that do not follow this pattern. For example, malignant melanoma, a malignant neoplasm of melanocytes, is not a benign tumor as its name would suggest. Glioma is used to refer to all tumors of the glial cells of the brain. Gliomas truly do not fit the terms of this classification system. They are benign in appearance and do not metastasize, but they are malignant (deadly) because

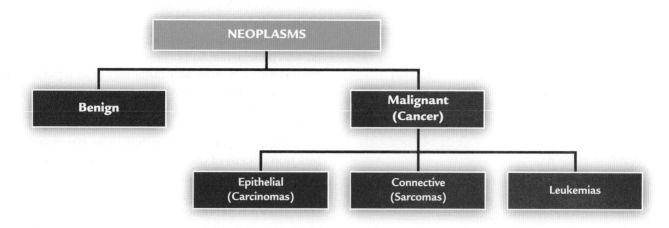

**FIGURE 3–2** Classification of neoplasms.

most are fatal. Examples of benign and malignant neoplasms are listed in Table 3–1.

## BENIGN AND MALIGNANT NEOPLASMS

Normal cells grow and function for a purpose. The growth of normal cells is regulated by several factors. First, the built-in genetic program of each cell regulates its growth pattern. Secondly, normal cellular growth is limited by contact with other cells. When two normal cells come in contact with one another, they tend to stick together and transmit a signal to each other to stop growing (Figure 3–3). Finally, normal cellular growth is regulated by growth-promoting or growth-inhibiting substances. Once the normal cells stop growing, they begin performing their specialized function. For example, epithelial cells begin functioning to cover and protect the organism while bone cells function to provide structure and support. This process of individual specialization is called **differentiation** (Figure 3–4).

Benign tumors may retain some normal structure and function. Cells of benign tumors often resemble cells of their origin, and even though they have an abnormal appearance, their appearance is uniform. These cells also may be able to function to some degree like normal cells. Benign tumors are encapsulated or covered with a capsule-like material that makes removal or excision easier. These tumor cells have a limited growth potential and are slower growing than metastatic neoplasms.

Benign tumors are expansive (grow and enlarge in the area), but are not invasive or metastatic. This does not mean that benign tumors are harmless. The presence and growth of any tumor can obstruct passageways such as those in the digestive and respiratory systems, leading to difficulty with eating or breathing.

Tumors also may exert pressure on nerves causing pain and loss of sensation or movement. Benign tumors affecting a gland may cause over- or undersecretion of hormones with resulting disorders. A benign tumor growing in an enclosed area such as the brain may place pressure on normal tissue,

**TABLE 3–1** Origin and Names for Benign and Malignant Neoplasms

| Cell or Tissue of Origin | Name of Benign Neoplasm | Name of Malignant Neoplasm |
| --- | --- | --- |
| Glandular epithelium | Adenoma | Adenocarcinoma |
| Squamous epithelium | Epithelioma | Squamous cell carcinoma |
| Adipose (fat) | Lipoma | Liposarcoma |
| Cartilage | Chondroma | Chondrosarcoma |
| Bone | Osteoma | Osteosarcoma |
| Glial | | Glioma |
| Blood | | Leukemia |

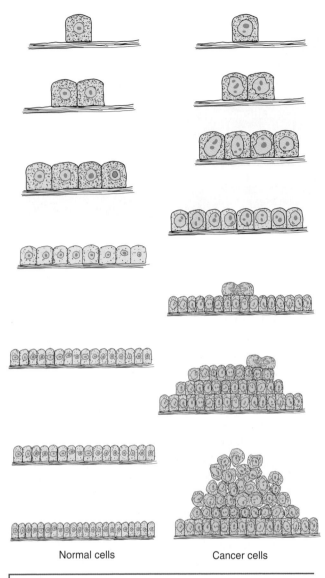

**FIGURE 3–3** Cellular growth patterns.

leading to death of the tissue and potentially, death of the individual.

Metastatic neoplasm describes cells whose growth pattern has no purpose and is uncontrollable. Neoplastic cells grow autonomously or independent of growth factors. These cells grow excessively without regard to normal regulatory factors like contact inhibition.

Neoplastic cells do not have the structure or function of cells of their origin. Unlike benign tumor cells, neoplastic cells do not look alike. Their structure is not uniform, but is haphazard and inconsistent. They are not differentiated and do not perform specialized functions. The surface area of the malignant neoplasm is not encapsulated. Rather, it is more crab-like in appearance with multiple claw-like extensions that invade surrounding tissue. A malignant neoplasm (cancer) also metastasizes to distant areas or organs. A comparison of benign and malignant tumors is listed in Table 3–2.

Cancer cells are fast growing. The entire metabolism of the cancerous cell is aimed at rapid reproduction and growth, far outpacing the growth of the normal cell. This increase in the metabolic needs of cancer cells leads to an increase in the need for nutrients and oxygen. To meet this need, **angiogenesis** (AN-jee-oh-**JEN**-eh-sis; angio = vessel, genesis = growth or new growth of blood vessels) occurs. This increase in blood flow provides increased nutrients to the neoplasm, allowing it to continue this rapid, uncontrolled growth. During this time, normal cells are deprived of needed nutrients, and the individual begins to lose weight and appear thin, frail, and weak. This condition is called **cachexia**.

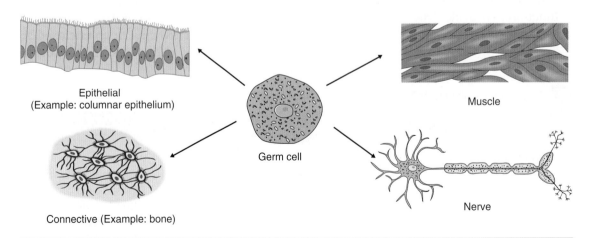

Epithelial
(Example: columnar epithelium)

Muscle

Connective (Example: bone)

Germ cell

Nerve

**FIGURE 3–4** The process of cell differentiation.

**TABLE 3–2** Comparison of Benign and Malignant Tumors

| Feature | Benign | Malignant |
|---|---|---|
| Growth | Slow, expansive | Fast, invasive, metastatic |
| Appearance | Symmetrical | Crab-like |
| Capsule | Yes | No |
| Tissue type | Resembles tissue of origin | Does not resemble tissue of origin |
| Cells | Differentiated | Undifferentiated |
| Surface | Smooth | Irregular, may ulcerate and hemorrhage |

## HYPERPLASIAS AND NEOPLASMS

It is important to note that there is another type of cellular growth that closely resembles a neoplasm. **Hyperplasia** (HIGH-per-**PLAY**-zee-ah; hyper = too much, plasia = growth) and neoplasia (neo = new, plasia = growth) are both overgrowths of cells that cause an increase in the size of the tissue. Both commonly produce masses that, once discovered, need to be identified as either hyperplasia or neoplasm, because the treatment of each is drastically different.

Hyperplasias and neoplasms differ in the cause and extent of their growth. Hyperplasia usually occurs in response to a stimulus and the growth stops when the stimulus stops. Neoplasm, as previously mentioned, grows independently, excessively, and usually unceasingly.

Hyperplasias may be caused by a variety of different stimuli. An example of a hyperplasia caused by tissue irritation is a skin callus on the foot. The stimulus is the irritation or rubbing of a shoe on that par-ticular area. When the shoe size is corrected, the stimulus is stopped, the hyperplasia stops, and the callus eventually disappears.

Hyperplasias may develop due to hormone excess or deficiency. An example of a hormone deficiency hyperplasia is the enlargement of the thyroid gland called goiter. Chronic inflammation may lead to hyperplasia as in lymph node hyperplasia or adenoid hyperplasia. Lastly, the hyperplasia may be caused by an unknown stimulus as in the case of prostatic hyperplasia in older men.

Hyperplasias and neoplasms both represent an increase in cell number due to an increase in mitosis (cellular division). Hyperplasias are an increase of cells that still look like cells of their origin. To simplify this concept, one might consider the cells as daughter cells that still look like their mother or the cell of their origin. Neoplasms are an increase in cell number, but the cells are new (neo = new) or different in their appearance than their cell of origin or their mother (Figure 3–5). This difference in appearance is important to the clinical pathologist

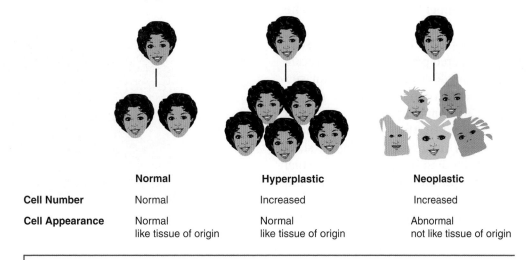

| | Normal | Hyperplastic | Neoplastic |
|---|---|---|---|
| **Cell Number** | Normal | Increased | Increased |
| **Cell Appearance** | Normal like tissue of origin | Normal like tissue of origin | Abnormal not like tissue of origin |

FIGURE 3–5　Comparison of hyperplasia and neoplasm.

who determines or diagnoses the mass as hyperplasia or neoplasm.

# DEVELOPMENT OF MALIGNANT NEOPLASMS (CANCER)

Genetic alteration is the basis for the development of malignant neoplasm or cancer. Cells throughout the body may undergo genetic alteration or mutation, but amazingly, few develop into cancer. A cell must undergo a change or series of changes in its DNA structure to acquire the altered growth pattern of cancer. Genetic mutation or change is brought about by a virus, chemicals, **radiation** (the process of using light, short waves, ultraviolet, or X-ray), or other biologic agent called a **carcinogen** (kar-SIN-oh-jen; carcino = cancer, gen = arising) or cancer-causing agent or substance.

Continued exposure to a carcinogen or to several carcinogens may increase or promote the abnormality of the cell. Abnormal cells may revert back to normal cells, appear as benign tumors, or digress to a malignant neoplasm. The body's immune system may prevent or reverse the development of cancer. Just removing or stopping the carcinogen may also reverse cancer development.

If development is not halted, abnormal cells begin to establish themselves in an effort to become cancerous. These cells must now grow rapidly enough to establish a site. They must fight for space and nutrition. The body and the abnormal cells are at odds with each other at this point. If the body wins, the abnormal cells may die out and disappear. If the abnormal cells get the upper hand, they may become established and thrive.

As long as the abnormal cells are not firmly established, they are considered preneoplastic or precancerous. If these cells are discovered at this point, surgical removal can be accomplished before cancer actually develops. Unfortunately, very few potential cancers are discovered at this stage. Squamous epithelial tissue often progresses through a slow series of changes including hyperplasia, abnormal hyperplasia called **dysplasia** (DIS-**PLAY**-zee-ah), and finally a stage called **carcinoma in situ**.

In carcinoma in situ, the atypical cells are "just sitting" in the epithelial layer of the tissue, and have not broken through the basement membrane and invaded the surrounding tissue. Carcinoma in situ commonly occurs in the uterine cervix, larynx, and mouth. Cancer can be avoided at this stage by surgical removal of the dysplasia or in situ tumor.

The final stage in cancer development is the invasion of the precancerous cells into the surrounding tissue. Local tissue invasion is the step that signifies a change from precancerous to malignant neoplasm. In epithelial tissue, this is the point where neoplastic cells (carcinomas) break through the basement membrane that separates the epithelium from the connective tissue below (Figure 3–6). Once this break occurs, the neoplastic cells can spread quickly, not only with local tissue invasion, but also via the lymphatic system (lymph fluid) and circulatory system (blood).

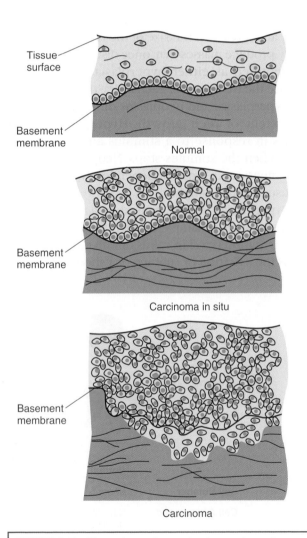

**FIGURE 3–6** Normal, carcinoma in situ, and carcinoma tissue.

# INVASION AND METASTASIS OF CANCER

Local invasion of cancer is similar to the way plants sink their roots into the soil. The finger-like projections of the neoplasms force themselves along the lines of least resistance. Pressure from the growing tumor occludes blood supply, leading to local tissue necrosis and weakening the tissue, which eases further spread of the neoplasm. Spread of cancer from this primary location or site to other secondary sites in the body is called metastasis.

Carcinomas, epithelial tissue neoplasms, commonly spread through the lymphatics or lymphatic system. Lymph nodes can catch or filter cancer cells. For this reason, lymph nodes are commonly removed surgically and examined for the presence of cancerous cells. Lymph nodes near the tumor are generally the first to filter cancerous cells. As more and more neoplastic cells spread into the lymphatic system, the filters fill with neoplastic cells. Eventually, the nodes become full and are unable to filter more cells. When this occurs, the neoplastic cells may spill over into the bloodstream.

Absence of lymph node involvement with cancer is a favorable sign and may mean that surgical cure is possible. Usually, the higher the number of lymph nodes involved, the poorer the chance of survival.

Sarcomas do not utilize the lymphatic system as readily as carcinomas (Table 3–3). These tumors shed neoplastic cells directly into the blood. Once cancerous cells enter the bloodstream, they may be widely distributed throughout the body. Common sites of bloodstream metastasis are the liver, lungs, and brain. Frequently, it is the secondary cancer site that is discovered first.

Metastasis may also occur by invasion and implantation within a serous cavity. Once neoplastic cells reach a serous cavity such as the pleural or peritoneal cavity, they may seed and implant freely within that cavity.

# GRADING AND STAGING OF CANCER

**Grading** and **staging** of malignant tumors are utilized to plan treatment and predict possibility of a cure. Grading determines the degree of abnormality of the neoplasm and staging considers the degree of spread.

Grading is the microscopic examination of the tumor to determine the degree of differentiation. The more differentiated the tumor, the more it looks like the tissue of its origin. The more abnormal the tissue appears in comparison to its normal tissue, the more undifferentiated or **anaplastic** (AN-ah-PLAST-ic) it is. The higher the degree of differentiation, the better the prognosis. Tumors that are undifferentiated or anaplastic do not resemble the tissue of origin, are highly malignant, and have a poor prognosis. Tumors are typically placed into grades I to IV. Grade I tumors are the less aggressive and serious whereas grade IV tumors are the most aggressive and serious in nature.

Staging is utilized to determine the extent of spread of the neoplasm. Clinical examination, X-rays, **biopsy** (BYE-op-see; removing a small piece of tissue for microscopic examination), and surgical exploration may be used to evaluate the degree of spread. Tumors may be placed in stages according to a numerical system (I to IV), much like the grading system described above.

A second, more detailed staging, is the **TNM** system. In this system, tumors are staged according to the size and extent of the primary **T**umor, number of lymph **N**odes involved, and **M**etastasis to other sites.

Grading and staging are two predictors of prognosis. Of the two predictors, staging is the better indicator.

**TABLE 3–3** Comparison of Carcinomas and Sarcomas

| Feature | Carcinoma | Sarcoma |
|---|---|---|
| Tissue | Epithelial | Connective |
| Occurrence | Very common | Less common |
| Growth | Slow | Rapid |
| Metastasis | Primarily through lymph | Primarily through blood |

## CAUSES OF CANCER

Unfortunately, the actual cause of most cancer is unknown. Cancer appears to occur due to a variety of circumstances, which suggests that more than one factor is involved in its development. One thing remains constant in the development of cancer: the genetic alteration that allows the cell to grow independently and uncontrollably. It is thought that cellular mutations actually occur frequently in humans. It is further theorized that the human immune system catches and destroys these abnormal cells as soon as they occur. So, in some respects, cancer may represent some failure of the immune system in the involved individual.

Prevention and cure of cancer will depend on finding the initiating agents that cause the genetic alteration in the cell or the event that causes an altered cell to become malignant. Currently, there are hundreds of carcinogenic compounds that have been identified. The process of **carcinogenesis** (KAR-sin-oh-**JEN**-eh-sis; cancer development) may take many years to develop, may stop and start, or may even be reversed, but usually there will be a continual progression of cellular changes from hyperplasia to dysplasia to **metaplasia** (MET-ah-**PLAY**-zee-ah) to neoplasia (Figure 3–7).

### Chemical Carcinogens

Chemical carcinogenesis is quite complex. The frequency of exposure and the strength or potency of the chemical are important factors in the development of cancer. Chemicals that do not cause a problem by themselves may enhance cancer development when used in combination with other chemicals. Chemical carcinogens abound in our environment. Exposure to certain chemicals used in industry may lead to cancer among workers. Naphthylamine, found in certain types of dye, has been found to cause bladder cancer. Asbestos, previously used in roofing and insulating materials, has been identified as a carcinogen leading to lung cancer. Miners of nickel ore have a high rate of nasal cancer. Farmers using arsenic as an insecticide often suffer from skin and lung cancers. Currently, chemicals used as food additives, cosmetics, and certain plastics are the focus of intensive research investigating the possible relationship of these chemicals to cancer.

### Hormones

Hormones may increase the incidence of cancer, yet at times, hormones may be used as a form of cancer treatment. The action of hormones as related to cancer is not clearly understood. For example, a benign mole never becomes malignant until sex hormones increase at puberty. Administration of diethylstilbestrol, a synthetic estrogen compound, to pregnant women during the 1940s and 1950s led to an increase in a rare vaginal adenocarcinoma in their female children and to testicular abnormalities in their male children. Excessive production of estrogen in the female may lead to cancer of the breast and uterus. Estrogen medication used to treat menopausal symptoms in women has been shown to lead to an increase in endometrial cancer. The ovaries are

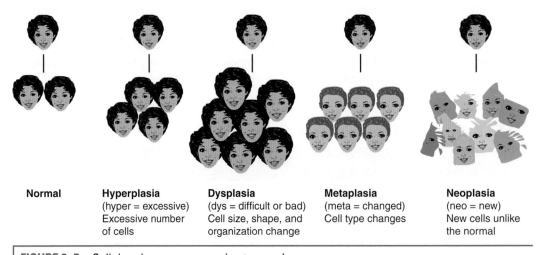

| Normal | Hyperplasia | Dysplasia | Metaplasia | Neoplasia |
|---|---|---|---|---|
| | (hyper = excessive) Excessive number of cells | (dys = difficult or bad) Cell size, shape, and organization change | (meta = changed) Cell type changes | (neo = new) New cells unlike the normal |

**FIGURE 3–7** Cellular changes progressing to neoplasm.

sometimes removed after a female has breast cancer in an effort to decrease stimulation of other possible tumors. Although much research had been done to correlate cancer with birth control pills, the findings are inconclusive. The most widely used "combination" pill, combining estrogen and progesterone, may actually decrease the risk of cancer.

Cancer of the prostate is stimulated by the male hormone testosterone, but slowed or inhibited by estrogen treatment. Males who suffer with prostatic cancer may undergo treatment with estrogen medication to counteract the effects of testosterone. Treatment to decrease testosterone production may also include an orchiectomy—removal of the testes—in an effort to decrease or slow the growth of the prostatic tumor, or decrease stimulation of other possible tumors.

## Radiation

Ultraviolet (UV) radiation, X-radiation, and radioactive materials are all known carcinogens. About one million cases of skin cancer are diagnosed each year (American Cancer Society, 2004). Sunbathers, farmers, fishermen, construction workers, mariners, and anyone else with an extended exposure to the UV rays of the sun or tanning lights have an increased risk of developing basal or squamous cell carcinomas. While basal and squamous cell carcinomas tend to occur due to cumulative exposure to the sun, melanoma occurs more frequently due to extreme, blistering burns at a young age. Fair-skinned people are at greatest risk for skin cancer because they lack the protective effects of melanin. UV-related skin cancer is uncommon among the black population.

X-rays have been used extensively as a diagnostic tool since discovery by Roentgen in 1895. Radiologists commonly developed cancers before the correlation of radiation and cancer. Roentgen, himself, developed skin cancer. In the late 1800s, radiation dosage was determined by taking repeated X-rays of the operator's hand. Soon after X-ray discovery, the development of the first hand cancer was reported. Presently, radiation is considered a professional risk for radiologists and those working in the field of radiology, but with proper use of protective clothing and equipment, the risk is minimal. High doses of radiation may be used as treatment for some cancers. This treatment does carry a risk of leading to the development of secondary tumors. These tumors usually develop after a lengthy

period of time (20 to 25 years), which makes the benefits of radiation therapy far outweigh its risk.

Radioactive materials that emit alpha, beta, and gamma rays are potential carcinogens. Most of these materials are used in medicine and research, and are under strict regulation. With the use of protective clothing, the risk to workers in these areas is minimal. The most devastating and dramatic link between radiation and cancer was the increase shown in leukemia and thyroid cancers in the survivors of the atomic bombs dropped on Hiroshima and Nagasaki in 1945.

## Viruses

Viruses have been proven to cause cancer in laboratory animals, but the proof is not as clear cut in humans. Some examples that are worth noting include the Epstein-Barr virus, which causes infectious mononucleosis. The Epstein-Barr virus has been associated with Burkitt's lymphoma, a malignant neoplasm seen primarily in Africa. Hepatitis B virus has been closely connected to liver cancer. Individuals with cervical cancer also tend to have the herpes simplex virus.

## Genetic Predisposition

There is some genetic predisposition for cancer as evidenced by the increased occurrence of certain types of cancers in the same family. This knowledge has led to intensive research. Discovery of certain cancer suppressor genes, and most recently a breast cancer gene, has aided research efforts, but complete understanding of the correlation of genetics and cancer has not yet been reached. It is known that colon and breast cancer have a higher incidence in certain families. A woman whose mother or sisters have or have had breast cancer runs a five-times greater chance of developing breast cancer than other women. Genetic testing is now available for the breast cancer gene.

## Personal Risk Behaviors

There are several personal behaviors common in our society that put an individual at increased risk for developing cancer. These behaviors include smoking cigarettes and use of other tobacco products, some dietary practices, alcohol use, and certain sexual behaviors.

**Smoking and Tobacco Products Use.** Cigarette smoking is carcinogenic. Approximately 160,000–170,000 deaths occur yearly from tobacco use (American Cancer Society, 2004). It is the major cause of lung cancer. Cancer of the lung is 15 times greater in smokers than nonsmokers. Smoking also doubles the incidence of cancer of the bladder and pancreas. Chemicals in cigarette smoke affect all organs of the body because the chemicals are absorbed from the lungs into the blood and circulated to all organs. These chemicals are found in increased concentrations in the urine of smokers. Second-hand smoke has now been proven to be detrimental to smokers and nonsmokers.

The chemicals in smokeless tobacco are absorbed into the blood and again circulate to the entire body, causing detrimental effects. Oral cancer occurs more frequently with smokeless tobacco use than in non-tobacco users.

**Diet.** Identifying the carcinogenic nature of dietary practices is difficult because many factors are involved. Diet seems to function over a period of time to place an individual at risk for cancer. There is a consistent relationship between increased weight in women and the risk of cancer, although there is not a relationship between the two for men. Obesity and a high consumption of dietary fat in women is a consistent risk factor for endometrial, breast, and colon cancer.

Much controversy exists concerning food additives, especially saccharin and nitrites. Saccharin has been shown to cause bladder cancer in rats, but this correlation has not been clear in humans. Nitrates are used as preservatives in meat and fish, and have been shown to produce stomach cancer in animals. Countries with high nitrite consumption, Japan for example, have high rates of gastric cancer.

Colon cancer rates are lower in countries that have a lower consumption of dietary fat and a higher consumption of dietary fiber than the United States. The western plains area of the United States is high in selenium and has the lowest colon cancer rates, thus supporting the concept of some correlation between selenium levels and colon cancer.

**Alcohol Use.** Cancer of the mouth, throat, and esophagus occurs more often in people who smoke and consume large quantities of alcohol. Alcohol has not been proven as a carcinogen per se, but recent studies have also shown a higher incidence of breast cancer in women who drink even moderate amounts (three drinks per week).

**Sexual Behavior.** The risk of developing cervical cancer is related to the age of first sexual intercourse and the number of sexual partners. The younger the female and the larger the number of sex partners, the greater the risk. Females who have only one sexual partner are at risk if that partner has had multiple partners. True virgins do not experience cervical cancer (Coleman, 1992). The factor causing the increased risk may be the human papilloma virus (HPV) transmitted between partners. The incidence of cervical cancer is two times greater in black women than in white, and is found more commonly in women from lower socioeconomic groups. Women marrying men whose previous sexual partners had developed cervical cancer also are at greater risk of developing cervical cancer. Pregnancy and childbirth appear to be protective mechanisms for women from cancer of the ovary, endometrium, and breast. Females who start menstrual cycles at a later age, have early menopause, and/or bear the first child at an early age are at decreased risk for breast cancer.

# CANCER PREVENTION

Cancer of the lung, breast, and colon are responsible for the majority of cancer deaths. Many of these cancers can be prevented by lifestyle changes. Smoking and tobacco use lead to approximately 30 percent of all cancers. Cigarette smoking is considered the single, most preventable cause of lung cancer, heart disease, and other diseases of the lung.

Diet and nutrition play a significant role in the prevention of cancer. **Preventive** measures include reduction of fat intake and an increase in consumption of fruits, vegetables, and fiber.

Americans' passion for a suntan encourages people to lie in the sun and use tanning lights. The most widespread cancer—skin cancer—can be prevented by avoiding unnecessary exposure to the sun and tanning lights. If exposure to the sun is necessary, the use of a sun block agent with 15 or higher SPF is recommended.

The American Cancer Society recommends the following preventive measures.

- Do not smoke. The risk of developing lung cancer is 15 times greater for smokers.

- Limit alcoholic intake. Heavy drinking increases the risk of cancer of the esophagus, mouth, throat, larynx, and liver.

- Protect skin from excessive sun exposure.

- Refuse needless X-rays. Special precautions must be taken to protect the unborn child if X-rays are necessary.

- Take hormone therapy to relieve menopausal symptoms only as long as necessary.

- Avoid heavily polluted air and long exposure to household solvent cleaners, paint thinners, and the like.

- Follow label instructions carefully when using pesticides, fungicides, and other home garden and lawn chemicals.

- Monitor caloric intake and exercise properly. Eat fewer fatty foods and more high-fiber food such as bran, whole grains, and fibrous vegetables and fruits.

- Women should regularly perform breast examinations.

- Men should regularly perform testicular examinations.

- Have regular checkups by physicians. For women over 50, the doctor may recommend a mammogram as part of the routine examination. Also, the **Pap test** (a test to screen for cervical cancer) should be performed at regular intervals. Men should be regularly checked for prostate cancer. A rectal examination should be part of every medical checkup for men and women, and stool samples should be examined for blood, which may be an indication of colon cancer.

According to the American Cancer Society (1999), the relative survival rate for 50 percent of newly diagnosed cancer cases is about 80 percent, but this could increase to 95 percent if all individuals participated in regular screening programs.

# FREQUENCY OF CANCER

Cancer is a focus of major concern for our society because it strikes over a million individuals per year. Cancer, along with heart disease, causes over half of all deaths in the United States. One in two men and one in three women will be diagnosed with cancer

## HEALTHY HIGHLIGHT

**Breast Awareness and Self-Examination**

Beginning in their 20s, women should be made aware of the benefits and limitations of breast self-examinations (BSEs). Women should know how their breasts normally feel and report any new breast changes to a health professional as soon as they are found. Finding a breast change does not mean that a cancer is present. By choosing to use a step-by-step, systematic approach, and a specific schedule to examine their breasts, women can detect any changes or abnormalities quickly and easily.

If you choose to do BSE, the following information provides a step-by-step, systematic approach for the examination. The best time for a woman to examine her breasts is when the breasts are not tender or swollen. Women who are pregnant, breast-feeding, or have breast implants can also choose to examine their breasts regularly. Women who examine their breasts should have their technique reviewed during their periodic health examinations by their health care professional. It is acceptable for women to choose not to do BSE or to do BSE occasionally.

If you choose not to do BSE, you still should be aware of your breasts and report any changes to your doctor without delay.

*(continued)*

**HEALTHY HIGHLIGHT —continued**

## How to Examine Your Breasts

1. Lie down and place your right arm behind your head. The exam is done while lying down, not standing up, because when lying down, the breast tissue spreads evenly over the chest wall and becomes as thin as possible, making it much easier to feel all the breast tissue.

2. Use the finger pads of the three middle fingers on your left hand to feel for lumps in the right breast. Use overlapping, dime-sized circular motions of the finger pads, to feel the breast tissue.

3. Use three different levels of pressure to feel all the breast tissue. Light pressure is needed to feel the tissue closest to the skin, medium pressure to feel a little deeper, and firm pressure to feel the tissue closest to the chest and ribs. A firm ridge in the lower curve of each breast is normal. If you are not sure how hard to press, talk to your doctor or nurse. Use each pressure level to feel the breast tissue before moving on to the next spot.

4. Move around the breast in an up-and-down pattern, starting at an imaginary line drawn straight down your side from the underarm. Move across the breast to the middle of the chest bone (sternum or breastbone). Be sure to check the entire breast area, going down until you feel only ribs and up to the neck or collar bone (clavicle). There is some evidence to suggest that the up-and-down pattern (sometimes called the vertical pattern) is the most effective pattern for covering the entire breast and not missing any breast tissue.

5. Repeat the exam on your left breast, using the finger pads of the right hand.

6. Stand in front of a mirror with your hands pressing firmly down on your hips. Look at your breasts for any changes of size, shape, contour, or dimpling. (The pressing down on the hips position contracts the chest wall muscles and enhances any breast changes.)

7. Examine each underarm while sitting up or standing, and with your arm only slightly raised so you can easily feel in this area. Raising your arm straight up tightens the tissue in this area and makes it very difficult to examine.

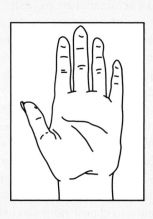

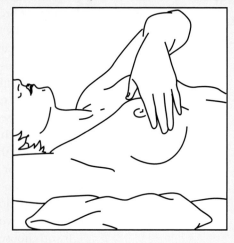

*Source: American Cancer Society website www.cancer.org.*
*Reprinted by the permission of the American Cancer Society, Inc.*

during their lifespan. Since 1990, over 11 million cases of cancer have been diagnosed with five million deaths occurring. One out of four deaths (1,500 per day) is due to cancer. It affects many lives, causing extreme grief, suffering, and financial loss. However, over seven and one-half million Americans who have or have had cancer are still alive.

The term cancer covers a large number of specific types of malignant neoplasms. Each of these types may vary considerably in behavior, treatment, and prognosis. The prognosis for these individual types will depend on the individual cancer's metastatic rate, the extent of spread when discovered, and the effectiveness of current treatments. In general, the overall survival rate of cancer is approximately 50 percent. Even though all malignant neoplasms may fit into a classification of carcinomas, sarcomas, leukemias, or lymphomas, there is a great difference in the way they behave. Some types, such as pancreatic carcinoma, are usually deadly, whereas skin carcinoma seldom is.

Cancer affects people of all ages, young and old, both male and female. The most common type of cancer is basal and squamous cell skin cancer. These neoplasms are seldom fatal because they are very visible, slow growing, and can be completely excised. Because these tumors are generally treated in a physician's office, they are difficult to track statistically and are usually excluded in statistical data. Malignant melanoma, on the other hand, is a deadly form of skin cancer that only comprises approximately 1 percent of all skin malignancies but is statistically recorded as skin cancer.

The most common types of cancer, excluding skin cancers, are cancers of the lung, colon, breast, uterus, and prostate. The common sites for cancer in the male and female are presented in Figures 3–8 and 3–9.

## DIAGNOSIS OF CANCER

The prognosis for the individual with a malignant neoplasm is best if the cancer is located and treated early. Routine screening can be very effective in discovery and early diagnosis of cancer. Screening measures include monthly breast self-examinations, regular Pap tests, and mammograms for females. Screening for males includes routine testicular self-examinations. Occult stool examinations after age 40 to screen for colon cancer is important for both sexes.

Lifetime Probability of Developing Cancer, by Site, Men, US, 1998–2000

| Site | Risk |
| --- | --- |
| All sites | 1 in 2 |
| Prostate | 1 in 6 |
| Lung & bronchus | 1 in 13 |
| Colon & rectum | 1 in 17 |
| Urinary bladder | 1 in 29 |
| Non-Hodgkin lymphoma | 1 in 48 |
| Melanoma | 1 in 55 |
| Leukemia | 1 in 70 |
| Oral cavity | 1 in 72 |
| Kidney | 1 in 69 |
| Stomach | 1 in 81 |

Source: DevCan: Probability of Developing or Dying of Cancer Software, Version 5.1 Statistical Research and Applications Branch, NCI, 2003. http://srab.cancer.gov/devcan

Lifetime Probability of Developing Cancer, by Site, Women, US, 1998–2000

| Site | Risk |
| --- | --- |
| All sites | 1 in 3 |
| Breast | 1 in 7 |
| Lung & bronchus | 1 in 17 |
| Colon & rectum | 1 in 18 |
| Uterine corpus | 1 in 38 |
| Non-Hodgkin lymphoma | 1 in 57 |
| Ovary | 1 in 59 |
| Pancreas | 1 in 83 |
| Melanoma | 1 in 82 |
| Urinary bladder | 1 in 91 |
| Uterine cervix | 1 in 128 |

Source: DevCan: Probability of Developing or Dying of Cancer Software, Version 5.1 Statistical Research and Applications Branch, NCI, 2003. http://srab.cancer.gov/devcan

**FIGURE 3–8** Lifetime probability of developing cancer by site and sex. *(American Cancer Society website www. cancer.org. Reprinted by the permission of the American Cancer Society, Inc.)*

Discovery of tumors may occur through routine screening or accidentally during other diagnostic procedures. X-ray examinations of the chest prior to surgery may reveal a mass. Annual physical examinations may lead to the discovery. Recognition of cancer warning signals by an individual is important. The American Cancer Society lists several of these signs, with the initial letters forming the

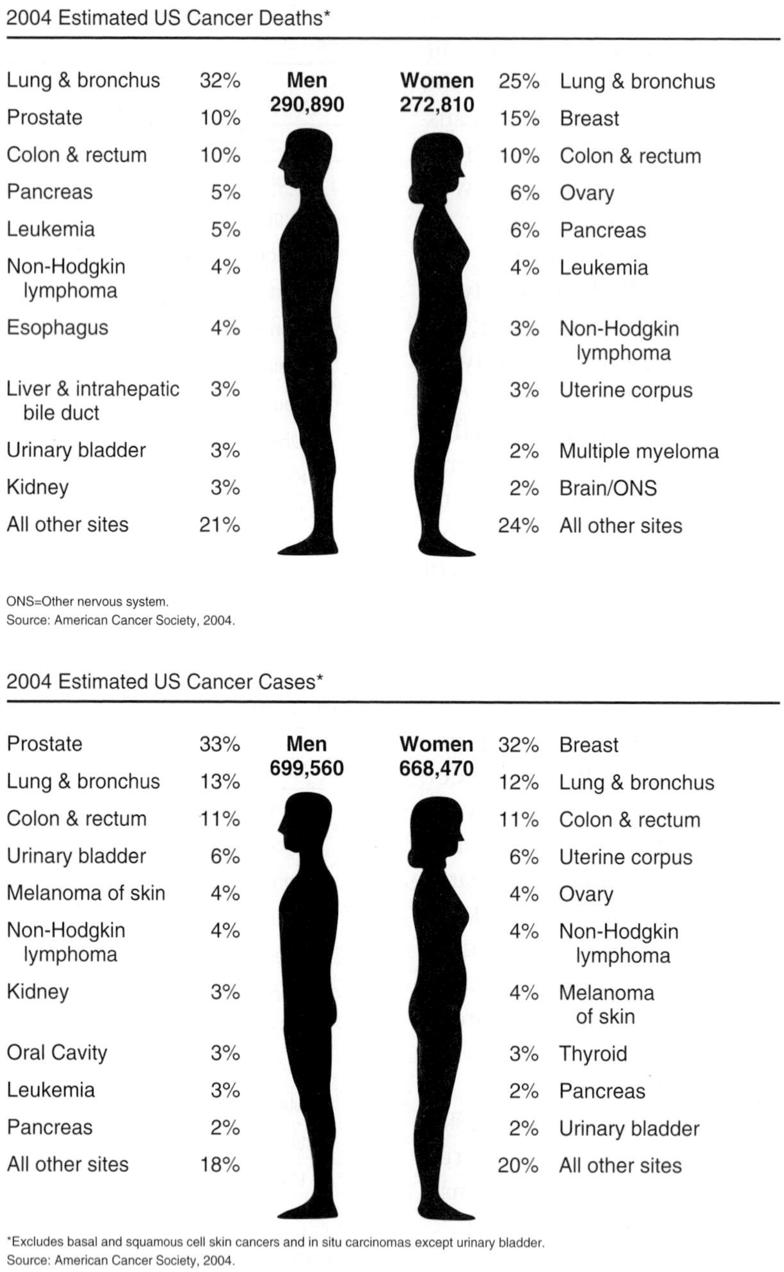

2004 Estimated US Cancer Deaths*

| | | Men 290,890 | Women 272,810 | | |
|---|---|---|---|---|---|
| Lung & bronchus | 32% | | | 25% | Lung & bronchus |
| Prostate | 10% | | | 15% | Breast |
| Colon & rectum | 10% | | | 10% | Colon & rectum |
| Pancreas | 5% | | | 6% | Ovary |
| Leukemia | 5% | | | 6% | Pancreas |
| Non-Hodgkin lymphoma | 4% | | | 4% | Leukemia |
| Esophagus | 4% | | | 3% | Non-Hodgkin lymphoma |
| Liver & intrahepatic bile duct | 3% | | | 3% | Uterine corpus |
| Urinary bladder | 3% | | | 2% | Multiple myeloma |
| Kidney | 3% | | | 2% | Brain/ONS |
| All other sites | 21% | | | 24% | All other sites |

ONS=Other nervous system.
Source: American Cancer Society, 2004.

2004 Estimated US Cancer Cases*

| | | Men 699,560 | Women 668,470 | | |
|---|---|---|---|---|---|
| Prostate | 33% | | | 32% | Breast |
| Lung & bronchus | 13% | | | 12% | Lung & bronchus |
| Colon & rectum | 11% | | | 11% | Colon & rectum |
| Urinary bladder | 6% | | | 6% | Uterine corpus |
| Melanoma of skin | 4% | | | 4% | Ovary |
| Non-Hodgkin lymphoma | 4% | | | 4% | Non-Hodgkin lymphoma |
| Kidney | 3% | | | 4% | Melanoma of skin |
| Oral Cavity | 3% | | | 3% | Thyroid |
| Leukemia | 3% | | | 2% | Pancreas |
| Pancreas | 2% | | | 2% | Urinary bladder |
| All other sites | 18% | | | 20% | All other sites |

*Excludes basal and squamous cell skin cancers and in situ carcinomas except urinary bladder.
Source: American Cancer Society, 2004.

**FIGURE 3–9** Leading sites of new cancers and deaths. *(Source: American Cancer Society website www.cancer.org. Reprinted by the permission of the American Cancer Society, Inc.)*

acronym **CAUTION**. They may be indicative of cancer development, so the individual with one or more of these signs should be evaluated immediately by a physician.

**C**hange in bowel or bladder habits

**A** sore that does not heal

**U**nusual bleeding or discharge

**T**hickening or lump in breast or elsewhere

**I**ndigestion or difficulty swallowing

**O**bvious change in a wart or mole

**N**agging cough or hoarseness

Once discovered, the tumor must be diagnosed by microscopic examination of the cells and tissue. Examination of cells is called **cytology** (sigh-TOL-

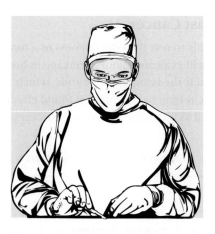

A small piece of tissue is surgically removed.

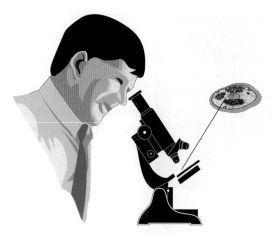

Pathologist views tissue under microscope looking for presence of disease.

**FIGURE 3–10** Tissue biopsy.

oh-jee; cyto = cell, ology = study) or a cytologic examination. Live tissue examination is a biopsy. A biopsy is the most definitive (clear-cut or without question) test used to diagnose a tumor.

A Papanicolaou or Pap test, so named after its developer Dr. George Papanicolaou, may be utilized to examine the cells. Although most people think of a Pap test as a test only for cervical cytology, in reality, this simple staining test can be utilized to examine other body fluids such as urine, feces, sputum, prostatic fluid, or vaginal fluids. Once the sample is stained, it is placed under a microscope and examined for abnormal cells.

To microscopically examine live tissue, a biopsy must be done. A biopsy may be obtained by aspiration, needle biopsy, endoscopy, or surgery. Aspiration biopsy utilizes a needle attached to a suction device to remove a small piece of tissue from the tumor. Needle biopsy is obtained by punching a needle through the tumor and using the tissue caught in the lumen of the needle for examination. If the size of the needle is quite small, the biopsy is called a fine needle biopsy. During endoscopy, the tissue is removed by use of the appropriate scope; for example, bronchoscope, colonoscope, or gastroscope. For surgical biopsy, the tissue is removed by cutting or incising the tissue (Figure 3–10).

Surgical biopsy may be performed with the patient's consent to surgically excise the tumor if it is found to be cancerous. Once the biopsy is obtained, it is sent immediately to the pathologist for diagnosis. The patient often remains in the surgical suite under anesthesia while the surgeon awaits these results. A technique called a **frozen section** enables the pathologist to make a rapid determination of the tumor condition: benign or malignant.

## SIGNS AND SYMPTOMS OF CANCER

Signs and symptoms of cancer are highly variable with the site and type of malignancy. Pain, obstruction, hemorrhage, anemia, fracture, infection, and cachexia may be manifestations of cancer. Any one of these or a combination may be present, but often, cancer is asymptomatic until late in its developmental stage, including metastasis.

Pain from cancer is usually not an early symptom. Cancer causes pain by growing to the point of causing destruction of normal tissue, obstructing the lumen of hollow organs like the intestine, placing pressure on nerve endings, and/or causing inflammation leading to discomfort.

Obstruction of a hollow organ may occur from a tumor growing inside the organ or from tumor growth outside the organ that compresses or pushes into the organ. Examples of obstruction could include the bronchus of the lung and any area of the intestine.

Hemorrhage may be caused by the cancerous tissue ulcerating and bleeding. This may lead to acute or chronic blood loss, and often results in anemia. Hidden blood in the feces may be detected by a Hemoccult stool test.

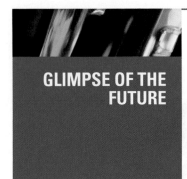

**Possible Vaccine against Breast Cancer**

Researchers have begun clinical trials to test the effectiveness of a tumor antigen for breast cancer. The study will evaluate tumor shrinkage in breast cancer patients. The antigen being studied is the telomerase peptide, which is found in almost all breast cancer tumors. The telomerase peptide, if found effective for shrinking the tumors, may then be used as a vaccine against breast cancer for women in the future.

*Source:* Biotech Week *(March 3, 2004).*

Anemia is very common in individuals with malignant neoplasm. The anemia may be the result of tumor hemorrhage as previously discussed. Anemia also may be due to a decrease in red blood cell production as a result of cancer treatments.

Pathologic fractures may occur if a tumor has invaded the bone and caused weakness at that site. A fracture occurring with a minimal injury may be indicative of a cancer, but in an older person, may also be due to osteoporosis. The bone tumor may be primary or secondary with cancer of the lung, breast, and prostate readily metastasizing to the bone.

Infection is common and may lead to the final demise of the individual. Tumor ulceration may allow entry of microorganisms causing infection. The individual may have impaired immunity due to **chemotherapy** (chemo = chemical, therapy = treatment) and radiation treatments, affecting the bone marrow and causing a decrease in production of white blood cells. Individuals with cancer often have a loss of appetite, leading to a poor nutritional state and increasing the chance of infection. Immune deficiency often leads to infection of the individual by a host of organisms such as fungi, viruses, protozoa, and bacteria that are not usually pathogenic.

Cachexia is a condition of general ill health and malnutrition often seen in the terminally ill patient (refer to Chapter 2, Figure 2–3). This condition is evidence of the demands placed on the body by the rapidly growing tumor and treatment modalities, coupled with poor nutritional intake.

## CANCER TREATMENT

New technological advances lead to ever changing treatment of malignant neoplasms. Treatment may be aimed at cure (**curative**), at relief of symptoms (**palliative**; **PAL**-ee-AY-tiv) or at prevention (preventive). The three major types of treatment include

## COMPLEMENTARY AND ALTERNATIVE THERAPY

**Cancer Patients and the Use of Complementary and Alternative Therapies**

Complementary and alternative therapies are frequently used by cancer patients. In fact, there is a recent increase in the use of these treatments as more herbal medicines and treatments are available over the counter in drug stores, grocery stores, and health food stores. In addition, treatments such as biofeedback, hypnosis, acupuncture, and aromatherapy are increasingly being offered in clinics and other offices. There are some significant safety issues that patients who choose to use these therapies need to consider. Although research has shown many of them to be effective, caution is necessary when using alternative therapies to prevent increased risk for the cancer patient.

*Source: Michaud, (2000).*

surgery, chemotherapy, and radiation. Hormone treatment may be the treatment of choice in some instances. The oncologist may recommend one of these treatments or a combination of them, depending on the type of cancer and treatment plan.

Surgery for cancer may be curative, palliative, or preventive. Curative surgery is aimed at complete removal of the tumor. Cancer of the lung, stomach, skin, breast, intestine, and female reproductive organs respond well to this type of surgery. Palliative surgery is usually indicated when cure is not possible, but when surgery will alleviate pain and discomfort. The intestine is an area commonly undergoing this type of surgery for obstruction, bleeding, or perforation. Surgery also may be performed to sever nerves in an effort to reduce pain. Preventive surgery may be performed to prevent development of cancer. Polyps in the colon may be removed if they are thought to be precancerous. A woman may undergo prophylactic mastectomy if she has been identified as one at high risk for breast cancer.

Chemotherapy may be the medication of choice, or used in combination with surgery and radiation therapy. Generally, chemotherapy is effective to treat rapidly growing metastatic neoplasms. Chemotherapy is aimed at rapidly growing neoplastic cells with the idea that it will kill or inhibit the growth of these cells while having minimal effect on normal cells. In some instances, the growth rate of normal cells and neoplastic cells is not varied enough and normal body cells suffer from the effects of the treatment. Rapid growing normal cells such as those found in the epithelium, hair, and bone marrow suffer the most, leading to nausea, vomiting, loss of appetite, hair loss, anemia, and impaired immunity.

Radiation is generally used to treat tumors that are not surgically accessible nor operable, and in treatment of residual neoplasm postoperatively. Palliative radiation treatments may shrink the tumor and relieve discomfort. Radiation treatment may be external with direct radiation or internal using radioisotope beads, seeds, or ribbons that are implanted inside the body. Both methods are aimed at disrupting DNA and interfering with cell growth and replication. The goal is to destroy as much of the tumor as possible without affecting the normal tissue surrounding it. Adverse effects generally occur in the skin, mucous membranes, and bone marrow, leading to nausea, vomiting, loss of appetite, hair loss, and impaired immunity.

Hormone therapy may cause regression in tumors of the breast and prostate. Administration of antagonistic hormones or excision of hormone-producing organs such as the ovaries and testes may be effective in prolonging life. Hormone therapy is generally used as a palliative treatment for metastatic tumors.

## SUMMARY

Neoplasms are new growths that can arise from cells almost anywhere in the body. They can be benign or malignant. Tumor is the term commonly used to describe a neoplasm, but not all neoplasms form tumors. Hyperplasias are similar to neoplasms because they are an overgrowth of cells, but they are like their cell of origin and neoplasms are not. Neoplasms that are malignant are usually called cancers. They are usually named for the type of tissue from which they developed. Metastatic cancers are those that spread to other parts of the body.

The cause of most cancer is unknown, but research has identified some carcinogens in the environment as well as high-risk behaviors that may contribute to cancer development. The American Cancer Society has recommended preventive measures and lists seven warning signs of cancer. Although cancer causes over half of all deaths in the United States, with early diagnosis and treatment, there is a good prognosis for most types of cancer.

# REVIEW QUESTIONS

## Short Answer

1. What is the difference between a neoplasm and a tumor?

2. How are neoplasms classified?

3. What is the largest group of malignant neoplasms?

4. When a malignant neoplasm moves to various parts or organs of the body, it is said to be a _____ tumor.

5. What is the difference between hyperplasia and neoplasms?

## True or False

6. T F Grading is the microscopic examination of the tumor to determine the degree of differentiation.
7. T F Tumors that are undifferentiated or anaplastic do not resemble the tissue of origin, are highly malignant, and have a poor prognosis.
8. T F Radioactive materials that emit alpha, beta, and gamma rays are not considered to be potential carcinogens.
9. T F There is no known genetic predisposition for cancer.
10. T F There are several personal risk behaviors common in our society that put an individual at increased risk for developing cancer.

## Matching

11. Match the term in the left column with the phrase that best describes it from the column on the right.

_____ Metastatic neoplasm

_____ Cancer of the lung, breast, and colon

_____ CAUTION

_____ Basal and squamous cell skin cancer

_____ Biopsy

_____ Liver, lungs, and brain

_____ Ultraviolet (UV) radiation, X-radiation, and radioactive materials

_____ Routine screening

a. known carcinogens

b. an acronym for the seven warning signs of cancer

c. microscopic examination of live tissue

d. responsible for the majority of cancer deaths

e. cells whose growth pattern has no purpose and is uncontrollable

f. common sites of bloodstream metastasis

g. the most common type of cancer

h. major types of cancer treatment

_____ Surgery, chemotherapy, and radiation

_____ Palliative

**i.** treatment aimed at relieving symptoms

**j.** very effective in the discovery and early diagnosis of cancer

## CASE STUDY

**Mr. Holloway** is a 65-year-old man who has made an appointment for a routine checkup. He has not complained of any unusual symptoms but feels he should have a yearly examination because of his age. What are some routine screening tests that should be done on Mr. Holloway because of his age and gender? What important cancer prevention strategies should you discuss with Mr. Holloway during his visit?

## BIBLIOGRAPHY

American Cancer Society (2004). *Cancer Statistics 2004.* www.cancer.org (accessed November, 2004).

Bostrom, B., Sandh, M., Lundberg, D., & Fridlund, B. (2004). Cancer related pain in palliative care: Patient's perceptions of pain management. *Journal of Advanced Nursing 45*(4), 410–419.

Caruso, F., & Rossi, M. (2004). Antitumor titanium compounds. *Initial Reviews in Medicinal Chemistry 4*(3)49–60.

Coker, A. L., Bond, S. M., Williams, A., Gerasimova, T., & Pirisi, L. (2002). Active and passive smoking, high-risk human papillomaviruses and cervical neoplasia. *Cancer Detection & Prevention 26*(2), 121–128.

Coleman, R. L. (1992). Cervical cancer. Causes and prevention. *Priorities 4*(3), www.acsh.org/41Ahealth issues/newsID.801/healthissue_detail.asp.

Coleman, E. A., Hall-Barrow, J., Coon, S., & Stewart, C. B. (2003). Facilitating exercise adherence for patients with multiple myeloma. *Clinical Journal of Oncology Nursing 7*(5), 529–535.

Continuing research should improve, may achieve cure of common neoplasms. (2004, January 5). *Health & Medicine Week*, 524–525.

Cullinane, C. A., Boreman, T., Smith D. D., Chu, D. Z. J., Ferrell, B. R., & Wagman, L. D. (2003, November 15). The surgical treatment of cancer. *Cancer: Diagnosis, Treatment, Research 98*(10), 2266–2274.

Di Paolo, A., Danesi, R., & Del Tacca, M. (2004). Pharmacogenetics of neoplastic diseases: New trends. *Pharmacological Research 49*(4), 331–342.

Findley, R. S. (2003, December 15). Overview of targeted therapies for cancer. *American Journal of Health-System Pharmacy 60*(24), 4–10.

Lobchuk, M. M. (2003). The memorial symptom assessment scale: Modified for use in understanding family caregivers' perceptions of cancer patients' symptom experiences. *Journal of Pain & Symptom Management 26*(1), 644–654.

Loerzel, V. W., & Dow, K. H. (2003). Cardiac toxicity related to cancer treatment. *Clinical Journal of Oncology Nursing 7*(5), 557–563.

Michaud, L. B. (2000). Complementary/alternative therapies. *Cancer Practice 8*(5), 243–247.

Purvis Cooper, C., Merritt, T. L., Ross, L. E., John, L. V., & Jorgensen, C. M. (2004). To screen or not to screen, when clinical guidelines disagree: Primary care physicians' use of the PSA test. *Preventive Medicine 38*(2), 182.

Risk of second malignant neoplasms increased after childhood neuroblastoma. (2004, January 5). *Health & Medicine Week*, 565.

Schwartz, L. M., Woloshin, S., Fowler, F. J., Jr., & Welch, H. G. (2004, January 7). Enthusiasm for cancer screening in the United States. *JAMA 291*(1), 71–79.

Sherry, V. W. (2002). Taste alterations among patients with cancer. *Clinical Journal of Oncology Nursing 6*(2), 1–5.

Shoulder girdle neoplasms can mimic frozen shoulder syndrome. (2003, December 16). *Cancer Weekly*, 162.

Skarin, A. T., Shaffer, K., & Wieczorek, T. (eds.). (2003). *Atlas of diagnostic oncology.* St. Louis, MO: Mosby.

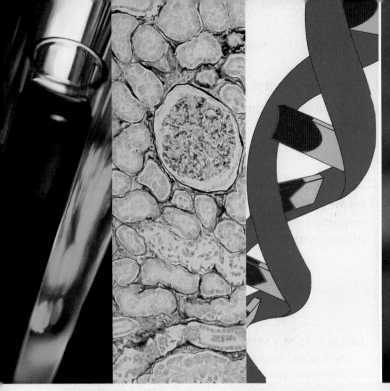
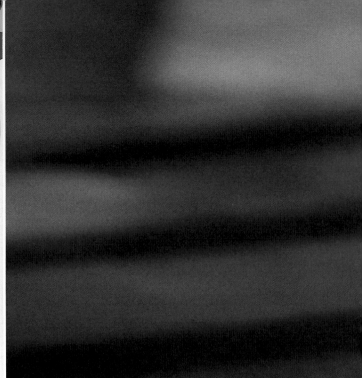

## OUTLINE

## KEY TERMS

# Inflammation and Infection

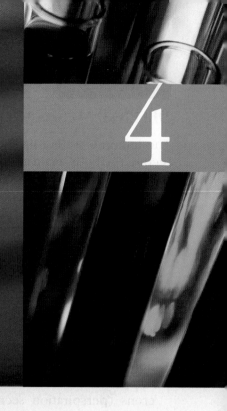

**4**

## LEARNING OBJECTIVES

*Upon completion of the chapter, the learner should be able to:*

1. Identify important terminology related to the defense mechanisms.

2. Describe the basic defense mechanisms in the body.

3. Explain the steps in the inflammatory process.

4. Describe the process of tissue repair and healing.

5. Identify complications of wound healing.

6. Describe the process of infection development.

7. Identify the common infectious microorganisms and the resulting diseases.

8. Identify the common laboratory test conducted to identify pathogenic organisms.

## OVERVIEW

*T*he human body is in a constant state of activity. The overall goal in the body's responses to foreign invaders or pathogens is to prevent trauma and maintain homeostasis. The defense mechanisms are responsible for this protection. Inflammation is a natural protective mechanism. When the protective mechanisms fail, the usual result is an infection. Infections are diagnosed and treated in a variety of ways. ■

## DEFENSE MECHANISMS

The immune system has the difficult job of protecting the body against foreign invasion. Defense may be nonspecific, protecting the body against any and all invaders; or it may be specific, identifying the invader prior to its demise. This system utilizes three basic lines of defense to accomplish this goal.

1. Physical or Surface Barriers (nonspecific)—An intact skin is the body's first line of defense. The skin is a physical barrier and the acidic surface is also antimicrobial. The normal bacterial flora of the skin acts as a placeholder, preventing habitation by other **bacteria** (microscopic, one-celled organisms). Sebaceous (oil secreting) and odoriferous (perspiration secreting) glands secrete antibacterial acids and enzymes. Mucous membranes serve to trap invaders.

2. Inflammation (nonspecific)—If physical barriers are broken and the foreign invader penetrates the cells and tissues, the inflammatory response occurs. This response begins within seconds of an unwanted invasion. It is a stereotypic vascular response. In other words, the process unfolds or follows the same pattern, regardless of the type of invader. The primary goals of the inflammatory response are to isolate or wall off the invader, destroy it, and clean up the debris, thereby promoting healing.

3. Immune Response (specific)—The third and last line of defense reacts to invasion much slower than inflammation, but with specific killing ability. All cells, even human body cells, have protein or saccharide markers on their surfaces that identify the cell. This marker is called an **antigen** (AN-tih-jen). During the immune response, the body actually identifies the invader by the antigen. Once the antigen is identified, antibodies are produced by lymphocytes. Antibodies link with the cell antigen, thus killing the cell or rendering it helpless. This immunologic defense has the unique ability to remember the invader and produce more antibodies if the invader returns (Figure 4–1).

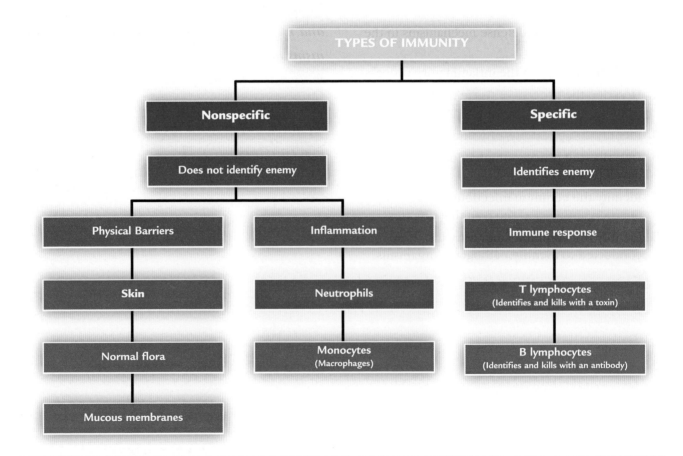

**FIGURE 4–1**  Immunity—lines of defense.

# INFLAMMATION

Inflammation is a nonspecific cellular and vascular reaction to any tissue **trauma** (TRAW-mah; injury). The primary goals of the inflammatory response are to isolate or wall off the invader, destroy it, and clean up the debris, thereby promoting healing. One limiting factor of inflammation is that it cannot occur in tissue that does not have a blood supply.

If tissue is destroyed by injury, the inflammatory process will only occur along borders of the injury where blood supply is maintained. Gangrene is an example of this process. In gangrenous tissue, inflammation cannot occur in the dead or necrotic tissue, but there is an observable reaction along its borders.

The fact that inflammation will only occur in vascularized (supplied with blood) tissue is important in forensic medicine. Evidence of inflammation in tissue confirms that an injury occurred while the individual was alive. If no evidence of inflammation exists, the pathologist can be assured that the person was dead when the injury was inflicted.

Inflammation is designed to be a beneficial, protective defense mechanism. In some instances, the reaction may become so intense that it becomes harmful to tissues. An acute hypersensitivity reaction may lead not only to local tissue damage, but also to anaphylactic shock and death of the individual. If the process goes awry, producing an autoimmune reaction, the body begins to basically destroy itself. Anti-inflammatory medications may be needed to stop the reaction if it becomes injurious.

# THE INFLAMMATORY PROCESS

When any tissue undergoes trauma (injury), regardless of the cause, inflammation will occur. The trauma may be due to physical injury, invasion of microorganisms, ischemia (decreased oxygen in cells), freezing, burning, electrocution, radiation, or chemical irritation to name a few.

**Mast cells**, also called tissue histocytes, are found in all tissues of the body and play a major role in the inflammatory process. When injured or irritated, these cells release **histamine**. Histamine causes local arterioles, venules, and capillaries to dilate, resulting in an increase in blood flow to the area. This increase in blood flow, called **hyperemia** (HIGH-per-EE-me-ah; hyper = increased, emia = blood), causes increased redness and heat in this area.

Hyperemia also brings increased numbers of leukocytes (white blood cells) to the area. The white cells that move into this area first and in the greatest numbers are neutrophils, also called *PMNs* (poly = many, morphic = shaped nucleus). These white cells line the endothelium of the vessels, awaiting the opportunity to move into the tissue.

As the capillaries dilate under the influence of histamine, vascular permeability occurs. In other words, the capillary becomes permeable or leaky as the endothelial cells are stretched apart. This permeability allows blood fluid called **exudate** (ECKS-you-dayt) to leak into the tissue. This leakage of fluid is the cause of the swelling or edema observed with inflammation.

As edema increases, more pressure is exerted on nerve endings, leading to increased pain. With increased pain and tenderness, the individual tends to guard this area and experiences loss of function. These vascular and cellular responses produce the five cardinal signs of inflammation: heat, redness, swelling, pain, and loss of function (Figure 4-2).

Vascular permeability also allows the awaiting neutrophils to escape into the tissue. The neutrophil extends a part of its body between the epithelial cells and squeezes through the capillary wall by a process called **diapedesis** (DYE-ah-pe-DEE-sis) (see Figure 4-2). The process of diapedesis is very effective, delivering millions of neutrophils to the area within a few hours.

Neutrophils can be considered the "foot soldiers" of the inflammatory process. They arrive first, they arrive in great numbers, and they readily move into action in the tissue. Neutrophils are drawn or directed to the injured area by a process called **chemotaxis**. One might think of this process as a "chemical taxi cab." Chemicals are released by a variety of things including bacteria, injured tissue, and plasma proteins. This chemical is detected through chemoreceptors on the neutrophil's outer membrane. This draws the neutrophil in the direction of the highest chemical concentration (see Figure 4-2).

Once the neutrophil arrives at the scene of the trauma, it begins the job of phagocytosis or cell eating. The neutrophil eats and destroys microorganisms, foreign materials, and dead cells. The life of the neutrophil is shortlived. Death of numerous neutrophils mixed with exudate or blood fluid make up, in part, the white fluid identified as **pus**.

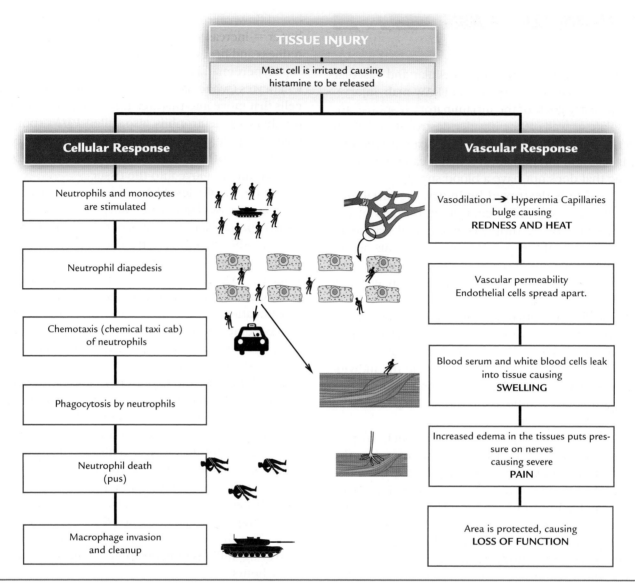

**FIGURE 4–2**   Acute inflammation—cellular and vascular response.

Approximately three to four days after the inflammatory process begins, large numbers of another type of white cell begin to arrive at the scene. This large, slow-moving cell is the monocyte. As the monocyte leaves the bloodstream and moves into the tissue, it becomes phagocytic and is called a **macrophage** (macro = large, phage = eat). As the name suggests, a macrophage is a large eater of microorganisms, foreign material, and dead cells. This cell might be considered the "tank" of the war because it is slower moving but has more killing power than the neutrophil. Another job of the macrophage is to act as the clean-up crew, cleaning up the dead neutrophils and tissue debris in the inflamed area.

Until this point, the **inflammation** is considered to be an acute (short-lived) situation. If the inflammation persists for a longer period of time, it is considered to be a chronic problem. This time period is difficult to establish because some chronic inflammations will exhibit periods of exacerbation (flare up), eliciting a new outpouring of neutrophils. Likewise, some acute inflammations will trigger the response of an unusually high number of macrophages.

After approximately seven to ten days, if the inflammatory process has not overcome the invader, the nuclear warheads of the defense system—the lymphocytes—are called on to respond. Lymphocytes are slow but powerful killers. They are part of the body's third line of defense: the immune response. They are specific killers. They identify the enemy, make an **antibody** to kill it, then remember the enemy and the killing process (see Figure 4–1). Refer to Chapter 5 for more detailed information on the immune system.

# CHRONIC INFLAMMATION

Generally speaking, a chronic inflammation may be considered to be one that lasts two weeks or longer. If the acute attack by neutrophils and macrophages is unsuccessful, the battle may become chronic. Microscopic examination of chronic inflammation will reveal a large number of macrophages and fewer neutrophils.

If macrophages are unable to overcome the invader and protect the host, the body may try to wall off and isolate the area by forming a granuloma. A granuloma is formed by macrophages and fibrous deposits of collagen, and may be hardened by calcium deposits. This granuloma protects the surrounding tissue and allows healing to begin. A classic cause of granuloma formation is tuberculosis. These granulomas may become quite large, form a fibrous rim, and eventually calcify. Another cause of granuloma is foreign body involvement. If foreign materials such as a wood splinter, gravel, suture, glass sliver, or metal fragments are embedded in the tissue, the body walls off the material to protect the adjacent tissue. This granuloma may become hardened with fibrous tissue and remain for the life of the individual.

# INFLAMMATORY EXUDATES

The duration and extent of an inflammatory **lesion** (LEE-zhun; any discontinuity of tissue) may be determined by direct visualization of the site. External inflammatory lesions are easily observed whereas internal inflammatory lesions in organs and cavities may require surgical or endoscopic examination. The appearance and amount of exudate or blood fluid may assist in identifying an acute or chronic condition.

Serous exudate is a clear serum-like fluid containing small amounts of protein. It implies a lesser degree of damage and occurs in the acute stage of inflammation. Examples of serous exudate include the fluid in skin blisters, cold sores, and injured joints to name a few. Serous exudate is easily reabsorbed once the inflammatory response is halted and healing begins.

Fibrinous exudate is composed of fluid and large amounts of fibrinogen. In comparison to serous exudate, the leakage of fibrinogen indicates a larger injury with more severe inflammation. Fibrinous exudate may be observed in strep throat or bacterial pneumonia, forming a mesh-like lesion. A superficial skin wound may be covered with dried fibrinous exudate commonly called a scab.

**Purulent** (PURR-you-lent) exudate is loaded with dead and dying PMNs or neutrophils, tissue debris, and **pyogenic** (PYE-oh-**JEN**-ick; pyo = pus, genic = arising) or pus-forming bacteria. Purulent exudate is commonly called pus. A localized collection of pus is called an **abscess**. An accumulation of pus in a body cavity is called **empyema** (EM-pye-**EE**-mah). For example, pus accumulated in the chest or thoracic cavity would be called thoracic empyema.

# INFLAMMATORY LESIONS

Any discontinuity or abnormality of tissue is called a lesion. Lesion is a broad term that includes wounds, ulcers, wheals, blisters, vesicles, pustules, or tumors to name a few. Lesions are due to physical or pathologic injury. Inflammatory lesions include abscesses, ulcers, and **cellulitis** (SELL-you-**LYE**-tis; inflammation of connective tissue).

## Abscesses

Abscesses are typically caused by streptococcal and staphylococcal (pyogenic) bacteria. During the inflammatory response, the body attempts to contain or stop the spread of the bacteria into adjacent tissue by forming a wall around the area. When this wall forms around a purulent exudate, an abscess is formed. Boils, furuncles, and pimples are examples of abscesses.

Typically, a small abscess shows signs of acute inflammation: redness, heat, swelling, and pain. When the central portion of the abscess softens or develops a "head," puncturing the head will cause an outpouring of pus, relief of pain, and onset of healing. Puncturing the abscess before the area is walled off and the head is soft may lead to a spread of the infecting organism.

A small abscess may rupture and heal spontaneously, but a large abscess may need to be surgically incised and drained. Draining an abscess speeds healing. Without drainage, the body must continue to battle the invading organisms. If the body is successful, it will eventually win the battle, reabsorb the exudate, and replace the area with fibrous tissue. A large abscess, if not contained, may spread and become fatal. An example of this process is the abscess formation occurring in appendicitis. If a large abscess ruptures, it tends to form a tract or opening to the surface of the body called a **sinus**. If this tract connects two organs or cavities to each other or to the surface of the skin, it is called a **fistula** (FIS-tyou-lah) (Figure 4–3).

## Ulcer

An **ulcer** is a crater-like lesion in the skin or mucous membranes. It is the result of an injury and the subsequent inflammatory response. The tissue in this

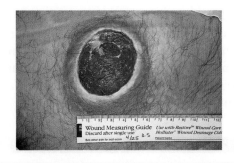

**FIGURE 4–4**   Pressure ulcer. *(Permission to reproduce this copyrighted material has been granted by the owner, Hollister Incorporated.)*

area becomes necrotic (dead) and sloughs off, leaving a crater or excavated area. Ulcers are commonly seen in the stomach and duodenum as a result of injury by bacteria and stomach acid. Pressure ulcers, commonly called bedsores or decubitus ulcers, are caused by excessive pressure on tissue. Pressure ulcers primarily appear over bony prominences of the body, especially those effected in the lying position such as the heel, sacrum, elbow, and scapula (Figure 4–4).

## Cellulitis

Cellulitis is a diffuse or widespread acute inflammatory process. It is usually seen in the skin and subcutaneous tissues. Cellulitis is characterized by general edema and redness. Cellulitis of the face primarily involves the cheeks and periorbital (peri = around, orbital = eye) areas. This type of cellulitis must receive special attention as it may spread to the sinuses of the brain. Cellulitis is often caused by streptococcus or staphylococcus bacteria, and is due to the body's inability to confine or wall off the causative organism. Cellulitis is potentially dangerous but usually can be treated effectively with antibiotics.

## TISSUE REPAIR AND HEALING

Tissue repair and healing is an ongoing process much like any other body process. Proper repair and healing occurs in most instances, but this process can be influenced by many other factors. Healing may be impaired or slowed when secondary diseases are present, the body is malnourished, or the immune system is compromised.

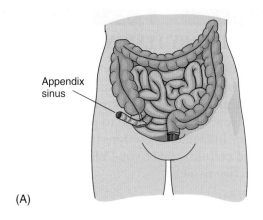

Appendix sinus

(A)

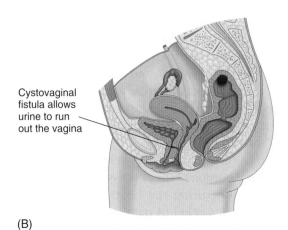

Cystovaginal fistula allows urine to run out the vagina

(B)

**FIGURE 4–3**   (A) sinus and (B) fistula.

# Tissue Repair

During the final phase of the inflammatory process, macrophages are responsible for cleaning up the area and producing growth factors that aid in the repair process. Repair of tissue also depends on cellular regeneration and the type of cells that make up the tissue. Some cells divide quite readily but others do not. Cellular proliferation or division can be grouped into three general categories.

1. Mitotic Cells—continuously divide throughout life. These cells are found in the skin and mucosa of internal organs. They readily replace damaged tissue.

2. Facultative Mitotic Cells—do not divide regularly, but can be stimulated to divide when necessary. These cells are found in such organs as the liver and kidney. Some part of these organs must remain intact for these cells to be available to divide and replace the lost tissue.

3. Nondividing Cells—do not divide under any condition. Cells of this type include nerves, brain cells, and heart muscle cells. Repair of these tissues is by fibrous scarring.

The body's two basic methods of repair involve healing by regeneration and fibrous connective tissue repair or **scar** formation. Regeneration is the best type of repair because it usually leads to restoration of normal function while fibrous connective tissue repair does not.

**Regeneration.** Regeneration involves mitotic cell division. During regeneration, the damaged tissue is replaced by cellular division of healthy tissue. For example, skin tissue is replaced by epithelial cell division, and bone tissue is replaced by osteocyte division. Regeneration can usually occur in internal organs if the major framework of the organ has not been destroyed. Complex structures such as lung tissue and glomeruli (in the kidney) do not regenerate. Regeneration is particularly important when there is damage to a large amount of tissue. Epithelial regeneration is very beneficial with massive burns. Bone cells have a remarkable ability to regenerate from a few remaining cells or may be transplanted from another individual by bone marrow transplant.

**Fibrous Connective Tissue Repair (Scar Formation).** Fibrous connective tissue repair or scar formation may occur in any tissue and produces the same result, no matter the location. The result is a tough fibrous tissue called a scar. A scar provides a bridge between the normal tissue and the wound, but it does not restore function. Wound repair of nerves, brain tissue, and heart muscle is by fibrous connective tissue repair (Figure 4-5).

# Tissue Healing

Tissue healing can be separated into categories of healing by primary union or secondary union. Categorization is determined by whether the wound edges are approximated (pulled together) or left separated during the healing process.

**Primary Union (First Intention).** **Primary union,** also called healing by first intention, involves approximating the edges of the wound. A classic example of healing by primary union is the healing process following a clean surgical incision. The wound edges are clean, there is minimal tissue damage, and the edges are approximated or brought together with sutures, staples, or tape.

Primary healing occurs in an orderly fashion. The steps of primary healing include the following:

1. The incisional line quickly fills with serum, forming a scab.

2. Within one to two days, new capillaries begin to bridge the gap between the wound edges.

3. In the next few days, fibroblasts grow across the deeper wound layers and begin to deposit collagen in this fibrous network. This tissue is called granulation tissue.

4. The collagen begins to contract, pulling the wound edges together and forming a scar.

After a few weeks, the incision may appear healed, but the deeper layers of tissue may not be healed for a month or more. Usually, an incisional scar will pale in color and shrink in size over a period of months or years.

**Secondary Union (Secondary Intention).** Large wounds and those infected by dirt, debris, and bacteria cannot be pulled together to heal by primary intention. The process of healing by **secondary union** is the same process as that of primary union, but involves a larger degree of tissue damage and more inflammation to resolve (Figure 4-6). To fill the wound, large numbers of capillaries, fibroblasts,

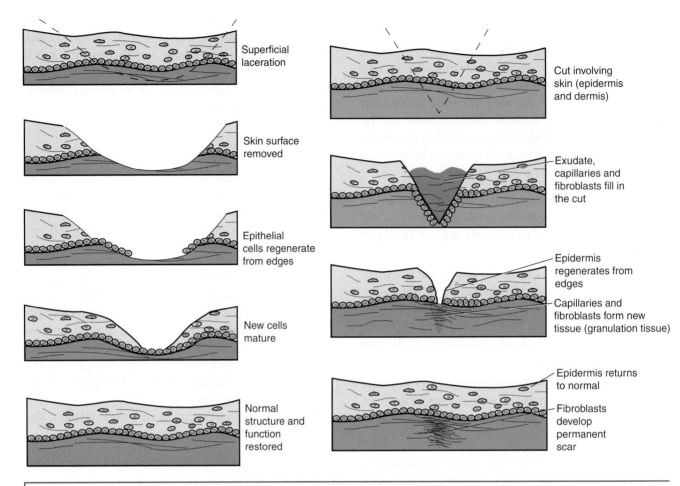

Superficial laceration

Skin surface removed

Epithelial cells regenerate from edges

New cells mature

Normal structure and function restored

Cut involving skin (epidermis and dermis)

Exudate, capillaries and fibroblasts fill in the cut

Epidermis regenerates from edges

Capillaries and fibroblasts form new tissue (granulation tissue)

Epidermis returns to normal

Fibroblasts develop permanent scar

**FIGURE 4–5** Tissue repair—complete regeneration and fibrous connective tissue repair.

and collagen must be produced. After a week or so, the new, soft red tissue is called granulation tissue. Granulation tissue is eventually replaced as more collagen is deposited in the area. The collagen contracts, pulling the wound edges together and beginning the formation of a scar. Healing time varies depending on the size of the wound. Large wounds may take a long time to heal by secondary union. Additional time will be needed for the scar to develop the strength of the surrounding tissue. If the wound is too large, the epithelium may not be able to bridge the gap and a skin graft may be needed.

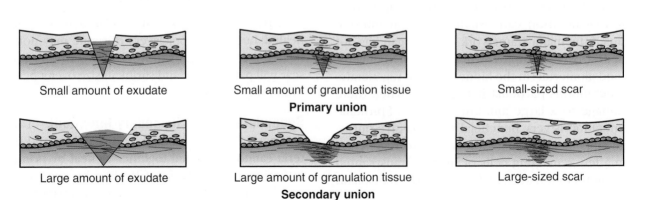

Small amount of exudate

Small amount of granulation tissue
**Primary union**

Small-sized scar

Large amount of exudate

Large amount of granulation tissue
**Secondary union**

Large-sized scar

**FIGURE 4–6** Tissue healing—primary and secondary union.

# Delayed Wound Healing

One of the greatest impediments to wound healing is the amount of dead tissue and debris in the wound. The debris may be dirt, bacteria, dead leukocytes, or a variety of other contaminates. It could take the body's leukocytes weeks or months to phagocytize (eat up) all the debris. In the meantime, bacteria may be producing dead cells and necrotic tissue as fast as the clean-up effort can advance. To speed healing, dirty wounds are cleaned and débrided. **Débridement** (day-breed-MON) is a process of washing or cutting away necrotic tissue and foreign material.

Other factors affecting healing time include the following:

1. Age—Younger people heal more rapidly than older people.

2. Size—Smaller wounds heal faster than larger ones.

3. Location—Epithelial tissue heals rapidly compared to other tissue types.

4. Nutrition—Good nutritional status promotes wound healing. Protein and vitamin C are essential to healing.

5. Immobility—Wound tissue heals more rapidly if it is kept immobile.

6. Circulation—Tissue with good blood supply heals more rapidly. Epithelial tissue heals more readily than cartilage. Individuals with diabetes have small blood vessel disease (diabetic microangiopathy), leading to ischemia of the tissue and poor wound healing.

7. Organism Virulence—Wounds infected with **virulent** (VIR-you-lent; poisonous) microorganisms are slower to heal than those that are not infected.

8. Steroids—Steroid therapy inhibits the inflammatory response, giving the invading offender the upper hand.

# Complications of Wound Healing

Prolonged wound healing may occur as a result of any one or a combination of the factors previously discussed. Other complications of wound healing involve poor or excessive scar formation. A scar that does not have adequate strength may lead to wound **dehiscence** (dee-HISS-ens) or separation of tissue margins. Excessive collagen formation often results in a hard raised scar called a **keloid** (KEE-loid) (Figure 4–7). Keloid scars are often unsightly but harmless, and occur more often in the black population. Surgical removal may result in the formation of another keloid.

Adhesions from scar tissue may be a complication of surgery, especially abdominal surgery. As normal fibrous scar tissue develops in the operative organ, a part of this tissue may cling to the surface of the adjoining organs. The fibrous band that develops is called an **adhesion** (ad-HE-zhun). Adhesions are often asymptomatic and cause no difficulties, but in some cases, they may become painful and may lead to obstruction of the adjacent organ. The intestine is an organ that is frequently obstructed by adhesions following abdominal surgery. Further surgery may be needed to release painful or obstructive adhesions.

# INFECTION

Chapter 2 briefly discusses the difference between inflammation and infection. Inflammation is a protective immune response and can occur without bacterial invasion. **Infection**, on the other hand, refers to the invasion of microorganisms into the tissue causing cell or tissue injury, thus leading to the inflammatory response.

Humans live with disease-causing microorganisms all around them. Some bacteria even live on the skin surface, in the respiratory tract, and in the intestine without causing illness, and some are actually beneficial. These bacteria are called normal flora.

Microorganisms that produce disease are called pathogenic. Normal flora may become pathogenic under certain conditions. When this occurs, the normal flora bacteria become **opportunistic** because they take the "opportunity" to cause infection in the host.

Certain conditions must be present for a microorganism to cause an infection in the host. Pathogens must have an area to enter, be resistant enough to survive, enter in great enough numbers to survive, and overcome the defenses of the individual.

First, the microorganism must successfully gain access into the body through a portal of entry. Any break in the skin allows entry of microorganisms. Common openings such as the nose, mouth, eyes, and ears are portals of entry. The most common port

**FIGURE 4–7**  Keloid. *(Courtesy of Mark L. Kuss.)*

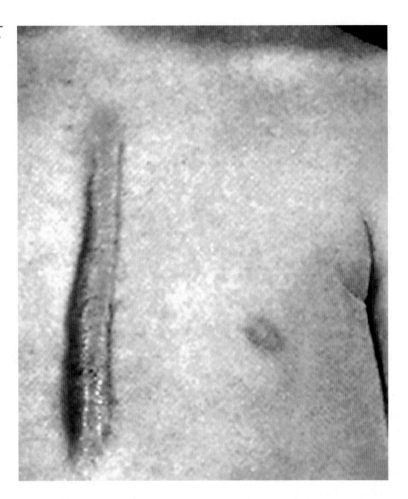

of entry is the respiratory system. Other portals include the digestive system, urinary tract, and reproductive tract.

Second, the pathogen also must be resistant to the defenses of the host. The ability of a microorganism to overcome the defense of the host is its virulence. A virulent microorganism has an aggressive or invasive nature. It also has the ability to produce a toxin or poison, which injures tissues. The degree of virulence of a microorganism varies. Generally speaking, organisms that come from an infected host are more virulent than those grown in laboratory conditions.

Third, the number of invading pathogens also plays a part in the conditions necessary for infection. Pathogenic organisms that are weak or not very virulent may cause infection if they invade in large enough numbers to overcome the body's defense system. Generally speaking, the higher the number of invading pathogens, the greater the risk of infection.

Finally, the condition of the individual or the host is a determinant of infection risk. An individual who is in good physical and emotional health, has good nutrition, practices risk-reducing living habits,

and is relatively young has a good chance of avoiding infection.

## Frequency and Types of Infection

Infectious diseases are the leading cause of death in the world. A country's ability to track and identify infectious diseases is an important weapon in the control of disease. In the United States, the Centers for Disease Control and Prevention (CDC), based in Atlanta, provide these services.

Respiratory infections, including upper respiratory infections, influenza-like infections, pneumonia, and bronchitis account for over 80 percent of all infections. Childhood infections, wound infections, viral infections, and other types of infection account for the remaining number of infections diagnosed.

Microorganisms that produce infection in humans include bacteria, **viruses**, **fungi**, **rickettsiae** (RIC-**KET**-see-ah), **protozoa**, and **helminths** (Table 4-1). These organisms can produce infections in the host that range from very mild to life threatening.

**TABLE 4–1** Some Common Infections Caused by Microorganisms in Humans

| Bacteria | Virus | Fungus |
| --- | --- | --- |
| *Staphylococcus* | Common Cold | Ringworm (Tinea) |
| *Streptococcus* | Herpes Simplex | Athlete's Foot |
| *Escherichia Coli* | Mononucleosis | *Candidiasis* |
| *Klebsiella* | HIV | Thrush |
| *Pseudomonas* | Measles | Vaginitis |
| *Shigella* | Mumps | Histoplasmosis |
| *Salmonella* | Rubella | *Coccidioidomycosis* |
| | Influenza (flu) | |

| Rickettsial | Protozoan | Helminths |
| --- | --- | --- |
| Rocky Mountain | Malaria | Roundworms |
| Spotted Fever | Giardiasis | Flatworms |
| | | Pinworms |
| | | Tapeworms |

**Bacteria.** Bacterial infections may occur as a primary or secondary disease. Primary bacterial infections occur when one is exposed to a pathogen. Secondary infection occurs after the onset of another disease process or condition. Secondary infections are very common. The most common cause for secondary infection is obstruction of a body passageway. For example, nasal obstruction may lead to sinusitis, and obstruction of the eustachian tubes may lead to otitis media or middle ear infection.

Bacteria normally live on or in the skin, mouth, nose, genital tract, and intestines of humans. These normal flora bacteria often become pathogenic when they gain access into the body or when the body's resistance is less than normal. *Staphylococcus* is a bacterium of the skin that often enters the body and can infect any organ. *Staph aureus* is an important member of the staphylococcus family because it has the ability to develop strains that are resistant to penicillin and other antibiotics. Methicillin resistant

## COMPLEMENTARY AND ALTERNATIVE THERAPY

**Herbal Medicines for Fighting Infections**

Herbal therapies for fighting infections may not be a well-accepted treatment in Western medicine, but historically, many medical practitioners have used a variety of herbal medicines for prevention and treatment of infections. Traditional Mayan and Native American cultures have used herbs for centuries, and still do today. Even some Western medicine practitioners now support the use of herbs for some ailments. Such preparations as cordyceps (*Cordyceps sinensis*) for strengthening the lungs, guduchi (*Tinospora cordifolia*) for enhancing antibody production, and astragalus (*Astragalus membranaceus*) for strengthening immunity are commonly used in other cultures. None of these potentially infection-fighting herbs should be taken without consulting a physician. Some herbal medicines may react with prescription medications.

*Source: Tarkan, (2003).*

## HEALTHY HIGHLIGHT

### Medication Precautions

**W**ARNING! Anyone taking a prescribed antibiotic medication should always take ALL of the medication. Even if the symptoms stop, the medication should be taken until it is completed. Antibiotics should not be "saved" for the next illness. Failure to complete antibiotic therapy may lead to the development of antibiotic resistant strains of bacteria. In other words, the first doses of medication may kill weaker bacteria and stun the stronger ones. If therapy is halted, the stronger bacteria may survive and reproduce strains that can resist the antibiotic. When this occurs, stronger and usually more expensive medications must be used to treat the same infection at a later date. Mismanagement of antibiotic therapy has led to development of strains of bacteria that now must be treated with stronger oral antibiotics or IV antibiotics.

---

*Staphylococcus aureus* (MRSA) is such a strain. These antibiotic-resistant strains are particularly dangerous because they are difficult to control and eliminate.

*Streptococcus* bacteria normally live on the skin and in the throat. Common infections caused by *streptococcus* bacteria include strep throat, scarlet fever, pneumonia, and meningitis. Strep throat in a select group of individuals may lead to rheumatic fever and glomerulonephritis.

Enteric bacteria are those living in the intestinal tract. Common enteric bacteria include *Escherichia coli* (*E. coli*), *Klebsiella, Pseudomonas, Shigella,* and *Salmonella. E. coli* causes enteritis in infants and adults, and may be the cause of travelers' diarrhea. *E. coli* and *Klebsiella* are common causes of urinary tract infections. *Pseudomonas* commonly infects wounds, and is associated with a foul odor and green pus production. *Shigella* and *Salmonella* infections cause diarrhea. *Salmonella* is the causative organism of food poisoning.

**Viruses.** Viruses are the smallest infective organisms and must be visualized by an electron microscope. Viruses cannot reproduce or live outside the cell. They must invade the cell and use it to reproduce their genetic information. Lymphocytes of the immune system are the body's primary defense against viruses. Some viruses have the ability to mutate or change so the body cannot develop just one antibody to kill that type of virus.

Viral infections cannot be treated easily. There are some antiviral agents that can be given to individuals with reduced resistance to infections to try

to prevent the viral infection. Antibiotic therapy does not kill a virus. Usually, supportive care is given by treating the symptoms that the virus causes. Symptoms may include fever, sore throat, runny nose, headache, and chest congestion. Antibiotics will help in treatment of a secondary bacterial infection occurring with the viral infection.

Viral infections of the upper respiratory system, including the common cold, far outnumber other viral diseases. Cold sores, also known as herpes simplex, are very common and affect many individuals. Infectious mononucleosis frequently affects adolescents and young adults. Human immunodeficiency virus (HIV) is the cause of acquired immune deficiency syndrome (AIDS) and has become the most noted virus due to its fatal outcome.

Immunizations are effective in preventing many viral diseases such as measles, mumps, rubella, and small pox. Influenza virus (flu) mutates and requires new vaccines, with each mutation. Some viruses are latent types meaning they live inside the cell causing no harm until the body becomes stressed or impaired. Latent viruses, like those in the herpes family, replicate and cause symptoms during stressful periods.

**Fungi.** Fungi are microscopic plant-like organisms that cause diseases referred to as mycoses. Fungi are larger than bacteria and only a few types are pathogenic. Single-celled forms of fungi are called yeast.

Fungal infections of the skin such as those of the tinea family (ringworm and athlete's foot) are common. Candida, commonly called candidiasis or yeast

## HEALTHY HIGHLIGHT

### Prevention for the Common Cold

The common cold virus has over 100 strains. The body must identify and kill each different strain as the body becomes infected. An individual will not suffer with the same cold virus twice. This explains why young children have more colds than adults. As we age, we have become ill with many cold viruses and have developed immunity to this greater number. Cold viruses are very contagious, entering the body primarily through the respiratory tract. **Good hand washing is the best preventive measure for the common cold.**

---

infection, often occurs in individuals with suppressed immune systems, anyone on long-term antibiotic therapy, and in individuals with diabetes. Candida is a superficial infection of the skin and mucous membranes, appearing commonly in the moist folds of the skin, the mouth (thrush), vaginal cavity (vaginitis), and genital area.

Other fungal infections include histoplasmosis and coccidioidomycosis. These infections are common to certain geographical locations, but are not common in the general populous. Fungal infections can be treated with antifungal and antibiotic medications, but often are difficult to cure and may require long-term therapy.

**Rickettsiae.** Rickettsiae are microscopic organisms that are intermediate between bacteria and virus. They must live in the host cell like a virus. Rickettsiae are spread by fleas, ticks, mites, and lice, and can cause fatal infections in humans. The most common rickettsial infection is Rocky Mountain spotted fever.

**Protozoa.** Protozoa are single-celled microscopic members of the animal kingdom. They are found in the soil, and live on dead or decaying material. Infection is by ingestion of spores or by infected insect bites.

Malaria is the most prevalent protozoan infection worldwide, but is uncommon in the United States. The protozoa causing malaria live in and destroy the red blood cell of the host. Malaria is spread by mosquitos. Giardiasis is an intestinal infection caused by the protozoan *Giardia lamblia*. It is caused by drinking infected water and is treated with antibiotic therapy.

**Helminths.** Helminths are any of the round or flatworms. Helminth infestation is common worldwide but not as common in the United States. Pinworms and tapeworms are the most common helminths. Pinworms cause anal itching but do not cause serious illness. Tapeworms may cause intestinal disease in humans. All tapeworms are acquired by eating uncooked or inadequately cooked meat.

## Testing for Infection

Symptoms of infection in an individual may include fever, **tachycardia** (TACH-ee-**KAR**-dee-ah; tachy = rapid, cardia = heart rate), and **malaise** (general ill feeling). Often, blood studies will reveal **leukocytosis** (leuko = white, cyto = cell, osis = condition) or an increase in the white cell count. Blood from an

---

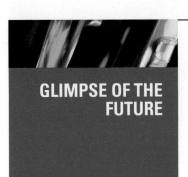

**GLIMPSE OF THE FUTURE**

### A Chinese Herbal Preparation May Be Used for Viral Diseases

The Chinese medicine zicao (purple gromwell, a dried root) has been found to inhibit the human immunodeficiency virus type 1 (HIV-1). The component in the medicine that has antiviral properties is called shikonin. The effect of shikonin on viruses is presently being studied at the National Cancer Institute. It has long been known that purple gromwell root (*Lithospermum erythrorhizon*) has a variety of biological effects. It may be used in the future as an anti-HIV agent.

*Source:* Health & Medicine Week (*October 20, 2003*).

individual with **septicemia** (SEP-tih-**SEE**-me-ah) will reveal the presence of the pathogen in the blood. Infection in the meninges, or meningitis, may show presence of pathogens in the individual's spinal fluid.

A culture is the process of growing pathogenic cells on or in a gelatin-like substance called media. Pathogenic organisms use this media for food (Figure 4–8). Media may be made of different nutrient agars. A common nutrient agar is sheep's blood agar. Laboratory studies of how the microorganism utilizes this food assist in the determination of the type of pathogen.

A culture is the most definitive test for organisms in a lesion or wound. Cultures are most commonly utilized for bacteria identification, but may also be utilized for identification of fungal infections. Most bacterial specimens are obtained from the throat, urine, sputum, purulent wound lesions, feces, blood, and spinal fluid.

A culture helps identify the pathogen. After identification of the pathogen, a sensitivity test is utilized to identify the type of treatment needed. The combined test for these is called a **culture and sensitivity** test. During a sensitivity test, the microorganisms are smeared on the nutrient agar and small antibiotic permeated disks are placed on the agar (Figure 4–9). After incubation, the agar plate is observed for killing zones around the disk. Disks that display a large kill zone are the most effective in treatment.

Specific antigen-antibody reactive tests may be utilized to determine the presence of pathogens. For example, a rapid diagnosis of strep throat may be made by testing for the presence of an antigen in a throat specimen. The streptococcus antigen will clot or clump when mixed with laboratory streptococcus antibody.

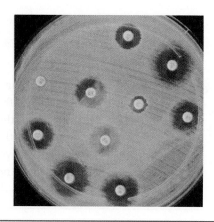

**FIGURE 4–9** Bacterial sensitivity.

Bacterial, rickettsial, and some other pathogenic infections may be determined by serologic testing. Serologic testing uses the individual's blood serum to test for antibodies against the pathogen.

Skin testing also utilizes antibody presence to determine exposure to pathogens. Tuberculosis (TB) skin testing is one of the most common skin tests. This test (also called the Mantoux test) involves the intradermal (under the skin) injection of tuberculin bacteria particles (antigen) (Figure 4–10). If an individual has been exposed to TB and has developed the TB antibody, this antibody will attack the antigen and cause an **induration** (**IN**-dur-RAY-shun; hardened tissue). Presence of an induration at the injection site is a positive skin test.

A positive skin test and serology testing may not indicate current infection or the degree of infection. These tests only indicate that the individual has been exposed to the pathogen and has developed antibodies. These are only a few of the many laboratory tests used in diagnosing pathogenic infections.

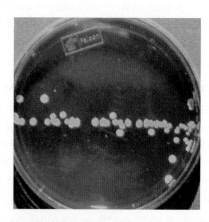

**FIGURE 4–8** Bacterial culture.

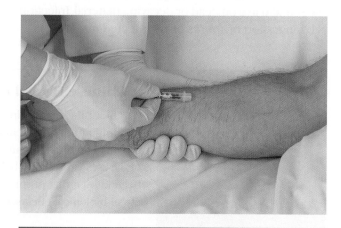

**FIGURE 4–10** Tuberculosis (TB) skin test.

## SUMMARY

The body responds to the invasions of pathogens by utilizing its defense mechanisms. Inflammation is a natural protective mechanism that occurs when physical barriers are broken and the invader penetrates the tissues. The inflammatory process consists of a series of events that eventually, if functioning properly, destroy the invading pathogen.

When this system of protection fails, infection may occur. Infections are caused by a variety of organisms, most commonly by bacteria and viruses. They are diagnosed and treated in a variety of ways. Several laboratory tests can be used to identify the organism and determine the appropriate therapy.

## REVIEW QUESTIONS

### Short Answer

1. What are the three defense mechanisms of the body? (Describe them.)

2. What are the steps in the inflammatory process?

3. How do inflammatory exudates and inflammatory lesions differ?

4. What are the five cardinal signs of inflammation?

5. What is the difference between a keloid and an adhesion?

6. Compare and contrast some microorganisms that produce infection in humans.

7. What type of testing is used to identify the organism causing an infection?

### Fill in the Blanks

8. Cellular proliferation can be grouped into the three categories of _____, _____, and _____.

9. The body's two main methods of repair involve _____ and _____.

10. Primary union is also called _____.

11. The process of secondary union involves a larger degree of _____ and more _____ to resolve than primary union.

12. The greatest impediments to wound healing are _____ and _____.

## CASE STUDY

**Mr. Jordan** has a sore throat and frequent cough, so he made an appointment with his physician for an evaluation. He was diagnosed with an upper respiratory infection. The physician prescribed an antibiotic for Mr. Jordan to be taken four times a day for ten days. What are some important points about taking the medication that Mr. Jordan should know? Although he already has an infection, is good handwashing still important? If so, why?

## BIBLIOGRAPHY

Caldwell, D. A., & Lovasik, D. (2002). Endocarditis in the immunocompromised. *American Journal of Nursing* (suppl.)*102*(5), 32–36.

Casillas, A. M., Nyamathi, A. M., Sosa, A., Wilder, C. L., & Sands, H. (2003). A current review of ebola virus: Pathogenesis, clinical presentation, and diagnostic assessment. *Biological Research for Nursing 4*(4), 268–275.

Coleman, E. A. (2001). Anthrax. *American Journal of Nursing 101*(12), 48–52.

Diabetic foot ulcers. (2003). *British Journal of Community Nursing 8*(9), S4.

Kennamer, M. (2002). *Basic infection control for health care providers*. Clifton Park, NY: Delmar Thomson Learning.

Michael, P. A. (2002). Preventing and treating meningococcal meningitis. *MEDSURG Nursing 11*(1), 9–12.

Nyamathi, A. M., Fahey, J. L., & Sands, H. (2003). Ebola virus: Immune mechanisms of protection and vaccine development. *Biological Research for Nursing 4*(4), 276–281.

Reilly, C. M., & Deason, D. (2002). Smallpox. *American Journal of Nursing 102*(2), 51–55.

Tarkan, L. (2003). Natural cold and flu fighters. *Natural Health 33*(9), 52–55.

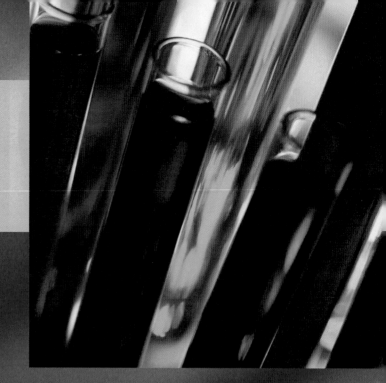

# UNIT

# II

# Common Diseases and Disorders of Body Systems

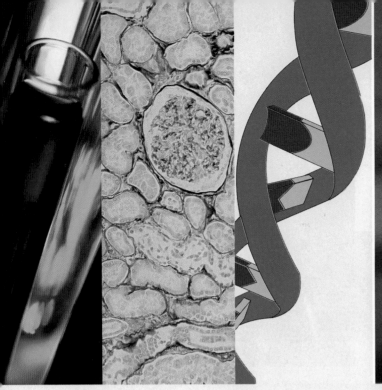
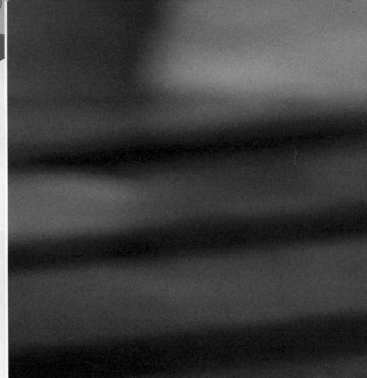

## OUTLINE

## KEY TERMS

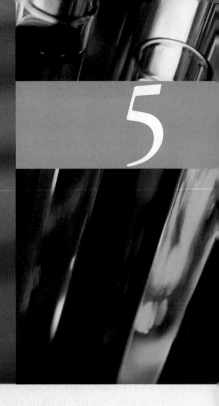

# Immune System Diseases and Disorders

# 5

## LEARNING OBJECTIVES

*Upon completion of the chapter, the learner should be able to:*

1. Define the terminology common to the immune system and the disorders of the system.

2. Discuss the basic anatomy and physiology of the immune system.

3. Identify the important signs and symptoms associated with common immune system disorders.

4. Describe the common diagnostics used to determine type and/or cause of an immune system disorder.

5. Identify disorders of the immune system.

6. Describe the typical course and management of common immune system disorders.

7. Describe the effects of aging on the immune system and the common disorders of the system associated with it.

## OVERVIEW

*The immune system provides protection for the body through the processes of defense, attack, and removal of pathogens. The immune system also helps the body by removing aged or dead cells and other debris. Diseases or disorders of the immune system may range from mild to severe. Many of the disorders of the system are extremely debilitating and require long-term therapy. Immune diseases can affect individuals of any age, race, or gender. If the immune system is not functioning properly due to disease or other influencing factors, the result may be a secondary disease of the body resulting from the compromised immune system.* ■

## ANATOMY AND PHYSIOLOGY

The immune system is made up of a complex group of cells and organs that are found throughout the body. The system includes primary organs such as the thymus gland and the bone marrow, and secondary organs such as the lymph nodes, spleen, liver, and the tonsils (Figure 5–1). The lymphocytes, the major cells of the immune system, arise and develop in the primary organs. The secondary organs are responsible for filtering foreign substances and providing the space for antigen reactions.

The cells of the immune system include four types of leukocytes: polymorphonuclear leukocytes, monocytes, macrophages, and lymphocytes. The polymorphonuclear leukocytes, also known as granulocytes and PMNs, are active in the inflammatory process. Some leukocytes react when infection threatens the body; others respond when there is an allergic reaction to prevent damage to cells and tissues. The monocytes and macrophages become phagocytic in the presence of pathogens and foreign substances. The lymphocytes are the major players in the immune response (Table 5–1).

Lymphocytes are formed in the bone marrow. Those remaining and maturing in the bone marrow become B lymphocytes. Others migrate and mature in the thymus and become T lymphocytes. Once

| **TABLE 5–1** | Types and Functions of Leukocytes |
| --- | --- |
| **Type** | **Function** |
| **Polymorphonuclear leukocytes** | |
| Neutrophils | Phagocytosis |
| Eosinophils | Allergic responses |
| Basophils | Release histamine |
| **Monocytes** | Become macrophages (phagocytosis) |
| **Macrophages** | Phagocytosis |
| **Lymphocytes** | |
| T lymphocytes | Cell-mediated immunity |
| B lymphocytes | Humoral immunity |
| Plasma cells | Antibody production |

mature, both B and T lymphocytes enter the blood, and circulate and colonize the lymphatic organs, predominately the spleen and lymph nodes.

T lymphocytes are responsible for the cell-mediated response. These cells destroy microorganisms that invade the body. These reactions do not require antibodies produced by the B cells because the T cells have been previously sensitized by circulating antigens. There are several different types of T cells functioning to stimulate B cells to produce antibodies, destroy foreign cells in the body, stop the immune response, and remember previous exposure to antigens.

B lymphocytes are responsible for humoral immunity. Humoral immunity is associated with circulating antibodies in contrast to cell-mediated immunity. The B lymphocytes enlarge and divide to become mature plasma cells. The plasma cells secrete antibodies into the blood and lymph to protect the body against infections and toxins produced by microorganisms.

There are two types of immune responses in the body: specific and nonspecific. Specific immune response is associated with antigens and the antibody reaction. It is the body's watch-guard system for foreign invaders. The antibody response occurs after exposure to an antigen. Antibodies may neutralize, kill, or cause clumping of the foreign microorganism. The complement system also works with the antibodies to destroy the invader. The complement system is a group of proteins that are formed

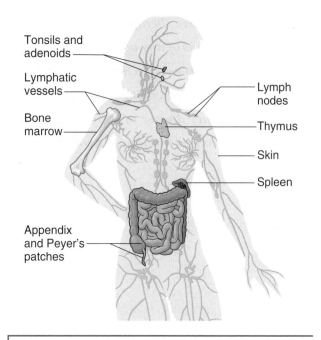

Tonsils and adenoids

Lymphatic vessels

Bone marrow

Appendix and Peyer's patches

Lymph nodes

Thymus

Skin

Spleen

**FIGURE 5–1** Organs of the immune system.

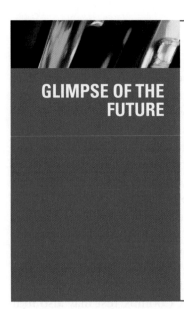

### Thymus Transplant Might Save Babies Born without an Immune System

Researchers have discovered that thymus tissue, normally discarded during cardiac surgery on infants, may be used to give life to babies with complete DiGeorge syndrome. This syndrome includes babies who are born without a thymus. The thymus normally rests atop the heart and functions as a "schoolhouse" for immune cells. As cells pass through the thymus, they become T cells, those white cells that specialize in fighting infection. Without a thymus, affected babies are destined to die.

Duke University, the only center in the world to offer experimental thymus transplantation procedures, has treated 12 children since 1993. Of these 12 children, 7 are alive and living at home. Without treatment, children with complete DiGeorge syndrome will live approximately one year.

*Source:* Health and Medicine Week, *(July 11, 2003).*

in the liver and circulate in the serum. They enhance the work of the antibodies.

The nonspecific immune response includes inflammation, phagocytosis, physical barriers (the skin and mucous membranes), and chemical barriers (acids and other secretions). These immune response defenses are the body's first line of protection against foreign invaders.

There are several ways to classify types of immunity, but the most common method used is to divide immunity into passive and active and natural and artificial. Table 5–2 outlines the types of immunity and gives examples of each. In addition, some classification systems use the term "natural resistance" when describing immunity. Natural resistance is the inherited immunity the individual may possess due to race, species, or ethnic background. Some races, species, or particular groups of populations are naturally resistant to certain diseases, just as some are more susceptible to certain diseases.

## COMMON SIGNS AND SYMPTOMS

In some cases a patient's concern may be considered as both a symptom and a sign. Some references call this an objective or observable symptom, while others state that it is also a sign. An example would be a patient complaining of a runny nose. The runny nose is the patient's symptom and because it is observable to the physician it is also a sign.

**TABLE 5–2** Types of Immunity

| Type of Immunity | Example |
| --- | --- |
| Active natural immunity | Having the disease (like mumps) |
| Active artificial immunity | Receiving a vaccination (like MMR) |
| Passive natural immunity | Antibodies produced by the body itself or received from maternal-fetus transmission |
| Passive artificial immunity | Injection of antibodies |

The common signs and symptoms related to the various immune system diseases are quite varied, depending on the organ or organ system that is affected. Symptoms common to allergic reactions include local or systemic inflammatory responses (redness, heat, swelling, and itching) and respiratory symptoms (runny nose, coughing, sneezing, and nasal congestion).

The classic clinical problem with immune deficiency disorders is the development of unusual and severe infections such as pneumonia, meningitis, or septicemia to name just a few. Also, the development of infections by microorganisms that are not usually pathogenic (opportunistic infections) may be indicative of an **immunodeficiency** (lack of immunity) disorder. The common signs and symptoms related to the various **autoimmune** (immunity against self) and **isoimmune** (immunity against other humans) disorders are also varied, depending on the organ or organ system that is affected, and the invading pathogen. For this reason, signs and symptoms of these diseases are identified in the discussion of the specific disease.

## DIAGNOSTIC TESTS

Determining the cause of an allergic reaction may be quite difficult. There are hundreds of possible **antigens (allergens)** that cause allergic reactions. Some of the more common allergens are house dust, pet hair, chocolate, ragweed, cigarette smoke, pollen, seafood, nickel, plants, paints, dyes, and chemical cleaners.

The most important test for diagnosing allergies is the skin test. A skin test may be performed by intradermal injection involving injection of a small amount of the suspected antigen under the skin. A skin patch test utilizes placement of a small antigen-soaked patch against the individual's skin. Another skin test is a scratch test, performed by placing a small amount of suspected antigen in a small scratch. All three types of tests are used to identify an allergen.

**Allergy** to the antigen is positive if an inflammatory response or wheal occurs at the injection site. The size of the wheal is usually indicative of the individual's sensitivity to the allergen. There are hundreds of allergic antigens that may be used in skin testing.

Once an antigen has been identified, a desensitization treatment may be attempted. Desensitization requires the injection of an increasing amount of allergen over a long period of time. The goal is to desensitize the body to the allergen. Other treatments include avoiding exposure to the allergen and antihistamine medications.

**Hypersensitivity** reactions to blood cells are usually identified by a blood count indicating low levels of red cells, white cells, and platelets. Antibodies may form against all these blood elements leading to anemia, leukopenia, and thrombocytopenia, respectively.

A Coombs' test will indicate the formation of antibodies on the red blood cell. This test can be used to determine blood type and diagnose certain **hemolytic** (HE-moh-**LIT**-ick; hemo = blood, lytic = destroying) anemias. A Coombs' test may also indicate the presence of maternal antibodies against the fetal blood type as occurs in erythroblastosis fetalis.

Autoimmune disorders may be diagnosed utilizing blood tests that measure for specific diseases. For example, individuals with systemic lupus erythematosus will have a positive ANA or antinuclear antibody test. Rheumatoid factor (RF) in the blood is often indicative of rheumatoid arthritis.

Immunodeficiency disorders are usually diagnosed by blood testing that reveals low white cell counts, specifically B and T lymphocytes. Presence of an antibody in the blood against a causative pathogen may also be utilized. Finding an antibody against the human immunodeficiency virus (HIV) is indicative of exposure to AIDS.

---

## COMPLEMENTARY AND ALTERNATIVE THERAPY

**Echinacea for Colds**

Common name: Purple Coneflower
Echinacea is one of the most popular herbs in America today. Native Americans may have used echinacea hundreds of years ago to treat infections, wounds, and as a general cure-all. Currently, echinacea is used primarily to reduce symptoms of the common cold, and to alleviate the associated symptoms of sore throat, fever, and cough. Herbalists also recommend echinacea to help boost the immune system and to help fight infection.

# COMMON DISEASES OF THE IMMUNE SYSTEM

Diseases of the immune system can be divided into two main groups: hypersensitivity disorders and immune deficiency disorders. There are several specific diseases within each grouping. Each of these has some unique problems associated with the disease, but some of the signs and symptoms may be quite similar.

## Hypersensitivity Disorders

Hypersensitivity disorders are the result of an overreaction of the immune system to an antigen or allergen. Hypersensitivity disorders can be further classified as those related to allergy, autoimmunity, and isoimmunity (Figure 5–2).

**Allergies.**   Allergies are among the most prevalent types of hypersensitivity problems. Millions of people suffer from some type of allergy. Hay fever, asthma (AZ-ma), **urticaria** (UR-tih-**KAR**-ree-ah; a reaction characterized by intense wheals and itching), and contact dermatitis are common allergic reactions. These reactions are usually just bothersome, but they can be a serious health threat. Severe asthma, for example, may be life threatening. Food allergies are also common in some populations, but may be difficult to diagnose.

**ETIOLOGY** Allergy is an acquired hypersensitivity. The individual with an allergy must first be exposed or sensitized to the antigen. Subsequent or repeated exposure leads to the reaction by the immune system identified as an allergy or an allergic reaction. Allergens may cause an immediate response like those identified with hay fever, asthma, or food allergy. Delayed response allergies are slower to react and are usually less harmful. An example of delayed response allergy would be contact dermatitis, caused by exposure to poison ivy.

**SYMPTOMS** Signs and symptoms of allergies include an elevated blood eosinophil (a white blood cell that responds in allergic conditions) level, along with local or systemic inflammatory responses such as redness, heat, swelling, and often itching of the tissues involved. Respiratory symptoms may include runny nose, coughing, sneezing, wheezing, and nasal congestion.

### ■ Hay Fever

Hay fever is a reaction in the mucous membranes of the nose and upper respiratory tract to an allergen.

**ETIOLOGY** The allergen is usually airborne and may be seasonal. Tree pollen, grasses, agricultural crops, and ragweed pollen may cause an increase in symptoms during the different seasons of the year. Nonseasonal hay fever may be the result of house dust, pet dander, or food allergies.

**SYMPTOMS** Symptoms include sneezing, watery eyes, runny nose, and itching.

**TREATMENT** Treatment of hay fever includes removal of the allergen or separation of the allergen and the hay fever sufferer. Individuals who suffer from hay fever may choose to permanently move to a different climate or to vacation in a different area when the pollen count is high in their area. An air-conditioned environment is beneficial as this filters much of the allergen. Antihistamines and other drugs

---

## COMPLEMENTARY AND ALTERNATIVE THERAPY

**Therapy for Immune System Problems**

A variety of physicians claim that all disease and health problems are related to a low immune system. Most health problems are transferred to us by genes that may be triggered by emotional, physical, or nutritional trauma. Treatment of a variety of diseases, including depression, colitis, allergies, and migraine headaches, can be accomplished by negative emotional release therapy, and permanent allergy and related diseases elimination technique.

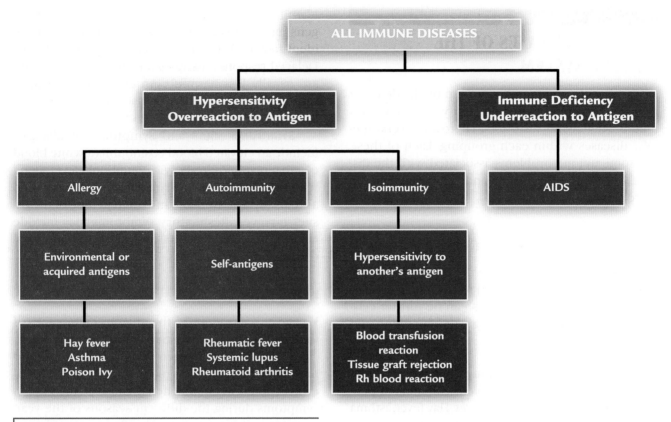

**FIGURE 5–2** Classification of hypersensitivity disorders.

are given orally—and in nose drops and sprays—in an effort to control symptoms. Allergy desensitization may be of benefit.

## ■ Asthma

This chronic allergic condition is also known as bronchial asthma. It affects 5–10 percent of children, making it the leading cause of chronic illness in childhood. Male children have asthma twice as often as girls prior to puberty. After puberty, the ratio is more equal.

**ETIOLOGY** When exposed to an allergen, the hypersensitive individual has episodes of wheezing due to **bronchospasm** (**BRONG**-ko-SPA-zm) or muscular constriction of the bronchi of the respiratory tract. The individual appears perfectly normal between episodes.

Asthma may be caused by allergens in the environment such as pollen, dust, pet dander, smoke, or various fumes. Other causes of asthma are nonallergic and include events that produce stress. Triggers for nonallergic asthma include respiratory infections like the common cold, changes in temperature and humidity, exercise, and emotional stress.

**SYMPTOMS** Symptoms of an attack are extreme shortness of breath, difficulty breathing, wheezing, and anxiety. Attacks vary in severity from mild to almost suffocating. Coughing during the attack usually begins with a mild, dry cough, but progresses to production of large amounts of mucus as the attack continues. Skin may be pale and moist in mild attacks, with cyanosis of the nail beds and lips occurring in more severe attacks. During an attack, asthmatics often assume a sitting position, leaning forward with hands resting on the knees. This position helps the individual breathe by utilizing all the respiratory muscles (Figure 5–3). A severe attack that lasts for several days is called **status asthmaticus** (**AZ**-MAH-ti-kus). This is a life-threatening medical emergency.

**TREATMENT** Treatment includes avoidance of causative allergens, desensitization, education, and medications to treat symptoms. Deep breathing exercises, maintenance of proper posture, and relaxation techniques are of benefit. A regimen of medications to relax and open the bronchi (bronchodilators), and to thin the excessive mucus (mucolytics) is important. There is no cure for asthma, but it can be controlled by a combination of

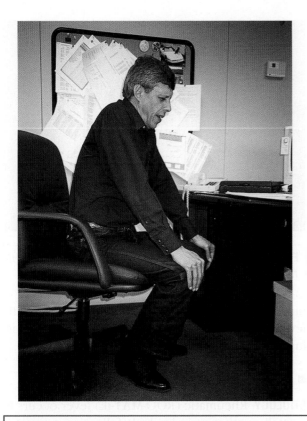

**FIGURE 5–3** Positioning in an asthma attack.

therapies including strict compliance to a medication regimen, relaxation techniques, exercise, and avoidance of allergens.

### ■ Urticaria

Commonly called hives or nettle rash, urticaria is a vascular reaction of the skin.

**ETIOLOGY** This condition is caused by contact with an external irritant such as insect bites, pollen, drugs, food, or plants.

**SYMPTOMS** It is characterized by slightly elevated lesions that are redder or paler than the surrounding skin, and is associated with severe itching. The elevated areas are called wheals or hives. Scratching or rubbing the hypersensitive area may lead to formation of larger or additional wheals (Figure 5–4).

**TREATMENT** Treatment includes antihistamines and avoidance of the allergen.

### ■ Anaphylaxis

This is a severe allergic response to an allergen, often leading to anaphylactic shock.

**ETIOLOGY** **Anaphylaxis** (AN-ah-fih-**LACK**-sis), also known as an anaphylactic reaction, is caused by

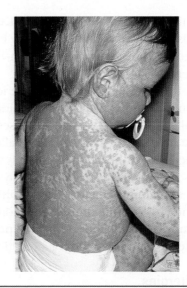

**FIGURE 5–4** Urticaria. (*Courtesy of Robert A. Silverman, MD, Pediatric Dermatology, Georgetown University*).

absorption of the antigen into the blood directly or through the mucous membranes. Substances that commonly cause anaphylaxis include antibiotics, anesthetics, codeine, insulin, hormones, iodinated X-ray contrast media, vaccines, antitoxins, foods, pollen, mold, animal dander, latex, and insect venom of wasps, bees, or hornets.

**SYMPTOMS** A local anaphylactic reaction may be mild and produce generalized itching, swelling, and urticaria. This reaction should be closely monitored as it may rapidly progress to systemic anaphylaxis. Systemic anaphylaxis is a true medical emergency involving the release of histamine throughout body tissues. Within minutes, the individual feels itching of the throat, tongue, and scalp. Edema or swelling of the face and airways leads to difficulty breathing. The individual suffers a huge drop in blood pressure (shock) and body temperature. Unconsciousness usually occurs with the drop in blood pressure. If these symptoms are not reversed with medical attention, death from respiratory and cardiac arrest may occur within 15 to 20 minutes.

**TREATMENT** Treatment during an attack may include performance of an emergency tracheostomy (TRAY-kee-**OS**-toh-me; trache = trachea, ostomy = new opening) or endotracheal (endo = within, trachea = windpipe) intubation with mechanical ventilation. Immediate administration of the medication epinephrine is necessary. Epinephrine (adrenalin) is a vasoconstrictor and a smooth muscle relaxant. Effects of epinephrine will raise the blood pressure, dilate the bronchi, and decrease laryngeal spasms.

Antihistamines and **corticosteroids** (**KORT**-ti-ko-STEHR-oyds; powerful anti-inflammatory hormones) are given to limit histamine production, thus slowing the allergic reaction.

Follow-up treatment would include identifying the allergen. The individual is taught to identify and avoid the allergen, and recognize the onset of a reaction. These individuals should wear an allergy identification necklace or bracelet. Individuals who experience this severe reaction should always carry an allergy kit containing Benadryl (an antihistamine), syringes, and vials of epinephrine. The individual and family members should understand and practice the appropriate steps in treatment of a reaction.

### ■ Food Allergies

Gastrointestinal food allergies are often difficult to diagnose. The process involves elimination of certain foods, then adding these to the diet one at a time.

**ETIOLOGY** Chocolate and shellfish are common food allergies. Often, the allergy is not to a specific food but to additives or preservatives in the food. Allergy to milk may not be a true allergy but rather an intolerance to the lactose in the milk. Lactose intolerance may be treated by taking lactose enzyme (lactase) before consumption of dairy products.

**SYMPTOMS** Symptoms of food allergies include cramping, diarrhea, and vomiting.

### ■ Contact Dermatitis

Contact dermatitis is an acute or chronic allergic reaction affecting the skin.

**ETIOLOGY** Often the allergen is some type of cosmetic, laundry product, plant, jewelry, paint, drug, plastic, or a variety of other agents. Often, it is difficult to determine the causative agent, and once found, complete avoidance may not be possible.

**SYMPTOMS** Allergic lesions may range from small red localized lesions to vesicular lesions that cover the entire body. A common example of contact dermatitis is poison ivy (Figure 5–5).

**Autoimmune Disorders.** Autoimmune disorders are hypersensitivities in which the body fails to recognize its own antigens or **self-antigen**. An individual's body cells have specific antigen on the cell surfaces. Failure to recognize this antigen as a self-antigen leads to the body attacking and destroying its own tissues. Several theories exist as to the cause of this type of disorder, but currently, the cause for autoimmune disorders is

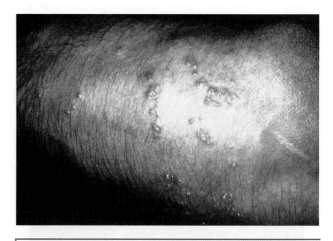

**FIGURE 5–5** Contact dermatitis. *(Courtesy of the Centers for Disease Control and Prevention, Atlanta, GA.)*

unknown. Autoimmune disorders include rheumatic fever, rheumatoid arthritis, myasthenia gravis, systemic lupus erythematosus, and multiple sclerosis.

### ■ Rheumatic Fever

**ETIOLOGY** Rheumatic (ROO-**MAT**-ik) fever occurs in a small number of individuals following a group A **streptococcal** (**STREHP**-toh-KAHK-al) infection, usually strep throat. In this select number of individuals, the proteins in their hearts and other connective tissue is similar to the protein of the strep bacteria. For this reason, rheumatic fever tends to run in families. Exposure to strep bacteria causes the immune system to make antibodies to fight the bacteria. These antibodies also attack the tissues of the heart and joints because they cannot distinguish the differences in the proteins. Rheumatic fever is characterized by myocarditis (myo = muscle, cardi = heart, itis = inflammation) and arthritis.

**SYMPTOMS** Rheumatic fever usually occurs one to four weeks after a streptococcal infection. Children and adolescents are most commonly affected. Onset of the disease may be sudden or gradual, and includes symptoms of fever, malaise, and joint pain. The first occurrence of rheumatic fever may be mild and resolve without any permanent damage. Further episodes are usually more severe and may lead to permanent scarring and deformity of the heart valves (Figure 5–6). Deformity of the mitral and aortic valve may eventually lead to heart failure.

**TREATMENT** Prompt and accurate diagnosis and treatment of group A streptococcal infections is the best preventive measure against rheumatic fever. Culturing for strep infections and prolonged treatment

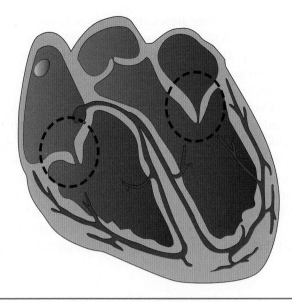

FIGURE 5–6   Valves affected in rheumatic fever.

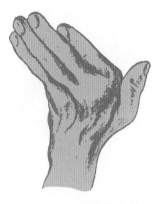

FIGURE 5–7   Ulnar deviation from rheumatoid arthritis.

(at least 10 days) with antibiotics is most effective. **Prophylactic** (pro-fil-LACK-tic; works to prevent) antibiotics may be given to susceptible individuals. Surgical replacement of the heart valves may be necessary for individuals with severe valve deformity.

### ■ Rheumatoid Arthritis

Rheumatoid arthritis is an autoimmune disease that causes chronic inflammation of connective tissue. Joint tissue is primarily affected, but any connective tissue of the body may be involved.

**ETIOLOGY**  The exact cause of rheumatoid arthritis is unknown, but it is associated with the production of an abnormal antibody that attacks or attaches to the body's own cells and tissues. Presence of the antibody called rheumatoid factor (RF) in the affected individual's blood is indicative of the disease.

**SYMPTOMS**  Commonly, metacarpal-phalangeal joints of the hands are initially affected with rheumatoid arthritis. This leads to a classic sign of rheumatoid arthritis called ulnar deviation of the fingers (Figure 5-7). As the disease progresses, involvement of other synovial joints may occur. Joints affected may include those of the fingers, wrists, elbows, feet, ankles, and knees. Symptoms of rheumatoid arthritis may vary in severity from mild to severe, and may go through periods of remission and exacerbation.

Rheumatoid arthritis begins with inflammation of the synovial lining of the joint leading to pain, stiffness, and joint deformity. Eventually, the cartilage of the joint is destroyed and replaced with a granula-

tion tissue, called pannus (PAN-nus). As the disease progresses, the entire joint surface is destroyed and replaced with fibrous tissue, making the joint less movable. Fusion or total loss of joint function is called ankylosis (ANG-kih-**LOH**-sis) (Figure 5–8).

In addition to joint changes, the individual may also have lesions in the collagen of the lungs, blood vessels, heart, and eyes leading to pleuritis (PLOO-**RIGH**-tis; pleura = pleura or lining of the lung, itis = inflammation), anemia, valvulitis (VAL-view-**LYE**-tis; valvu = valve, itis = inflammation), and glaucoma (glaw-KOH-mah), respectively. Rheumatoid nodules characteristically appear in the subcutaneous tissue around the fingers, toes, and elbows (Figure 5–9). Individuals with rheumatoid arthritis often appear

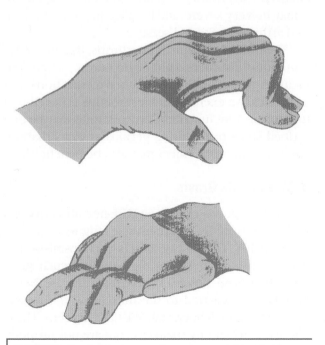

FIGURE 5–8   Joint changes from rheumatoid arthritis.

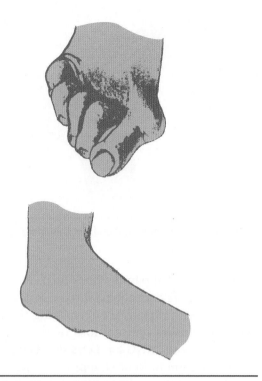

FIGURE 5–9   Rheumatoid nodules.

frail and chronically ill. Anemia and infection are common secondary problems.

This chronic disease affects both sexes and all ages, but onset is most common in women between the ages of 20 and 40. Women are affected three times more often than men. Rheumatoid arthritis in children usually affects infants to children aged 16. It may be very severe, and is called juvenile rheumatoid arthritis or Still's disease.

**TREATMENT** Rheumatoid arthritis, like other autoimmune disorders, cannot be cured. Treatment includes use of anti-inflammatory medications and analgesics. An exercise and rest routine is developed to maintain joint function. Corticosteroids may be prescribed short term during periods of exacerbation. Surgical joint replacement may also be beneficial.

### ■ Myasthenia Gravis

Myasthenia gravis (MY-uh-**STHEE**-nee-uh GRAV-iss) is characterized by severe muscle fatigue.

**ETIOLOGY** This disease affects the transmission of nerve signals to muscle at the neuromuscular junction. There is no muscle or nerve tissue disease. Nerve impulses are carried to the muscle by the neurotransmitter acetylcholine (ah-SEE-til-**KOH**-leen). These impulses are sent by the nerve, but are not properly received by the muscle. This error in transmission is due to antibodies attacking the muscle receptors, which blocks the transmission by acetylcholine (Figure 5–10). This poor transmission of information to the muscle leads to weak muscle contractions and fatigue.

There are approximately 36,000 Americans affected with myasthenia gravis. The estimated annual incidence is about 2 in 1,000,000 individuals so it is considered to be a rare disorder (Shah, 2004). Myasthenia gravis can be categorized as an autoimmune, musculoskeletal, or neurologic disease because it has characteristics of problems in each of these systems.

**SYMPTOMS** Onset of the disease is usually slow and diagnosis may be difficult as it may affect any

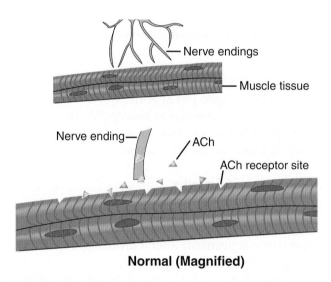

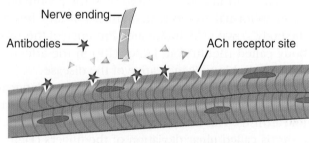

Nerves do not touch muscle tissue to stimulate movement. Nerve endings secrete a neurotransmitter, acetylcholine (ACh), that sticks to muscle tissue receptor sites causing muscle contraction.

Antibodies produced with myasthenia gravis block these receptor sites thus blocking muscle stimulus and movement.

FIGURE 5–10   Blocking of receptor sites in myasthenia gravis.

muscle of the body. Commonly, facial muscles are the ones initially affected, leading to diplopia (dip-PLOHP-ee-ah; double vision), ptosis (TOE-sis; drooping eye-lids), dysphagia (dys-FAY-jee-ah; difficulty swallowing), dysphonia (dys-FOH-nee-ah; difficulty talking), and difficulty with facial expressions, which may leave the individual with an expressionless facial appearance. Other symptoms relate to fatigue of all voluntary muscles and include difficulty rising from a sitting position, lifting the arms, standing, and walking.

The degree of weakness varies with the time of day and activities. Generally, these individuals feel stronger in the morning due to a buildup of acetyl-choline, and become weaker as the day progresses because acetylcholine stores diminish. Short rest periods are necessary to help restore muscle function.

Periods of exacerbation and remission do occur. During exacerbation, complete bed rest may be necessary.

**TREATMENT** Treatment may include cholinergic medications that do not allow the normal breakdown of the neurotransmitter acetylcholine. These drugs allow a buildup of the neurotransmitter, thus improving neuromuscular transmission. Plasma exchange to remove the circulating antibodies provides some improvement in the condition. Recent advances in care and treatment have reduced the mortality rate to 3 to 4 percent. Death is usually due to muscle weakness, leading to respiratory failure.

## ■ Type 1 Diabetes Mellitus (Insulin-Dependent Diabetes Mellitus)

Type 1 diabetes mellitus, formerly known as insulin-dependent diabetes mellitus or IDDM, is a disease that alters the body's carbohydrate or sugar metabolism.

**ETIOLOGY** It is believed to be caused by an auto-immune disorder triggered by a viral infection. The most common viral infections that may lead to diabetes include rubella, mumps, and influenza. The infecting virus inflames insulin-producing beta cells of the pancreas. The inflammatory process, for reasons that remain unclear, seems to stimulate the beta cells to produce an abnormal cell antigen. Lympho-cytes recognize the abnormal antigen as non-self and destroy it along with the beta cells. Without insulin-producing beta cells, the individual becomes dependent on insulin injections to manage carbohydrate utilization.

The normal antigens in the cells of the pancreas are histocompatibility locus antigens (HLAs). Indi-viduals genetically inherit the HLAs of the pancreas. The tendency to develop an autoimmune response, and thus diabetes mellitus, is considered hereditary in nature.

There are other types of diabetes that are not caused by autoimmunity. Because all types of dia-betes affect the endocrine system, they will be dis-cussed and compared in detail in Chapter 14.

## ■ Lupus Erythematosus

The term lupus originally referred to any chronic, destructive type of skin lesion. The Latin word *lupus* means wolf, and erythematosus refers to redness. The term lupus erythematosus has been used since the thirteenth century because physicians of that time thought the shape and color of the skin lesions resembled a wolf bite. The word lupus is often used to refer to lupus erythematosus, although used alone, this term truly has no meaning. There are several forms of lupus including lupus pernio, lupus vul-garus, drug-induced lupus, and lupus erythematosus.

There are two types of lupus erythematosus: cutaneous (discoid) and systemic (diffuse). Cuta-neous or discoid lupus erythematosus (DLE) is lim-ited to skin or cutaneous involvement. DLE does not affect multisystems as does systemic (SLE). A classic sign is the presence of a persistent red facial butterfly-shaped rash across the bridge of the nose and cheeks. DLE may be thought of as a type of systemic lupus because cause, testing, and treatment are sim-ilar for cutaneous involvement. DLE is the less serious type of lupus erythematosus.

**ETIOLOGY** Systemic lupus erythematosus is an autoimmune disorder in which B lymphocytes pro-duce autoantibodies that attack body cells. Individu-als with SLE have a high number of antinuclear anti-bodies (ANA). These antibodies attack the body's own cell nuclei, destroying the RNA and DNA of the cell. Detection of ANA by microscopic immunofluo-rescence supports the diagnosis of SLE.

**SYMPTOMS** Systemic lupus erythematosus often affects the skin, and a number of other organs or sys-tems. A common sign is the previously described butterfly-shaped facial rash (Figure 5–11). Sympto-matic individuals often complain of fever, joint pain, weight loss, and facial rash. Joint, kidney, and muscle involvement may lead to complaints of arthritis, glomerulonephritis (inflammation of the glomeru-lus or filtering unit of the kidney), and atrophy,

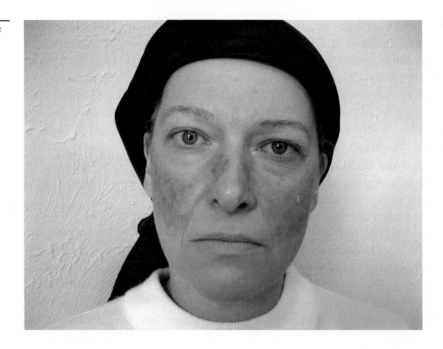

**FIGURE 5–11** Butterfly rash of systemic lupus erythematosus (SLE). *(Courtesy of Ruth Tannehill-Jones.)*

respectively. Heart valve deformities and abnormal blood composition are not unusual findings.

SLE affects approximately 1 in 2,400 people. It is primarily a disease that affects women, occurring 10 times more frequently in women than men. Onset is usually between age 30 and 40, but it may appear at any age. The disease is most severe among individuals of African-American descent.

**TREATMENT** SLE is a chronic disease that goes through periods of exacerbation and remission. Complete remission is very rare. Treatment is symptomatic. Nonsteroidal anti-inflammatory, antipyretic, and analgesic medications may be used to treat symptoms. Life-threatening exacerbations are often treated with corticosteroids. There is no cure for SLE. Prognosis depends on which organs are affected and the severity of the infection. Ten-year survival rates approximate 75 percent, but long-term survival rate is less than 15 years. Renal insufficiency, bacterial endocarditis, cardiac failure, sepsis, and pneumonia commonly lead to death.

## ■ Scleroderma

Scleroderma (skle-ro-DER-mah; sclero = hardening, derma = skin) is a chronic autoimmune disorder characterized by hardening, thickening, and shrinking of the connective tissues of the body, including the skin.

**ETIOLOGY** It is thought that this autoimmune reaction begins with the skin and connective tissues attracting lymph cells. These lymph cells stimulate the production of collagen, leading to the disorder.

Milder forms of scleroderma include those limited to the skin, face, and extremities. The more severe form of scleroderma is systemic or diffuse. This type affects not only the skin but also internal organs including the heart, lungs, and kidney. These tissues become hardened, thickened, and often limited in function.

Like many other chronic diseases, scleroderma may exhibit periods of remission and exacerbation. There is generally a slow progression of the disease that allows the individual a reasonably long life. If the disorder progresses rapidly, affecting vital organs, early death may result. Death is usually related to kidney failure.

The milder forms of scleroderma commonly affect women 30 to 50 years of age. The more severe forms usually affect men and older persons. Diagnosis is difficult because this disease initially mimics other disorders like bursitis and arthritis.

**SYMPTOMS** Characteristically, individuals with scleroderma have thick, leather-like, shiny, taut skin, and joint contractures. The first symptom is usually Raynaud's phenomenon, an episodic vasoconstriction affecting the hands. The mouth area often becomes wrinkled with a tight purse-lipped appearance, leading to difficulty eating. Diagnosis may be confirmed by clinical examination and tissue biopsy.

**TREATMENT** Currently, there is no treatment to cure or stop the progression of scleroderma. Treatment with anti-inflammatory medications, immunosuppressives, and antibiotics may be of some help. Muscle stretching and strengthening exercises may be beneficial to maintain muscle strength and joint mobility.

**Isoimmune Disorders.** Isoimmunity refers to a hypersensitivity of one individual to another individual's tissues. Examples include blood type reactions, tissue rejections, and maternal/fetal reactions.

## ■ Blood Transfusion Reaction

As previously stated, all body cells have a specific antigen that identifies them. Red blood cells have surface antigens. Transfusion of blood from one individual to another is in a sense a type of tissue transplant. RBCs have to be typed and cross-matched to properly identify antigens and prevent rejection.

The blood types are identified by antigens and can be divided into four groups: A, B, AB, and O. Types O and A are the most common. Each red blood cell has an antigen and a corresponding antibody. Blood type A has an A antigen and anti-B antibody. B type has a B antigen and anti-A antibody. O has no antigen

and both anti-A and anti-B antibody. AB has an A and B antigen and no antibody. These antigen-antibody patterns make type O the universal blood donor and type AB the universal blood recipient (Figure 5–12).

**ETIOLOGY** If a blood type with an antigen is given to a type that has antibodies against that antigen, the antibodies will attack the antigen and break down the donor RBCs. For example, if type A (with antigen A and anti-B antibody) is given to type B (with antigen B and anti-A antibody), the anti-A antibody in the B type recipient's blood will attack the A antigen and break down the type A donor blood (see Figure 5–12).

As antibodies react with the antigen, they also cause clumping of the blood, leading to microthrombi (microscopic sized blood clots). These microthrombi can lead to multiple organ emboli and have fatal consequences.

**SYMPTOMS** Symptoms of transfusion reaction include chills, shivering, and fever.

**TREATMENT** The transfusion must be discontinued immediately to avoid fatality.

## ■ Erythroblastosis Fetalis

Erythroblastosis fetalis (eh-RITH-roh-blas-**TOH**-sis feh-**TAH**-lis) is an isoimmune condition where antibodies in a mother's blood attack and destroy the antigen on

| Type | Percent of Population with Type | Antigen | Antibody | Color Jar Example | Donate Blood To: | Receive Blood From: |
|------|--------------------------------|---------|----------|-------------------|------------------|---------------------|
| A | 41 | A | B | RED | A and AB | A and O |
| B | 12 | B | A | BLUE | B and AB | B and O |
| O | 44 | None | A and B | CLEAR | A, B, AB, O | O |
| AB | 3 | A and B | None | PURPLE | AB | A, B, AB, O |

To understand the concept of transfusion reaction with antigen and antibodies, consider this example. The particular blood type can give blood to any type that does not change the color in the jar and receive blood from any type that does not change the color in the jar. For example, A can give blood to AB because adding red to purple will not change the purple color. However, A cannot give to B because giving red to blue will change the color. Since O is in the clear jar, it can give to all types but could not receive from anything but O or the clear color would change.

**FIGURE 5–12** Blood types for donors and recipients.

the baby's red blood cells, ultimately killing the unborn fetus. This condition is also known as hemolytic (hemo = blood, lytic = breaking or crushing) disease of the newborn.

Antigens on the red blood cells give each type of cell a special identity. In addition to antigens that determine blood type, 85 percent of Americans have another antigen called the Rh factor. This group is collectively called Rh positive (Rh+) because they have the factor or antigen. Those who do not have the factor—approximately 15 percent of the population—are Rh negative (Rh−). Cross-match for transfusions must not only match an appropriate type, but also a compatible factor. The common rule is, "those who don't have it don't want it; those that have it don't care." In other words, Rh− individuals cannot receive Rh+ blood. On the other hand, Rh+ individuals "don't care," so they can receive Rh+ or Rh− blood. Blood type and factor are genetically determined or received from an individual's mother or father.

Because blood type and factor is determined by one's mother or father, it is possible for a mother to be pregnant with a baby of different blood type and factor (received from the father) (Figure 5-13). Mothers pregnant with babies of different blood types do not have a problem because red blood cells do not cross the placenta. Oxygen and nutrients simply diffuse across placental membranes to nourish the baby. RBCs do not normally exchange between the mother and the infant. Mothers who are Rh− and "don't want" Rh+ factor may have difficulty with Rh+ babies.

**ETIOLOGY** Rh− mothers pregnant with Rh+ babies usually do not have a problem with the first baby. During the first pregnancy, the mother's blood has not had the opportunity to identify the antigen because there has been no exchange of blood cells or antigens. However, there may be some slight mixing of blood during the birthing process. As this blood intermingles, the Rh+ antigen is picked up by the mother's blood. The mother's immune system recognizes this antigen as a foreign invader and builds antibodies to destroy it. Subsequent Rh+ babies are not as fortunate as the first Rh+ baby.

If this Rh− mother becomes pregnant with another Rh+ baby, antibodies against the Rh factor that she has built up in her blood do cross the placental membranes. These antibodies attack the blood of the unborn child, breaking down the RBCs, and leading to anemia and possible death of the baby.

This condition only affects Rh+ babies carried by Rh− mothers. Rh+ mothers "don't care" about the factor. Rh+ mothers have the antigen, so they do not build up antibodies against it.

**TREATMENT** Treatment for erythroblastosis fetalis is exchange transfusion of the baby's blood with Rh− blood at birth. This treatment stops the destruction of the baby's red blood cells. Over a period of time, the transfused Rh− blood is replaced by the

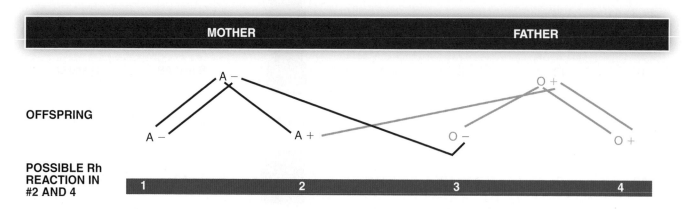

The offspring of this mother and father have the possibility of four different blood types. Since this is an Rh− mother, there is a possibility of an Rh reaction with the two Rh+ children. If the father was also Rh−, all offspring would be Rh− and no reaction would occur in any of the children. If the mother were Rh+ no Rh reaction could occur in any of the offspring since Rh+ mothers are not sensitive to the Rh antigen.

**FIGURE 5–13** Blood type in inheritance patterns and identification of possible Rh reactions.

baby's own blood. If erythroblastosis fetalis is a possibility in an Rh− mother, the baby's condition may be monitored by amniocentesis. Babies who are mildly affected may be allowed to be carried to full term. Severe cases may indicate the need to induce labor and premature delivery of the baby to begin lifesaving treatment.

Historically, an Rh factor marital mismatch may have been the reason why queens or wives of royalty were beheaded when unable to produce living heirs to the throne. If the king was Rh+ and the queen Rh−, every child after the first would have been at successively higher risk of fetal death. Erythroblastosis fetalis rarely occurs in the modern world. The development of RhoGAM, a special immune globulin, has halted this condition. RhoGAM is an injectable medication given to Rh− females to prevent the development of antibodies against Rh+ factor. This medication is given prophylactically after the delivery of the first fetus.

### ■ Organ Rejection

Organs such as the liver, kidney, heart, and lungs could be easily transplanted if not for the human immune system.

**ETIOLOGY** The immune system recognizes transplanted tissue as foreign and attacks it. This attack by lymphocytes brings about donor tissue destruction recognized as tissue or organ rejection.

**SYMPTOMS** Transplant rejection may be hyperacute in nature and actually occur during the surgical procedure. Acute rejection occurs within the first few weeks whereas chronic rejection occurs over a period of time, usually months to years. Chronic rejection occurs slowly and is due to vessel damage that decreases blood flow to the donor tissue. Decreased blood flow causes chronic ischemia, and ultimately, death of the donor organ.

**TREATMENT** Donated organs are matched to possible recipients. The closer the donor antigen matches that of the recipient, the less chance the organ will be rejected. Administration of immunosuppression medications also decreases the possibility of rejection. Immunosuppression medications must be taken prior to transplantation surgery and for the remainder of the organ recipient's life. This medication suppresses or decreases the body's ability to wage war against the donor tissue.

## Immune Deficiency Disorders

The second classification of immune disorders is immunodeficiency. These disorders represent an inability of the immune system to protect the individual against disease. This deficiency may be congenital due to a genetic disorder, or it may be acquired during the individual's lifetime. Acquired disorders are the most common type and may be due to disease therapies. Chemotherapy and radiation treatments often lead to immunodeficiency by suppressing bone marrow, thus decreasing leukocyte production. Medications given to organ transplant recipients purposefully suppress the immune system. The most common and fatal disorder is acquired immunodeficiency syndrome (AIDS).

The classic clinical problem with immunodeficiency disorders is the development of unusual and severe infections such as pneumonia, meningitis, or septicemia to name a few. Also, the development of infections by microorganisms that are not usually pathogenic (opportunistic infections) may be indicative of an immunodeficiency disorder. Other signs and symptoms are numerous and varied, depending on the organs or organ systems affected and the invading pathogen. Specific signs and symptoms will be included in the discussion of the disorder.

### ■ Acquired Immunodeficiency Syndrome (AIDS)

The name of this disease briefly describes its pathology. It is an acquired disease that causes the immune system to be deficient in its ability to protect the body, leading to a syndrome of symptoms or secondary diseases. The cause of AIDS is a virus called human immunodeficiency virus or HIV. The Joint United Nations Programme on HIV/AIDS (UNAIDS) and the World Health Organization (WHO) 2004 estimates that by year's end 2004, 39 million people were infected with HIV (AIDS epidemic update, 2004).

**ETIOLOGY** The wicked characteristic of HIV is that its battle plan is to wipe out the individual's lymphocytes, thus leaving the body defenseless against attack by all pathogenic organisms. The primary target is the T lymphocyte, but macrophages are affected as well. HIV is **cytotoxic** (cyto = cell, toxic = killing). Ultimately, the HIV-infected individual will have a low T lymphocyte cell count, indicative of a positive diagnosis of AIDS.

AIDS was first diagnosed in the United States in the early 1980s. The first diagnosed cases were a group of homosexual men who became ill with a series of opportunistic diseases and eventually died. These individuals had surprisingly suppressed immune systems. Further research led to the discovery of the virus and mode of transmission.

**SYMPTOMS** Previously, HIV was staged as four separate clinical presentations. Those stages were Asymptomatic carrier, Latency, AIDS Related Complex (ARC), and Full-Blown AIDS. Currently, HIV infection is known to be a continuous disease process. Staging this disease may be helpful for medical intervention. The new stages of HIV infection are acute infection, asymptomatic HIV, symptomatic HIV, and advanced disease.

1. Acute infection—This stage begins about one to three weeks after initial infection. During this time, the virus undergoes massive replication. Signs and symptoms include fever, sore throat, headache, and malaise. At this stage, HIV infection may be misdiagnosed as influenza.

2. Asymptomatic HIV—No chronic signs or symptoms are displayed during this stage. Lymphadenopathy (lymph = lymphatic, adeno = gland, opathy = disease) and headache may occur intermittently. If blood testing is utilized during this stage, the T lymphocyte count may be dropping by 40 to 80 cells per microliter per year (normal T cell count is 750–1000 cells per microliter). T cell count is a useful indicator of disease progression. This count is utilized in studying the effects of antiviral drugs and predicting the potential for opportunistic infections. This stage may last for 10 to 12 years, depending on drug therapy and individual resistance.

3. Symptomatic HIV—This stage is divided into early and late phases. During the early phase, the individual becomes symptomatic with a variety of symptoms or diseases affecting any or all of the body organs. Fever is a common symptom along with oral *Candida albicans*, recurrent herpes simplex lesions, and night sweats. The chronic diarrhea of this phase leads to dehydration and cachexia. Individuals are considered to be in the late phase when T cell count drops below 200 cells per microliter. At this point, the individual has met the criteria set by the CDC for a diagnosis of AIDS. Common diseases and disorders experienced during this phase include gastric ulcer, esophagitis, colitis, hepatitis, pancreatitis, fungal infections, neurologic disorders, herpes zoster, dermatitis, nausea, and vomiting to name just a few. In this phase, the individual experiences severe weight loss, weakness, persistent diarrhea, and usually at least one opportunistic disease. These opportunistic infections include:

- **Pneumocystis carinii** (NEW-moh-**SIS**-tis kah-RYE-nee-eye) pneumonia—an infection of the lungs with a protozoan. This organism has never been documented as a cause of pneumonia in persons with normal immune systems.

- **Kaposi's sarcoma** (KAP-oh-seez sar-KOH-mah)—a blood vessel cancer that causes reddish-purple skin lesions (Figure 5–14).

4. Advanced HIV—This stage is determined by a T cell count of less than 50 cells per microliter. In this stage, mortality increases significantly. Commonly, more virulent and persistent infections occur that are more resistant to treatment. Symptoms at this stage include seizures, confusion, urinary and fecal incontinence, blindness, hemiparesis (hemi = one side, paresis = weakness), and coma.

**TREATMENT** Once AIDS is diagnosed, life expectancy is approximately three to five years. Currently, AIDS is 100 percent fatal. Life can be extended by

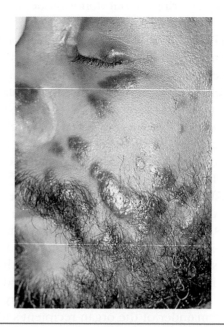

**FIGURE 5–14** Kaposi's sarcoma *(Courtesy of Robert A. Silverman, MD, Pediatric Dermatology, Georgetown University.)*

vigorous treatment of infections. In late-stage AIDS, every possible symptom or disease may be present because the individual's immune system is crumbling and incapacitated (Figure 5–15). Ultimately, super infections and massive diarrhea may be the cause of death. Antiviral medication like zidovudine (AZT) may slow HIV replication and thus slow the progression of the disease to some extent.

### ■ Transmission of AIDS

HIV is transmitted from one individual to another through intimate contact and sharing of body fluids. The virus must enter the body and bloodstream to infect the individual. The human immunodeficiency virus is a fragile virus that is easily killed by temper-

ature changes. There are many misconceptions and fears about the transmission of AIDS still prevalent in society today. An individual *cannot* get HIV infection from toilet seats, doorknobs, furniture, water fountains, and other objects. An individual *cannot* get HIV from social kissing, coughing, sneezing, or even sharing eating utensils. HIV is *not* transmitted through air, food, urine, feces, or water. HIV is primarily transmitted or spread in three ways:

1. Sexual intercourse—semen and vaginal secretions carry HIV. Transmission rate is higher from male to female because females may have microscopic vaginal tears during intercourse. Transmission rate is very high with anal intercourse because the internal lining of the rectum is very

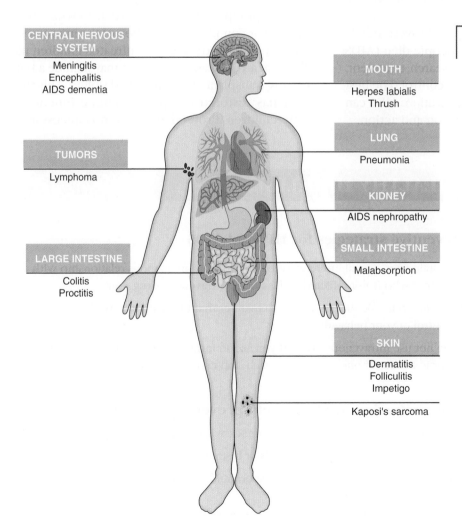

**FIGURE 5–15** Pathologies associated with AIDS.

**CENTRAL NERVOUS SYSTEM**
Meningitis
Encephalitis
AIDS dementia

**TUMORS**
Lymphoma

**LARGE INTESTINE**
Colitis
Proctitis

**MOUTH**
Herpes labialis
Thrush

**LUNG**
Pneumonia

**KIDNEY**
AIDS nephropathy

**SMALL INTESTINE**
Malabsorption

**SKIN**
Dermatitis
Folliculitis
Impetigo

Kaposi's sarcoma

thin. Approximately 75 percent of infected individuals in the United States contract AIDS through sexual intercourse.

2. Sharing of hypodermic needles—HIV infected blood is injected into the body by the sharing of needles. This type of transmission accounts for 18–25 percent of infected individuals in the United States.

3. In utero from infected mother to unborn child—HIV passes across the placenta to infect the baby. This accounts for 1–3 percent of AIDS cases.

Transmission of HIV through blood transfusions has been virtually eliminated due to effective screening methods. Health professionals following appropriate precautions are at very little risk of contracting HIV.

### ■ AIDS Prevention

AIDS is currently a worldwide epidemic or pandemic. In 2004, the Joint United Nations Programme on HIV/AIDS estimated the number of people worldwide infected with HIV at 39 million. In that same year approximately 4.9 million people were newly diagnosed and another 3 million people died (AIDS epidemic update, 2004). Costs for research, treatment, and prevention are escalating out of control. The best weapon available against AIDS is education. AIDS can be stopped with preventive education and action.

## TRAUMA

Trauma to the immune system is generally limited to treatments or medications that suppress the system. Chemotherapy and radiation treatments often lead to immunosuppression. Individuals on corticosteroid medications often have undetected infections because this medication suppresses the protective inflammatory response. Graft and organ recipients take immunosuppression medications to purposefully traumatize the system in hopes of protecting the transplanted graft or organ.

## RARE DISEASES

### Severe Combined Immunodeficiency Disease (SCID)

SCID is a group of inherited disorders in which there is partial or complete dysfunction of the immune system, or complete deficiency. Untreated children usually die at a young age. Treatment may include a bone marrow transplant from a matched sibling. This treatment has restored complete immune function in some children. Protective isolation is necessary to

 **HEALTHY HIGHLIGHT**

**Preventive Strategies for HIV and AIDS**

**Preventive strategies for HIV and AIDS**

- Abstain from sexual intercourse, or develop a monogamous relationship with a partner who is not infected and is not an intravenous drug user

- Do not abuse alcohol or drugs in a manner that prevents you from being in control of your behavior

- Do not use intravenous drugs. If you are an intravenous drug user, always use a sterile needle or one soaked in bleach, and do not share your needles

**Other behaviors that will help prevent the spread of HIV**

- Refrain from multiple sex partners or sex with intravenous drug users

- Refrain from sex with homosexuals or bisexual men

- Always use a latex condom with a spermicide and virucide if you are uncertain about your partner's sexual history prevent lethal infections. This protected environment has led to these children being called "bubble babies."

# EFFECTS OF AGING ON THE IMMUNE SYSTEM

Presently, not all age-related changes in the immune system are well understood. It is known that the thymus gland degenerates with age. The thymus reaches its maximum size in early childhood and then slowly decreases in size after puberty. As the gland decreases in size, so does the number of T cells because they originate in the cortex of the thymus. The remaining

T cells do not function as well, increasing the chance of developing invasive diseases (like cancer) as an individual ages. There also are some defects in lymph cells that occur in the aging process.

The B cell levels remain stable throughout life, but the antibodies in older persons may not function as well as in younger years. Thus, infections are common in the older population. The antibodies are more likely to attack the body's own tissue (autoantibodies) as a result of loss of tolerance to self-antigens. General resistance to disease seems to decrease with age, but this may be due to many other factors such as general nutrition, exercise, medications, and psychosocial influences rather than changes in the immune system.

## SUMMARY

The immune system consists of organs such as the thymus gland, bone marrow, lymph nodes, spleen, liver, and tonsils, and major cells such as the lymphocytes. The immune system is an important defense system for the body. A malfunctioning or compromised immune system leaves the body with weakened defenses against invading microorganisms. Many secondary disorders such as infections are due to a compromised immune response. Primary diseases or disorders of the immune system are categorized as hypersensitivity disorders or immune deficiency disorders. Hypersensitivity disorders include allergies, autoimmune disorders, and isoimmune disorders. The immune deficiency disease AIDS is one of the most common and debilitating fatal conditions of the immune system. Diagnostic testing for immune disorders includes skin testing, complete blood cell counts, and some specific antibody studies. Treatment for immune disorders varies with the specific problem. Some immune disorders are quite mild, whereas others are severe and require long-term therapy.

## REVIEW QUESTIONS

### Short Answer

1. What are the functions of the immune system?

2. Which signs and symptoms are associated with common immune system disorders?

3. Which diagnostic tests are most commonly used to determine the type and/or cause of an immune system disorder?

## Matching

4. Match the disorders listed in the left column with the correct category of immune system diseases in the right column. (Right-hand column categories may be used more than once.)

_____ Hay fever

_____ AIDS

_____ Anaphylaxis

_____ Rheumatic Fever

_____ Erythroblastosis Fetalis

_____ Organ Rejection

**a.** allergies

**b.** autoimmune disorders

**c.** isoimmune disorders

**d.** immune deficiency disorders

## Multiple Choice

5. Which of the following behaviors may contribute to increasing the risk for HIV transmission?

   **a.** Donating blood

   **b.** Sharing intravenous needles

   **c.** Failure to wash hands after toileting

   **d.** Unprotected sex

   **e.** Sharing eating utensils

   **f.** Direct contact with body fluids

   **g.** Frequent use of laxatives and enemas

## True or False

6. T F The immune system is the body's only defense system against invading organisms.

7. T F Signs and symptoms of hypersensitivity disorders may include rash, redness, heat, swelling, nasal congestion, coughing, and sneezing.

8. T F The Coombs' test is used to detect certain antibodies in the blood.

9. T F Autoimmune disorders are hyposensitivities in which the body fails to recognize its own antigens.

10. T F The effects of aging put the older adult at an increased risk for immune system problems.

## CASE STUDY

**Terry Stephens** is a 26-year-old male who has been diagnosed as HIV positive. He has told you that he and his girlfriend have unprotected sex. You have been close friends for many years. What are some strategies you could use to inform Terry about the danger of this behavior? Should you also talk to his girlfriend? When Terry was hospitalized, you noticed his caregivers wore gloves when starting his IV and drawing blood. Was this because he is HIV positive?

## BIBLIOGRAPHY

AIDS epidemic update: 2004. Joint United Nations Programme AIDS Information Centre. 20 Avenue Appia, 1211 Geneva 27, Switzerland. www.unaids.org or www.niaid.nih.gov/aids.

Aschenbrenner, D. (2003). New drug option for invasive aspergillosis. *American Journal of Nursing 103*(5), 90–91.

Bone marrow transplant program offers "mini-transplant." (2003, December 17). *Immunotherapy Weekly*, 83.

Chronic infection and regulation in the immune system. (2003). *Immunology Supplement 110*, 26-32.

Data support initiation of program to boost immune system to fight HBV. (2003, August 22). *Drug Week*, 234-234.

Davidson, B. T. & Donaldson, T. A. Immune system modulation in the highly sensitized transplant candidate. (2004). *Critical Care Nursing Quarterly 27*(1), 1-8.

Gravallese, E. M. (2003). Erratum. *Journal of Clinical Investigation 112*(2), 147-149.

Help for overactive immune systems. (2003). *Consumer Reports on Health 14*(10), 8.

Huizinga, R. (2002). Update in immunosuppression. *Nephrology Nursing Journal 29*(3), 261-267.

IBM to help find genetic links to immune system diseases. (2003, September 10). *Immunotherapy Weekly*, 57.

Immune system stages of eliminating viral infections, cancer cells discovered. (2003, July 2) *Immunotherapy Weekly*, 6-8.

Jones, J. (2003). Stress responses, pressure ulcer development and adaptation. *British Journal of Nursing* (suppl.), *12*(11), S17-S21.

Langone, J. (2003, July 7). At immune system's mercy. *New York Times 152*(52531), F7.

Marcos, A., Nova, E., & Montero, A. (2003). Changes in the immune system are conditioned by nutrition. *European Journal of Clinical Nutrition (suppl.), 57*(9), 66.

Otto, S. E. (2003). Understanding the immune system: Overview for infusion assessment. *Journal of Infusion Nursing 26*(2), 79-87.

Persistent infection impairs the immune system. (2003, October 27). *Health & Medicine Week*, 455.

Rogge, M. M. (2002). The case for an immunologic cause of obesity. *Biological Research for Nursing 4*(1), 43-53.

Shah, A. K. (2004). *Myesthenia Gravis.* emedicine.com.

Thymus transplant might save babies born without immune system. (2003, July 11). *Health and Medicine Week*, 140-143.

Weber, R. (2003). Our innate immune system: Barking at the doorbell. *Nursing 15*(5), 471.

Zinkernagel, R. M. (2003). On natural and artificial vaccination. *Annual Review of Immunology 21*(1), 515.

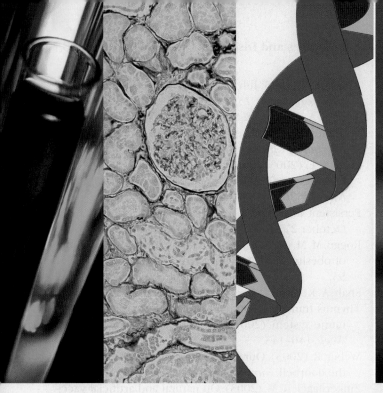
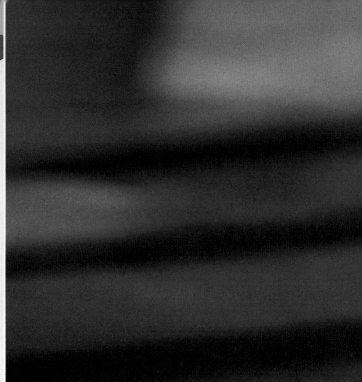

## OUTLINE

## KEY TERMS

# Musculoskeletal System Diseases and Disorders

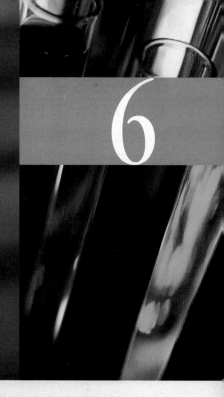

**6**

## LEARNING OBJECTIVES

*Upon completion of the chapter, the learner should be able to:*

1. Define the terminology common to the musculoskeletal system and the disorders of the system.

2. Discuss the basic anatomy and physiology of the musculoskeletal system.

3. Identify the important signs and symptoms associated with common musculoskeletal system disorders.

4. Describe the common diagnostics used to determine type and/or cause of a musculoskeletal system disorder.

5. Identify the common disorders of the musculoskeletal system.

6. Describe the typical course and management of the common musculoskeletal system disorders.

7. Describe the effects of aging on the musculoskeletal system and the common disorders of the system.

## OVERVIEW

The musculoskeletal system provides the structure and movement function for the individual. Because the muscles and bones run throughout the body, disorders of the system may affect any other system, and disorders of other systems frequently affect the musculoskeletal system. The system includes bones, joints, ligaments, muscles, and tendons. Each of these has a unique function, but also interacts with the other components of the system to support the person and provide for mobility. Problems with the musculoskeletal system frequently affect the individual's independence and thus the quality of life. ■

## ANATOMY AND PHYSIOLOGY

The skeletal component of the musculoskeletal system is made up of bones and joints. The bones are responsible for providing the framework to support the body. They also produce blood cells, store fat and minerals, protect soft tissues (like the brain), and help create body motion. Bones are very vascular. Blood circulates through bone, picking up or storing body minerals such as calcium, phosphorus, magnesium, and sodium. Osteoblasts are active bone-building cells, osteoclasts are cells that reabsorb bone, and osteocytes are mature bone cells.

Bones are often classified by shape and composition. For example, the skeletal system is composed of long bones such as the femur in the leg, short bones such as the metacarpal bones or bones in the fingers, flat bones such as the sternum or skull, and irregular bones such as the vertebrae or pelvic bones (Figure 6–1). The composition of bone is either cortical or cancellous. Cortical bone is dense, smooth, and compact, whereas cancellous bone is spongy, with many open spaces throughout. The ligaments are fibrous connective tissue that connect bones to other bones and joints.

Bone can be damaged and repair itself. The steps of bone repair include (1) bleeding at the site of injury with clot and granulation tissue formation; (2) proliferation of cells at the site, forming a callus (soft bony deposit) over the injury or fracture; (3) cells becoming bone (osteoblasts) or cartilage at the site; (4) the bone calcifying (hardened) by the deposit of inorganic salts at the site; and (5) the remodeling of the bone to the shape necessary to complete its designated function. Bone repair is dependent on many

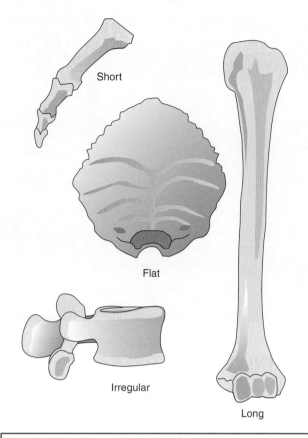

**FIGURE 6–1**   Examples of types of bones.

factors. The general health status of the individual will affect the healing process as well as age, degree of injury, circulation to the site, and presence of other diseases or infection.

The joints are where two or more bones meet. They are usually classified as to the amount of movement of the joint, but they also may be classified by their structure. The classification of joints by move-

## COMPLEMENTARY AND ALTERNATIVE THERAPY

**Herbal Medicine for Bone Growth**

The herbal medicine *Angelica sinensis* has been promoted in the past as a treatment to improve blood circulation. It is being studied for its ability to increase bone reformation. In Chinese medicine, *Angelica sinensis* is often included in compounds given by prescription for bone injuries. Scientists are now trying to understand how it actually helps bone growth. In laboratory tests, it directly stimulated bone cell proliferation.

*Source: Yang, Q., Populo, S.M., Zhang, J., Yang, G. And Kodama, H. (2002).*

**TABLE 6–1** Classification of Joints by Movement

| Classification | Amount of Movement | Example of Joint |
| --- | --- | --- |
| Synarthrosis | No movement | Suture of the skull |
| Amphiarthrosis | Some movement but very limited | Pelvis |
| Diarthrosis | Complete movement | Knee, hip, elbow |

ment is described in Table 6–1. Classification of joints by structure includes fibrous (such as the joints of the skull), cartilaginous (such as the joints of the vertebrae), and synovial (such as the joints of the knee). The synovial joints are those separated by a fluid-filled cavity.

The major movements of joints are flexion (bending), extension (reaching out or spreading out), abduction (away from the body), adduction (toward the body), rotation (turning on an axis), circumduction (circular movement), and elevation (lifting).

Cartilage is collagen tissue that supports articulating (adjoining) bones. It provides protection and a cushion to prevent friction between bones. Carti-

lage also acts like a shock absorber to reduce stress on the bone surface.

The functions of the muscles of the body are to provide structure, movement, and produce heat (Figure 6–2). The muscles of the musculoskeletal system are called "striated" because they look striped or banded under a microscope. They are also called voluntary muscles because most are moved by conscious control as opposed to other muscles, like cardiac, that move involuntarily. Skeletal muscles move in response to signals from the central nervous system. Connective tissue holds the muscle fibers together. Tendons are long, fibrous, nonelastic connective tissues that attach muscle to bone.

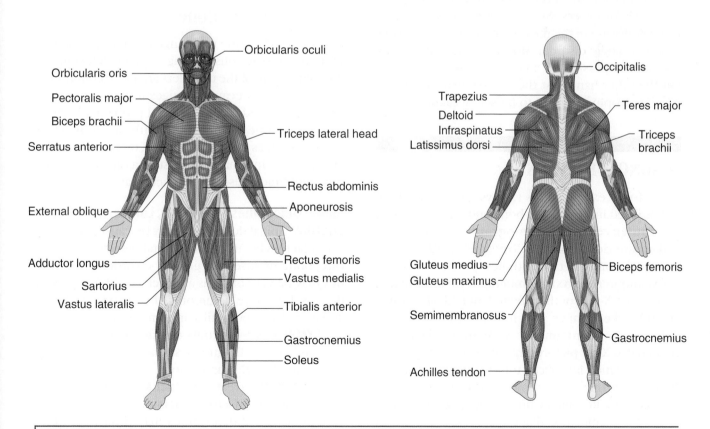

**FIGURE 6–2** The skeletal muscles.

Each muscle fiber in the body contains myofibrils. The myofibrils are composed of sarcomeres that are the contracting and relaxing component of the muscle. This contracting and relaxing characteristic provides the smooth, elastic movement of the muscle.

The source of energy for the movement of muscles is the metabolism of adenosine triphosphate (ATP) in the cell. ATP is produced from available glucose and glycogen (stored glucose) in the cells. Oxygen is necessary for parts of this process as well as adequate stores of glucose.

## COMMON SIGNS AND SYMPTOMS

The most common signs and symptoms of bone and joint disease are pain, swelling, decreased mobility, and deformity. Most fractures are associated with pain due to a disruption of the periosteum and related sensory nerves. Many fractures are easy to recognize due to the obvious displacement and related deformity. **Nondisplaced** (not out of place or position) fractures are not as easy to recognize, but may cause pain just the same.

Weakness is the most common sign or symptom of muscle disorders. Weakness may be related to a primary disease of the muscle or it may be secondary to a neurologic disorder. Muscle tissue will atrophy if weakness persists for an extended length of time. On the other hand, just the reverse may occur, and muscle atrophy will lead to muscle weakness.

## DIAGNOSTIC TESTS

**Radiologic** examinations (X-rays) are the primary tool utilized in diagnosing bone and joint disorders. **Computerized Axial Tomography (CAT or CT)** and **Magnetic Resonance Imaging (MRI)** may be needed for more detailed studies.

Computerized Axial Tomography involves taking specialized X-rays of the affected individual in a special tube-like scanner. The individual must be able to lie still for approximately 30 minutes. The results are detailed X-ray pictures that appear to cut the area of consideration into slices, thus the name tomogram (tomo = cutting, gram = picture) (Figure 6–3).

Magnetic Resonance Imaging is another detailed X-ray type examination that utilizes a large magnet to make electromagnetic images. Individuals must be able to lie still and must not wear any type of metal during the test. MRI is more expensive to perform but takes more detailed images of soft tissue than a CT scanner.

Blood studies including calcium, phosphorus, and an enzyme (alkaline phosphatase) also may prove helpful with metabolic disorders. Infectious disorders may be cultured. Often, the specimen for culture is obtained during surgical procedures like débridement.

Muscle disorders are often evaluated by **electromyography** (EMG). This is accomplished by inserting a small needle into muscle tissue and recording the electrical activity. Electromyography can assist in determining if the disorder is muscular or neurologic in nature. Muscle tissue biopsy may be performed on difficult cases. Biopsy is the most definitive means of determining cause of muscle disorder. Biopsy is also the most reliable test for tumors of the musculoskeletal system.

## COMMON DISEASES OF THE MUSCULOSKELETAL SYSTEM

### Diseases of the Bone

Diseases of the bone may range from mild to severe with the most serious causing extreme deformity or disability. Many of the disorders are more common in the older adult because changes in the system may lead to increased risk for skeletal problems. Individuals with bone disease frequently need assistive devices such as crutches, walkers, or canes to maintain mobility. Internal devices such as artificial joints, pins, and braces also may be necessary.

**Spinal Deformities—Kyphosis, Lordosis, Scoliosis.**
**ETIOLOGY** Spinal deformities may be caused by a variety of factors including congenital defects, poor posture, bone disease, and growth disorders. Deformities may be very obvious at onset as with congenital defects, but more commonly, they progress slowly and are unnoticed until symptoms arise.

**SYMPTOMS** Symptoms commonly include back pain and fatigue. Diagnosis is generally confirmed by X-ray and clinical examination.

**TREATMENT** Treatment includes eliminating or treating causative factors, bracing, and spinal surgery. Untreated spinal deformities may progress to life-threatening conditions when cardiac and respiratory function are compromised.

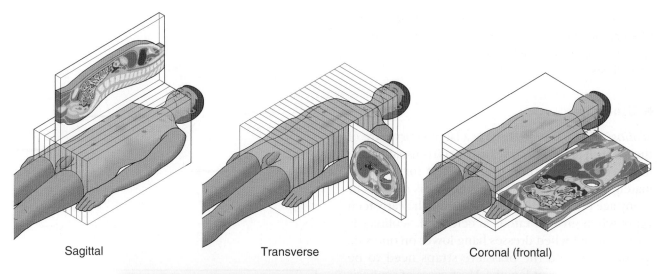

Sagittal                    Transverse                    Coronal (frontal)

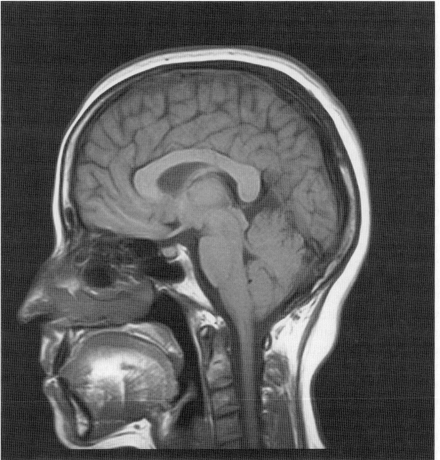

**FIGURE 6–3**    (Top) CT of chest and abdomen, (Bottom) MRI of head.

## ■ Kyphosis

*Kyphosis* (kie-FOE-sis) is a humped curvature of the thoracic spine, commonly called humpback or hunchback. Kyphosis often appears in postmenopausal osteoporitic females.

## ■ Lordosis

*Lordosis* (lor-DOE-sis) is an exaggerated anterior or inward curve of the lumbar spine, and is also called swayback. It normally occurs with pregnancy as the individual compensates for the increased size of the abdomen. When compared to the normal spine, lordosis results in a protruding abdomen and buttocks, and a swayed lower back. Obesity is a common cause of lordosis.

## ■ Scoliosis

*Scoliosis* (SKOLE-lee-**OH**-sis) is a lateral curvature of the spine. It affects both sexes, but girls usually have more severe curvatures and account for approximately 90 percent of the cases. Scoliosis may occur at any age but is usually noticed during the early teen years when growth rate is accelerated. Scoliosis is often noticed when dresses hang lower on one side or the other, and the brassiere straps need to be adjusted to different lengths. Most cases of scoliosis can be corrected if detected early, and treated properly and promptly. Treatment often includes bracing. Compliance with brace-wearing for female adolescents is often poor, leading to the need for further treatment. Scoliosis screening in school-aged children was initiated in the 1960s and is now mandated by law in some states. Screening involves observation of the spine as the individual bends forward. Scoliosis is suspected if the spine curves to the side and the scapula shifts upward (Figure 6–4).

### Osteoporosis.
Osteoporosis (OS-tee-oh-por-**OH**-sis) is a metabolic bone disease that causes a porosity or Swiss cheese appearance of the bone, leading to a decrease in bone mass. It is the most prevalent bone disease worldwide. It is estimated that osteoporosis causes major orthopedic problems in approximately one-third of the women in the United States.

**ETIOLOGY** There are many causative factors that play a part in osteoporosis. Age-related osteoporosis affects both men and women equally, and is due to normal age-related bone loss. Osteoporosis occurs secondary to diseases that affect mobility. For example, quadriplegia may lead to a loss of 30–40 percent of bone mass after six months of immobility. The most common type of osteoporosis is seen in women who are postmenopausal and estrogen-deficient. It is believed that this osteoporosis is due to a combination of factors including a decrease in estrogen, calcium, and exercise.

Osteoporosis is a slow, progressive disease that robs skeletal bone of its mass and strength. It may be decades before the bone becomes weak enough to fracture. Most fractures in women over age 50 are related to osteoporosis. Diagnosis may be con-

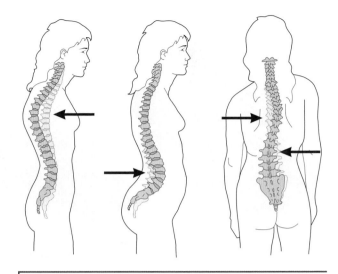

**FIGURE 6–4**   Spinal deformities: kyphosis, lordosis, and scoliosis (S curvature).

firmed by clinical examination, X-rays, CT scans, and bone **densitometry** (measurement of bone thickness).

**SYMPTOMS** Early signs of osteoporosis include **compression** (bone mashed down on itself, common in vertebra) fractures of the spine and pathologic wrist fractures. Compression fractures of the spine lead to a decrease in height, and pain in the thoracic and lumbar spine. Over a period of time, the individual may lose four to five inches of height, decreasing the thoracic and abdominal cavity size. This decrease in chest cavity size leads to decreased activity tolerance due to shortness of breath. A decrease in the abdominal cavity size leads to feelings of fullness after eating only small amounts of food and a constant bloated feeling. Other symptoms are kyphosis and the appearance of a **Dowager's hump** (abnormal curvature in the upper thoracic spine; Figure 6–5). Wrist fractures, especially of the distal radius, commonly occur in osteoporitic individuals with only a slight fall. As the disease progresses, the individual has an increased risk for fracturing a hip. More than one million hip fractures occur annually in the United States. Hip fractures in frail, older women often lead to complications that result in mortality (Figure 6–6).

**TREATMENT** Currently, there is no treatment to reverse osteoporosis because bone mass is not replaced in older adults, although administration of the drug alendronate (Fosimax) appears quite promising in increasing bone mass. The progression of osteoporosis can be slowed and bone mass

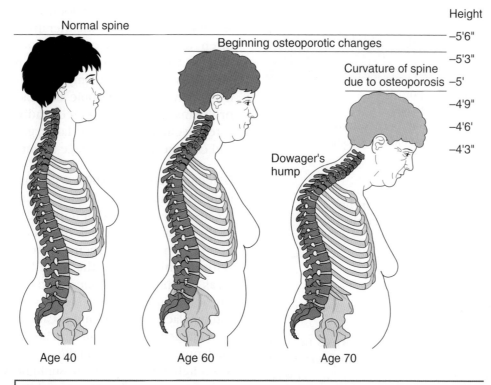

**FIGURE 6–5** Osteoporosis: loss in height and the Dowager's hump.

levels maintained by a combination of therapies. Reduction of risk factors includes decreasing alcohol and caffeine consumption, and not smoking (Table 6–2). Other therapies include increasing estrogen, increasing calcium and vitamin D intake, and a daily exercise routine that includes weight-bearing exercise. Much controversy exists concerning the use of estrogen replacement therapy because it is associated with an increase in breast and gynecologic malignancies. An increase in calcium levels also may lead to the formation of kidney stones. These treatments must be considered on an individual basis. The one treatment that is agreed on by most practitioners is the need for daily exercise.

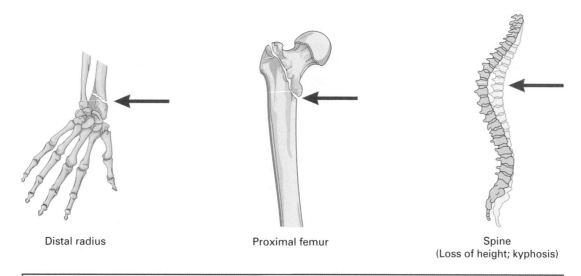

Distal radius      Proximal femur      Spine
(Loss of height; kyphosis)

**FIGURE 6–6** Fracture site related to osteoporosis.

| TABLE 6–2 Risk Factors for Osteoporosis |
|---|
| **The following are considered factors that increase the risk of developing osteoporosis:** |
| ■ Family history of osteoporosis |
| ■ Age—risk increases with age |
| ■ Medications—tetracycline, corticosteroids, aluminum antacids, some diuretics, some anticonvulsants |
| ■ Female, white or Asian |
| ■ Lack of exercise |
| ■ Lack of calcium in diet or supplements |
| ■ Oophorectomy (removal of ovaries)—risk increases postsurgery |

Regular exercise has been shown to reduce the rate of hip fractures by 50 percent.

Preventive measures for osteoporosis need to begin early because bone mass is built prior to age 30. Young women should be encouraged to exercise daily, eat a balanced diet, quit smoking, and limit caffeine and alcohol consumption. Entering menopausal years with good bone mass and maintaining as much of the bone as possible is the best weapon against osteoporosis.

**Osteomyelitis.** **ETIOLOGY** Osteomyelitis (OS-tee-oh-MY-ull-**LIE**-tis; osteo = bone, myel = marrow, itis = inflammation) is an inflammation of the bone commonly caused by infection. *Staphylococcus aureus* is the responsible organism in approximately 90 percent of the cases. This bacterium may enter the bone through a wound, spread from an infection nearby, or come from a skin or throat infection. Osteomyelitis usually affects the long bones of the arms and legs. It most often occurs in children and adolescents as a result of a throat infection. In severe cases, it may affect the growth plate of the bones, leading to shortening of the limb.

**SYMPTOMS** Symptoms of osteomyelitis may include sudden onset of high fever, chills, tenderness over the affected bone, leukocytosis (leuko = white, cyto = cell, osis = condition of increase), and bacteremia (bacteria = microscopic organism, emia = blood, bacteria in the blood). In adults, osteomyelitis often occurs following a traumatic accident involving the bone or following bone surgery, especially when implants such as screws, plates, or other hardware are needed.

**TREATMENT** Treatment for osteomyelitis is aggressive intravenous antibiotic therapy. Affected bone is often débrided surgically to speed the healing process. Surgical hardware is often removed for this same reason. Acute osteomyelitis, if not treated effectively, may become chronic and lead to a lifetime of problems for the affected individual. Chronic osteomyelitis may lead to large, gaping scar tissue and chronic wound drainage (Figure 6–7).

**Osteomalacia.** **ETIOLOGY** Osteomalacia (OS-tee-oh-muh-**LAY**-shuh; osteo = bone, malacia = softening) is caused by decreased or impaired **mineralization** of the bone due to a lack of vitamin D. Mineralization of bones causes their characteristic hardness. Without this process, the bone becomes soft and weak. To mineralize, bones need calcium, phosphorus, and vitamin D. Bone softness in adults is called osteomalacia; in children it is called rickets.

Deficiency of vitamin D in adults may be due to inadequate nutritional intake, inadequate exposure to sunlight (skin exposed to sunlight synthesizes vitamin D), or a malabsorption problem.

**SYMPTOMS** Symptoms and signs of osteomalacia include bone pain, loss of height, bending, and deformity in weight-bearing bones such as the spine, pelvis, and legs.

**TREATMENT** Correction of the deficiency potentially cures the problem. Bones that have bowed, shortened, or flattened may not regain normal appearance and function.

## Diseases of the Joints

Most of the diseases of the joints occur as a slow, degenerative process, so they tend to be more common with age. As with diseases of the bones, diseases of the joints often result in the individual requiring assistive devices or artificial parts to maintain mobility. Frequently, damage to joints occurring during youth is not apparent until middle or older adulthood.

**Arthritis.** Arthritis (arthro = joint, itis = inflammation) and rheumatism are terms commonly used to describe a variety of conditions that cause pain and stiffness in the musculoskeletal system. Both are terms that cover a broad group of conditions, but arthritis is a condition of inflammation in a joint whereas rheumatism is a condition of stiffness. Arthritis is any inflammation of a joint. Everyone at some time or

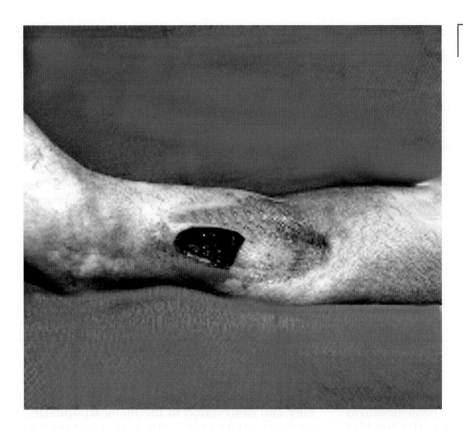

**FIGURE 6–7** Chronic osteomyelitis scar of the lower leg. *(Courtesy of Mark L. Kuss.)*

another has had arthritis; for example, a sprained ankle or jammed finger are arthritic conditions. Arthritis can be divided into two main groups: osteoarthritis and rheumatoid arthritis. Osteoarthritis is the most common form of arthritis, but rheumatoid arthritis is the more serious and debilitating type.

## ■ Osteoarthritis or Degenerative Joint Disease

**ETIOLOGY** Osteoarthritis is a degenerative process or a "wearing out" of a joint. It may begin in the early 20s with 90 percent of all adults showing some radiologic changes. The amount or degree of wear is associated with several factors (Table 6–3). Sports injuries speed the wear and tear on the joints, leading to osteoarthritis at a younger age.

**SYMPTOMS** Older adults are usually symptomatic with this type of arthritis. It often affects frequently used joints like those in the hands, and joints that are weight-bearing such as those of the spine, hip, and knee. Affected joints of the hands often swell and are painful. The distal and proximal **interphalangeal** (inter = between, phalangeal = finger bones) joints are often affected, and may lead to a crooked deformity of the fingers. The **metacarpophalangeal** (meta = beyond, carpo = wrist, phalangeal = finger bones) joints are usually not affected (Figure 6–8).

| **TABLE 6–3** | **Risk Factors for Osteoarthritis** |
|---|---|

| **The following are considered factors that increase the risk of developing osteoarthritis:** |
|---|
| ■ Family history of osteoarthritis |
| ■ Excessive wear and tear, or injury to joints |
| ■ Obesity |
| ■ Age—risk increases with age |
| ■ Female |

Osteoarthritis that affects weight-bearing joints often affects the spine, hips, and knees. As the joints of the spinal column are affected with arthritis, individuals may become symptomatic with back pain. Osteoarthritis affects the hips and knees by wearing away the **articular** (are-TICK-you-lar) cartilage at the end of the long bones where bones articulate or meet. Eventually, the entire surface of the cartilage may be worn away, exposing areas of raw bone. When this occurs, new bone forms in and around the joint, causing the bone ends to thicken. Fragments of this new bone are called bone spurs and often lead to a decrease in joint motion. X-ray examination may reveal the spurs and only small patches of cartilage on the bone ends. This is called a "bone on bone" condition. At this point,

## HEALTHY HIGHLIGHT

### Knuckle Cracking

"Will knuckle-cracking cause arthritis in my joints?" This is a commonly asked question by those who have developed the habit of knuckle-cracking. This cracking sound is made by the rush of synovial fluid from one area of the joint to another as the joint is forcefully pulled apart. Research supports the fact that this action does not cause an increase in osteoarthritis, but it also supports the fact that individuals who crack their knuckles eventually have decreased grip and hand function. Research does not rule out the idea of knuckle-cracking causing joint damage. Knuckle-crackers may not have to worry about an increase in osteoarthritic pain due to chronic knuckle-cracking, but they may still develop long-term pain from chronic ligament inflammation. Some researchers feel that chronic joint pain, whether related to arthritis or not, is still chronic joint pain, and thus recommend that knuckle-crackers stop this behavior. Interestingly, related research found that knuckle-crackers are also more likely to bite their fingernails, smoke, and drink alcohol.

individuals are often candidates for total hip or knee replacement surgery. Osteoarthritis peaks in the fifth to sixth decade of life with approximately 80 percent of individuals showing symptoms by age 70.

**TREATMENT** Treatment for osteoarthritis includes rest, nonweight-bearing exercise like swimming and biking, heat, and use of analgesics and anti-inflammatory medications. Severe osteoarthritis may be treated by steroid injections into the joint capsule to relieve pain. Total surgical joint replacement may be recommended.

### ■ Rheumatoid Arthritis

**ETIOLOGY** Rheumatoid arthritis was discussed in Chapter 5 as an autoimmune disorder that not only affects the joints, but also affects the connective tissues of the entire body. Rheumatoid arthritis often affects the lungs, heart, and blood vessels, causing the individual to appear chronically ill. This type of arthritis often affects people in the prime of life and affects women more often than men. It is a debilitating, chronic disease that destroys the joints.

**SYMPTOMS** A noticeable difference in the way osteoarthritis and rheumatoid arthritis affect the joints can be observed in joints of the hand. Osteoarthritis, as previously discussed, affects the working joints of the hand (primarily the distal and proximal interphalangeal joints), causing swelling and pain. All joints of the hand may be affected in

rheumatoid individuals, often with noticeable deformity and destruction in the metacarpophalangeal joints (see Figure 6–8). Also, refer to Chapter 5 for more information on rheumatoid arthritis.

**Gout.** Gout is often called gouty arthritis because this condition leads to inflammation of the affected joints.

**ETIOLOGY** Gout is caused by a metabolic alteration in the breakdown of certain protein foods. Individuals with gout deposit uric acid crystals in joints of the body.

**SYMPTOMS** The primary joint that is affected is the **metatarsophalangeal** (meta = between, tarso = foot, phalangeal = toe bones) joint of the big toe. These uric acid crystals have razor sharp edges that irritate the joint, causing an acute inflammatory response. Symptoms are redness, heat, swelling, and pain in the joint.

Gout primarily affects males as approximately 95 percent of gout patients are male. Onset is usually after age 30. Chronic gout may be characterized by uric acid deposited in subcutaneous tissue as well. These deposits appear as small whitish nodules called **tophi**, and are commonly seen around a joint and in the soft tissue of the ear (Figure 6–9). Kidney dysfunction and an increase in the occurrence of kidney stones is common with chronic gout.

**TREATMENT** Treatment may include dietary adjustments to decrease the amount of protein consumed,

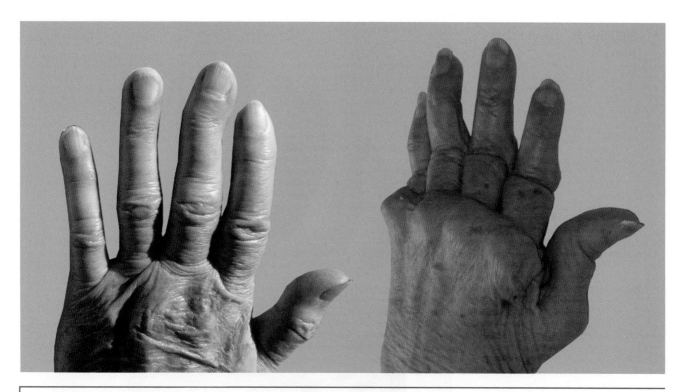

**FIGURE 6–8**   Comparison of (left) osteoarthritis and (right) rheumatoid arthritis: hands and joints. *(Courtesy of Ruth Jones.)*

and anti-gout medication (probenecid and allopurinol [Zyloprim]). Weight loss in obese patients also may be beneficial.

**Hallux Valgus.**   Hallux (big toe) valgus (bent outward) is a deformity affecting the metatarsophalangeal joint of the big toe. It is more commonly called a bunion. This condition occurs more frequently in women and tends to run in families.

**ETIOLOGY** Bunions may be the result of congenital conditions or other disease processes like rheumatoid arthritis. More commonly, bunions are the result of wearing pointed-toe shoes, especially with high heels. This type of shoe forces the great toe into a valgus position and increases the pressure on the metatarsophalangeal joint. Over a period of time, this chronic irritation leads to a buildup of soft tissue and bone in the joint area (Figure 6–10).

**SYMPTOMS** Symptoms and signs include redness, pain, and swelling in the area, and often the inability to wear pointed-toe or high-heeled shoes.

**TREATMENT** Mild cases may be resolved by changing to a properly fitting low-heeled shoe. Analgesic and anti-inflammatory medications may be benefi-

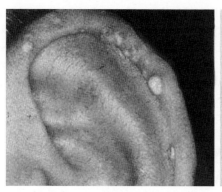
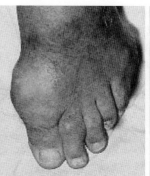
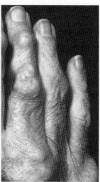

**FIGURE 6–9**   Common sites of tophi. *(Courtesy of Mark L. Kuss.)*

**FIGURE 6–10** Hallux Valgus (Bunion).

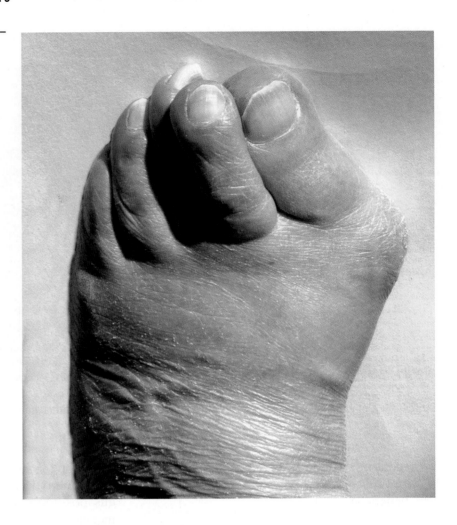

cial in pain relief. More severe cases may need surgical intervention with bunionectomy.

**Temporomandibular Joint Syndrome (TMJ).** **ETIOLOGY** TMJ may be due to joint tissue lesions, overbite, malocclusion, or improperly fitted dentures or dental work.

**SYMPTOMS** Severe headaches and pain in the "jaw" joint may be indicative of TMJ. This pain may be made worse by chewing. Classic signs include marked decrease in the ability to open the mouth and a clicking sound made during chewing motion.

**TREATMENT** Treatment includes correction of the causative factor, often leading to surgical intervention.

## Diseases of the Muscles and Connective Tissue

Diseases of the muscles and connective tissue, unlike many of the bone disorders, are quite common in very young or young adult individuals. Some of these disorders, such as the muscular dystrophies, are chronic, progressive, and devastating to families because they usually result in early death. Other disorders of the muscles and connective tissue are considered to be rather minor, and can be treated medically or surgically.

### ■ Muscular Dystrophy (MD)

**ETIOLOGY** Muscular dystrophy is an inherited genetic disorder that affects skeletal muscle. There are many types of dystrophies, but the most common type is Duchenne's MD that primarily affects male children.

**SYMPTOMS** Duchenne's MD is characterized by a wasting away of shoulder and pelvic girdle muscles. Survival beyond age 20 is rare. This disorder is discussed in detail in Chapter 19.

### ■ Ganglion Cyst

A ganglion cyst is a fluid-filled benign tumor that usually develops on a tendon sheath near the wrist area.

**ETIOLOGY** The cause of these cysts is unknown, although some feel that they may be associated with a repetitive injury.

**SYMPTOMS** A cyst is commonly a single, smooth, round lump just under the skin (Figure 6–11). It may be quite small, or grow to the size of a dime or quarter. Usually, these are painless but are unsightly. Cysts may disappear gradually over a period of months.

**TREATMENT** If they are painful or unsightly, the physician may choose to rupture the cyst or drain it. Ganglionectomy or, surgical removal, also may be performed.

### ■ Tetanus

Tetanus, also called lockjaw, is an acute, infectious, life-threatening disease characterized by painful, uncontrolled contractions of skeletal muscle.

**ETIOLOGY** A toxin produced by the bacillus bacterium, *Clostridium tetani*, causes tetanus. This bacterium is commonly found in animal feces, and when excreted, lives as spores in the soil. The number of these spores is especially high in barnyards, pastures, or garden areas fertilized with animal manure. When this infectious bacterium enters the body in an **anaerobic** (ana = without, erobic = air) wound like a puncture wound, it grows and produces a dangerous toxin. This toxin travels in the blood and attaches to motor or muscle neurons. The toxin irritates the nerve, producing the stimulus for skeletal muscle contraction. Because of the neurological involvement, tetanus also may be categorized as a nervous system disorder.

**SYMPTOMS** The bacterial toxin affects the nervous system rather slowly. The further the distance between the wound and the spinal cord, the slower the progression. One to three weeks may pass before the onset of symptoms. The jaw muscles are often the first muscles affected with **tetany** (TET-ah-nee) or

rigid muscle contraction. The individual may not be able to open the mouth, hence the term "lockjaw." Eventually, muscles of the esophagus, neck, back, arms, and legs are affected. Other symptoms are a high fever, tachycardia (rapid pulse rate), dysphagia (difficulty swallowing), and intense pain.

**TREATMENT** Treatment is a prompt and immediate cleansing of wounds with special consideration given to puncture-type wounds. Immunization may be needed depending on the individual's immunization history. If the individual has not received a tetanus toxoid injection in the past five years, an antitoxin may be given. Tetanus toxoid injection will cause the immune system to build antibodies. Initially, tetanus toxoid should be administered to children as part of basic immunization DPT (diphtheria, pertussis, and tetanus). Tetanus antibodies need to be "boosted" approximately every seven to ten years throughout life. Individuals with low tetanus antibody levels are susceptible to tetanus. An antitoxin may be given to prevent tetanus following an injury because the body does not have time to build up its own antibodies. Following this episode, it is usually recommended that the individual follow up with the proper tetanus toxoid booster.

Care of an individual with tetanus includes symptomatic treatment, often including respiratory, nutritional, and hydration support. Antibiotics and muscle relaxants also may be administered. Even with the best of care, tetanus is usually fatal due to respiratory failure. If the individual survives, the disease process usually lasts six to eight weeks. Surprisingly, the disease usually does not leave any permanent disability, but it also does not confer any lasting immunity to tetanus.

## Neoplasms

Primary neoplasms of the musculoskeletal system are uncommon. Typically, neoplasms of this system are secondary, metastasizing from the lungs, breast, and prostate. The most common primary tumor of bone is osteosarcoma. Primary tumors of the bone marrow include myeloma or multiple myeloma, and Ewing's sarcoma. Myeloma is the most common marrow tumor. It affects the pelvis, vertebrae, and long bones of adults. Ewing's sarcoma primarily affects long bones in children and teens. It is highly malignant and quickly metastasizes to nearly every organ of the body. Kaposi's sarcoma affects soft tissue of primarily immunosuppressed individuals. Rhabdomyosarcoma is a very rare but highly malignant tumor of skeletal muscle.

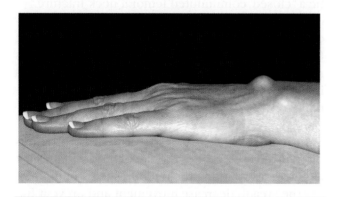

**FIGURE 6–11** Ganglion cyst. *(Courtesy of Mark L. Kuss.)*

Symptoms of musculoskeletal tumors may include pathologic fracture and bone pain. Clinical examination followed by radiologic studies, CT scan, blood studies, and biopsy often confirm the diagnosis. Treatment of malignant tumors of the musculoskeletal system may include radiation, chemotherapy, and surgery. Surgical procedures often involve excision and amputation. Even with aggressive therapy, prognosis for these malignant neoplasms is often very poor.

# TRAUMA

Trauma is the main cause of problems in the musculoskeletal system. Fractures are by far the most common and frequent injury to bone. Tennis elbow is the most frequent ailment of the upper body. Treatment for sprains and strains is among the top 10 reasons that patients seek medical attention for acute disease. Low back pain is in the top 10 for chronic disease.

## Fracture

A fracture is any discontinuity of a bone. A fracture and a "break" are synonymous, although a **stress** (related to too much weight-bearing or pressure) fracture or incomplete fracture may not "break" the bone in two. Fractures may be caused by trauma (injury) or may be **pathologic** (caused by weakness from another disease).

**Types of Fractures.** Fractures may be classified in a number of ways. One method of classification is based on the condition of the overlying skin. If the bone has protruded through the skin or an object has punctured the skin, making an opening through the skin to the fracture site, it is an **open** fracture. Open fractures are also called **compound** fractures because the fracture, plus the open skin, is compounding the problem. An open fracture is always an emergency, due to the high risk of bone infection. Patients with open fractures are taken to surgery for cleaning and débridement. If there is no opening in the skin, it is called a **closed** or **simple** fracture.

Another method of classification considers the condition of the bone. If the fracture goes completely through the bone, it is a **complete** fracture. If the bone is fractured but not in two, it is an **incomplete** fracture. A common incomplete fracture that occurs in children is called a **greenstick** fracture, because

it appears to have broken partially like a sap-filled green stick.

Fractures also may be described by the number of fragments or the position of the fragments. A **displaced** fracture is one in which fragments are out of position, whereas nondisplaced means the fragments are still in correct position. If there are more than two ends or fragments, the break is a **comminuted** fracture. Bone appearing to be mashed down is a compression fracture. A common site of a compression fracture is in the vertebrae. An **impacted** fracture is one characterized as a bone end forced over the other end. **Avulsion** fracture describes a separation of a small bone fragment from the bone where a tendon or ligament is attached.

The position of the fracture line as compared to bone position may also describe the fracture. A **longitudinal** fracture runs the length of the bone; a **transverse** fracture runs across or at a 90-degree angle. **Oblique** fractures run in a transverse pattern; while **spiral** fractures twist around the bone. **Stellate** fractures form a star-like pattern.

Location may be used to describe the fracture. An articular fracture involves a joint surface. **Intracapsular** and **extracapsular** describe fractures inside or outside the joint capsule, respectively. **Intertrochanteric** describes fractures in the trochanter of the femur, and **femoral neck** and **subcapital** fractures describe fractures located on the femur. Finally, fractures may be named by the physician who first described them; for example, **Colles'** (Figure 6-12) and **Pott's** fractures are fractures of the wrist and ankle respectively.

To be very specific, a fracture may be more clearly defined by using several descriptive names. For example, a diagnosis of a "closed fracture" is a broad diagnosis covering many different fractures. A more descriptive diagnosis would be a "closed, comminuted fracture." An even clearer diagnosis would be a "closed, comminuted femoral neck fracture."

Sites and causes of fractures vary by age and gender. Children commonly fracture their arms during falls. Teen males commonly have long bone fractures related to MVAs (motor vehicle accidents) or sports injuries. Older females suffer with hip fractures generally related to falls and osteoporosis.

**Treatment of Fractures.** Treatment of fractures often involves first aid at the site of the accident. First aid includes splinting the fracture site by immobilizing the area to decrease movement and prevent fur-

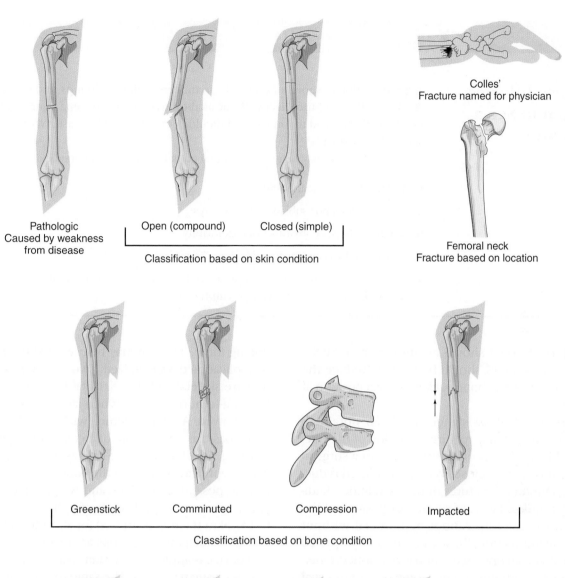

Pathologic
Caused by weakness
from disease

Open (compound)    Closed (simple)

Classification based on skin condition

Colles'
Fracture named for physician

Femoral neck
Fracture based on location

Greenstick    Comminuted    Compression    Impacted

Classification based on bone condition

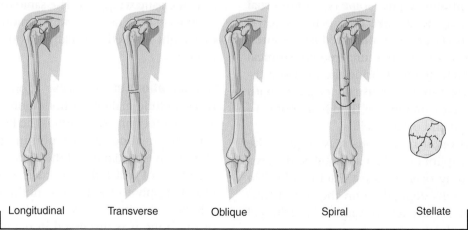

Longitudinal    Transverse    Oblique    Spiral    Stellate

Classification based on position of fracture line

**FIGURE 6–12**  Types of fractures.

### Sports Injuries—When to See a Doctor

Participation in sports often results in numerous "lumps, bumps, and bruises." Often, these injuries heal without medical treatment, but some injuries, left unattended, may lead to long-term difficulties. Often, individuals ask, "When should I see a doctor?"

The following may be used as general guidelines for seeking medical attention.

- Any injury in or near a joint
- Pain that does not subside after 10 days
- Any time there is obvious bone deformity
- Injury that has not improved in 5 to 7 days
- Any sign of infection: temperature of 101°F or greater, presence of pus, red streaks in the tissue, or swollen lymph glands

ther injury. A splint should be applied in an "as is" position. No attempt should be made to reduce the fracture or place the bone back in normal position at this time.

Once medical assistance has been obtained, proper treatment may require reduction of the fracture. If this can be accomplished without a surgical incision, it is called a closed reduction. Closed reduction is common in fractures of the extremities. Radiography is utilized to confirm proper position of the bones. If the fracture cannot be reduced without internal manipulation, the area is surgically opened or incised, and an open reduction is performed. Open reductions commonly require some type of internal fixation or holding device like pins, plates, screws, or rods. This procedure is an open reduction, internal fixation (**ORIF**). Open fractures require surgical intervention to clean and débride the involved tissue. An open fracture site is usually cleansed with copious (excessive) amounts of fluid in an effort to prevent infection and osteomyelitis.

Closed and open reductions may require the application of a splint or cast to immobilize the area during the healing process. Most fractures heal in four to eight weeks depending on the site of fracture, the type of fracture, and the age and nutritional status of the involved individual.

The application of traction may be beneficial to relieve muscle spasms, to hold a fracture in correct position, or to stretch the muscles, allowing bone fragment ends to separate, and thus reducing pain and further tissue damage. Traction involves the application of a device to maintain alignment and apply a

pulling force. Traction may be classified by the type of application device utilized. Two basic types of traction are skeletal and skin. Skeletal traction is utilized for long-term traction or when large muscle groups are involved. A femur fracture, with resultant quadriceps spasm, is an example of a condition commonly utilizing skeletal traction. Skeletal traction involves placement of a pin through the bone distal to the fracture. Ropes, pulley devices, and weights are used to apply traction or pull to the fracture site (Figure 6-13). Skin traction is utilized for short-term traction or when small muscle groups are involved. The traction device is applied to the skin with the use of adhesive or elastic wrapping. The same ropes, pulleys, and weights may be used for skin traction, but the amount of weight applied is usually less than with skeletal traction.

**Complications of Fractures.** Complications of fractures include mal-union, nonunion, avascular necrosis, and infection. Mal-union is the healing of the fracture in an abnormal or nonfunctional position. Nonunion is the failure of the bone to heal. The complication of avascular necrosis occurs when the blood supply to the bone is not adequate to maintain bone health and the bone tissue dies. Infection of the bone was discussed in detail under the section Osteomyelitis (see page 92).

## Strains and Sprains

**ETIOLOGY** A strain is an overstretching injury of a muscle.

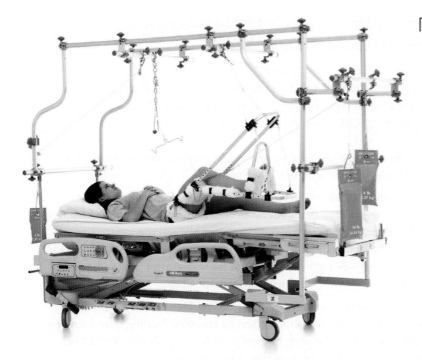

**SYMPTOMS** Symptoms include soreness, pain, and tenderness. Individuals commonly have lumbar strains from lifting too much weight, lifting improperly, or lifting repetitively. Strained backs are common after a weekend of activity by an individual not in adequate physical condition.

**TREATMENT** Treatment includes rest, moist heat, and the use of analgesics and anti-inflammatory medications. A strain is less serious than a sprain.

**ETIOLOGY** A sprain is a traumatic injury to a joint with partial or complete tearing of ligaments. The ankle joint is commonly affected and may become so painful that the joint cannot be used. The degree of ligament tearing, plus involvement of associated tendons, muscles, and blood vessels, determines the degree of injury. Severe sprains may exhibit complete tearing of the ligaments.

**SYMPTOMS** Symptoms include varying degrees of swelling, pain, heat, and redness to purple or dark blue discoloration from blood vessel hemorrhage (Figure 6–14).

**TREATMENT** Treatment for sprains includes the concepts **RICE**: rest, ice, compression, and elevation. Severe sprains may be X-rayed to rule out fractures.

## Dislocations and Subluxations

**ETIOLOGY** Dislocation is the complete separation of a bone from its normal position in a joint. A subluxation is a partial separation (Figure 6–15). Disloca-

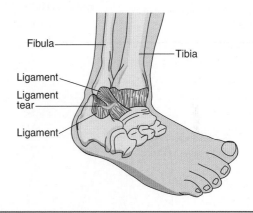

**FIGURE 6–14** Sprained ankle.

tions occur with major traumatic injuries like MVAs, contact sports, or falls. A dislocation injury also may cause a fracture. Dislocations also may be related to joint abnormalities or disease. In the case of disease, the dislocation may occur frequently and without cause.

**SYMPTOMS** Dislocation causes acute pain and obvious joint deformity. In ball and socket joints, the ball may be totally anterior or posterior to the socket. The joint tissue rapidly swells, making reduction difficult.

**TREATMENT** Because of the swelling, a dislocated joint should be reduced or repositioned by a physician immediately. Even with emergency treatment, general anesthesia may be needed for the reduction procedure.

## HEALTHY HIGHLIGHT

### RICE

**R**ICE, an acronym for **R**est, **I**ce, **C**ompression, and **E**levation, can be used effectively for almost all types of injuries from a sprained ankle to a broken bone. When an injury occurs, RICE should be followed for the first 24 hours.

**REST**—Immediate nonweight-bearing rest will prevent further damage. Rest includes use of splints, slings, and crutches.

**ICE—** Application of ice slows bleeding and swelling by causing vasoconstriction. The more blood that collects in an area, the longer the healing time. Ice should not be applied directly to the skin. Wrap the ice pack in a towel before application. Alternating ice treatment—30 minutes on and 15 minutes off—is a general rule. Heat is applied after 24 hours to improve vascular flow and carry away tissue debris.

**COMPRESSION**—Application of a compression stocking or ace wrap will provide support and limit swelling, thereby speeding healing time. Compression devices should be snug but not so tight as to cut off circulation, which could lead to increased pain and numbness.

**ELEVATION**—Place the injured area at a height above the heart to allow gravity to assist venous flow to further reduce swelling.

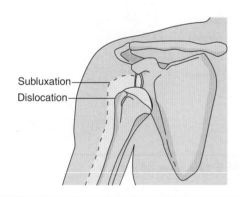

**FIGURE 6–15**　Dislocation and subluxation.

Individuals who suffer with recurrent dislocations and subluxations may be taught how to reduce the joint. If the joint ligaments become weakened with repeated dislocations, surgery may be necessary to tighten the ligaments, thus strengthening the joint.

## Low Back Pain (LBP)

**ETIOLOGY** The low back or lumbar area of the spine is very susceptible to stress or strain. This stress may be increased by such factors as obesity, poor posture, weak abdominal muscles, and constant or improper lifting. These factors are more likely to cause low back pain in individuals who have spinal deformities or diseases affecting the spine.

Some disorders that affect the spine and often lead to LBP include spinal deformities, osteoarthritis, rheumatoid arthritis, osteoporosis, and bone cancer to name just a few. X-ray examinations are usually helpful in determining the cause of LBP, but further detailed study with a CT scan or MRI may be needed.

**SYMPTOMS** Low back pain is a very common disorder of the musculoskeletal system. This pain may be acute and resolve in a few days, or it may be a chronic discomfort that lasts a lifetime.

**TREATMENT** Treatment of acute LBP is usually rest, warm moist heat, analgesics, and anti-inflammatory medications. Lumbar **spasms** (uncontrolled muscle contractions) are common and are very painful. These spasms often twist the back out of normal position. Muscle relaxants may be prescribed for acute attacks, but rest and application of heat are usually adequate to control spasms. Once the acute attack subsides, a daily exercise program including aerobic walking is very beneficial in building muscle tone and decreasing the risk of further attacks. One of the most common causes of LBP is a herniated intervertebral disk or herniated nucleus pulposus.

### ■ Herniated Nucleus Pulposus (HNP)

HNP is commonly called herniated disk or disc, ruptured disk, slipped disk, or bulging disk. All these different terms are very similar.

**ETIOLOGY** HNP is the protrusion of the soft center (nucleus pulposus) of a disk on the spinal cord or spinal nerve (Figure 6–16).

**SYMPTOMS** Pressure on the spinal nerve may cause pain in the sciatic nerve, called **sciatica**, which radiates down the back side of the leg.

Diagnosis involves physical examination, often confirmed by a CT scan, MRI, or **myelogram**. A myelogram involves injecting dye into the spinal canal and taking pictures to reveal compression on the spinal cord or spinal nerves.

**TREATMENT** Treatment of HNP is often the same as for LBP. Extensive exercise therapy may reduce the size of the protrusion and relieve the associated LBP. If pain persists after therapy, or if the disk is found to be causing severe spinal cord or spinal nerve compression, surgery for disk removal may be needed. Surgery to remove the disk or to cut away vertebra to open the area around the nerve is called a **diskectomy** or **laminectomy**, respectively.

## Bursitis

**ETIOLOGY** Bursitis (ber-SIE-tis) is the inflammation of a bursa or small fluid-filled sac near joints. Bursae help reduce friction during movement. Repetitive motions often lead to irritation of the bursa, resulting in bursitis. Any joint may be affected, but bursitis of the shoulder is the most common type. Bursitis that occurs in the elbow is commonly called tennis elbow.

**SYMPTOMS** Symptoms include severe pain that limits motion in the joint.

**TREATMENT** Rest, application of moist heat, and use of analgesics and anti-inflammatory medications will usually resolve the condition. If bursitis persists, further treatment of the bursa includes injection with corticosteroids, draining, and surgical excision. Active range-of-motion exercises are needed after pain subsides to regain and maintain joint motion.

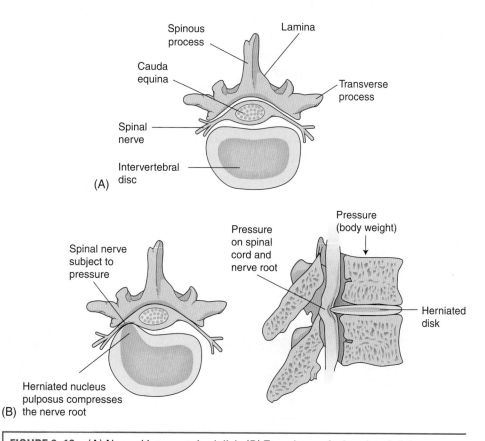

**FIGURE 6–16** (A) Normal intervertebral disk. (B) Two views of a herniated disk.

## ■ Tennis Elbow

**ETIOLOGY** Tennis elbow is a type of bursitis that affects the elbow area. This bursitis is not always caused by playing tennis, as its name suggests. Tennis elbow is a repetitive motion injury.

**SYMPTOMS** Diagnosis may be confirmed by eliciting increased pain when the middle finger is pushed backward or extended against resistance.

**TREATMENT** Treatment is the same as with bursitis. Application of a wide strap just below the elbow will change and support muscle movement in the forearm, thus reducing some of the pain.

## Tendonitis

**ETIOLOGY** Tendonitis is inflammation of a tendon or the connective tissue that attaches muscle to bone. Tendonitis may occur in any tendon, but most often, it affects the shoulder. It may be due to calcium deposits or to repetitive motion injury. Athletes in baseball, basketball, swimming, and tennis are often affected. Tendonitis also may occur in association with bursitis.

**TREATMENT** Treatment is rest, application of ice (that may irritate bursitis), and use of analgesics and anti-inflammatory medications. Active range-of-motion exercises may be initiated once the pain subsides to restore motion. If joint adhesions have developed, surgical intervention may be necessary to free the joint and restore mobility.

## Carpal Tunnel Syndrome

**ETIOLOGY** Carpal tunnel syndrome is a repetitive motion injury affecting the hands and commonly seen in individuals who complete computer data entry, work at manufacturing jobs, or do any task that requires continuous, repetitive finger and wrist motions.

The blood vessels, tendons, and nerves that feed or innervate the hands pass through a tunnel in the wrist area formed by the carpal tunnel ligament (Figure 6–17). The repetitive motion causes inflammation of the tendons, resulting in pressure on the medial nerve.

**SYMPTOMS** Symptoms of carpal tunnel syndrome often include numbness, pain, swelling, coolness, and discoloration in the affected hand and fingers. Diagnosis is confirmed by history, physical examination, and testing.

**TREATMENT** Treatment consists of stopping the repetitive motion, resting the hand, splinting, administration of anti-inflammatory medications, and physical therapy. Carpal tunnel syndrome not relieved by these measures may require surgery to split the carpal ligament, enlarging the tunnel and relieving pressure on the median nerve. Prevention of carpal tunnel syndrome is the best plan, and can be accomplished by ergonomic principles and job rotation to improve hand positions and provide adequate rest periods.

## Plantar Fasciitis

Plantar fasciitis (FAS-ee-**EYE**-tis) is also called calcaneal spur or heel spur. The plantar **fascia** is a thick, fibrous connective tissue that runs the length of the bottom or plantar surface of the foot. The plantar fascia attaches to the heel or **calcaneal** area of the foot, and helps develop the arch of the foot (Figure 6–18).

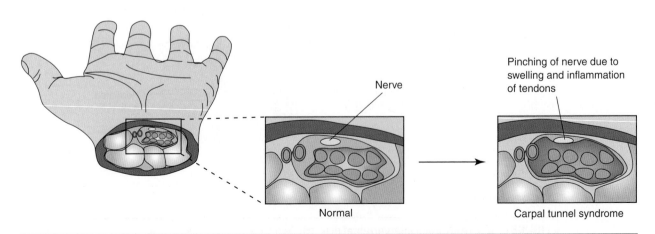

**FIGURE 6–17** Carpal tunnel syndrome.

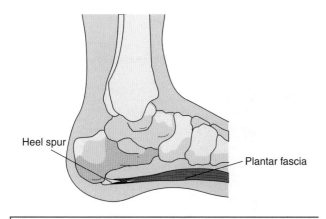

Heel spur

Plantar fascia

**FIGURE 6–18** Plantar fasciitis.

**ETIOLOGY** Plantar fasciitis is often seen in runners due to the repeated pressure placed on the fascia during running. This constant pressure causes inflammation and pain at the point of attachment to the calcaneus. It is not uncommon for individuals to have a small heel spur at this point of attachment, but it becomes more noticeable and more painful with this condition. Heel spurs do not cause the problem; they are the result of the problem.

**SYMPTOMS** The common symptom of plantar fasciitis is an intermittent pain in the heel that is worse when taking the first few steps after sitting or standing for some time, when getting out of bed, or at the beginning of an exercise routine. Plantar fasciitis develops more often in individuals who have a sudden increase in activity or weight. Other factors include individuals who are flat-footed, toe runners, overweight, have high arches, and who have poor shoe support.

**TREATMENT** Treatment includes rest, application of ice, use of analgesics and anti-inflammatory medication, and use of a heel pad that will relieve pressure on the heel. After pain subsides, exercises to strengthen the foot may help prevent reinjury. Surgery to remove the heel spur and release the plantar fascia has proven ineffective in most instances.

## Torn Rotator Cuff

The rotator cuff is comprised of a group of muscles that hold the head of the humerus in the shoulder socket area.

**ETIOLOGY** Tears are commonly traumatic injuries of baseball, basketball, and tennis.

**SYMPTOMS** Tears in the tendons that hold these muscles to the bone produce a snapping sound, followed by acute pain, and the inability of the individual to abduct (move away from midline) or raise the arm.

Diagnosis is made by physical examination and may be confirmed with a CT scan or arthroscopy.

**TREATMENT** Acute rotator cuff tears are surgically repaired to restore motion of the shoulder. Postoperatively, the individual is placed in a shoulder immobilizer for three to four weeks. Analgesics and anti-inflammatory medications may be administered for acute pain. Active rehabilitation exercise is needed postoperatively to restore shoulder function.

## Torn Meniscus

There are two semilunar cartilages in each knee joint, forming a lateral and medial meniscus. The meniscus (meh-NIS-cuss) is attached to the top of the tibia and provides cushion for the distal femur.

**ETIOLOGY** Athletes participating in football, baseball, soccer, and tennis commonly suffer with this injury. The tear usually results from a sudden twisting of the leg while the knee is flexed (Figure 6–19).

**SYMPTOMS** Symptoms include acute pain with weight bearing on the affected knee. The individual may feel that the knee is "locking" or "giving." Full flexion or extension of the knee may not be possible due to increased pain. X-ray or MRI may be needed to confirm the diagnosis.

**TREATMENT** Treatment is immobilization, elevation, and application of ice to decrease inflammation and pain. Analgesics and anti-inflammatory medications also may be needed. If surgical treatment is needed, it is commonly done arthroscopically or with the use of a scope to look into the knee. An extensive exercise rehabilitation program is begun postoperatively.

## Cruciate Ligament Tears

Cruciate (shaped like a cross) ligaments are located inside the knee joint. They work as a pair (the anterior cruciate ligament and the posterior cruciate ligament) and form a cross, giving the knee front to back and rotary stability.

**ETIOLOGY** These ligaments are often injured when the leg is twisted, or hit from the front or back while in a planted or weight-bearing position. Diagnosis involves clinical examination, joint stability testing, and possible CT scanning.

**TREATMENT** Treatment depends on the degree of injury, and may vary from immobilization to surgical intervention (Figure 6–19).

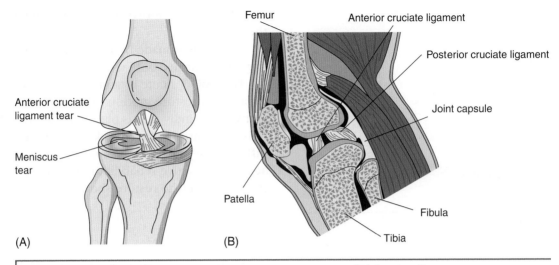

**FIGURE 6–19**   (A) Meniscus and anterior cruciate ligament tear. (B) Cruciate ligaments.

## Shin Splints

**ETIOLOGY** Shin splints is a term used to describe an overuse injury to the periosteum and extensor muscles of the lower leg. Shin splints occur routinely with a sudden increase in activity or a new exercise routine. This disorder commonly occurs in runners, joggers, and high-impact aerobics enthusiasts. Running on hard surfaces may also cause the problem. Diagnosis is usually based on clinical examination, but X-ray examination may be utilized to rule out a stress fracture.

**SYMPTOMS** Pain and tenderness along the inner aspect of the tibia, worsening with exercise and disappearing with rest, are common symptoms.

**TREATMENT** Rest, analgesics, anti-inflammatory medications, and alternating ice and heat treatments are usually beneficial. Proper conditioning, stretching exercises, and padded exercise shoes assist in preventing this disorder.

## RARE DISEASES

## de Quervain's Disease

de Quervain's disease is a repetitive use tendonitis affecting the thumb. Pain may radiate up the forearm several inches and down into the thumb. Pain is increased if the individual attempts to pull the thumb and little finger together while the fingers are point-ing upward. Physical examination and testing confirms the diagnosis.

## Tuberculosis of the Bone

The bacterium *Mycobacterium tuberculosis* primarily affects the lungs, but it may enter the bloodstream and travel to other organs of the body. Tuberculosis (TB) of the bone generally affects the arms and legs, and the knee is a common site for infection. Just as it does in the lungs, TB causes the development of cavities in the tissue, leading to bone weakness and pain. Antibiotic treatment is generally effective. A special form of TB in the vertebra or back of children is called Pott's disease.

## Paget's Disease

Paget's (PAJ-ets) disease, also known as osteitis deformans, is a chronic metabolic bone disease that affects bone formation. Normally, bone is broken down and replaced at a consistent rate. Paget's is characterized by an overgrowth of new bone that outpaces the breakdown of old bone. The new bone is thicker than the old, but much weaker, increasing the possibility of fracture. Radiologic examination reveals a mosaic bone pattern that is easily recognized as Paget's.

Paget's disease often affects the pelvis and long bones of the legs in individuals over age 40, and becomes more common with advancing age. Paget's may be asymptomatic, in which case no treatment is necessary or beneficial. When symptomatic, individuals may complain of bone pain that becomes worse at night. Bones may fracture easily or become deformed, leading to bowed legs and curvature of the spine. If the disease affects bones of the ear, hearing may become impaired. A secondary problem or complication of Paget's is the development of osteosarcoma or bone cancer. The cause of Paget's is idiopathic. Treatment is primarily symptomatic although a high-protein diet with calcium and vitamin D supplements may be beneficial.

## Myasthenia Gravis

Myasthenia gravis (MY-uh-**STHEE**-nee-uh GRAV-iss) is an autoimmune disorder characterized by muscle weakness and fatigue that is somewhat relieved with rest. The problem is related to blocking of the neurotransmitter acetylcholine by antibodies in the neuromuscular junction. For more details about myasthenia gravis, see Chapter 5.

## Systemic Lupus Erythematosus

Systemic lupus erythematosus is an autoimmune disorder that affects the connective tissue throughout the body. One of the main characteristics is a butterfly patterned rash across the nose and face. For more details, see Chapter 5.

## EFFECTS OF AGING ON THE SYSTEM

Normal changes that occur in bones, joints, and muscles cause a variety of problems in the older adult.

Bone density decreases with age as calcium is reabsorbed from the bone. This causes greater brittleness of the bone with increased risks for fractures. Osteoporosis is a common problem in the older adult, especially in older females because of its association with decreasing estrogen levels in the blood.

As the individual ages, muscles decrease in strength and mass. Some muscle cells atrophy and decrease in total number. Arm and leg muscles lose tone, and become somewhat flaccid and flabby in appearance.

Changes in height and curvature of the spine occur from changes in the vertebral disks and compression of the vertebrae. As muscles waste and joints stiffen, some loss of flexibility and agility is also common, along with an overall decreased mobility. Research has demonstrated the benefits of weight training and exercise classes for the older adult to prevent some of the muscle wasting, decreases in bone density, and loss of flexibility.

Musculoskeletal diseases, especially the debilitating ones such as arthritis, are extremely difficult for the older adult. Healing, such as after a fracture, is slower and often impaired by other chronic disorders common to the older adult. Pain associated with these disorders and changes in the system tend to decrease the individual's mobility and independence even more. Safety issues are of utmost importance when musculoskeletal system disorders are present because falls are one of the most common causes of injury in the older adult.

## SUMMARY

The musculoskeletal system consists of bones, joints, muscles, ligaments, and tendons. It is the body's main framework and is responsible for all movements. Movements are the result of contraction and relaxation of the muscle fibers. The muscles are stimulated by responses from the nervous system. Most muscle movements are voluntary movements. The most common symptoms of musculoskeletal system disorders are pain, immobility, and disability. Diagnosis of a musculoskeletal system problem is usually made by assessment and X-ray, or magnetic resonance imaging. However, other specific tests such as bone scans or endoscopy also may be utilized. Although fractures are a major group of musculoskeletal system disorders, many other diseases are common to the system. Some of these are short-term, but many are long-term, debilitating disorders. Individuals with musculoskeletal system diseases frequently need assistive devices such as crutches or walkers to maintain mobility. Changes in the musculoskeletal system in the older adult often leads to increased risk for fractures and disability.

## REVIEW QUESTIONS

### Short Answer

**1.** What are the major functions of the musculoskeletal system?

**2.** What are the common signs and symptoms associated with musculoskeletal system disorders?

**3.** What are the most common tests used to diagnose musculoskeletal system disorders?

### Fill in the Blank

Fill in the blanks in the following statements:

**4.** The musculoskeletal system is composed of _____, _____, _____, _____, and _____.

**5.** _____ attach muscle to bone.

**6.** _____ joints are ones that have full movement.

**7.** The most common disorder of the system is _____.

**8.** _____ _____ is the most serious form of arthritis but _____ is the most common type of arthritis.

### Matching

**9.** Match the fracture-related term in the left column with the appropriate description in the right column.

| | |
|---|---|
| ____ comminuted | **a.** Bone fragments are in correct position |
| ____ nondisplaced | **b.** One bone end is forced over another |
| ____ transverse | **c.** More than two ends or fragments are present |
| ____ greenstick | **d.** Bone has protruded through the skin |
| ____ stress | **e.** An incomplete fracture common in children |
| ____ impacted | **f.** Fracture runs across or at a 90-degree angle |
| ____ compound | **g.** Caused by too much weight-bearing or pressure |

## CASE STUDY

**Estella Gore** is a 77-year-old resident of a local nursing home. She fell four weeks ago and fractured her left hip. She is now in rehabilitation therapy, and is walking with the assistance of a physical therapy aide and a rolling walker. She states she is very frightened to walk and would rather use her wheelchair for mobility. What should you tell Ms. Gore about the importance of continuing to walk, even if she needs the assistance of a walker or other personnel? Why is it important for her to be as mobile as possible? What are the overall effects of immobility? How does immobility affect other body systems?

# BIBLIOGRAPHY

Barton, E., & Morris, C. (2003). Mechanisms and strategies to counter muscle atrophy. *Journals of Gerontology Series A: Biological Sciences & Medical Sciences 58*(10), 923-927.

Cisternas, M., Yelin, E., Murphy, L., & Helmick, C. G. (2003, November 21). Direct and indirect costs of arthritis and other rheumatic conditions—United States, 1997. *MMWR: Morbidity & Mortality Weekly Report, 52*(46) 1124-1128.

Conaghan, P. G., Marzo-Ortega, H., & Emery, P. (2003). Gout: An update. *Rheumatology 22*(4), 87-90.

Farley, R., Clark, J., Davidson, C., Evans, G., MacLennan, K., Michael, S., Morrow, M., & Thorpe, S. (2003). What is the evidence for the effectiveness of postural management? *International Journal of Therapy & Rehabilitation 10*(10), 449-456.

Holick, M. F. (2003). Vitamin D deficiency: What a pain it is. *Mayo Clinic Proceedings, 78*(12), 1457-1460.

McConville, A. (2003). Building a future of healthy bones. *Orthopaedic Nursing 22*(5), 321.

Mosher, T. J. (2003). Imaging in diagnosis of musculoskeletal diseases. *Current Opinion in Orthopaedics 14*(5), 334-341.

Osteoarthrosis. (2003). *Rheumatology 22*(4), 97-99.

Rheumatic disease. (2003). *Postgraduate Medicine 114*(5), 9.

Ruzek, K. A., & Wenger, D. E. (2004). The multiple faces of lymphoma of the musculoskeletal system. *Skeletal Radiology 33*(1), 1-8.

Schofield, C. (2004). What is osteonecrosis? *Nursing 34*(1), 29.

Surgical obesity treatment reduces risk of musculoskeletal pain. (2003, October 29). *Biotech Week*, 409.

Wongworawat, M. D., Schnall, P. D., Moon, C., & Schiller, F. (2003). Negative pressure dressings as an alternative technique for the treatment of infected wounds. *Clinical Orthopaedics & Related Research 2003*(414), 45-49.

Yang, Q., Populo, S. M., Zhang, J., Yang, G. And Kodama, H. (2002). Effect of Angelica Sinensis on the proliferation of human bone cells. *International Journal of Clinical Chemistry 324*(1-2), 89-97.

Ziran, B. H. (2003). A dedicated team approach enhances outcomes of osteomyelitis treatment. *Clinical Orthopaedics & Related Research 2003*(414), 31-37.

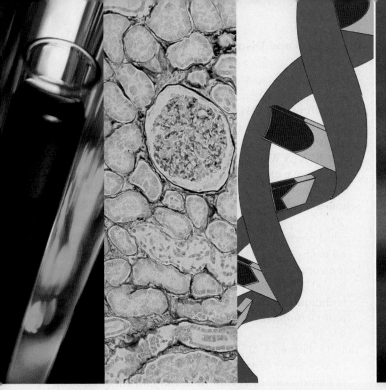
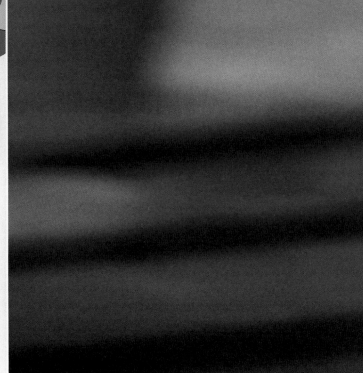

## OUTLINE

## KEY TERMS

# Blood and Blood-Forming Organs Diseases and Disorders

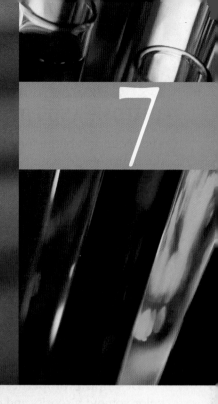

7

## LEARNING OBJECTIVES

*Upon completion of the chapter, the learner should be able to:*

1. Define the terminology common to the blood and blood-forming organs, and the disorders of the blood and blood-forming organs.

2. Discuss the basic anatomy and physiology of the blood and blood-forming organs.

3. Identify the important signs and symptoms associated with common blood and blood-forming organ disorders.

4. Describe the common diagnostics used to determine the type and/or cause of blood and blood-forming organ disorders.

5. Identify the common disorders of the blood and blood-forming organs.

6. Describe the typical course and management of the common blood and blood-forming organ disorders.

7. Describe the effects of aging on the blood and blood-forming organs and the common disorders of the system.

## OVERVIEW

*The blood and the blood-forming organs make up the individual's hematologic system. The blood is the body's life fluid. It is responsible for transporting nutrients to cells and removing wastes. The blood-forming organs are the lymph nodes, bone marrow, spleen, and liver. Disorders of the system may have severe effects on other systems because of the responsibilities of the blood and blood-forming organs. Altered nutrition, medications, and diseases of other systems, in turn, can greatly affect the functioning of the hematologic system.* ■

## ANATOMY AND PHYSIOLOGY

The blood and blood-forming organs are also called the hematologic system. The major function of the blood is to transport necessary nutrients to the cells and to aid in the removal of wastes. The blood also transports hormones secreted by the endocrine system. In addition, the white blood cells (leukocytes) are important in infection prevention. The blood is composed of a variety of substances. The plasma portion of the blood is a straw-colored liquid and makes up about 55 percent of the total. The formed elements constitute the other 45 percent of the total. They include the erythrocytes (red blood cells or RBCs), leukocytes (white blood cells or WBCs), and platelets (clotting fragments) (Figure 7–1).

Descriptive properties of the blood include its color, volume, viscosity, and pH. Blood is bright red in the arteries due to its oxygen content. Blood in the veins is a dark red (often depicted as blue) due to the absence of oxygen. The average adult has about 75 ml/kg of body weight of circulating blood (five to six liters or approximately one and a half gallons). The viscosity or density of blood is about three or more times greater than water. Blood is slightly alkaline (pH 7.35–7.45).

The erythrocytes transport oxygen from the lungs to the tissues. The normal erythrocyte count is 4.2 to 6.3 million. Their life span is only about 120 days. Erythrocytes actually formed in the bone marrow do not reproduce. Erythrocyte production increases when oxygen needs increase. During their life span, the red cells become worn and often ragged from bumping and bouncing into the vessel walls of the circulatory system. The worn RBCs are filtered out of circulation by the spleen and liver. These organs are responsible for breaking down the RBCs and saving the iron component for reuse in the development of new RBCs.

Hemoglobin, a component of the red blood cell, is important in the transport of oxygen. A low level of hemoglobin in the blood reduces the level of circulating oxygen. The normal level of hemoglobin for an adult male is 13.5–18g/100 ml and 12–16g/100 ml for an adult female.

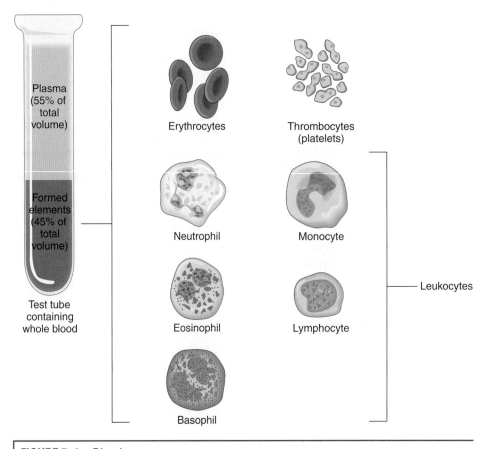

Plasma
(55% of
total
volume)

Formed
elements
(45% of
total
volume)

Test tube
containing
whole blood

Erythrocytes

Neutrophil

Eosinophil

Basophil

Thrombocytes
(platelets)

Monocyte

Lymphocyte

Leukocytes

**FIGURE 7–1** Blood components.

Leukocytes are concerned with protecting the individual from infections. The average white blood cell count for an adult is 4,500–11,000/cu mm. A count higher than 11,000 usually indicates the presence of an infection. See Chapters 4 and 5 for more information about leukocytes.

Platelets (also called thrombocytes) produce the thrombokinase used in the clotting process. The average number of platelets in adults is 150,000–350,000/mm$^3$ of blood.

The plasma portion of blood is composed of 91 percent water and 9 percent plasma proteins. The plasma proteins include (1) albumin, responsible for maintaining osmotic pressure; (2) globulin, responsible for infection fighting; (3) fibrinogen, responsible for a part of the clotting process; and (4) prothrombin, also responsible for a part of the clotting process.

Blood coagulation (clotting) occurs in phases. In the first phase, the platelets, in association with several plasma proteins, agglutinate (clump) at the site of injury or blood loss, and thromboplastin is formed. In the second phase, prothrombin is converted to thrombin in the presence of calcium. In the third phase, thrombin and fibrinogen form fibrin. With the presence of calcium, a fibrin clot is formed. In the fourth phase, the clot is removed through the process of fibrinolysis.

Blood is classified by the antigens in the red blood cells and the antibodies in the plasma. The antigens are A and B and the antibodies are anti-A and anti-B. In addition, a factor called Rh is also used in the classification system (see Chapter 5 under erythroblastosis fetalis and blood transfusion reaction for more information). Blood is typed as A, B, AB, and O. Type A blood has A antigens and anti-B antibodies, type B blood has B antigens and anti-A anti-bodies, type AB blood has A and B antigens and does not have anti-A or anti-B antibodies, and type O blood has neither A nor B antigens but has both anti-A and anti-B antibodies. The Rh designation is based on 12 different antigens. Rh positive blood has this antigen present while Rh negative does not. Because of these designations and blood properties, blood transfusion recipients must have a type and crossmatch of blood to be certain a reaction will not occur (Table 7–1).

The blood-forming organs include the lymph nodes, bone marrow, spleen, and liver. The lymph nodes are found throughout the body along the lymphatic vessels. The lymph system is important for protection from pathogens. The nodes filter the lymph, and produce lymphocytes and antibodies.

The bone marrow is found in the center part of long bones and in the spongy part of other bones. The bone marrow is the major blood cell producing organ in the body.

The spleen is found in the upper left quadrant of the abdomen. It produces lymphocytes, plasma cells, and antibodies, and filters microorganisms from the blood. It also removes old blood cells from the body.

The liver is a large organ found in the right upper quadrant of the abdomen. It has multiple responsibilities for many body systems. The liver functions as a blood-forming organ in intrauterine life, and is active the rest of the individual's life as a producer of prothrombin and fibrinogen for blood clotting.

## COMMON SIGNS AND SYMPTOMS

Signs and symptoms of this system include those related to increases and decreases in the number of

**TABLE 7–1** Blood Donor and Recipient Chart

| | | Recipients | | | |
|---|---|---|---|---|---|
| | **Blood Types** | **O** | **A** | **B** | **AB** |
| **Donors** | O | YES | YES | YES | YES |
| | A | NO | YES | NO | YES |
| | B | NO | NO | YES | YES |
| | AB | NO | NO | NO | YES |

YES = This type (row) can donate blood and this type (column) can receive the blood.
NO = This type (row) cannot donate blood and this type (column) cannot receive the blood without a transfusion reaction.

blood cells. Diseases affecting the blood-forming organs (primarily spleen, bone marrow, and lymph nodes) may lead to decreased or increased production of cells. Diseases that hemolyze, destroy, or use up the cells will also lead to a decrease in cell number and volume.

**Erythrocytopenia** (erythro = red, cyte = cell, penia = decrease) leads to **anemia** (an = without, emia = blood). Anemia does not mean without any blood; it means low or decreased blood volume. Signs and symptoms of anemia may be minor to major or asymptomatic to life threatening, depending on cause. Common signs and symptoms include a low erythrocyte count, headache, fatigue, pallor, and shortness of breath.

**Erythrocytosis** (erythrocyte = red cell, osis = condition) is a condition of increased red blood cells. Common signs and symptoms include a high red blood cell count, reddened skin tones, bloodshot eyes, increased blood volume and pressure, and an increase in the workload of the heart.

**Leukocytopenia** (leuko = white, cyte = cell, penia = decrease) is a decrease in white cell count. Leukocytopenia weakens the immune system because these cells are primary players in the defense system. **Neutropenia** (neutrophil decrease) and **lymphopenia** (lymphocyte decrease) may be associated with chronic infection as the numbers are "used up" during a long-term battle. Signs and symptoms are related to the particular type of infection.

**Leukocytosis** (leukocyto = white cell, osis = condition of) is an increase in white cell count. This condition is a normal response to acute infection. If leukocytosis is related to a tumor, these numbers may be extreme as in the case of leukemia (leuk = white, emia = blood).

**Thrombocytopenia** (THROM-boh-SIGH-toh-**PEE**-nee-ah; thrombocyte = platelet, penia = decrease) is a decrease in platelets leading to a coagulation problem. Signs and symptoms include small hemorrhages in the skin called **petechiae** (pee-TEE-kee-eye), large areas of bruising or hemorrhage called **ecchymoses** (ECH-ih-**MOH**-ses), and **epistaxis** (EP-ih-**STACK**-sis; nosebleeds). Bleeding lesions in the mouth, gums, and mucous membranes are also common.

**Thrombocytosis** (THROM-boh-sigh-**TOE**-sis; thrombocyte = platelet, osis = condition of) is an increase in platelets. This condition is uncommon and usually has no serious side effects (Table 7–2).

---

**TABLE 7–2**   Blood Cell Abnormalities and Associated Symptoms

**RED BLOOD CELLS**

INCREASED—Erythrocytosis: reddened skin, increased blood pressure, increased workload on the heart
DECREASED—Erythrocytopenia: anemia

**WHITE BLOOD CELLS**

INCREASED—Leukocytosis: usually asymptomatic
DECREASED—Leukocytopenia: weakened immune system

**THROMBOCYTES (PLATELETS)**

INCREASED—Thrombocytosis: increased clotting
DECREASED—Thrombocytopenia: increased bleeding

---

# DIAGNOSTIC TESTS

Diagnostic tests for blood and blood-forming organ disorders include complete blood count (CBC) with differential and indices. Biopsy of the blood-forming organs also may be helpful in diagnosing disorders of the spleen, lymph nodes, and bone marrow.

A **complete blood count** (CBC) identifies the number of red blood cells (RBCs), white blood cells (WBCs), and platelets per cubic millimeter (Table 7–3). A CBC may be utilized in the determination of most blood diseases. Red blood cell count and indices can assist in the determination of the different anemias, polycythemia, and erythrocytosis. A **differential** is a more detailed count identifying the number of each type of leukocyte. A white blood cell count and differential may assist in determination of inflammation and infection, or tumors of white cells. **Hematocrit** (Hct) reflects the amount of red cell mass as a proportion of whole blood. **Hemoglobin** (Hgb) reflects the amount of hemoglobin or oxygen-carrying potential available in the blood. Special measurements of red cells are called indices and include:

- MCV—mean corpuscular volume; reflects average size of the red cell

- MCH—mean corpuscular hemoglobin or average hemoglobin content

- MCHC—mean corpuscular hemoglobin concentration, or average hemoglobin concentration

The morphology of each of the cells and platelets may be observed by performing a blood smear. A blood smear is performed by placing a drop of blood on a glass slide, smearing it to spread the cells to a thin layer, and staining and examining it microscopically for abnormal cell morphology or shape. Adding a staining solution to the slide helps in the identification of granular and agranular WBCs. A blood smear may be helpful in determining the cause of anemia, especially sickle cell disease.

A **bleeding time** may assist in determining platelet disorders such as hemophilia, thrombocytopenia, and disseminated intravascular coagulation. A bleeding time test is performed by pricking the earlobe of the involved individual, and measuring the amount of time it takes for the area to clot or stop bleeding. Prothrombin time (PT) and partial thromboplastin time (PTT) are both blood tests that measure the ability of the blood to clot related to clotting factors.

Biopsy of blood-forming organs may be helpful in diagnosing diseases and disorders. A bone marrow biopsy is performed by boring a needle into the bone of the iliac crest of the hip to obtain tissue. This tissue is prepared and microscopically examined. Lymph node biopsy may be performed to determine proper functioning of the marrow, detect anemias, and diagnose neoplasms.

**TABLE 7–3** Complete Blood Count (CBC) Normal Values

| Cells | Values |
|---|---|
| Erythrocytes | **Males** 4.6–6.3 million/mm$^3$ |
| | **Females** 4.2–5.4 million/mm$^3$ |
| Hematocrit | **Males** 40–54% |
| | **Females** 38–47% |
| Hemoglobin | **Males** 13.5–18 g/dl |
| | **Females** 12–16 g/dl |
| Red Blood Cell Indices | |
| MCV | 80–96 μm$^3$ |
| MCH | 27–31 pg |
| MCHC | 32–36% |
| Leukocytes | 4500–11,000 million/mm$^3$ |
| Differential | |
| Myelocytes | 0/mm$^3$ |
| Band neutrophils | 1500–3000/mm$^3$ |
| Segmented neutrophils | 300–500/mm$^3$ |
| Lymphocytes | 50–250/mm$^3$ |
| Monocytes | 15–50/mm$^3$ |
| Eosinophils | 15–50/mm$^3$ |
| Basophils | 15–50/mm$^3$ |
| Platelets | 150,000–350,000/mm$^3$ |
| Reticulocytes | 25,000–75,000/mm$^3$ |

Key:
mm$^3$ = cubic millimeter
g/dl = grams per deciliter
pg = picograms

## COMMON DISEASES OF THE BLOOD AND BLOOD-FORMING ORGANS

The most common problem related to this system is anemia. Anemia is a decrease in red blood cell mass that may be caused by a number of different disease processes. Anemia is generally a sign of a disease, but is commonly used as a diagnosis until the cause is discovered. Anemia may be serious if the cause is not determined or cannot be corrected.

Disorders of white blood cells are usually secondary to other diseases rather than as a primary disease. Infections demand an increased need for WBCs as they are used up while fighting the invader. This may lead to leukocytopenia or a decrease in white blood cell number.

Any disorders of the blood-forming organs (spleen, bone marrow, and lymph nodes) may lead to secondary disorders of this system. Leukemias, lymphomas, and myelomas are the primary tumors affecting the system.

# Disorders of Red Blood Cells

Any increase or decrease in number or size of red blood cells will affect the mass or volume. Red cell mass is important because it directly affects the amount of hemoglobin available (oxygen-carrying potential). Commonly, the problem is not enough red cell mass leading to anemia. Too much red cell mass is called erythrocytosis. The most common type of erythrocytosis is a condition called polycythemia.

**Anemia.**    Any decrease in oxygen-carrying ability of the red blood cell is **anemia**.

**ETIOLOGY** This is commonly due to a low number of RBCs or a decrease in hemoglobin in RBCs. Acute hemorrhage or chronic bleeding may lead to a low number of circulating RBCs, and thus anemia.

Any disease of the liver, spleen, or bone marrow may also lead to anemia. If the cells are broken down (**hemolyzed**) too soon, this may lead to a decrease in cell number. If cells are not formed quickly enough to replace the worn cells, the number of circulating cells will be low. If cells are formed abnormally, their ability to carry oxygen may be impaired. In this case, the number of cells may be adequate, but oxygen-carrying ability is not adequate. Dietary deficiencies may lead to an inadequate supply of needed nutrients to make RBCs.

**SYMPTOMS** Despite the cause, the symptoms of anemia are fairly common. The individual suffering from anemia commonly is pale or has a condition of **pallor**. Facial paleness may be difficult to determine, but further examination of the mucous membranes of the mouth and conjunctiva of the eyes will reveal definite paleness. The nail beds also may be noticeably pale in color.

Anemic individuals are weak and suffer with fatigue due to poor oxygenation of muscle tissue. Shortness of breath, **dyspnea** (DISP-nee-ah; dys = difficult, pnea = breathing), **tachycardia** (TACH-ee-**KAR**-dee-ah; tachy = fast, cardia = heart), and **tachypnea** (TACK-ihp-**NEE**-ah; tachy = fast, pnea = breathing) are common as the heart and lungs attempt to meet the body's oxygen need. Headache, irritability, and **syncope** (SIN-koh-pee; fainting) also may be symptoms.

**TREATMENT** Determining the cause of anemia is very important because treatment is directed at the cause. Complete blood counts often will indicate low cell number, and low hemoglobin and hematocrit. Blood indices and chemistries also may be helpful.

Treatment for anemia varies, depending on cause or type of anemia. Some anemias may be cured with treatment whereas others, like sickle cell anemia, are not curable.

## ■ Iron Deficiency Anemia

**ETIOLOGY** Iron deficiency anemia may be due to a loss of iron or an inadequate intake of iron. Chronic blood loss may lead to loss of iron and, therefore this type of deficiency anemia. Chronic blood loss may be due to bleeding hemorrhoids, gastrointestinal bleeding, and heavy or prolonged menstrual flow. Low dietary intake of iron also may lead to this type of anemia. Iron deficiency anemia is commonly seen in females during times of increased iron demand. Increased iron is needed during pregnancy and with breast-feeding. During their menstrual years, females often have a combination of iron loss due to menstruation and inadequate dietary intake of iron.

**TREATMENT** Treatment is aimed at the cause and may include increasing dietary intake of iron.

## ■ Folic Acid Deficiency Anemia

Folic acid is a B complex vitamin that is needed for the maturation of red blood cells.

**ETIOLOGY** Deficiency of folic acid may be related to poor diet, overcooking vegetables, or as a consequence of alcoholism. The deficiency may occur during times of high folic acid need like those associated with infancy and pregnancy.

**TREATMENT** Treatment is aimed at increasing dietary intake of folic acid by eating green and yellow vegetables.

## ■ Pernicious Anemia

**ETIOLOGY** Pernicious anemia has an unusual cause. The mucosa or lining of the stomach secretes a protein called intrinsic factor. This factor is needed for vitamin $B_{12}$ to be absorbed in the small intestine. Vitamin $B_{12}$ is essential for red blood cell formation. Pernicious anemia is due to a lack of intrinsic factor leading to inadequate absorption of vitamin $B_{12}$, thus anemia. Increasing the dietary intake of vitamin $B_{12}$ will not alleviate the problem.

**TREATMENT** Treatment is a monthly injection of vitamin $B_{12}$ for the life of the individual. Pernicious anemia usually affects older individuals and is thought to be related to an autoimmune disorder.

## ■ Hemolytic Anemia

**ETIOLOGY** Hemolytic anemia is characterized by increased destruction of red blood cells. It may be related to an antigen-antibody reaction as with Rh factor in blood transfusion reaction or erythroblastosis fetalis (see Chapter 5 for detailed information). Hemolytic anemia also may occur due to a disorder of the immune system leading to destruction of one's own erythrocytes. This type of anemia may be severe and lead to the death of the individual. Hemolytic anemia may be brought on by exposure to chemicals such as Benzene, medications including aspirin and penicillin, and bacterial toxins.

**TREATMENT** Treatment may include prompt exchange transfusion (removal of the individual's blood and replacement by donor blood). A splenectomy also may be of some benefit.

## ■ Sickle Cell Anemia

**ETIOLOGY** Sickle cell anemia is a hereditary anemia found in the black race that causes an abnormal sickle shape of the erythrocyte. The sickle cell has abnormal hemoglobin that causes it to elongate or sickle when deoxygenated or as it loses the oxygen load. The cell regains its normal shape once it is reoxygenated or picks up an oxygen load (Figure 7–2). The sickle shape causes a problem because it does not allow the cell to travel smoothly through small blood vessels. Sickle cells tend to stick and clump together in small vessels, leading to occlusion of the vessel, ischemia, and infarction. This occlusion may occur

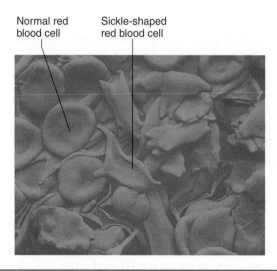

Normal red blood cell    Sickle-shaped red blood cell

**FIGURE 7–2** Sickled erythrocytes. (*Courtesy of Philips Electronic Instrument Company.*)

in any vessel, causing multiple thrombi (clots) and emboli (traveling clots) formations that may lead to infarctions throughout the body, including the vital organs.

**SYMPTOMS** Symptoms of the disease may vary from mild to severe. Individuals suffering severe symptoms often die in infancy or childhood. Few severely affected individuals live beyond age 20. Even mildly affected individuals usually die before age 50. Interestingly, sickle cell disease is thought to have developed as a defense mechanism against malaria. The parasite that causes malaria does not grow in cells that sickle, giving these individuals a health advantage in countries where malaria is prevalent.

**TREATMENT** There is no cure for sickle cell disease. Treatment is symptomatic. An increase in fluid intake to two times the normal amount may be beneficial. Additional fluids increase blood volume and improve sickle cell movement.

## ■ Hemorrhagic Anemia

**ETIOLOGY** Acute loss of large amounts of blood leads to hemorrhagic anemia. This may lead to **hypovolemia** or low blood volume. Severe hypovolemia may lead to life-threatening shock (low blood pressure). If the loss is not severe, blood fluid will be replaced within a few hours, decreasing the risk of shock. The decreased number of circulating erythrocytes will stimulate the bone marrow to step up production of erythrocytes. Bone marrow has the potential of replacing large numbers of blood cells, thus correcting this type of anemia.

**TREATMENT** If the individual is symptomatic, blood transfusions may be the treatment of choice.

## ■ Aplastic Anemia

**ETIOLOGY** Aplastic anemia is characterized by failure of the bone marrow to produce blood components. A severe decrease or total absence of erythrocytes, leukocytes, and thrombocytes, called **pancytopenia** (pan = all, cyto = cell, penia = decrease), is commonly seen. This anemia is due to injury or destruction of the blood-forming area of the bone marrow. Causes include chemotherapy, radiation, viruses, and chemical toxins.

**SYMPTOMS** This decrease in blood cells leads to anemia, infection, and hemorrhage respectively.

**TREATMENT** Severe cases of aplastic anemia have a poor prognosis with 50 percent fatality. Treatment includes discontinuing or avoiding the causative agent. Other treatment may include bone marrow transplantation and blood transfusions.

**Polycythemia.**   Polycythemia is also called primary polycythemia or polycythemia vera. It is a condition of too many blood cells.

**ETIOLOGY** Primary polycythemia is caused by hyperplasia (hyper = excessive, plasia = growth) of the cell-forming tissues of the bone marrow, leading to an increase in the production of erythocytes, leukocytes, and thrombocytes. This disease has an unknown etiology.

**SYMPTOMS** The increase in erythrocytes leads to an increase in blood volume. Increased blood volume raises blood pressure and causes an increase in the workload of the heart. The spleen, an organ of blood cell storage, is enlarged. The mucous membranes are reddened in color and the eyes often appear bloodshot. The palms of the hands are noticeably a deeper red color.

**TREATMENT** Treatment is to reduce the red cell count and thus blood volume. Phlebotomy or donating blood at regular intervals will reduce the volume, and is a common treatment.

Another type of polycythemia is called secondary polycythemia or erythrocytosis (erythocyte = red cell, osis = condition of).

**ETIOLOGY** Secondary polycythemia differs from primary polycythemia in that only red cell numbers are increased. Erythrocytosis is a protective mechanism of the body to meet the need for extra oxygen. This is a normal compensatory mechanism for people in high altitudes where oxygen content of air is low. Also, highly trained athletes may have erythrocytosis to meet the high oxygen demands of the body's muscle tissue. Certain respiratory and circulatory conditions cause a decrease in oxygen supply to the tissues and thus stimulate erythrocytosis. When the condition for extra oxygen is returned to normal, the erythrocytosis disappears. For example, if people living in high altitudes move to a lower altitude, the red cell count will return to a normal level.

## Disorders of White Blood Cells

Disorders of white blood cells are common problems of the hematologic system, especially among certain age groups. For example, mononucleosis is common in teenage populations. The common symptom of white blood cell disorders is a compromised immune response, leaving the individual susceptible to infections.

**Mononucleosis.**   **ETIOLOGY** Mononucleosis is a viral infection that primarily affects children and young adults. It is somewhat contagious and is commonly called "kissing disease."

**SYMPTOMS** Symptoms include fatigue, sore throat, and swollen lymph glands. Diagnosis is confirmed by a white blood cell count showing a marked elevation in monocytes.

**TREATMENT** Treatment is symptomatic, and includes rest, analgesics, and throat gargles.

**Leukemia.**   **ETIOLOGY** Leukemia is a malignant neoplasm of the blood-forming organs (bone marrow, lymph nodes, and spleen). It is characterized by an abnormally high production of leukocytes that are immature and function abnormally. This increase of white cells in the blood-forming organs causes a decrease in the production of erythrocytes and platelets.

Leukemia may be classified as acute or chronic. Acute forms commonly affect children, progress rapidly, and may be fatal. Chronic forms occur more commonly in older adults, are often asymptomatic, and may not be the cause of death. Leukemia is also classified as myelogenous (affecting the bone marrow) and lymphocytic (affecting the lymph nodes). The cause of leukemia is unknown. It is usually diagnosed by clinical history and blood studies. A bone marrow biopsy is the most definitive test for confirming the diagnosis.

**SYMPTOMS** Symptoms of leukemia include fatigue, headache, sore throat, dyspnea, bleeding of the mucous membranes of the mouth and gastrointestinal system, bone and joint pain, and enlargement of lymph nodes, liver, and spleen. Infections are common because white cells are not functioning properly. Bleeding disorders and anemia are due to erythrocytopenia and thrombocytopenia, respectively.

**TREATMENT** Treatment includes aggressive chemotherapy utilizing several neoplastic agents. Once in remission, a bone marrow transplant to replace the neoplastic tissue with normal tissue may be performed. Pain from enlargement of lymph nodes, spleen, and liver may be treated with analgesics. Complete remission occurs approximately 50 percent of the time, depending on the type of leukemia and the individual's tolerance of the treatment.

## Lymphoma.

Lymphoma refers to several types of neoplasms that affect lymphoid tissue (lymph nodes, tonsils, spleen, and lymph fluid). There are many types of lymphoma, but all affect normal lymphocyte production, leading to an impaired immunity.

### ■ Hodgkin's Disease

Hodgkin's disease is the most common lymphoma.

**ETIOLOGY** The cause is thought to be viral in nature.

**SYMPTOMS** It is characterized by painless enlargement of the lymph nodes in the neck, weight loss, and fever. Hodgkin's primarily affects young adults with an average age of 35 years. Men are affected with Hodgkin's at a slightly higher rate than women. Diagnosis is made when a large connective tissue cell called **Reed-Sternberg cell** is present in lymphatic tissue. The diagnosis may be confirmed by lymph node and bone marrow biopsy.

**TREATMENT** Treatment with radiation and chemotherapy is usually effective in bringing about remission. If the disease is kept in remission for five years or longer, complete cure may be possible. Mortality rate is approximately 20 percent.

### ■ Non-Hodgkin's Lymphoma (NHL)

Non-Hodgkin's lymphoma (NHL) is a group of lymphomas not containing the Reed-Sternberg cell characteristic of Hodgkin's. NHL is more widespread than Hodgkin's.

**SYMPTOMS** Usually, there is painless enlargement of lymph nodes in the neck, axilla, and inguinal areas. Other symptoms include fever, night sweats, and weight loss. NHL affects more older adults than Hodgkin's disease with the average age of 50 years. Men are affected one and a half times more often than women. The cause of NHL is unknown, but individuals receiving, or who have received, immunosuppressive medications, have more than a 100 times greater chance of developing NHL.

**TREATMENT** Treatment and prognosis depends on the type of NHL, but some combination of radiation and chemotherapy is usually of benefit.

## Multiple Myeloma.

**ETIOLOGY** Multiple myeloma is a malignant neoplasm of plasma cells or B-lymphocytes. The plasma cells multiply abnormally in the bone marrow, causing weakness in the bone leading to pathologic fractures and bone pain (Figure 7-3). Multiple myeloma occurs increasingly with age, peaking in the 70s, and is more common in men. It is one of the most common neoplasms affecting the bone.

**SYMPTOMS** Overgrowth of plasma cells leads to a decrease in other blood components causing anemia, leukocytopenia, and thrombocytopenia. The breakdown of bone leads to hypercalcemia (hyper = excessive, calc = calcium, emia = blood) or excessive blood calcium levels. Antibodies secreted by the plasma cells attach to kidney tubules, causing tissue damage leading to kidney failure.

Diagnosis is confirmed by:

■ X-ray exhibiting a honeycombed bone pattern due to tumor involvement

■ Hypercalcemia due to the tumor breaking down bone

---

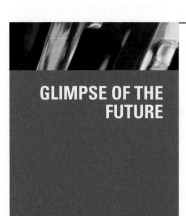

**GLIMPSE OF THE FUTURE**

### Treating Cancer by Stopping Blood Vessel Development

Blood vessel development, angiogenesis, is one way cancer growths metastasize. If tumors cannot get oxygen and nutrients that are provided by new blood vessels, they cannot continue to grow. Antiangiogenesis is the process of stopping the new growth of blood vessels, thus cutting off the lifeblood of a tumor. Researchers are studying antiangiogenic therapies using a variety of compounds that inhibit blood vessel growth. This process may be used in the future to reduce tumor growth if it proves successful in the clinical trials (see Complementary and Alternative Therapy, page 120).

*Source: Camp-Sorrell, D. (2003).*

## COMPLEMENTARY AND ALTERNATIVE THERAPY

### Honoliol from Magnolia Trees—An Antitumor Compound

Scientists are studying the effects of honoliol, a compound extracted from the southern magnolia tree, for use in cancer treatment. This active component of the magnolia cones inhibited the growth of new blood vessels in laboratory situations. It also cut growth of tumors by 50 percent. The antiangiogenesis property of honoliol may be beneficial in cancer treatment in the future. Honoliol has historically been used in tea products in Japan. It is reported to have calming effects on the person who drinks the tea.

*Source: Biotech Week ( July 6, 2003).*

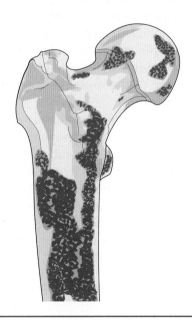

**FIGURE 7–3** Multiple myeloma—extensive bone destruction caused by disease.

- Evidence of **Bence Jones protein** (a special protein), found in the blood and urine
- A bone marrow biopsy confirming the presence of an excessive number of plasma cells

**TREATMENT** Prognosis is poor for multiple myeloma. Chemotherapy and radiation are not very effective, and death is usually within two to three years as the result of infection and kidney failure.

## Disorders of Platelets

Platelet disorders are varied in terms of cause, severity, treatment, and prognosis. However, they all share the common symptom of bleeding. The bleeding may be mild or severe, depending on the particular condition. Many disorders of platelets are inherited diseases.

**Hemophilia.** **ETIOLOGY** Hemophilia (hemo = blood, philia = lover) is an X-linked hereditary bleeding disorder. The characteristic inability to clot blood makes hemophiliacs "love blood" or realistically, need transfusions. There are several types of hemophilia but the most common is Type A. Hemophilia commonly occurs in male children and is passed on to these children—often by their mother—who is usually asymptomatic and unaffected. Hemophiliacs lack a blood protein that plays a part in clot formation.

**SYMPTOMS** Symptoms of frequent epistaxis (nosebleeds), bruising, and prolonged bleeding in a male child may be indicative of hemophilia. Diagnosis is confirmed by blood testing and clinical history of the involved individual.

This condition may vary from mild to severe. A hemophiliac may experience severe and prolonged bleeding with a minor injury. Severe hemophilia often leads to **hemarthrosis** (hem = blood, arthro = joint, osis = condition) or bleeding into joints. This is extremely painful. Recurrent episodes often lead to joint deformity.

**TREATMENT** There is no cure for hemophilia. Treatment is aimed at prevention of injury and treatment of symptoms. Whole blood transfusions may be needed along with a concentrated form of the needed clotting protein.

**Thrombocytopenia.** **ETIOLOGY** Thrombocytopenia, also known as thrombocytopenia purpura, is a decrease in platelets that leads to an inability to normally clot blood. Thrombocytopenia may be due to inadequate or abnormal platelet production or destruction. In the case of abnormal destruction, platelet life may be reduced to hours instead of days. The cause of this disorder is frequently unknown. In these cases, the condition may be called idiopathic thrombocytopenia purpura.

**SYMPTOMS** This condition is characterized by abnormal bleeding in the skin, mucous membranes, and internal organs. The skin may exhibit small hemorrhagic spots called petechiae or larger purplish hemorrhagic spots called ecchymoses. This purple coloring of the skin leads to another descriptive term, **purpura** (PUR-pew-rah; purplish color of the skin caused by hemorrhaging). Symptoms of thrombocytopenia include gastrointestinal hemorrhages, frequent epistaxis (nosebleeds), and **hematuria** (HEM-ah-**TOO**-ree-ah; hema = blood, uria = urine, blood in the urine).

Diagnosis is made utilizing individual clinical history along with platelet count and bleeding time.

**TREATMENT** Treatment includes avoiding tissue trauma to reduce the potential for bleeding, administration of vitamin K to improve clotting, and transfusion of platelets. If the disorder persists, a splenectomy may alleviate symptoms since the spleen is the main site of platelet destruction. Splenectomy is usually the last treatment of choice but is very effective.

### Disseminated Intravascular Coagulation (DIC).

**ETIOLOGY** Disseminated intravascular coagulation is a condition of abnormal clotting, followed by abnormal bleeding. It usually follows some major trauma such as complicated childbirth, major surgery, trauma involving major tissue destruction, septicemia, snakebite, and shock.

**SYMPTOMS** Multiple microscopic clots form mostly in the capillaries, causing infarctions throughout the body with resulting consequences. Clotting factors are used up during the formation of all the microthrombi. Reduced clotting factor leads to the inability to clot blood, resulting in multiple hemorrhages. The individual with DIC often oozes blood-forming petechiae, ecchymosis, hematoma, and hematuria. Other symptoms include gastrointestinal bleeding that causes **hematemesis** (HEM-ah-**TEM**-eh-sis; hema = blood, emesis = vomiting), blood in the stool, and symptoms associated with anemia.

Diagnosis is made on the basis of history of traumatic injury and blood studies.

**TREATMENT** Treatment includes heparin, an anticoagulant medication, to halt the formation of thrombi, and platelet administration to stop hemorrhage or increase clotting ability. This disorder is very difficult to manage as one administers agents to clot and thin blood at alternating intervals. The condition is usually life threatening and leads to death.

## TRAUMA

Any traumatic injury to the bone marrow, spleen, or lymph nodes may lead to a decrease in the production of blood cells. Enlargement of the spleen or splenomegaly may lead to premature breakdown of blood cells. Chemotherapy and radiation treatments affecting bone marrow often lead to symptoms of anemia and infection related to decreased production of red cells and white cells, respectively.

## RARE DISEASES

### Thalassemia

Thalassemia is a hereditary hemolytic anemia that primarily affects people of Mediterranean descent. The red blood cells are fragile and thin, and form defective hemoglobin. These RBCs do not function normally and lead to symptoms of anemia. One form of thalassemia is called Cooley's anemia or Thalassemia major. This is the most severe form of the disease and presents in childhood.

### Von Willebrand's Disease

Von Willebrand's disease is a hereditary congenital bleeding disorder caused by a deficiency in clotting factor and platelet function. This disorder is also called angiohemophilia. It affects females as well as males.

### Lymphosarcoma

Lymphosarcoma is a type of lymphoma also known as non-Hodgkin's lymphoma. Symptoms are similar to those found in Hodgkin's disease. Lymphosarcoma occurs more frequently in males of all age groups.

Prognosis is good if treatment leads to remission. Without remission, the prognosis is poor.

# EFFECTS OF AGING ON THE SYSTEM

Older adults may be more prone to developing diseases of the hematologic system because of the age-related changes occurring in other systems such as the immune or digestive system, leaving them more susceptible to infections and nutritionally related blood disorders. However, total serum iron, total iron-binding capacity, and intestinal iron absorption all decrease with age. Aging does not change the number of lymphocytes, but their functioning decreases to some degree over time.

The most common disorder of the blood in the older adult is anemia. This is not usually due to a defect in the system, but rather to poor nutrition (iron deficiency anemia) or inability to absorb the needed nutrients (pernicious anemia). The anemia problem often complicates other chronic diseases of the affected individual.

Some types of leukemia are more common in the older adult. Problems can arise during treatment for the condition due to decreased gastric motility and impaired circulation. These age-related changes can reduce the effectiveness of some therapies and increase the chance of experiencing side effects of the treatment.

## SUMMARY

The blood and blood-forming organs (hematologic system) form the body's life fluid by transporting oxygen and nutrients to cells, removing wastes, and helping to prevent infection. The main components of the system include the blood, lymph nodes, bone marrow, spleen, and liver. Common signs and symptoms of diseases of the blood and blood-forming organs are fatigue, shortness of breath, bleeding, lesions, pain, and increased susceptibility to infections. The most common disorder of the system is anemia. Although there are several types of anemia, they all have some common symptoms. White blood cell disorders include mononucleosis and leukemia as the most common. Disorders of platelets include the major bleeding diseases of the blood and blood-forming organs such as hemophilia. The older adult may develop problems of the hematologic system such as anemia, but it is usually due to other problems or disorders in other systems.

## REVIEW QUESTIONS

### Multiple Choice

1. Which of the following are major functions of blood? (Select all that apply.)

   a. transportation of nutrients

   b. metabolism of nutrients

   c. removal of wastes

   d. protection from infection

   e. production of lymphocytes

   f. production of erythrocytes

2. Which of the following are common signs and symptoms of disorders of the blood and blood-forming organs? (Select all that apply.)

   **a.** inflammation

   **b.** fatigue

   **c.** shortness of breath

   **d.** paralysis

   **e.** urinary frequency

   **f.** bleeding

   **g.** pain

   **h.** lesions

3. The individual with a bleeding disorder should avoid which of the following activities?

   **a.** shaving with a straight razor

   **b.** using mouthwash

   **c.** eating solid foods

   **d.** jogging

4. The purpose of the screening test for sickle cell anemia is to determine:

   **a.** if the individual is a carrier of the sickle cell trait.

   **b.** the presence of the sickled hemoglobin.

   **c.** the severity of the disease.

   **d.** if the individual will eventually develop sickle cell anemia.

5. Bone marrow biopsies are done to:

   **a.** determine the presence and number of platelets.

   **b.** diagnose cancers, anemias, and bone marrow functional disorders.

   **c.** diagnose vitamin $B_{12}$ deficiency.

   **d.** test for antigens to prevent antigen/antibody reactions.

6. Foods recommended for the individual with a folic acid deficiency would include:

   **a.** milk and cheeses.

   **b.** beef and chicken.

   **c.** green and yellow vegetables.

   **d.** breads and grains.

7. In which of the following ways does primary polycythemia differ from secondary polycythemia (erythrocytosis)?

   **a.** The most common symptom of the primary type is shortness of breath, and fatigue is the most common symptom of the secondary type.

   **b.** The primary type disease responds to phlebotomy while the secondary type does not.

   **c.** The primary form of the disease is considered to be a type of cancer but the secondary form is not.

   **d.** Both red and white cell numbers are increased in the primary type, but just red cell numbers are increased in the secondary type.

8. Which of the following statements is true about hemophilia?

   **a.** It is most common in the older adult.

   **b.** It results in continuous minor bleeding internally.

   **c.** It is caused by a deficiency of clotting factor.

   **d.** It is found in male children of mothers who carry the defective gene.

9. Which of the following statements is true about leukemia?

   **a.** It is considered to be a group of disorders with a cancerous development occurring in the bone marrow.

   **b.** It is the most common cause of death in young children.

   **c.** Chemotherapy is ineffective against leukemia.

   **d.** There are several types of leukemias, but most types are diagnosed in the young or middle-aged adult.

## Short Answer

10. List some of the common tests used to diagnose disorders of the blood and blood-forming organs.

11. List some diseases of the blood or blood-forming organs that are transmitted through an inherited trait.

12. Describe the common effects of a hemorrhagic disorder on an individual.

13. Why would an individual with Hodgkin's disease be instructed to avoid individuals with coughs, colds, and fever?

14. What diagnostic test would probably be used to diagnose leukemia?

15. Why are older adults more susceptible to infections if there is a hematologic disorder present?

## CASE STUDY

**Ms. Sloan** is a 27-year-old who is complaining of fatigue, shortness of breath, stomach pain, and overall weakness. She is diagnosed with iron deficiency anemia. What could you tell her about this condition? What specific nutritional needs does she have based on her diagnosis, gender, and age?

# BIBLIOGRAPHY

Angerio, A. D., Allan, D., & Lee, N. D. (2003). Sickle cell crisis and endothelin antagonists. *Critical Care Nursing Quarterly 26*(3), 225–229.

Apostolopoulou, E., Katsaris, G., & Katostaras, T. (2003). Risk factors for nosocomial bloodstream infections. *British Journal of Nursing 12*(12), 718–725.

Baldwin, P. D. (2003). Thrombocytopenia. *Clinical Journal of Oncology Nursing 7*(3), 349–352.

Barker, D. (2002). Standing and moving. *Nursing Older People 14*(6), 39.

Braun, L., Cooper, L. M. Malatestinic, W. N., & Huggins, R. M. (2003). A sepsis review. *Dimensions of Critical Care Nursing 22*(3), 117–124.

Camp-Sorrell, D. (2003). Angiogenesis: The fifth cancer treatment modality? *Oncology Nursing Forum 30*(6): 934–944.

Derivan, M., Ferrante, C., Hawkins, R., & Camp-Sorrell, D. (2001). Aplastic anemia. *Clinical Journal of Oncology Nursing 5*(5), 1–3.

Diroll, A., & Hlebovy, D. (2003). Inverse relationship between blood volume and blood pressure. *Nephrology Nursing Journal 30*(4), 460–461.

Emde, K., & Rush, C. (2001). Suspecting pulmonary embolism. *American Journal of Nursing 101*(9), 19–24.

Ferri, R. S., & Safer, D. (2002). Predicting nosocomial infections in trauma patients. *American Journal of Nursing 102*(11), 21.

Ferri, R. S. (2003). Prehypertension? *American Journal of Nursing 103*(9), 18.

Flounders, J. A. (2003). Superior vena cava syndrome. *Oncology Nursing Forum 30*(4), E84–E90.

Fort, C. W. (2002). Get pumped to prevent DVT. *Nursing 32*(9), 50–52.

Gobel, B. H. (2003). Disseminated intravasculsr coagulation. *Clinical Journal of Oncology Nursing 7*(3), 339–340.

Kennedy, M. S. (2002). Heart disease and stroke prevention. *American Journal of Nursing 102*(2), 20.

Kragsbjerg, P., Jurstrand, M., & Fredlund, H. (2004). Similar inflammatory response in human whole blood to live streptococcus pneumoniae of different serotypes. *Clinical Microbiology & Infection 10*(2), 174–177.

Myths and facts. (2003). *Nursing 33*(7), 74.

Scientists find antitumor compounds in magnolia cones. (2003 July 6). *Biotech Week*, 145–147.

Turkowski, B. B. (2003). Tired blood. *Orthopaedic Nursing 22*(3), 222–227.

Willoughby, S., Holmes, A., & Loscalzo, J. (2002). Platelets and cardiovascular disease. *European Journal of Cardiovascular Nursing 1*(4), 273–276.

Woodrow, P. (2003). Assessing blood results in older people: Haematology and liver function tests. *Nursing Older People 15*(3), 29–31.

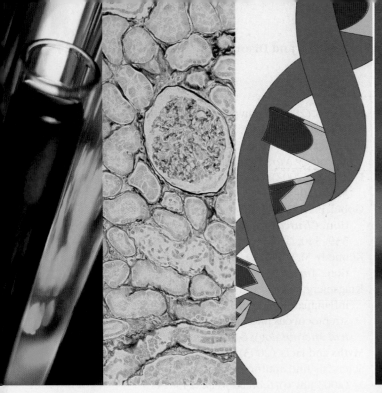
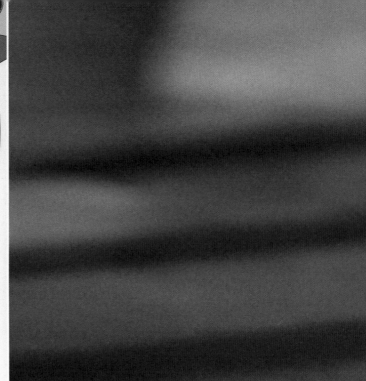

## OUTLINE

## KEY TERMS

# Cardiovascular System Diseases and Disorders

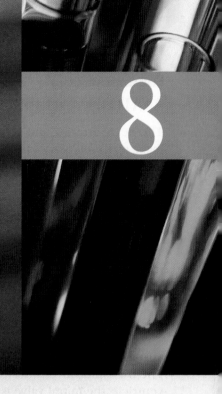

**8**

## LEARNING OBJECTIVES

*Upon completion of the chapter, the learner should be able to:*

1. Define the terminology common to the cardiovascular system and the disorders of the system.

2. Discuss the basic anatomy and physiology of the cardiovascular system.

3. Identify the important signs and symptoms associated with common cardiovascular system disorders.

4. Describe the common diagnostics used to determine the type and/or cause of the cardiovascular system disorders.

5. Identify the common disorders of the cardiovascular system.

6. Describe the typical course and management of the common cardiovascular system disorders.

7. Describe the effects of aging on the cardiovascular system and the common disorders of the system.

## OVERVIEW

*The cardiovascular system is often regarded as the major body system because the individual cannot live without a functioning heart and circulatory system. The heart is responsible only for pumping blood while the vascular system transports the blood throughout the body. Disorders of the system often share common symptoms and problems. Other systems are affected when the cardiovascular system is malfunctioning because it is responsible for delivering necessary nutrients and oxygen to the body. Diseases of the cardiovascular system are a major cause of morbidity and mortality in all ages, but especially in older adults.* ■

## ANATOMY AND PHYSIOLOGY

The heart, arteries, and veins, along with the blood, make up the cardiovascular system. The heart is a four-chambered muscular structure. It is about the size of a man's fist and weighs about 300 grams. The heart is situated approximately in the middle of the chest, slightly to the left, behind the sternum (breastbone). The heart is composed of the pericardium, the chambers, and the valves. The pericardium is a two-layer sac with fluid between the layers. The wall of the heart is divided into three layers. The epicardium is the outermost layer, the myocardium is the middle layer, and the endocardium is the innermost layer.

There are four chambers in the heart: the right atrium, right ventricle, left atrium, and left ventricle. The tricuspid valve is between the right atrium and ventricle; the mitral valve is between the left atrium and ventricle; the pulmonary valve is between the right ventricle and pulmonary artery; and the aortic valve is between the left ventricle and the aorta.

Blood enters the heart from the superior vena cava, then passes through the right atrium and the tricuspid valve into the right ventricle. It then passes through the pulmonary valve into the pulmonary artery, and travels to the lungs where carbon dioxide is exchanged for oxygen. The oxygenated blood returns to the heart through the pulmonary vein, and is pumped into the left atrium through the mitral valve and into the left ventricle. It then passes through the aortic valve into the aorta and to the body (Figure 8-1). The heart itself is supplied with blood by the coronary arteries.

Cardiac muscle normally contracts continually throughout one's lifetime. Designated areas of the heart produce electrical stimulation, causing the heart muscle to contract and pump the blood to the body. This sequence of events is termed the cardiac cycle. It begins in the sinoatrial (SA) node, then passes to the atrioventricular (AV) node to the bundle of HIS and the Purkinje fibers (Figure 8-2).

One sequence of the conduction pathway is one cardiac cycle. This is represented on the electro-

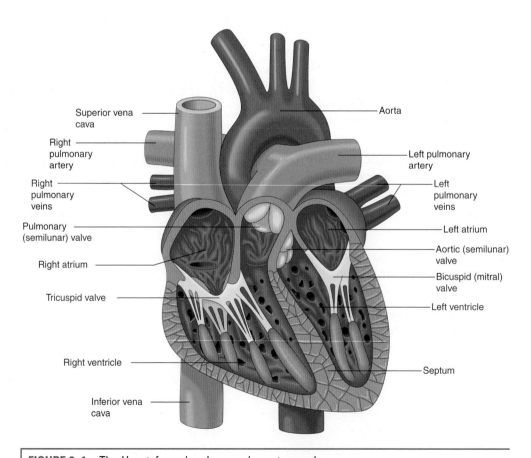

**FIGURE 8-1**  The Heart: four chambers and great vessels.

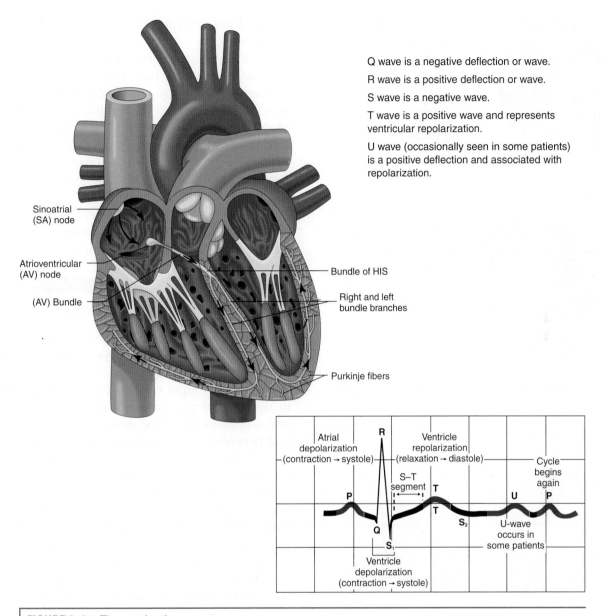

Q wave is a negative deflection or wave.

R wave is a positive deflection or wave.

S wave is a negative wave.

T wave is a positive wave and represents ventricular repolarization.

U wave (occasionally seen in some patients) is a positive deflection and associated with repolarization.

Sinoatrial (SA) node

Atrioventricular (AV) node

(AV) Bundle

Bundle of HIS

Right and left bundle branches

Purkinje fibers

Atrial depolarization (contraction → systole)

Ventricle repolarization (relaxation → diastole)

S–T segment

Ventricle depolarization (contraction → systole)

Cycle begins again

U-wave occurs in some patients

**FIGURE 8–2**   The conduction system.

cardiogram as the PQRST segment. The P wave represents the electrical stimulation beginning and passing over the atria (depolarization). The QRS wave is caused by the stimulation passing over the ventricles. The T wave represents the recovery of the ventricles (repolarization). The cardiac cycle repeats itself approximately 60-100 times per minute in the average adult. One cycle is one heartbeat. The pulsation (heartbeat) felt with the hand over the chest or the fingertips placed over an artery (such as at the wrist or neck) is called the pulse (Figure 8-3). The pulse rate is the number of pulsations felt in a

minute. The closing of the heart valves produces the sounds heard when listening with a stethoscope over the heart.

The circulatory component of the cardiovascular system includes the arteries and veins (Figure 8-4). The three major subsystems include the portal unit, the pulmonary unit, and the systemic unit. Each of these circulatory subsystems have special functions in addition to delivering blood to the body. The portal unit or subsystem includes the circulation to the stomach, spleen, intestine, and pancreas. Blood from these organs goes through the liver before returning

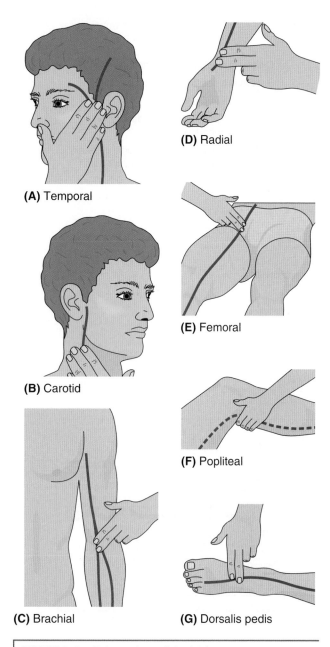

**(A)** Temporal

**(B)** Carotid

**(C)** Brachial

**(D)** Radial

**(E)** Femoral

**(F)** Popliteal

**(G)** Dorsalis pedis

**FIGURE 8–3**　Pulse points of the body.

to the heart. The pulmonary subsystem includes the pulmonary artery and its divisions, leading from the heart to the lungs, the circulation through the lungs, and the pulmonary vein leading from the lungs back to the heart. In this subsystem, nonoxygenated blood from the systemic circulation passes through the lungs where an exchange of carbon dioxide for oxygen occurs. The oxygenated blood returns to the heart to be pumped throughout the body. The systemic subsystem includes all the arteries and veins, and their capillaries not already included in the previous subsystems. This subsystem carries the oxy-

gen and nutrients to the body cells and removes waste products.

The level of pressure of the blood pushing against the walls of the vessels as it is delivered throughout the body is referred to as blood pressure. Most individuals are familiar with the arterial blood pressure taken in the arm over the brachial artery. The pressure measured with a sphygmomanometer is divided into two parts. The systolic pressure, caused by the contraction of the ventricles, is the first number recorded. The second number is the diastolic pressure, reflecting the relaxation of the ventricles. The average adult pressure is 120/80 mm Hg (millimeters of mercury).

## COMMON SIGNS AND SYMPTOMS

Common symptoms of heart disease include chest pain, **dyspnea** (DISP-nee-ah; dys = difficult, pnea = breathing), fatigue, and **tachycardia** (TACH-ee-**KAR**-dee-ah; tachy = rapid, cardia = heart). Chest pain may be described as a severe, crushing pressure like someone is crushing the chest, or the pain may be milder and described as a constant feeling of indigestion. Pain also may radiate down the left arm or into the jaw. Dyspnea is also a common symptom as a lack of oxygen to the tissues stimulates the respiratory system. Individuals with heart disease often feel fatigued and experience episodes of tachycardia. Other symptoms include **cardiac palpitations** (an unusually strong, rapid, or irregular heart rate that is so abnormal that the individual "can feel" it), sweating, edema in the extremities, and nausea and vomiting.

Pain, edema, and cyanosis are symptoms of diseases of the vascular system. Pain is often associated with poor blood perfusion to the tissues, leading to **ischemia** (iss-KEE-me-ah; lack of oxygen) of the organ. Edema of the extremities is commonly due to poor venous return, leading to congestion of blood and fluids in the tissues. Tissues that lack oxygen often exhibit a characteristic blue color called **cyanosis** (SIGH-ah-**NO**-sis; cyano = blue, osis = condition).

## DIAGNOSTIC TESTS

Noninvasive procedures of the cardiovascular system involve listening to the heart and movement of blood in the vessels. This is accomplished by use of a stethoscope in a procedure called **auscultation**

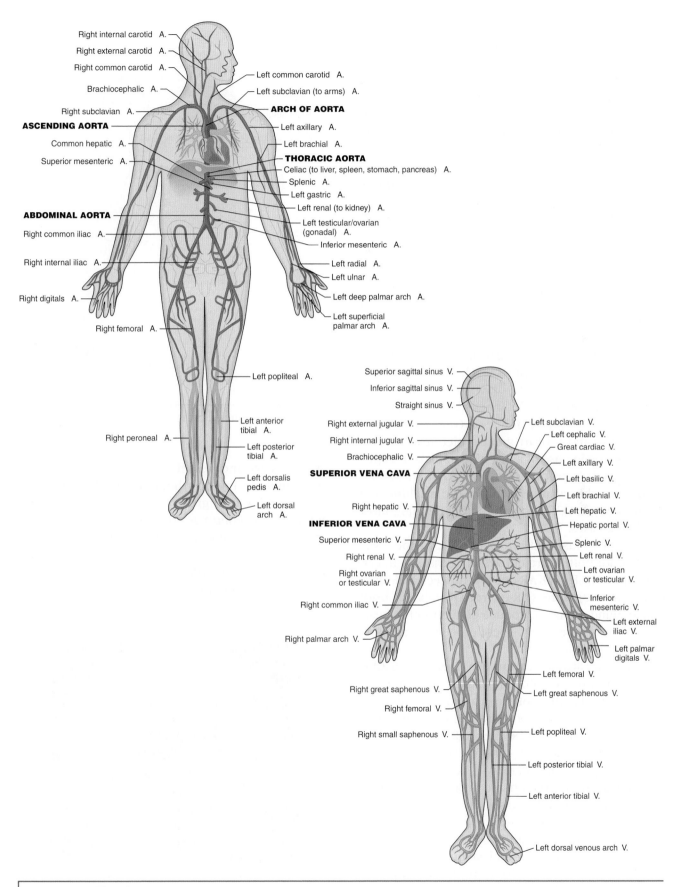

**FIGURE 8–4** The circulatory system.

(AUS-kul-**TAY**-shun). During auscultation, the stethoscope may be placed on the chest to listen to the heart and over various arteries to listen for blood flow. Murmurs may be auscultated in the heart area and indicate abnormal flow through the heart valves. A **Doppler** device may be placed over arteries to magnify the sound of blood flow. Decreased blood flow may be due to heart and/or vessel disease.

Arterial blood pressure is simply referred to as blood pressure and is measured by a sphygmomanometer. A sphygmomanometer is a cuff and pressure gauge used to measure pressure when the heart beats (**systolic**; sis-TALL-ick) and when it rests (**diastolic**; dye-as-TOL-ick). Venous blood pressure is an important measure of the heart's pumping ability and may be determined by examining the individual for edema. Edema in the extremities and distention of the jugular veins in the neck are common indicators of increased venous pressure.

The action of the heart may be drawn or graphed by an electrocardiograph, a machine that receives electrical information and draws heart action. The picture produced is an **electrocardiogram** (ECG or EKG) (ee-LECK-troh-**KAR**-dee-oh-GRAM; electro = electrical, cardio = heart, gram = picture). The procedure involving use of a machine to make this picture is called electrocardiography. ECG or EKG is also used as an abbreviation to name the machine and the procedure. ECG is helpful in determining most cardiac diseases.

Use of ultrasound for diagnostic purposes is valuable for both heart and vessel diseases. Echocardiography (ECK-oh-KAR-dee-**OG**-rah-fee) and ultrasound arteriography (AR-tee-ree-**OG**-rah-fee) both utilize sound waves to produce pictures of the heart and arteries, respectively. These procedures are noninvasive.

**Cardiac catheterization** (KATH-eh-ter-eye-**ZAY**-shun) is an invasive procedure used to sample the blood in the chambers of the heart to determine the oxygen content and blood pressure in the chambers. Cardiac output also may be checked. This procedure involves passing a small plastic catheter into the heart through a vein or artery. A vein is utilized for right-sided catheterization and an artery is used for a left-sided approach. Vessels of the arms and legs are commonly used (Figure 8–5).

X-rays of the heart and vessels may be beneficial in determining normal structure, size, and **patency** (openness). These procedures involve injecting dye into the system and taking pictures

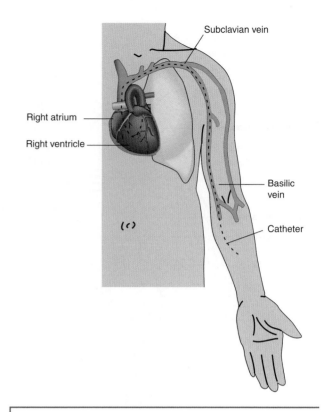

**FIGURE 8–5** Cardiac catheterization.

of the heart and vessels. Common X-ray procedures include angiocardiography (AN-jee-oh-KAR-dee-**OG**-rah-fee; angio = vessel, cardio = heart, graphy = procedure), arteriography (arterio = artery, graphy = procedure), and venography (veno = vein, graphy = procedure). The X-ray pictures produced are called angiocardiograms, arteriograms, and venograms, respectively (Figure 8–6).

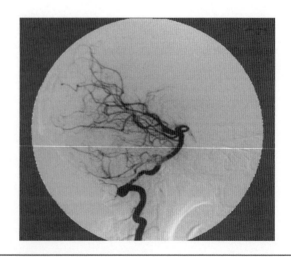

**FIGURE 8–6** Arteriogram.

Blood tests of this system include enzyme studies that assist in determining if the individual has had a myocardial infarction (heart attack). As the heart muscle dies, enzymes are released. The enzyme levels help determine the time and degree of the infarction. Common enzymes are creatinine phosphokinase (CPK) and lactic dehydrogenase (LDH).

# COMMON DISEASES OF THE CARDIOVASCULAR SYSTEM

Cardiovascular disease is the leading cause of death in the United States today (Figure 8–7). More than 2,600 Americans die each day due to cardiovascular diseases. Over 64,400,000 individuals have some form of cardiovascular disease. High blood pressure accounts for most of these cases, but coronary heart disease, rheumatic heart disease, and other forms of cardiovascular disease also contribute to these staggering numbers (American Heart Association, 2004). Education about lifestyle behavioral changes has helped decrease some individuals' risk for cardiovascular disease.

## Diseases of Arteries

Arterial disorders are the most common among all the cardiovascular diseases. High blood pressure (hypertension) accounts for the largest incidence of

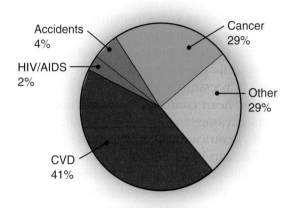

**FIGURE 8–7** Mortality statistics comparing cardiovascular diseases to other diseases.

arterial disorders, but coronary artery disease (coronary heart disease) is the single leading cause of death overall.

**Hypertension.** Most people are familiar with the basic concept that hypertension is high arterial blood pressure. Other concepts include the fact that hypertension is not only a disease process, but also serves as an indicator of the development of cerebrovascular, cardiovascular, and kidney disease. Hypertension is a chronic disease and is the leading cause of stroke and heart failure. Life expectancy in all individuals,

---

 **HEALTHY HIGHLIGHT**

**Prevention of Cardiovascular Disease**

To help reduce the risk of developing cardiovascular disease, practice the following lifestyle behaviors:

- Decrease intake of fats, especially saturated fats.
- Decrease intake of salt.
- Participate in a regular program of moderate exercise at least three times weekly.
- Keep weight within normal limits for age and body structure.
- Have blood pressure checked routinely. If necessary, take prescribed medications to reduce hypertension.
- Do not smoke.
- Decrease stress by participating in stress reduction activities.

regardless of age and sex, is reduced when diastolic hypertension is greater than 90 mm Hg.

Blood pressure varies from individual to individual, but average adult blood pressure is considered to be less than 120/80 mm Hg. The top number (120) is the systolic pressure and measures the highest amount of pressure in the artery when the ventricles of the heart contract. The lower number is the diastolic pressure and measures the artery pressure when the ventricles relax. If one could view the arteries as the heart beats, one would see a wavelike pattern of blood flow related to the heart beating and resting (Figure 8–8). Medical parameters for diagnosing high blood pressure are a systolic blood pressure of 140 mm Hg or greater and diastolic pressure of 90 mm Hg or greater.

In addition to heartbeat, blood vessel resistance also helps determine blood pressure. One might compare the heart and vessels to a water pump and hose. The amount of water the pump pumps and the width of the hose help determine the amount of water flow or water pressure. In the same way, the amount of blood the heart pumps and the resistance of the vessel or size of the **lumen** (LOO-men; inner open space or width) will help determine blood pressure. The larger the lumen or the more patent the vessel, the easier it is for the heart to pump blood and, generally speaking, the lower the blood pressure.

Specialized nerve receptors in the body help control pressure by bringing about vasoconstriction and vasodilatation at appropriate times. For example, when an individual stands up suddenly, the blood pressure to the head drops, often causing momentary dizziness. To correct this situation, nerves react and constrict blood vessels, raising blood pressure

and restoring normal pressure in the head. If blood pressure is too high, these nerve receptors dilate vessels leading to the kidneys. This increased blood flow leads to greater urine formation and output. Increased urine production decreases blood volume and thus lowers blood pressure. In this way, the kidneys play a vital role in blood pressure. If pressure is too low—as often occurs in shock—blood flow to the kidneys is diminished, urine output is minimal, blood fluid is maintained, and blood pressure is maintained or restored.

**ETIOLOGY** Because blood pressure and the kidneys have such a close relationship, any disease of the kidneys may cause an alteration in blood pressure. On the other hand, any change in blood pressure may have an adverse effect on the kidneys. The kidneys play a vital role in elimination of salt and water, two substances that also have a great effect on blood pressure. Retention of salt and water increases blood pressure whereas elimination of these substances reduces blood pressure. Hypertension, caused by kidney disease or some other type of disease process, is called secondary hypertension. Only 10 percent of all hypertensive cases are due to secondary problems.

Primary or essential hypertension accounts for approximately 90 percent of all hypertensive cases. This type of hypertension is due to an unknown cause and usually has a gradual onset over a number of years.

**SYMPTOMS** Symptoms usually do not occur until significant heart and vessel damage has already occurred. For this reason, blood pressure screening is very important in diagnosing hypertension before the cardiovascular system is damaged. A random blood pressure of greater than 140/90 may be physiologic; thus, screening with frequent blood pressure readings under varied conditions is needed to confirm the diagnosis.

Primary hypertension is idiopathic, but there are some identified genetic and environmental risk factors. These include:

- Heredity—hypertension affects black individuals twice as often as whites

- Diet—high salt and fat intake increases the risk of hypertension

- Age—blood pressure tends to rise with age

- Obesity—causes an increased workload on the heart

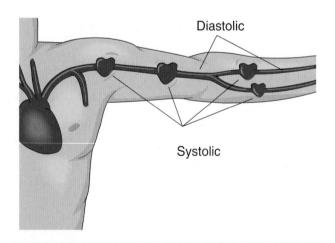

**FIGURE 8–8** Systolic and diastolic blood pressure.

- Smoking—vasoconstriction is caused by nicotine

- Stress—causes a rise in blood pressure due to vasoconstriction

- Type A personality—tends to experience more stress

The effects of hypertension may take years to develop, but ultimately—if untreated—high blood pressure overworks the heart. Because the left ventricle works harder to pump blood, it is the area most often affected, leading to left ventricle hypertrophy or muscle enlargement. The vascular system or blood supply to the left ventricle does not increase with this enlargement of muscle. As a result, this extra tissue does not have adequate blood supply, often leading to bouts of angina or chest pain due to ischemia. This condition often leads to myocardial infarction (MI) or heart failure, and death.

Hypertension not only affects the heart, but also adversely affects the vessels. Over a period of years, the vessels become hardened (sclerotic) and lose elasticity, a contributing factor in arteriosclerosis (arterio = artery, scler = hardened, osis = condition of ). Sclerotic (hardened) vessels are also more likely to form thrombi and to rupture. The results of thrombus or rupture may cause damage or death to the involved organs.

**TREATMENT** Treatment of hypertension depends on the degree of hypertension and the number of risk factors involved. If blood pressure is extremely high, antihypertensive medications may be prescribed immediately. If hypertension is discovered in a milder form, lifestyle changes or reduction of risk factors may be the initial treatment. A low-salt, low-fat diet, stress reducing exercise, and smoking cessation may solve

the problem (see *Healthy Highlight* on page 133). If this treatment is ineffective or inadequate, the individual may be placed on diuretic medications. Diuretics increase urine output, thus lowering blood pressure. If further control is needed, other antihypertensive medications may be prescribed. Patient compliance with hypertension is often a factor in the treatment of this chronic disease. Difficulty with lifestyle changes and following the medication regimen for the rest of one's life is often difficult for the individual to manage.

**Arteriosclerosis and Atherosclerosis.** Arteriosclerosis is a group of diseases that are characterized by a loss of elasticity and a thickening of the artery wall. Atherosclerosis is the most common form of arteriosclerosis. For this reason, these terms are often used interchangeably. Hardening of the arteries is a lay term describing this condition. The common result of arteriosclerosis is the gradual narrowing of the vessel lumen (Figure 8-9). This narrowing leads to a slowing or complete stoppage of blood flow to the organs supplied by those vessels. Without proper blood supply, these organs become ischemic and eventually may die if blood supply is not restored.

An artery has a very smooth endothelium (inner lining). The lining may be thought of as having a nonstick finish. As with nonstick cookware, food particles normally do not stick to the surface. If the endothelium is damaged, then blood material begins sticking to the inner lining of the artery just as food particles begin sticking to scratched cookware. The artery wall surrounds this endothelium. Atherosclerosis is a condition characterized by deposits of fatty or lipid material in the wall of the artery (see Figure 8-9). These

---

## COMPLEMENTARY AND ALTERNATIVE THERAPY

### Tai Chi for Lowering Blood Pressure

Tai Chi, also known as Tai Chi Chuan, is said to be a physical presentation and demonstration of the philosophy of Taoism. It is an exercise program combined with some relaxation and concentration. It has been shown in research studies to help lower blood pressure in patients with mild hypertension. The exercise program includes a 10-minute warm-up with a 30-minute session of Tai Chi exercises, followed by a 10-minute cool-down period. The exercise program also reduces anxiety in the participants.

*Source: Tsai, J. et al. (2003).*

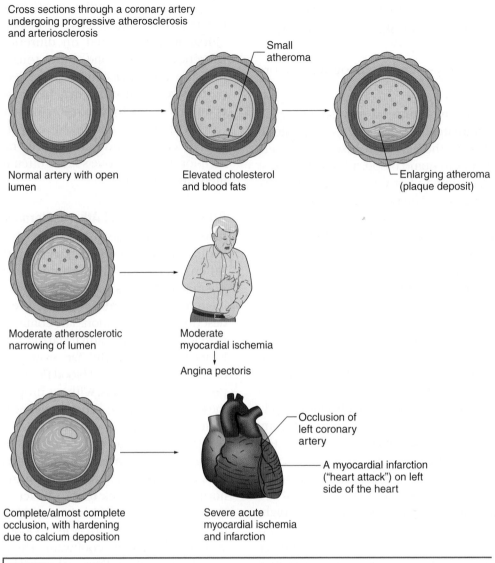

Cross sections through a coronary artery undergoing progressive atherosclerosis and arteriosclerosis

Small atheroma

Normal artery with open lumen

Elevated cholesterol and blood fats

Enlarging atheroma (plaque deposit)

Moderate atherosclerotic narrowing of lumen

Moderate myocardial ischemia

Angina pectoris

Complete/almost complete occlusion, with hardening due to calcium deposition

Occlusion of left coronary artery

A myocardial infarction ("heart attack") on left side of the heart

Severe acute myocardial ischemia and infarction

**FIGURE 8–9** Atherosclerosis: narrowing of arterial lumen.

fatty, cholesterol-containing deposits called **plaque** damage the artery and interrupt blood flow by:

■ pushing into the endothelium, thus damaging the inner lining. Damage to this lining allows blood material to stick to the inner lining and occlude the lumen.

■ causing the artery wall to harden or lose elasticity. This loss of elasticity increases blood pressure and increases workload on the heart. A hardened vessel is not able to expand and accommodate the surge of blood caused by the beat of the heart.

■ thickening the artery wall to the point that the lumen is partially or completely occluded.

■ leading to formation of plaque that often ulcerates or breaks loose, forming an **embolus** (EM-boh-lus; material floating in the blood) that may stick in a vessel and occlude or stop blood flow, leading to ischemia or death of the organs supplied by that vessel.

Narrowing of the lumen of the artery in all the aforementioned ways increases blood pressure, increases workload on the heart, and decreases blood supply to the organs. Increased blood pressure stretches the hardened arteries, causing further artery damage and further increasing workload on the heart.

Atherosclerosis may affect all arteries in the body. There are four major areas that are often affected by

## AFFECTED SITE

## COMPLICATION

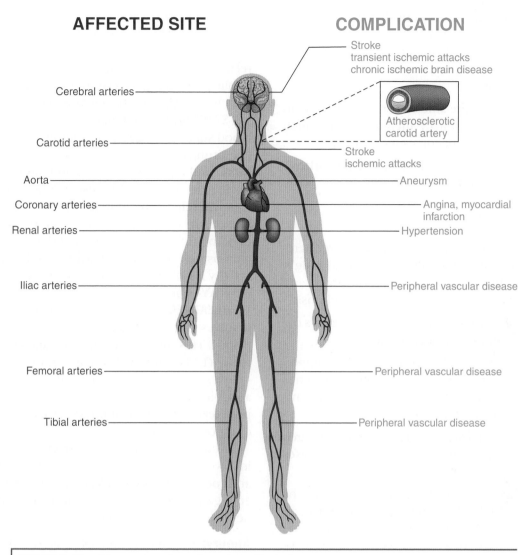

**FIGURE 8–10**  Atherosclerosis: major areas affected.

atherosclerosis, many times leading to disability or mortality (Figure 8-10).

The areas affected are the:

1. Coronary arteries—These arteries feed the muscle tissue of the heart. Atherosclerosis of these arteries leads to coronary artery disease, also called coronary heart disease. Consequences of coronary artery disease may include myocardial infarction or heart attack.

2. Cerebral arteries—These arteries feed brain tissue. Atherosclerosis of these arteries may lead to a cerebrovascular accident (CVA), commonly called a stroke.

3. Aorta—This artery is the largest artery in the body and is responsible for carrying blood to the general circulatory system. Atherosclerosis of this artery in any area may lead to aneurysms.

4. Peripheral arteries—Peripheral arteries primarily feed the extremities (arms and legs). Atherosclerosis of these arteries may lead to peripheral vascular disease.

**ETIOLOGY**  The cause of atherosclerosis is unknown, but it is thought to be the result of a combination of factors. Some of the factors are not controllable, but many are and may be altered by a change in lifestyle. Important risk factors include the following:

### Noncontrollable Factors.

■ Heredity—Atherosclerosis appears to run in families. This may be related to common diet, or in some instances, a clear genetic tendency to develop hypercholesterolemia (hyper = increased, cholesterol, emia = blood).

■ Age—Atherosclerosis is considered a degenerative disease because all adults over the age of 30 have some degree of plaque formation. In general, the older the person, the more atherosclerosis is present.

■ Sex—Men have more atherosclerosis present than women until after female menopause, at which time, the incidence becomes more equal.

■ Diabetes—Diabetics have more existing atherosclerosis than nondiabetics.

### Controllable Factors.

■ Diet—Obese individuals have more atherosclerosis present than individuals in the normal weight range. The higher the diet in carbohydrates and fats, the higher the incidence of atherosclerosis.

■ Sedentary lifestyle—Lack of exercise increases the risk of development of atherosclerosis.

■ Cigarette smoking—This is one of the most important risk factors. Stopping smoking is 10 times more effective in reducing risk than a combination of exercise and diet control.

■ Stress—Stress increases blood pressure, but research does not support the idea that stress increases atherosclerosis.

■ Hypertension—The higher the blood pressure, the greater the risk for development of atherosclerosis. It is difficult to determine which of these diseases occurs first. Atherosclerosis causes an increase in blood pressure, and hypertension leads to an increase in atherosclerosis. Often, hypertension and atherosclerosis occur simultaneously, each complicating the treatment of the other.

**SYMPTOMS** Symptoms of atherosclerosis appear late in the disease process and vary, depending on the area affected.

Diagnosis of atherosclerosis is by blood pressure measurement, arteriograms, and X-ray. Doppler studies to determine blood flow also may be utilized.

**TREATMENT** Treatment is aimed at treating symptoms as they arise. Surgery to bypass occluded arteries and remove plaque is commonly utilized. Prevention of atherosclerosis includes exercise, estrogen medication postmenopause, and changing lifestyle to reduce risk factors.

### Peripheral Vascular Disease (PVD). ETIOLOGY
Peripheral vascular disease is caused by atherosclerotic plaque, primarily in the arteries supplying blood to the legs. The occlusion by the plaque may be chronic or acute. Chronic occlusion is generally related to a progressive narrowing of the femoral and popliteal arteries. As these arteries become occluded, the blood supply to the leg muscles is decreased.

**SYMPTOMS** Individuals with PVD have adequate blood supply to leg muscles during minimal activity like sitting or slow walking. If activity is increased to brisk walking or running, blood supply becomes inadequate, causing leg muscle cramps. Resting the legs will relieve the muscle cramps. Rest allows the muscles to once again receive the needed amount of blood flow. This condition of developing muscle cramps that are relieved with rest and increase with activity is called **intermittent claudication** (KLAW-dih-**KAY**-shun).

**TREATMENT** Treatment of chronic PVD often involves opening the artery and cleaning out the plaque. This surgical treatment is called **endarterectomy** (END-ar-ter-**ECK**-toh-me; endo = inside, arter = artery, ectomy = excision). If the artery is damaged, it may be bypassed with a graft. A femoral popliteal graft may be utilized to treat the symptoms of chronic occlusion.

Acute occlusion of the peripheral arteries often involves smaller arteries supplying blood to the feet and toes. This type of PVD often leads to necrosis and gangrene. Amputation or resection may be needed to treat acute occlusion.

### Aneurysm.
Aneurysm (AN-you-rizm) is a weakening in the wall of an artery that allows the vessel to bulge or rupture (Figure 8–11).

**ETIOLOGY** This weakening is often due to atherosclerosis, but also may be due to a congenital defect or injury.

**SYMPTOMS** Aneurysms are usually asymptomatic, and are often discovered accidentally during physical examinations or X-rays. The most common area affected is the abdominal aorta. Rupture of an aneurysm is a medical emergency, often causing death due to massive hemorrhage and shock.

**TREATMENT** Treatment is aimed at repairing the aneurysm before rupture. Surgical resection and grafting is commonly performed (Figure 8–12).

### Coronary Artery Disease.
Coronary artery disease (CAD), often called coronary heart disease, is the narrowing of arteries that supply blood to the myocardium or heart muscle. It is the single leading cause of death in the United States today.

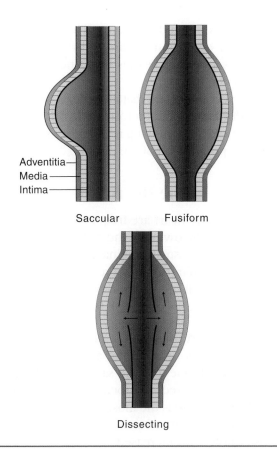

Adventitia—
Media—
Intima—

Saccular      Fusiform

Dissecting

**FIGURE 8–11**   Three types of aneurysm.

**ETIOLOGY** This disease is commonly due to atherosclerosis.

**SYMPTOMS** Progressive or slow narrowing of the arteries leads to ischemia of the heart muscle and symptoms of angina. Some muscle cells may actually die and be replaced with scar tissue. This scar tissue cannot function like muscle tissue, causing an increase in the workload of the remaining heart muscle. Congestive heart failure often results.

If a coronary artery becomes blocked to the point that oxygen demands by the heart muscle cannot be met, the heart muscle dies. Occlusion may progress slowly as plaque builds up in the vessel, or it may develop suddenly as a result of a **thrombus** (THROM-bus; a blood clot attached to a vein or artery) or embolus (traveling blood clot, free in the circulatory system, more dangerous than a thrombus). This dead muscle is called an infarct or myocardial infarct. The process of the myocardium dying is called myocardial infarction.

Slow, progressive occlusion of the arteries often leads to development of collateral arteries that extend into ischemic tissue. Collateral circulation provides some protection against ischemia and infarction. For this reason, infarction caused by slow occlusion oftentimes has a better outcome than infarction caused by sudden occlusion of a vessel.

Diagnosis of coronary artery disease is made by a history of symptoms, EKG, and angiograms. Symptoms

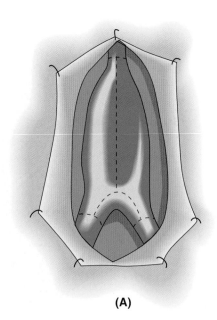
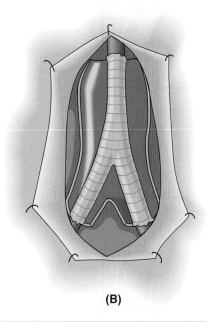

(A)                  (B)

**FIGURE 8–12**   Abdominal aneurysm surgical resection (A) and grafting (B).

usually do not develop until the vessels are at least 70 percent occluded.

**TREATMENT** Treatment of coronary artery disease is aimed at increasing blood flow or decreasing oxygen needs. Angina is often treated with rest and vasodilators. A coronary artery **angioplasty** (AN-jee-oh-**PLAS**-tee; angio = vessel, plasty = surgical repair) may be attempted to open the vessel. Angioplasty involves passing a catheter into the artery and inflating a balloon on the catheter to push the plaque against the vessel wall, thus widening the lumen of the vessel (Figure 8–13). Another common surgical treatment for coronary artery disease is a coronary artery bypass graft, commonly called a CABG (pronounced cabbage). This procedure bypasses the occlusion (Figure 8–14). Mammary vessels and saphenous vessels from the legs are often used for the bypass.

It is very important that individuals with coronary artery disease reduce atherosclerotic risk factors. Diet, exercise and a no-smoking regimen are prescribed to slow the progression of the disease.

## Diseases of the Heart

Diseases of the heart are frequently due to the atherosclerotic narrowing of the coronary arteries. The result of this is usually angina and/or a heart attack (myocardial infarction). Decreasing lifestyle behaviors that contribute to the development of atherosclerosis decreases one's risk for heart disease.

**Coronary Heart Disease.** Coronary heart disease, coronary artery disease, and arteriosclerotic heart disease are all one and the same. This disease was previously discussed as coronary artery disease. Coronary heart disease is the most common type of heart disease in the United States. The risk of this disease rises rapidly with increased age.

**Angina Pectoris.** Angina pectoris (an-JIGH-nah PECK-toh-riss) is commonly called chest pain.

**ETIOLOGY** It is caused by lack of oxygen to the myocardium or heart muscle. Angina is commonly a symptom of impending myocardial infarction.

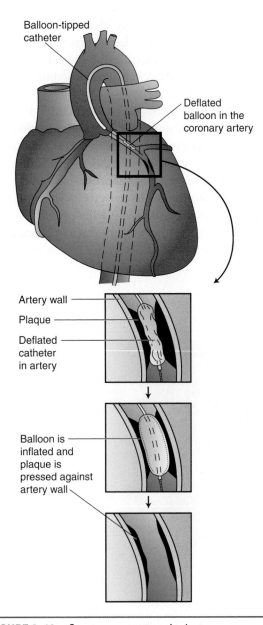

FIGURE 8–13 Coronary artery angioplasty.

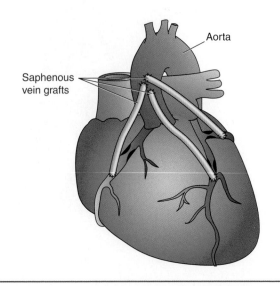

FIGURE 8–14 Coronary artery bypass graft (CABG).

**SYMPTOMS** During an attack, the individual may complain of a suffocating tightness in the chest that radiates to the left arm, neck, and jaw (Figure 8–15). Angina usually occurs during periods of increased workload on the heart, like those experienced with physical exercise, emotional stress, or digestion of a large meal.

**TREATMENT** Treatment of angina is to decrease workload on the heart by stopping the aggravating activity and to increase blood flow to the heart muscle. Vasodilatation of the coronary arteries or those that supply the heart muscle will improve blood flow and help relieve the oxygen deficit. Nitroglycerin is a vasodilator that is commonly used. It is administered sublingually (under the tongue) and usually provides immediate relief. Individuals suffering with angina need medical attention.

## Myocardial Infarction.

**ETIOLOGY** Myocardial infarction (MY-oh-**KAR**-dee-al in-FARK-shun) occurs when the heart muscle does not get adequate oxygen due to a decrease in blood supply, an increase in oxygen need, or a combination of both. The decrease in blood supply is most commonly caused by the atherosclerotic plaque of coronary artery disease. Any activity that increases the oxygen need of the heart beyond the supply level may lead to a myocardial infarct. Activities may include shock, hemorrhage, stress, or excessive physical exertion.

**SYMPTOMS** Classic symptoms of a myocardial infarction include severe chest pain with diaphoresis (sweating) and nausea. Often, the symptoms are not as obvious, and may include referred pain in the left arm, neck, and jaw, along with a discomfort similar to bad or unrelieved indigestion. Severity of symptoms may depend on the size of the infarction. If the area is small, symptoms may be mild and the infarction may be labeled as a "silent" MI. If the infarcted area is large, symptoms may include cardiogenic shock and death. Mortality from myocardial infarction is approximately 35 percent.

**TREATMENT** Treatment of a myocardial infarction involves immediate attention to prevent shock, relieve respiratory distress, and decrease workload on the heart. The individual should be assisted into a lying position. Tight or restrictive clothing should be loosened to improve respiratory function. If cardiac arrest has occurred, appropriate CPR (cardiopulmonary resuscitation) should be administered immediately and the individual should be immediately transported to a medical facility.

Medical treatment involves the administration of oxygen and pain medication. Medication to treat arrhythmias is often needed. Intravenous thrombolytic or "clot busting" therapy using a tissue plasminogen activator (TPA) or streptokinase may be utilized to open the occlusion and restore blood flow. Education following a myocardial infarction is aimed at prevention by possible changes in lifestyle to reduce risk factors. Smoking cessation, changes in diet, and exercise are usually recommended.

The main site involved in a myocardial infarction is the left ventricle. This is the hardest working area of the heart and has the greatest need for oxygen.

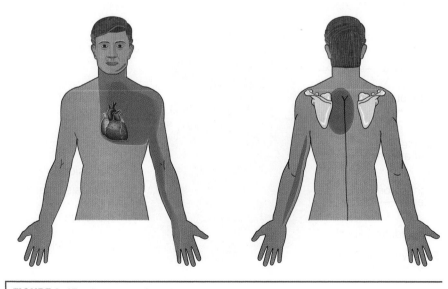

**FIGURE 8–15** Patterns of angina.

Tissue changes that appear with an infarction depend on the degree or extent of oxygen deprivation suffered by the cells. Under microscopic examination, the infarcted area may take on a bull's eye appearance (Figure 8–16). The central core is made up of cells that are dead or necrotic. Severely damaged cells surround this core. These cells may regain function within a few weeks or they may die, thus extending the infarcted area. On the outer border of the bull's eye pattern are cells that suffered from ischemia. These cells usually live and may regain function.

Death of myocardial cells brings about a release of certain enzymes (CPK and LDH) into the general circulation. Blood tests to measure the levels of these enzymes assist in determining the amount of dead or necrotic tissue, the severity, and time of the attack. Blood enzyme levels, along with an EKG, history, and physical examination often confirm the diagnosis of myocardial infarction.

Tissue infarction and injury naturally cause the inflammatory response. With this response comes an outpouring of PMNs and macrophages. Within the first five to seven days, macrophages phagocytize the dead tissue, often leaving a thin, weak myocardial layer. Possibility of rupture and sudden death is greatest at this time. Any activity that increases the workload of the heart or increases blood pressure should be avoided. Rest is essential during this time.

Within two weeks, the infarcted area is healing with granulation tissue. This tissue is not made of muscle tissue; it is scar tissue. This scar or patch will not stretch or contract like muscle, and it will never function as normal heart tissue. The inability of this scarred area to function increases workload on the remaining heart muscle cells for the rest of the individual's life.

Risk factors for myocardial infarction are the same as coronary artery disease, and primarily include hypertension, cigarette smoking, a sedentary lifestyle, obesity, and a high-cholesterol diet.

**Hypertensive Heart Disease.** **ETIOLOGY** Hypertensive heart disease is the result of long-term hypertension. Any disease or disorder that causes a chronic elevation in blood pressure may lead to hypertensive heart disease. Essential hypertension, arteriosclerosis, atherosclerosis, and kidney diseases are common causes.

**SYMPTOMS** As previously discussed, chronic hypertension leads to increased workload on the heart, causing cardiac hypertrophy and eventually, heart failure.

**TREATMENT** Treatment of hypertensive heart disease is related to treating the cause of hypertension. If the hypertension cannot be cured as with essential hypertension, then controlling blood pressure is necessary. Hypertensive heart disease, like hypertension, is not cured, only controlled.

**Rheumatic Heart Disease.** Rheumatic heart disease refers to the cardiac symptoms related to rheumatic fever. Rheumatic fever was discussed in Chapter 5 as an autoimmune disorder.

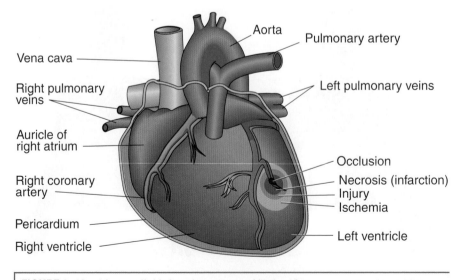

**FIGURE 8–16** Myocardial infarction: areas of ischemia.

**ETIOLOGY** One may recall that rheumatic fever is commonly caused by a streptococcal throat infection. The immune system in a select group of individuals builds antibodies that attack the bacteria and the heart tissue. All layers of the heart may be affected, along with the valves of the heart.

**SYMPTOMS** Valvular damage may lead to stenosis (narrowing) of the mitral and aortic valves, then to murmurs.

**TREATMENT** Treatment is aimed at prevention and proper treatment of streptococcal infections. Valvular stenosis increases the workload of the heart and may cause further heart disease. During acute carditis, treatment includes bed rest to reduce the workload on the heart and other symptomatic treatment. Severe valve damage may lead to the need for valve surgery to correct the deformity or replace the valve.

## Congestive Heart Failure.
Congestive heart failure (CHF) is a condition in which the heart fails to pump an adequate amount of blood to meet the body's needs. The cardiopulmonary and general vascular system gradually become "congested."

**ETIOLOGY** Congestive heart failure develops slowly and usually follows any type of cardiac condition that increases the workload of the heart. Such diseases include myocardial infarction, hypertension, coronary artery disease, and rheumatic heart disease to name a few.

**SYMPTOMS** The individual experiences a gradual increase in dyspnea (dys = difficult, pnea = breathing). Tachycardia (tachy = rapid, cardia = heart) and tachypnea (TACH-ihp-NEE-ah; tachy = rapid, pnea = breathing) occur as the body tries to compensate for decreased blood flow. As CHF progresses, fluid builds up in the vascular system, leading to neck vein distention, and edema in the ankles and lower legs. Right-sided heart failure leads to congestion of the liver and spleen. Left-sided failure leads to congestion and edema of the lungs (pulmonary edema) (Figure 8–17).

Diagnosis is made after a thorough history and physical examination combined with chest X-ray and EKG.

**TREATMENT** Treatment is aimed at decreasing the workload of the heart. Diuretic medications, low-salt diet, and fluid restrictions may be prescribed to increase urine output and limit fluid retention, thus reducing blood fluid volume. Cardiac medications may be prescribed to strengthen and slow the heartbeat. Digitalis is a common medication given for this purpose.

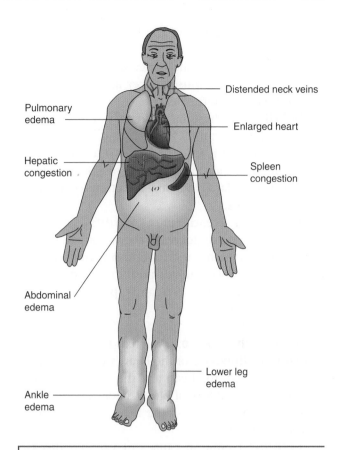

**FIGURE 8–17** Signs of congestive heart failure.

## Cardiomyopathy.
Cardiomyopathy (KAR-dee-oh-MY-OP-ah-thee; cardio = heart, myo = muscle, opathy = disease) is a general term describing disease of the heart muscle. This is a primary disease, not secondary to problems like hypertension or coronary artery disease. The heart muscle may be dilated or enlarged (dilated or congestive cardiomyopathy), characterized by a thin, flabby heart muscle.

**ETIOLOGY** The cause of this type of cardiomyopathy is often idiopathic, but a high number is seen in association with alcoholism. The heart muscle also may be enlarged and thick (hypertrophic cardiomyopathy). Hypertrophic cardiomyopathy is an inherited disease and runs in families. Lastly, the heart muscle may be restricted in movement due to some type of infiltrate (restrictive cardiomyopathy).

**TREATMENT** Cardiomyopathies are incurable and often lead to congestive heart failure, myocardial infarction, and death.

## Carditis.
Carditis (kar-DYE-tis) is a general term describing inflammation of the heart. Forms of carditis include pericarditis, myocarditis, and endocarditis,

depending on the area of the heart involved. Pericarditis affects the serous membrane on the outside of the heart as well as the pericardial sac. Myocarditis affects the heart muscle layer, and endocarditis affects the inside of the heart.

**ETIOLOGY** All these inflammatory states may be due to unknown causes, bacteria, and viruses, or as a result of rheumatic fever. Carditis is often secondary to a respiratory tract, urinary tract, or skin infection. It also may be related to dental infections or diseases of other systems.

**TREATMENT** Treatment of carditis generally includes bed rest to decrease the workload on the heart. Other treatments depend on the cause of the disease and may include antibiotics, analgesics, and antipyretics (anti = against, pyro = heat, or against fever).

## Valvular Heart Disease.

Valvular heart disease is related to malfunction of the heart valves. The purpose of a valve in the heart and the vascular system is to prevent backflow of blood. Backflow of blood causes extra workload on the heart as it has to re-pump the blood.

**ETIOLOGY** Common causes of valvular disease may be congenital anomalies or malformations, rheumatic fever, or endocarditis. Malfunction of a valve may be due to the valvular opening being too narrow (stenotic), or being too large to properly close (valvular insufficiency). Both of these problems may affect all the heart valves and lead to heart murmurs. A heart **murmur** is an abnormal sound in the heart or vascular system. One complication of all valve defects is the vascular tendency to form clots (thrombus) on the affected areas. If the thrombus breaks loose and becomes an embolus, it may occlude arteries leading to major organs such as the lungs, brain, liver, or kidneys. Another common problem of valvular heart disease is congestive heart failure due to the increased workload on the heart.

## Arrhythmias.

Arrhythmias (ah-RITH-me-ahs) are abnormalities in heart rhythm due to a disturbance in the conduction system of the heart.

**ETIOLOGY** Often, the cause of these is unknown. Known causes include medications, ischemia of the heart muscle, and a previous myocardial infarction. Auscultation and electrocardiography can diagnose arrhythmias.

**SYMPTOMS** Normal heart rhythm is often called "normal sinus rhythm," and indicates that the rate is between 60 and 100 beats per minute, is regular, and is originating normally from the SA node. An unusually fast (up to 350 beats per minute) but regular heart rate is called flutter. If the rhythm is wild and uncoordinated, it is an arrhythmia called **fibrillation** (FIH-brih-**LAY**-shun). Fibrillations may affect the atria or the ventricles. Atrial fibrillations are usually not serious in nature. Ventricular fibrillations, commonly abbreviated as V fib, are serious cardiac arrhythmias that require emergency defibrillation by electrical shock.

Heart block is another group of arrhythmias caused by an interruption in the conduction system. Heart block is divided into first, second, and third degree, depending on the seriousness of the blockage. Third-degree block is treated with insertion of an artificial pacemaker.

Premature or early contractions may affect the atria or the ventricles. Premature ventricular contractions are commonly abbreviated as PVCs. Treatment is usually unnecessary as long as the number per minute is minimal and the individual is asymptomatic.

# Diseases of the Veins

Diseases of the veins are more common in older adults. Age-related changes in the vessels and valves, along with other changes in the circulatory system, contribute to the overall general weakness of the vessels. Fluid often pools in the extremities, causing edema. Disorders of the veins are usually more serious in individuals with other chronic disorders such as diabetes mellitus.

## Phlebitis.

Phlebitis (fleh-BYE-tis; phlebo = vein, itis = inflammation) is relatively common, especially in the veins of the arms and lower legs. Phlebitis commonly refers to inflammation of superficial (near the skin surface) veins (Figure 8–18).

**ETIOLOGY** The cause of phlebitis is often unknown, but known causes may include injury, obesity, poor circulation, prolonged bed rest, and infection. Injury to a vein is often a known cause of phlebitis. Intravenous medications and catheters may cause vein injury in the arms. Pooling of blood, as occurs with varicose veins or physical injury to the vessel, may lead to phlebitis in the legs.

**SYMPTOMS** Symptoms of phlebitis include pain, swelling, and often the appearance of a red cord-like hardening that extends along the vein from the area of injury upward toward the heart. Occasionally, phlebitis in the lower leg occurs after childbirth in

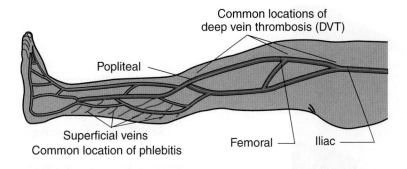

Common locations of
deep vein thrombosis (DVT)

Popliteal

Superficial veins
Common location of phlebitis

Femoral     Iliac

**FIGURE 8–18**   Superficial vs. deep veins in development of phlebitis and thrombus.

association with the onset of milk production. This form of phlebitis is commonly called "milk leg."

**TREATMENT** Treatment of superficial phlebitis often includes analgesics and warm compresses to reduce pain and improve circulation. Elevation of the area above heart level will improve venous return and decrease edema. To improve venous return in the lower extremities, the use of elastic or compression stockings and exercise may be prescribed.

### ■ Thrombophlebitis

A complication of phlebitis is the development of a clot in the inflamed vessel. This condition is called thrombophlebitis. Clots in superficial veins rarely embolize (break loose and travel), but clots in deep veins often do, making this condition in a deep vein of serious concern. Thrombophlebitis in the deep veins is called deep vein thrombosis (DVT).

### ■ Deep Vein Thrombosis

Deep vein thrombosis (DVT) primarily occurs in the lower legs, thighs, and pelvis (see Figure 8–18). Clots occurring in the femoral and pelvic veins commonly embolize.

**ETIOLOGY** Risk factors for DVT include:

■ Immobility—early postoperative ambulation (walking) is encouraged. Prolonged bed rest greatly increases risk

■ Dehydration—increases blood viscosity (thickness) and increases risk of thrombus formation

■ Varicose veins—veins already weakened with disease are more likely to develop a thrombus

■ Leg or pelvic surgery, obesity, and pregnancy—alter venous blood flow and increase risk

**SYMPTOMS** These clots are generally asymptomatic until embolization occurs, often causing a pulmonary embolism. Pulmonary embolism is often fatal.

**TREATMENT** Treatment of DVT is aimed at reducing the formation of more clots and preventing embolization. Bed rest with elevation of the affected area is essential to improve blood flow. Anticoagulants are given to decrease potential thrombus formation. Anticoagulants will not dissolve clots, only prevent formation of new ones.

**Varicose Veins.** Varicose veins (VAR-ih-kohs VAYNS) are dilated, tortuous, and elongated veins commonly found in the legs. Blood in the legs must move upward against the pull of gravity. Leg muscles are primarily responsible for this movement by contracting and relaxing. This action pushes against the vessel wall and pushes blood upward. Valves are necessary to prevent backflow of blood. With varicose veins, the flow of blood is slowed and/or collects in the veins, causing increased pressure on the vessel walls and the valves, and eventually leading to incompetent valves (Figure 8–19). Prolonged pooling of blood in the veins stretches the vessel wall and leads to the formation of varicosities.

**ETIOLOGY** Development of varicosities may be due to any activity that slows return flow and increases venous pressure. Such activities as prolonged sitting, standing, pregnancy, and obesity tend to increase the risk of developing of varicose veins. Heredity also plays a part in this disorder, as there appears to be an inherited vessel wall weakness.

**SYMPTOMS** Varicose veins develop gradually. Initial symptoms may include leg fatigue and leg cramps. Veins often become thick, hardened, and unsightly. Poor venous blood flow causes edema and congestion of fluid in the extremities. This congestion slows

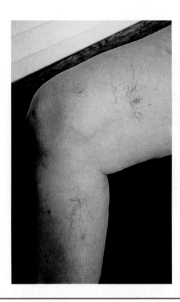

**FIGURE 8–19** Varicose veins. *(Courtesy of the Armed Forces Institute of Pathology.)*

arterial flow, leading to stasis dermatitis and ulceration. Stasis dermatitis is characterized by edema, dry and scaly skin, and small pinpoint hemorrhages. The skin also turns brown in color as blood pigment accumulates in the connective tissue. Stasis ulcers do not heal well and may lead to amputation of the affected area.

**TREATMENT** Treatment includes improving vascular flow by elevating legs, walking, and use of support or elastic hose. Surgery may be indicated to relieve discomfort and avoid recurrent thrombosis. Surgical treatment involves tying off the vessel and removing it. This procedure is commonly called vein stripping. There are numerous superficial veins, so blood return to the heart from this area is through alternate venous routes.

# TRAUMA

## Hemorrhage

Hemorrhage (hemo = blood, orrhage = burst forth) is an abnormal loss of blood. Hemorrhagic blood loss may be external or internal. Blood loss also may be acute (sudden onset) or it may be chronic.

**ETIOLOGY** Acute blood loss is usually related to trauma whereas chronic loss is more often related to disease processes.

External and internal blood loss, if severe enough, may lead to **exsanguination** (loss of circulating blood volume) and death. Internal blood loss may cause filling of body cavities. An example of internal bleeding into a cavity would be **hemothorax** (hemo = blood, thorax = chest, blood in the chest cavity). Internal bleeding may not be noticeable until a large amount of blood has been lost and the individual begins to show signs and symptoms of shock.

**SYMPTOMS** Hemorrhage may affect different vessels and have varying results. Hemorrhage of low-pressure vessels (the capillaries and veins) into the tissues leads to reddish to dark purple spots on the skin and mucosa. These discolorations are called petechiae, ecchymosis, or purpura, depending on the size or cause of the discoloration. Petechiae (pee-TEE-kee-ee) are small pinpoint hemorrhages. Ecchymosis (ECK-ih-**MOH**-sis) is a larger area of purplish color commonly called a bruise. Purpura (PUR-pew-rah) is spontaneous bleeding into the tissues related to a hemorrhagic disease that may be characterized by both petechiae and ecchymosis. Hemorrhage of the high-pressure vessels (the arteries) leads to forceful squirting of bright red (highly oxygenated) blood. The squirting of arterial blood is directly related to the beat of the heart.

Large venous and arterial hemorrhages, if not controlled, may be fatal. Blood volume varies with body size. The average adult has about five liters (approximately five quarts) of blood. Adults may lose approximately 500 ml (approximately one pint) of blood without any problems. This amount is equal to the amount given during a blood donation. Loss of one liter of blood may result in hypovolemic shock. Greater losses, 1,500 ml and up, are usually lethal. Hemorrhaging in a closed cavity also may cause organ damage due to increased pressure. For example, bleeding in the head may lead to brain tissue damage and/or death from the resulting increase in intracranial pressure.

Chronic hemorrhage, such as those occurring in the gastrointestinal tract and female reproductive tract, commonly lead to anemia. Normal menstrual bleeding is approximately 70-80 ml. As discussed in Chapter 7, replacement of the lost iron also may lead to iron deficiency anemia.

## Shock

Shock can be defined in many ways, but basically it is extremely low blood pressure that leads to decreased tissue **perfusion** (to pour through or supply with blood).

**ETIOLOGY** This low blood pressure may be caused by one of three mechanisms:

1. not enough blood volume

2. inadequate pumping of blood by the heart

3. vasodilatation that allows blood to pool in the vessels, thereby reducing circulating blood volume. Remember, the vascular system is composed of thousands of miles of vessels. If all these vessels were to open at the same time, the circulating volume of blood would be zero.

Shock may be caused by a variety of situations. Every injury brings about some degree of shock and should be treated appropriately. No matter the cause, shock leads to inadequate perfusion of tissues with blood. Inadequate tissue perfusion may cause tissue hypoxia, anoxia, ischemia, and necrosis as discussed in Chapter 2. Types of shock include:

■ Cardiogenic—the leading cause of death due to shock. This type of shock results from the inability of the heart to pump blood adequately, often due to myocardial infarction. Treatment may involve cardiopulmonary resuscitation, and administration of cardiotonic and vasoconstrictor medications (vasoconstrictor medications cause muscle contraction of vessels, increasing blood pressure).

■ Septic—the second most common cause of death due to shock. Septic shock usually results from an overwhelming septicemia (bacteria or microorganisms in the blood). Treatment may involve administration of antibiotics and vasoconstrictor medications.

■ Hypovolemic—results from low fluid volume and may be due to hemorrhage (often called hemorrhagic shock), severe burns leading to loss of blood plasma, severe vomiting, and diarrhea. Treatment may involve blood transfusions and intravenous fluid volume replacement.

■ Neurogenic—results from generalized vasodilatation, and may be due to highly emotional situations such as fear, surprise, pain, and unpleasant sights. Medications and spinal anesthesia also may lead to neurogenic shock. Treatment may involve vasoconstrictor medications.

■ Anaphylactic—results from severe allergic reactions, and may be due to allergens such as contrast dyes for diagnostic tests, bee stings, medications, and blood transfusion reaction. Treatment may involve removing the allergen and administering antihistamines and bronchodilators.

**SYMPTOMS** Signs and symptoms of shock vary, depending on the degree of the situation, and may include facial pallor, cool and clammy skin, cyanosis, tachycardia, tachypnea, altered mental status, syncope (fainting), unconsciousness, oliguria, and anuria.

**TREATMENT** Treatment depends on the type of shock. Other treatment measures include laying the individual in a supine (on the back) position, keeping the individual warm and quiet, and elevating the feet and legs above heart level to improve vascular return.

# RARE DISEASES

## Malignant Hypertension

Malignant hypertension is a form of essential hypertension that is considered a medical emergency. Diastolic blood pressure may reach 130 to 170 mm Hg. Symptoms include headache, blurred vision, and dyspnea. Without treatment, malignant hypertension is fatal.

## Cor Pulmonale

Cor pulmonale is right-sided heart failure related to acute or chronic pulmonary disease. Increased pulmonary blood pressure causes hypertrophy of the right ventricle, leading to decreased pumping ability. Polycythemia develops as the body tries to compensate for hypoxemia. This increase in red blood cell number increases the viscosity of the blood, further increasing workload on the heart. Treatment involves treating the lung disease and may also include phlebotomy to decrease blood viscosity.

## Raynaud's Disease

Raynaud's disease is a vasospastic disorder primarily affecting the fingers and toes. This idiopathic disease occurs most frequently in young women, and is usually related to cold temperature and emotional stress. During vasospasm, the extremities may turn pale and then cyanotic before returning to normal color. As the disease progresses, small ulcers may develop on the extremities, and may lead to contractures and chronic disability of the hands. Treatment is avoidance of cold and application of warmth to the extremities. Cigarette smoking is discouraged as nicotine causes further vasoconstriction.

## Buerger's Disease

Buerger's disease is also known as thromboangiitis (thrombo = clot, angi = vessel, itis = inflammation) obliterans and is an inflammation of the peripheral vessels with clot formation. The affected individual often has pain in the legs and feet that is made worse with activity and improves with rest. Progression of the disease leads to muscle atrophy, ulcers, and gangrene. The primary cause of Buerger's disease is cigarette smoking. Treatment involves cessation of smoking, exercises to improve circulation, and vessel bypass surgery.

## Polyarteritis Nodosa

Polyarteritis nodosa is a vasculitis that is characterized by inflammatory, necrotizing lesions in many different vessels. This rare autoimmune disease is usually fatal as a result of occlusion and rupture of the involved vessels.

## EFFECTS OF AGING ON THE SYSTEM

Heart and blood vessel diseases are a significant cause of death and disability in the older adult. As the individual ages, the heart muscle loses some of its contractility, causing a decreased cardiac output and/or an increased heart rate to compensate for the changes.

The vessels lose elasticity, and become more rigid and narrowed. The valves also lose some functioning, and become thick and sclerotic. These changes add to the workload of the heart by increasing the heart rate and the blood pressure. The older adult may become tachycardic with minimal exercise. Although many of the changes in the system are due to the normal aging process, other changes observed in the older adult are directly due to lifestyle. Many individuals have smoked for years, been overweight, eaten a high-fat diet, endured a stressful job, and lived a fairly sedentary life. These modifiable behaviors contribute to the adverse changes in the cardiovascular system, and increase the risk of chronic and acute problems in the system over time. Most older adults are at risk for hypertension, myocardial infarction, angina, arrhythmias, congestive heart failure, varicosities, and other cardiovascular problems.

With age, the arteries become more rigid, causing decreased blood flow to organs and distal body tissues. The vein valves lose some of their competency, reducing good blood flow even further. Decreased peripheral circulation often results in cool and/or pale extremities, improper healing, and pooling of fluid (edema) in the legs and feet. Medications may not be as efficiently transmitted to the body with these changes in circulation. This can affect the therapeutic regimen for the individual.

Many older adults have postural hypotension, which can be a significant safety problem. Postural hypotension is the decrease or drop in blood pressure that occurs when the individual rises to a sitting or standing position from a reclining position. The individual usually feels very dizzy on rising and may fall. Prevention strategies should be in place to prevent injuries due to postural hypotension.

## SUMMARY

The cardiovascular system is responsible for pumping the blood throughout the body, delivering nutrients and oxygen to cells, and removing waste products. Cardiovascular disease affects over 64 million Americans. It is a significant cause of mortality, especially in the older adult. The risk for developing many diseases of the system can be reduced by lifestyle behavioral changes. Common symptoms of cardiovascular disease include pain, fatigue, difficulty breathing, tachycardia, cyanosis, and edema. Some of the most common disorders of the system include hypertension, coronary artery disease, arteriosclerosis, and varicosities. Older adults are at greatest risk for developing heart disease. It is the number one cause of death in the older population.

# REVIEW QUESTIONS

## Multiple Choice

1. Which of the following risk factors are controllable or modifiable?

   **a.** heredity    **d.** stress

   **b.** diet       **e.** smoking

   **c.** age        **f.** exercise

2. Which of the following statements *are correct* in relation to coronary artery disease?

   **a.** It is often called coronary heart disease.

   **b.** Slow, progressive occlusion of arteries often leads to development of collateral arteries that extend into ischemic tissue, providing some protection against infarction.

   **c.** It will always lead to a myocardial infarction.

   **d.** Diagnosis of CAD is made by evaluating the history, EKG, and angiograms.

   **e.** CAD is not usually diagnosed in the older adult.

   **f.** The disease is commonly due to atherosclerosis.

3. Define the following terms related to hemorrhage.

   **a.** Petechiae

   **b.** Ecchymosis

   **c.** Purpura

## Short Answer

4. What are the functions of the cardiovascular system?

5. Which signs and symptoms are associated with common cardiovascular system disorders?

6. Which diagnostic tests are most commonly used to determine the type and/or cause of cardiovascular system disorders?

7. What symptoms are usually seen in congestive heart failure?

8. What is the difference between phlebitis and thrombophlebitis?

**9.** What are the most common signs and symptoms of shock?

**10.** What are some of the changes occurring in the cardiovascular system with age?

## CASE STUDY

**Mr. Winston** is a 72-year-old who has been diagnosed with congestive heart failure. He is a middle-class gentleman with a fairly broad educational background. He is a college graduate who has managed a business for 30 years. He asks you to explain his condition to him and his wife. How would you explain congestive heart failure to them? In addition, he wants to know why he is so short of breath at times, why he has pitting edema in his ankles in the evenings, and why the physician ordered a low-sodium diet. How would you answer those questions?

## BIBLIOGRAPHY

Bro, S. (2003). How abnormal calcium, phosphate, and parathyroid hormone relate to cardiovascular disease. *Nephrology Nursing Journal 30*(3), 275–283.

Burke, L. E., & Fair, J. (2003) Promoting prevention. *Journal of Cardiovascular Nursing 18*(4), 256–266.

Fair, J. M. (2003). Cardiovascular risk factor modification. *Journal of Cardiovascular Nursing 18*(3), 161–168.

Ferri, R. S. (2003). Prehypertension? *American Journal of Nursing 103*(9), 18.

Ferri, R. S., & Sofer, D. (2003). A new "crystal ball" for cardiac health? *American Journal of Nursing 10*(2), 19.

George, E. L. (2003). Predicting heart disease with c-reactive protein. *Nursing 33*(5), 70–71.

Haskell, W. J. (2003). Cardiovascular disease prevention and lifestyle interventions. *Journal of Cardiovascular Nursing 18*(4), 245–255.

Hughes, S. (2003). Novel cardiovascular risk factors. *Journal of Cardiovascular Nursing 18*(2), 131–138.

Initial hypertension treatment. (2003). *American Journal of Nursing 103*(5), 56.

Kennedy, M. S. (2002). Heart disease and stroke prevention. *American Journal of Nursing 102*(2), 20.

King, J. E. (2003). Could my patients have deep vein thrombosis? *Nursing 33*(9), 24.

Lifestyle and BP control. (2003). *Australian Nursing Journal 111*(1), 18.

Mennen, A., & Garner, K. (2003). Recent advances in the management of cardiothoracic patients. *Australian Nursing Journal 11*(3), 19–22.

Miracle, V. A. (2003). The latest in cardiac nursing. *Dimensions of Critical Care Nursing 22*(6), 251–252.

Mohacsi, A., Magyar, J., Banyasz, T., & Nanasi, P. P. (2004). Effects of endothelins on cardiac and vascular cells: New therapeutic target for the future? *Current Vascular Pharmacology 2*(1), 53–63.

Moore, A. (2003). After HRT: What now? *Nursing 33*(6), 13–15.

More evidence needed for "salt assault". (2004, January 11). Medical Letter on the CDC & FDA, 33–34.

New guidelines lower "normal" BP. (2003). *Nursing 33*(8), 34.

Nicolls, C., & Sani, M. (2003). The treatment of cardiovascular disease in older people. *Nursing Older People 15*(7), 31–32.

Oken, K., & Fletcher, G. (2003). Benefits of aggressive drug therapy. *Journal of Cardiovascular Nursing 18*(2), 7954.

Poor fitness in young adults associated with development of CVD risk factors. (2004, January 2). *Drug Week*, 280–281.

Rodgers, J. M., & Reeder, S. J. (2002). Managing heart failure. *Nursing Management 33*(10), 48A-56A.

Shellman, J. (2000). Promoting elderly wellness through a community-based blood pressure clinic. *Public Health Nursing 17*(4), 257-263.

Speck, B. J., & Harrell, J. S. (2003). Maintaining regular physical activity in women. *Journal of Cardiovascular Nursing 18*(4), 282-291.

Spivak, J. (2004). Daily aspirin—only half the answer. *New England Journal of Medicine 350*(2), 99-101.

Take it to heart. (2004). *Better Nutrition 66*(1), 30.

The low down on cholesterol. (2003). *Nursing 33*(6), 16-17.

Tsai, J., Wang, W., Chan, P., Lin, L., Wang, C., Tomlinson, B., Hsie, M., Yang, H., & Liu, J. (2003). The beneficial effects of Tai Chi Chuan on blood pressure and lipid profile and anxiety status in a randomized controlled trial. *Journal of Alternative and Complementary Medicine 9*(5), 747-754.

Whiteman, K., & Kress, T. (2003). Help me catch my breath! *Nursing 33*(12), 32-34.

Willoughby, S., Holmes, A., & Loscalzo, J. (2002). Platelets and cardiovascular disease. *European Journal of Cardiovascular Nursing 1*(4), 273-276.

Wingerter, L. (2003). Vascular access device thrombosis. *Clinical Journal of Oncology Nursing 7*(3), 345-348.

Women take heart. (2003). *American Journal of Nursing 103*(12), 18.

Woodrow, P. (2003). Assessing pulse in older people. *Nursing Older People 15*(6), 3840.

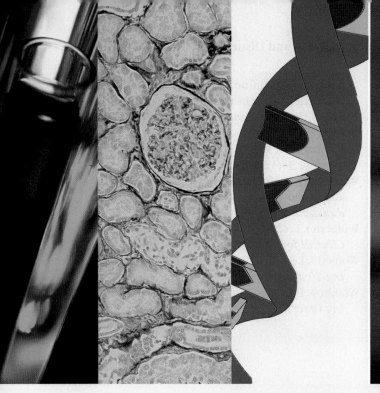
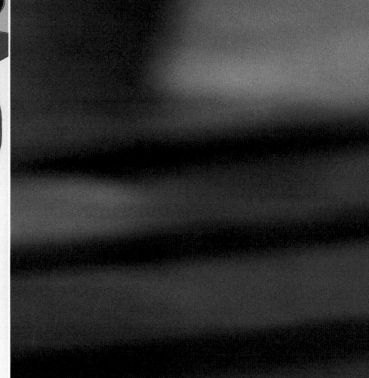

## OUTLINE

## KEY TERMS

# Respiratory System Diseases and Disorders

## LEARNING OBJECTIVES

*Upon completion of the chapter, the learner should be able to:*

1. Define the terminology common to the respiratory system and the disorders of the system.

2. Discuss the basic anatomy and physiology of the respiratory system.

3. Identify the important signs and symptoms associated with common respiratory system disorders.

4. Describe the common diagnostics used to determine type and/or cause of the respiratory system disorders.

5. Identify the common disorders of the respiratory system.

6. Describe the typical course and management of the common respiratory system disorders.

7. Describe the effects of aging on the respiratory system and the common disorders of the system.

## OVERVIEW

*The respiratory system includes the chest, lungs, and internal airway structures. To continue life, the individual must breathe and have a continuous exchange of oxygen for carbon dioxide. Breathing and the exchange of gases that takes place within the system are complex processes involving the respiratory system, as well as the neurological and circulatory systems. Diseases of the respiratory system include some of the most well-known disorders such as the common cold and pneumonia. Respiratory diseases affect all ages, but older people are the most susceptible to both chronic and acute disorders of the system.* ■

## ANATOMY AND PHYSIOLOGY

The respiratory system consists of the chest (thorax), lungs, and conducting airways. The chest or thorax is the structure that houses the lungs and the mediastinum (includes heart and vessels). The respiratory system structures in the thorax include the lungs, 12 pairs of ribs, part of the vertebral column, and the sternum. The diaphragm, a large muscle of respiration, separates the thorax from the abdomen (Figure 9-1). The lungs are two spongy organs divided into three lobes in the right lung and two lobes in the left lung. The lungs lie in the pleural cavity in the thorax. This cavity is lined with a membrane called the pleura. The lungs are also covered with a second membrane or pleura. Between the two pleural membranes is a lubricating liquid that prevents friction as the process of breathing and lung expansion occurs.

Usually, the airways of the respiratory system are divided into two parts. The upper respiratory system includes the nose (nasal cavities), mouth, sinuses, pharynx, and larynx. The lower respiratory system includes the trachea, bronchi, and bronchioles. The alveoli are found at the distal end of the terminal bronchioles. They are grape-like clusters of air sacs that are surrounded by capillaries (Figure 9-2). This is where the oxygen-carbon dioxide gas exchange in the lungs occurs.

The mechanism of ventilation and gas exchange is a complex process. Ventilation is the movement of air into and out of the respiratory system. This requires both inhalation and exhalation to occur. Ventilation is controlled by chemosensory receptors in spinal fluid, and in the carotid and aortic arteries, arterial carbon dioxide tension and oxygen deficiency. As the receptors detect increases or decreases in carbon dioxide and/or oxygen, ventilation is increased or decreased as needed to meet body requirements. This process can be altered by respiratory or neurologic disease because the respiratory control center is located in the medulla of the brain.

The exchange of gases occurs both in the lungs and throughout the body at the tissue level. In the

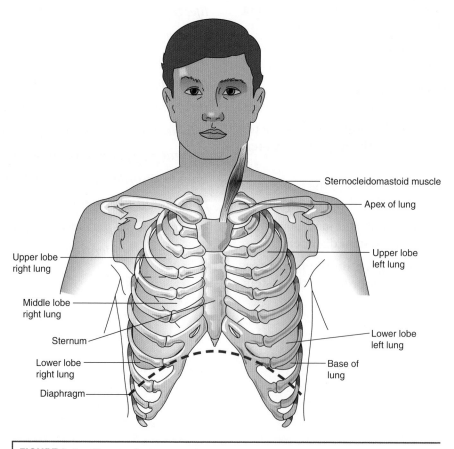

Upper lobe right lung

Middle lobe right lung

Sternum

Lower lobe right lung

Diaphragm

Sternocleidomastoid muscle

Apex of lung

Upper lobe left lung

Lower lobe left lung

Base of lung

**FIGURE 9–1**    The respiratory system.

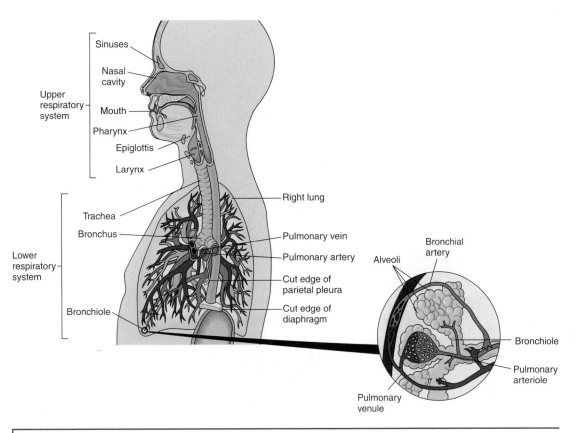

**FIGURE 9–2**  Airway divisions and terminal bronchiole/alveoli.

lungs, carbon dioxide is released from the capillary beds into the alveolar spaces by the process of diffusion. In the same way, oxygen moves from the air spaces into the capillaries for transport to the tissues. This process is reversed at the tissue level throughout the body where oxygen moves from the bloodstream into the tissues, and carbon dioxide moves from the tissues into the blood for transport to the lungs and removal from the body (Figure 9–3).

## COMMON SIGNS AND SYMPTOMS

There are many common signs and symptoms of respiratory disease. These symptoms can range from mild (the common cold) to severe (pneumonia). Dyspnea, orthopnea, apnea, wheezing, coughing, and nasal discharge are some of the most common symptoms.

**Dyspnea** (DISP-nee-ah; dys = difficulty, pnea = breathing) is a common sign of respiratory disease. Dyspnea may be in the form of **orthopnea** (or-THOP-nee-ah; ortho = straight, pnea = breathing) where an individual has difficulty breathing in a lying position

or is able to breathe with less difficulty when standing or sitting "straight" up. **Apnea** (ap-NEE-ah; a = without, pnea = breathing) for an extended amount of time is a life-threatening emergency. Dyspnea caused by a partial obstruction of the airways will produce **wheezing**. Severe dyspnea may lead to **hypoxemia** (high-POX-**SEE**-me-ah; hypo = not enough, ox = oxygen, emia = blood) or low blood oxygen level. A common sign of hypoxemia is **cyanosis** (SIGH-ah-**NO**-sis; cyano = blue, osis = condition) or a blue color often observed in the nail beds and lips.

Coughing is another common symptom caused by irritation of the airways or a buildup of fluid in the lung tissue. **Sputum** (SPYOU-tum) is fluid or secretions coughed up from the lungs, not to be confused with saliva or spit from the digestive system. A **productive cough** is one in which sputum or excessive mucus is brought up and expelled. Coughing up blood is called **hemoptysis** (he-MOP-tih-sis; hemo = blood, ptysis = saliva) and may be a sign of serious respiratory disease.

Nasal discharge is frequently present in infections, inflammation, and in allergic respiratory reactions. It

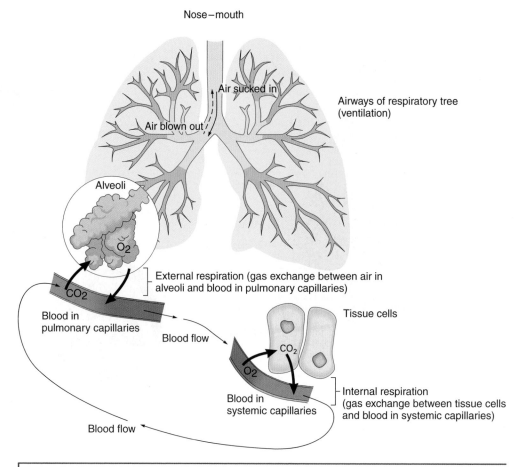

Nose—mouth

Air sucked in

Air blown out

Airways of respiratory tree (ventilation)

Alveoli

$O_2$

$CO_2$

External respiration (gas exchange between air in alveoli and blood in pulmonary capillaries)

Blood in pulmonary capillaries

Blood flow

Tissue cells

$CO_2$

$O_2$

Internal respiration (gas exchange between tissue cells and blood in systemic capillaries)

Blood in systemic capillaries

Blood flow

**FIGURE 9–3**   Gas exchange in the lungs and tissues.

is the most frequent symptom of the common cold, but it is also present in other respiratory disorders and may be a serious symptom of a chronic problem.

Hiccoughs, commonly called "hiccups," are the result of a sudden spasm of the diaphragm. They commonly occur after eating or drinking, and can be stopped by a variety of techniques including holding the breath and drinking water through a straw. Hiccoughs may accompany disease, and in this instance, are more difficult to eliminate.

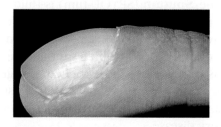

**FIGURE 9–4**   Clubbing. (*Courtesy of Robert A. Silverman, M.D., Pediatric Dermatology, Georgetown University.*)

Chronic respiratory conditions often lead to abnormal, permanent signs such as clubbing and barrel-chested appearance. **Clubbing** is a condition of unknown pathogenesis, but it usually is related to poor distal circulation and oxygenation. It affects the distal portion of the finger and is characterized by soft tissue enlargement and an abnormal curvature of the nail (Figure 9-4). A barrel chest appears as the individual uses accessory chest muscles over a long period of time in an effort to improve breathing.

## DIAGNOSTIC TESTS

A physical examination including auscultation (listening to the chest with a stethoscope) should be completed to assess for abnormal breathing quality and rate. **Tachypnea** (TACK-ihp-**NEE**-ah; tachy = rapid, pnea = breathing) or rapid breathing, and abnormal breath sounds including wheezes, rales, and rhonchi are common with respiratory diseases. **Rales** are abnormal musical sounds heard on inspiration and are often called crackles. **Rhonchi** are dry rattling sounds in the bronchi due to obstruction of the airways.

A chest roentgenogram (X-ray) is a major diagnostic tool utilized to diagnose lung diseases such as tumors, tuberculosis, abscesses, and pneumonia. Sputum cultures are effective in determination of infectious disease. A tissue biopsy may be obtained as a definitive test for lung disease. Tissue biopsy is often obtained during a **bronchoscopy** (brong-KOS-koh-pee; broncho = bronchus or lung passageways, oscopy = procedure to look into the bronchus) (Figure 9–5). Lung tissue may be biopsied utilizing a fine needle technique.

The best indicator of lung function is measurement of the amounts of carbon dioxide (waste) and oxygen in the blood. This measurement is done on arterial blood and is called **arterial blood gases** (ABGs). Normal arterial blood gases should be high in oxygen and low in carbon dioxide. Parameters for normal ABGs are oxygen ($PaO_2$) 70–100 mm Hg and carbon dioxide ($PaCO_2$) 35–45 mm Hg. The reverse of these readings is indicative of poor pulmonary function. Another important ABG is oxygen saturation ($O_2Sat$) with normal levels of 95–100%.

Pulmonary function tests (PFT) are a group of tests that measure volume and flow of air by utilizing a spirometer (Figure 9–6). PFTs are valuable in

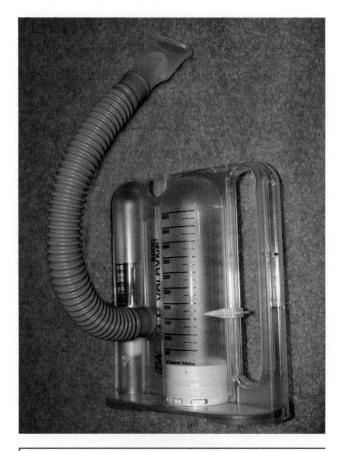

**FIGURE 9–6** Spirometry: used for pulmonary function tests. (Voldyne 5000 Incentive Spirometer. Photo courtesy of Hudson, RCI. Voldyne is a registered trademark of Hudson RCI.)

the diagnosis of a respiratory problem. PFTs may also be performed before and after brochodilation treatment to measure treatment effectiveness. PFTs are measured against a norm for the individual's age, height, and sex.

## COMMON DISEASES OF THE RESPIRATORY SYSTEM

Diseases of the respiratory system range from simple to very serious. The symptoms of the various disorders are often similar in the early stages, with most conditions manifesting in shortness of breath, coughing, and/or wheezing. However, some disorders may not present symptoms until late in the disease development. Smoking is the number one risk behavior for developing chronic respiratory disease.

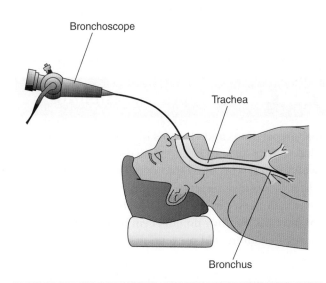

Bronchoscope

Trachea

Bronchus

**FIGURE 9–5** Bronchoscopy.

## Diseases of the Upper Respiratory Tract

Respiratory illnesses, which are mostly viral infections, account for approximately 50 percent of all acute illnesses. Respiratory infections account for over 80 percent of all infections (Figure 9–7). Most disorders of the upper respiratory tract are not life threatening.

**Upper Respiratory Infection (URI).** Upper respiratory infection is a broad term referring to several infectious diseases of the upper respiratory tract. These infections are the most common cause for lost days of work for adults.

**ETIOLOGY** Most URIs (not to be confused with UTI—urinary tract infection) are caused by viruses. The most common is a group called rhinovirus.

**TREATMENT** General treatment for viral diseases includes rest, drinking increased amounts of fluids,

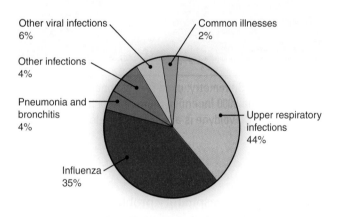

Other viral infections 6%
Common illnesses 2%
Other infections 4%
Pneumonia and bronchitis 4%
Upper respiratory infections 44%
Influenza 35%

**FIGURE 9–7** Frequency of infectious diseases.

taking **antipyretics** (anti = against, pyretic = fever), and **analgesics** (an = without, algesic = pain). Antibiotics are not effective with viral infections, but may be needed for secondary bacterial infection. The common cold is the most frequent URI and often leads to secondary infectious diseases.

### ■ Common Cold (Acute Rhinitis)

The common cold is an acute inflammation of the mucous membranes of the upper respiratory tract.

**ETIOLOGY** There are several hundred different virus strains that cause a cold. Developing immunity to one strain does not provide immunity to others.

**SYMPTOMS** Most individuals are very familiar with the symptoms of runny nose (**rhinorrhea**, rhino = nose, orrhea = run through), watery eyes, stuffy head, sore throat, sneezing, and fever.

A cold is very contagious, and is usually passed from one individual to another through touch and air droplets. Good hand washing is the best preventive measure against a cold. Many individuals believe that getting chilled and/or wet is the cause of a cold. In actuality, these actions do not directly cause a cold; they merely lower an individual's resistance to invasion by a cold-causing virus. Children, older people, and individuals in generally poor health are at increased risk of contracting a cold.

### ■ Hay Fever (Allergic Rhinitis)

Allergic rhinitis is an inflammation of the mucous membranes due to allergies. This sensitivity to an allergen tends to run in families. Ragweed and grasses are two common allergens. Hay fever was discussed in detail in Chapter 5.

## COMPLEMENTARY AND ALTERNATIVE THERAPY

**Vitamin and Herbal Preparations for Colds**

There are a variety of herbal preparations and vitamins that are advertised as cold remedies. Research has shown some to be ineffective such as Vitamin C, but others have not been well studied. The latest studies on zinc as a cold remedy have not shown consistently positive results. Herbal preparations such as goldenseal and elderberry have not been proven to reduce the symptoms of a cold or shorten the length of the cold, but they do not seem harmful either. Echinacea has demonstrated some benefit in cold prevention, especially in children (see Chapter 5.)

*Source: Carmichael, M. (January 12, 2004).*

## ◼️ Sinusitis

Sinusitis is an inflammation of the mucous membrane lining the sinuses. The sinuses are air-filled cavities in the bony tissue of the head. The membranes that line the nose extend into the sinuses.

**ETIOLOGY** For this reason, acute rhinitis often leads to sinusitis. It is also believed that blowing the nose too hard actually spreads infection into the sinuses. Other causes of sinusitis include tooth infections, air pollution, and nasal deformities.

**SYMPTOMS** As mucous membranes become swollen, the drainage system becomes blocked. Mucus accumulates in the sinuses, causing increased pressure, and often leading to sinus headaches, dizziness, and difficulty breathing.

**TREATMENT** Treatment often includes antibiotics and decongestants. Because sinusitis may lead to more serious infections like mastoiditis and encephalitis, aggressive treatment is necessary.

## ◼️ Pharyngitis

Pharyngitis is an inflammation of the throat (pharynx = throat, itis = inflammation) commonly called a "sore throat."

**ETIOLOGY** The most common cause is viral infection. Bacterial infection by streptococcus may also occur and is more common in children. Irritation to the mucous membranes may also lead to pharyngitis. Irritants may include breathing extremely hot or cold air, chemical fumes, or smoke.

**TREATMENT** Treatment may include throat lozenges, antiseptic or salt-water gargles, and analgesics. Bacterial infections need antibiotic treatment also. Chronic pharyngitis due to tonsillitis and adenoiditis may be treated by surgical removal of the tonsils and adenoids, called a tonsillectomy and adenoidectomy (T&A), respectively.

## ◼️ Laryngitis

Laryngitis is an inflammation of the larynx (lar-INKS) and vocal cords.

**ETIOLOGY** Laryngitis may be caused by viral or bacterial infections, or by breathing irritants such as extremely hot or cold air, chemical fumes, and smoke. Laryngitis frequently follows other URIs such as the common cold, pharyngitis, and sinusitis. Another cause may be overuse of the voice for an extended time.

**SYMPTOMS** Most individuals are familiar with the hoarse voice quality caused by laryngitis. Other symptoms include difficulty swallowing (dysphagia), throat pain, and fever.

**TREATMENT** Treatment may include voice rest, increased fluid intake, analgesics, throat lozenges, and removal of causative factors.

## Diseases of the Bronchi and Lungs

Diseases of the bronchi and lungs are usually more severe than diseases of the upper respiratory system. Many of these can be life threatening such as influenza, especially in the older population.

**Asthma.** Asthma is a hypersensitivity reaction that causes constriction of the bronchi, leading to difficulty breathing.

**ETIOLOGY** Asthma, also called bronchial asthma, was discussed in detail as a hypersensitivity disorder in Chapter 5.

**SYMPTOMS** Asthma is characterized by episodes of wheezing and dyspnea.

**TREATMENT** Treatment is aimed at identification and control of allergic factors, and use of bronchodilators.

**Acute Bronchitis.** Acute bronchitis is inflammation of the mucous membrane lining of the bronchus. It often involves the trachea (tracheobronchitis).

**ETIOLOGY** Acute bronchitis is a short-term disorder commonly following an upper respiratory infection. Inhaling fumes, smoke, dust, cold air, and other irritants also may cause acute bronchitis.

**SYMPTOMS** Symptoms include fever, a tight feeling behind the sternum, and a dry cough that later progresses to a productive cough (coughing up or expectorating mucus or sputum).

**TREATMENT** Treatment consists of rest, drinking increased amounts of fluids to help liquefy secretions, cough syrup, analgesics, and antipyretics. Antibiotics are helpful only if secondary bacterial infections occur. Prognosis is generally good for most individuals. Infants and small children may become seriously ill because the bronchioles are very small, and may become obstructed by swollen tissue or mucus plugs. Older people and the chronically ill may have a poor prognosis because they have an increased risk for developing secondary bacterial infections like pneumonia.

**Influenza (Flu).** Influenza is an acute, highly contagious respiratory infection.

**ETIOLOGY** Influenza is a viral infection commonly spread by coughing of respiratory secretions. There are many strains of influenza virus. The primary strains are identified as A, B, and C. Substrains or subtypes include H0N1, H1N1, H2N2, H3N2, and several others. The flu virus also has great genetic variation. The number of strains and variations help explain how this virus causes epidemics year after year. Unfortunately, like the common cold, immunity to one viral strain does not provide immunity to another; for this reason, an individual may have the flu multiple times. Flu epidemics commonly occur in the winter and early spring.

**SYMPTOMS** Influenza is characterized by sudden onset of fever, chills, headache, and back muscle pain. Other symptoms may include cough, runny nose, sore throat, sneezing, hoarseness, nausea, vomiting, and diarrhea.

**TREATMENT** Treatment of influenza is symptomatic and may include bed rest, analgesics, and antipyretics. Antibiotics are not indicated unless secondary bacterial infections occur. Complications related to bacterial infection include those affecting the sinuses, ear, and lungs. Pneumonia in the very young, old, and chronically ill may be fatal. For this reason, influenza vaccination should be given to older people and those individuals with chronic disease. Generally, the prognosis is good if complications do not occur.

**Chronic Obstructive Pulmonary Disease (COPD).** Chronic obstructive pulmonary disease is the name for a group of pulmonary diseases characterized by the inability to get air into or out of the lungs.

**ETIOLOGY** Ninety percent of the time, these problems are due to cigarette smoking. The two most common diseases classified as COPD are chronic bronchitis and emphysema. Because the etiology is the same—cigarette smoking—these two diseases usually coexist. There can be pure forms of either, but usually, the individual has predominantly one or the other coexisting with the second. For this reason, the diagnosis of COPD may describe the condition more adequately.

Individuals with COPD often become debilitated in the final stages of the disease. Loss of normal respiratory response is not unusual. Normally, individuals are stimulated to breathe by an increase of carbon dioxide in the blood. A secondary or backup stimulus is a decrease of oxygen in the blood. Individuals with COPD commonly have high levels of carbon dioxide in the blood. Initially, the body attempts to correct this by increasing breathing in an effort to blow out excessive $CO_2$. When this effort fails, the respiratory system adapts to the high $CO_2$ levels and begins responding to the secondary system, low

 **HEALTHY HIGHLIGHT**

## Influenza Immunization or "Flu Shots"

Because influenza is a viral infection, there is no treatment other than supportive treatment of symptoms. An individual is dependent on the immune system to build antibodies to kill the virus. Antibiotics may be helpful for secondary bacterial infections but do not kill the influenza virus.

The best course in dealing with flu is prevention. Prevention includes frequent hand washing to remove virus, avoiding crowds of people during flu season or when there is a local epidemic, avoiding individuals infected with influenza, and leading a healthy lifestyle to keep resistance high.

An immunization is available and is recommended for older people, those with chronic diseases, pregnant women, and health care workers. Reactions to the flu immunization are rare but do occur. Individuals allergic to eggs should not take the immunization as the virus is grown in eggs. Allergic hypersensitivity reactions usually occur immediately after receiving the injection. A reaction to the antigen may occur six to twelve hours after the injection. Reaction symptoms mimic the flu and include fever, muscle pain, and malaise.

blood oxygen levels. Giving oxygen to these individuals may be fatal because high oxygenation removes the stimulus to breathe.

Diagnosis of COPD is made by history and physical examination, and by ruling out other pulmonary diseases. Chest X-rays, pulmonary function tests (PFT), and arterial blood gases (ABGs) help confirm the diagnosis. There is no cure for end stage COPD. Cessation of smoking may slow or reverse the disease in the early stages, and will ease symptoms in the later stages.

**TREATMENT** Symptomatic treatment includes use of bronchodilator medications, inhalers, mucolytics, and cough medications. Avoiding exposure to individuals with respiratory tract infections is important because these diseases aggravate COPD. Influenza vaccination is recommended. Prognosis is poor due to progressive deterioration of pulmonary function, often leading to respiratory failure and death.

## ■ Chronic Bronchitis

Chronic bronchitis is a long-term inflammation of the mucous membranes of the bronchus. It is characterized by increased mucus production with a productive cough. Chronic inflammation leads to hypertrophy of the mucus-secreting glands, thickening of the mucous membrane, and **bronchiectasis** (BRONG-kee-**ECK**-tah-sis) or a chronic dilatation of the bronchus.

**SYMPTOMS** Bronchiectasis allows mucus to pool in the bronchus, producing a foul smelling cough. Chronic bronchitis may be mild in nature for many years. This form is commonly called a "smoker's cough" and occurs primarily in the morning hours. As the disease progresses, obstruction of the bronchi and bronchioles becomes more pronounced, leading to difficulty getting air into the lungs. Coughing, dyspnea, and **hypoxia** (HIGH-**POCK**-see-ah; hypo = low, oxia = oxygen) occur. During bouts of hypoxia, the individual often becomes cyanotic and may clinically be called "blue bloater." In the final or end stage, the symptoms are more continuous, causing lung damage, debilitation of the individual, and eventual death.

## ■ Emphysema

Emphysema comes from the Greek word *emphysana* meaning "to inflate". This chronic disease is characterized by an increased production of mucus, causing trapping of air in the tiny alveoli or air sacks of the lung. As air becomes trapped in the alveoli, they become overinflated, leading to destruction of the alveoli wall. Destruction of the alveoli wall allows the alveoli to fuse with another alveoli, forming a larger air sack and trapping more air (Figure 9-8).

**SYMPTOMS** The individual with emphysema is able to get air in, but the air becomes trapped and must be forced out before more air can be taken in. These enlarged alveoli have a decreased surface area, thus decreasing oxygenation of the blood. Air trapping and decreased oxygen exchange lead to dyspnea, tachypnea, wheezing, and coughing.

Individuals with emphysema often lean over a table or chair to more adequately use accessory respiratory muscles in an effort to blow out the trapped air. Pursing of the lips also helps hold the alveoli open while pushing the air out (Figure 9-9). This extra pressure often causes the face and skin to become reddened. For this reason, these individuals are clinically called "pink puffers." Extra pressure on the chest muscles also produces a characteristic "barrel chest" appearance.

Individuals with emphysema use large amounts of energy in their respiratory efforts. For this reason, a supplemented diet is often needed. The diet is eaten in small, frequent feedings to allow time for respiratory efforts. Even with a supplemented diet, these individuals are often unable to get adequate nutrition and commonly are physically very thin.

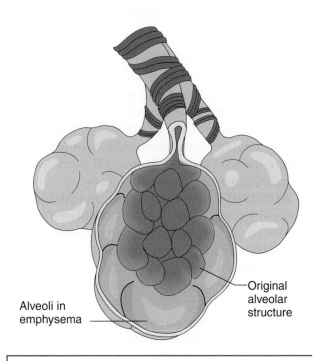

Alveoli in emphysema

Original alveolar structure

**FIGURE 9-8** Normal versus emphasematous alveoli.

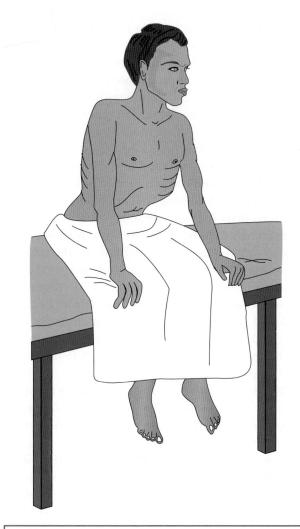

**FIGURE 9–9** Pursed lips and barrel chest of emphysema.

**Atelectasis.** Atelectasis is the collapse or airless state of part or all of a lung. More commonly, it affects only a small section of the lung.

**ETIOLOGY** Atelectasis is often related to inadequate breathing patterns related to pain. Surgical pain and fractured ribs often cause inadequate breathing, leading to atelectasis. Blockage of the airway by a mucus plug may also cause atelectasis.

**SYMPTOMS** Dyspnea, cyanosis, and anxiety are common symptoms. Diagnosis is confirmed after a positive chest X-ray and physical examination.

**TREATMENT** Prevention is aimed at relieving the cause if possible. Analgesics for pain, ambulation (walking), and frequent deep breathing and coughing help open the airway, expand the alveoli, and avoid atelectasis. Prognosis is good if complications do not occur. Pneumonia is a common complication.

**Pneumonia.** **ETIOLOGY** Pneumonia is an inflammation of the bronchioles and alveoli due to infection by bacteria, virus, or other pathogens. Pneumonia is the term specifically related to infection. Inflammation without infection is termed pneumonitis. Pneumonitis is inflammation generally caused by a hypersensitivity to dusts and chemicals.

Pneumonia may be identified in several ways. The cause may be included in the name as in pneumococcal, aspiration, and tuberculous. The location may be identified in the name as in lobar, bilateral, and double pneumonia. Secondary pneumonia indicates a connection to another cause. Often, the location and cause may be combined to describe the pneumonia as in bilateral pneumococcal pneumonia. No matter the cause and location, pneumonia affects approximately four million individuals each year. It is the most common cause of infectious death in the United States.

Pneumonia may range from mild to life threatening. Actions that inhibit the normal protective mechanisms of the respiratory system may lead to pneumonia. Such actions include smoking, immobility, general anesthesia, and endotracheal intubation. Pneumonia occurs more often among older people, the chronically ill, and those who are immunosuppressed, and is a significant cause of death in these individuals.

Pathogens may reach the lung tissue through the respiratory system or through the blood as a result of septicemia. Invasion of pathogens into the alveoli leads to inflammation of the alveolar tissue. Inflammation causes the classic outpouring of blood fluid and white cells from the capillaries into the tissues, filling the alveolus. This filling of the alveolus causes a decrease in gas exchange, leading to hypoxia (Figure 9–10).

**SYMPTOMS** Symptoms of pneumonia are related to the area involved and the amount of tissue involved. Symptoms include dyspnea, weakness, fever, chills, chest pain, and cough. Diagnosis is made after completion of a chest X-ray, history and physical examination, and sputum culture.

**TREATMENT** Treatment depends on cause. Bacterial infection is treated with antibiotics. Viral infection is treated symptomatically. Rest, analgesics, oxygen therapy, increased fluid intake, and high calorie diet are common for all types of pneumonia.

**Pulmonary Abscess.** Pulmonary abscess, also called lung abscess, is a collection of infectious material contained within a capsule (Figure 9–11). Abscess formation was discussed in detail in Chapter 4.

**ETIOLOGY** Abscess formation may be a complication of bacterial pneumonia, or aspiration of food or foreign objects.

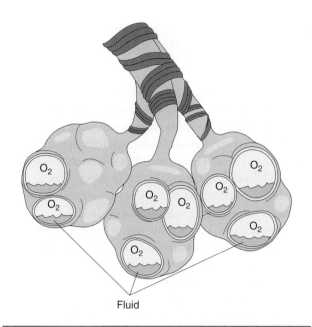

**FIGURE 9–10** Pneumonia: alveoli filling with fluid.

**SYMPTOMS** Symptoms include chills, fever, chest pain, and cough. Coughing of bloody or foul smelling sputum and foul smelling breath may also be indicative of a pulmonary abscess. Diagnosis is made by completion of a history and physical examination, chest X-ray, and sputum cultures.

**TREATMENT** Pulmonary abscesses are commonly treated with long-term antibiotic therapy. Surgical resection may be indicated if the abscess is quite large or if antibiotic therapy is unsuccessful.

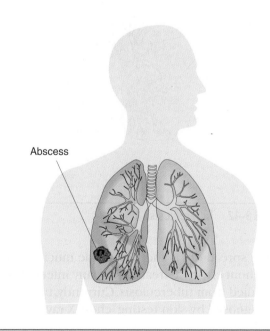

**FIGURE 9–11** Pulmonary abscess.

## Pulmonary Tuberculosis (TB).
Pulmonary tuberculosis is often called tuberculosis or TB. The pulmonary system is the one most often affected although the disease may spread to the kidneys, bones, and brain.

**ETIOLOGY** TB is a bacterial infection caused by *Mycobacterium tuberculosis*. It is acquired by breathing air that is infected with the bacteria, and is spread by coughing and sneezing.

**SYMPTOMS** Tuberculosis in an otherwise healthy individual often is asymptomatic. For this reason testing is needed to determine the presence of the disease. If symptoms appear, they are often vague and include loss of weight, energy, and appetite. As the disease progresses, the individual may become symptomatic with a chronic productive cough, dyspnea, fever, and night sweats.

*Mycobacterium tuberculosis* is protected in a strong coating that enables it to live outside the body for a lengthy amount of time. Infected droplets that are coughed or sneezed may dry up and remain on inanimate objects as dust. The tuberculosis bacteria can be killed by bactericidal solutions or by direct sunlight. TB is often prevalent in areas of overcrowding and poor sanitation. The incidence of tuberculosis was greatly reduced decades ago with the introduction of effective antibiotics. More recently, the number of TB cases in the United States has seriously risen due to the influx of high numbers of infected immigrants, the homeless, individuals with AIDS who have a poor resistance to infection, and the development of drug-resistant bacteria.

The infection begins with a primary lesion in the lungs. *Mycobacterium tuberculosis* does not attract PMNs and thus does not cause an acute inflammation. Lymphocytes and macrophages are attracted to these encapsulated bacteria. These immune cells begin producing antibodies and walling off the infection by forming a type of granuloma called a tubercule, hence the name tuberculosis. The inside of the tubercule contains dead bacteria, lung tissue, and immune cells that together exhibit a cheesy appearance called caseous necrosis.

After necrosis, the tubercules change by fibrosing and calcifying. If the immune system is effective in walling off the bacteria, the disease may be arrested or rendered inactive for a long period of time (months to years). During this time, the individual is often asymptomatic and not aware that he or she has tuberculosis. If the disease is not arrested, the individual will become symptomatic with progressive primary tuberculosis. The antibodies that are produced during this

## HEALTHY HIGHLIGHT

### Tuberculosis Skin Test (PPD)

TB skin testing works on the principle that once an individual is exposed to *Mycobacterium tuberculosis*, the immune system will develop antibodies. These antibodies will be present in all cells of the body (cellular immunity) from that point on. Introduction of the bacillus or a derivative, through injection or re-exposure, will cause a cellular reaction. The Mantoux (man-TOO) test utilizes this principle. A small amount of Purified Protein Derivative (PPD) is injected intra-dermally. PPD contains modified tuberculin bacteria that are no longer infectious. If the individual has been exposed to TB and has developed antibodies, the immune system will react. A reaction will also occur if the individual has been previously immunized with BCG (Bacille-Calmette-Guerin) tuberculin vaccine. A reaction is shown by the formation of an intradermal wheal. An 8–10 mm wheal within 72 hours of injection is considered a positive test.

Once an individual has a positive skin test, that individual will always react. For that reason, a skin test is no longer beneficial in determining if the individual has active TB. Individuals with a positive skin test need to be educated as to the symptoms of TB. They include unexpected weight loss, persistent cough, night sweats, and malaise. If these symptoms occur and persist, the individual will need a chest X-ray and possible sputum culture to determine the presence of disease.

time will circulate in the blood for the remainder of the infected individual's life in readiness to attack future tuberculosis bacteria. These circulating anti-bodies are the basis for the positive reaction of a TB skin test.

Secondary tuberculosis occurs when an individual is reinfected with *Mycobacterium tuberculosis* or the primary disease is reactivated due to a decline in the individual's resistance. Antibodies formed during the primary stage of the disease activate quickly and lead to larger areas of necrosis in the lung tissue. During secondary tuberculosis, the individual becomes symptomatic. The tubercule mass becomes liquified and is coughed up, leaving a cavity in the lung tissue (Figure 9–12). Frequent coughing often ruptures capillaries in the lung tissue, leading to hemoptysis or coughing and/or spitting of blood. Coughing by the infected individual fills the surrounding air with contagious bacteria, thus increasing the spread of the disease.

As large cavities are formed in the lung tissue, the ability of the tissue to oxygenate the blood is decreased. The individual becomes dyspneic and cachectic with a general appearance of being "consumed" by the disease. For this reason, historically, this disease was called consumption. During that time, individuals were placed in sanitariums to pre-

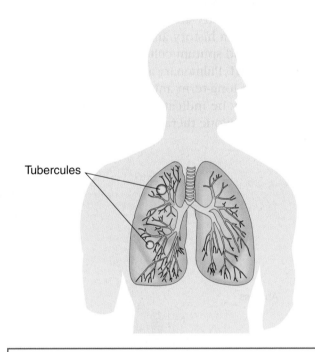

Tubercules

**FIGURE 9–12**  Tuberculosis.

vent the spread of TB and to provide much needed rest. Without effective treatment, many infected individuals died from tuberculosis. Currently, tuberculosis is diagnosed by skin testing, chest X-ray, and sputum culture.

**TREATMENT** Extended antibiotic therapy is needed to rid the individual of the infection.

## Adult Respiratory Distress Syndrome (ARDS).
Adult respiratory distress syndrome is also called "shock lung."

**ETIOLOGY** It often follows an episode of severe trauma such as shock, near drowning, fat embolism, aspiration pneumonia, or major burns. Following the trauma, the individual may be progressing smoothly when a sudden life-threatening attack of ARDs occurs.

**SYMPTOMS** ARDS is characterized by fluid escaping the vascular system and filling the alveoli, leading to acute respiratory failure.

**TREATMENT** Individuals suffer extreme dyspnea and need mechanical ventilation. Even with prompt and proper treatment, ARDs has a high mortality rate. Approximately one-third of the affected individuals dies within days, another third dies within weeks, usually due to pneumonia and heart failure. Approximately one-third recovers, but many of these individuals have permanent respiratory damage and are more prone to respiratory related illnesses.

## Sudden Acute Respiratory Syndrome (SARS).
Sudden acute respiratory syndrome (SARS) is the first severe, easily transmissible new disease to emerge in the twenty-first century. SARS is a respiratory illness that infected people in Asia, Europe, and North America starting in early 2003. Public health officials worked quickly to halt the spread of the disease, and actually contained it by July 2003. There are still gaps in our knowledge of this disease and although it has been contained, it is possible that outbreaks of SARS may reoccur as this disease may be seasonal and appear only during the winter months.

**ETIOLOGY** World experts have determined that SARS is caused by a previously unknown type of coronavirus, a family of viruses that usually causes only mild to moderate illness such as the common cold. This new virus has been named the SARS coronavirus.

The SARS virus appears to be spread by respiratory droplets. Persons who have close person-to-person contact with an infected individual are most at risk. Close contact is defined as having cared for or lived with someone with SARS, or having direct contact with the respiratory secretions of a person with SARS. Examples of close contact include sharing drinking and eating utensils, kissing, hugging, touching, or talking to someone within three feet. Close contact does not include walking past an infected individual or briefly sitting across from the person in a waiting room.

The SARS virus is thought to be easily spread when an infected individual coughs or sneezes, and spreads the infected respiratory droplets into the air as far as three feet. Infection may occur when these droplets fall on or are inhaled onto the mucous membranes of the mouth, nose, and eyes of persons nearby. The virus also may spread when a person touches an infected surface or object, then touches his or her mouth, nose, or eyes. Prevention includes avoiding contact with infected individuals and use of isolation procedures if contact is necessary. Respiratory isolation—including the use of gown, gloves, goggles, and an approved respiratory mask—are essential.

**SYMPTOMS** The most common symptoms of SARS include fever, malaise, chills, headache, myalgia, dizziness, rigors, cough, sore throat, and runny nose. Incubation of the SARS virsus appears to be approximately 7–10 days. In many cases, patients present with headache, dizziness, and myalgia. Temperature rises and becomes excessive as the disease progresses. In more acute cases, there is rapid deterioration with low oxygen saturation and acute respiratory distress requiring ventilatory support. Chest X-ray findings typically begin with small patchy shadows and then progress to generalized interstitial infiltrates. Adult Respiratory Distress Syndrome has been observed in a number of patients in end stage disease.

**TREATMENT** Treatment of SARS has included multiple antibiotic therapy although no clinical improvement has been demonstrated. The antiviral agent Ribavirin, given intravenously in combination with corticosteroids, may be somewhat effective. Early diagnosis, intensive care, mechanical ventilation, and symptomatic care with or without antiviral medications have improved prognosis. Fatality ratio for SARS is 0–50 percent, depending on the age and health of the persons affected, with an overall estimate of approximately 15 percent fatality rate.

## Lung Cancer.
Lung cancer is the leading cause of cancer deaths in the United States.

**ETIOLOGY** It is rare among those under 40, and in most cases, is caused by cigarette smoking. Ninety percent of lung cancer victims are smokers. Men are affected more commonly than women, although the increase in female smokers after World War II has increased the number of female lung cancer victims.

**SYMPTOMS** Lung cancer is often asymptomatic until metastasis has occurred. Metastasis to the brain,

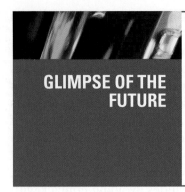

### Vaccine for Lung Cancer

Several cancer vaccines are in the trial stages and others are being tested in laboratory settings. A clinical trial is in progress testing a vaccine for lung cancer. Patients with non-small cell lung cancer are the subjects in this trial study. The vaccine contains a protein antigen that is showing some success in inducing an immunological response in the study subjects. The researchers are trying various approaches to develop a vaccine to prevent lung cancer in the future.

*Source:* Drug Week *(March 19, 2004).*

bone, and liver are common. Often, the first symptoms are those related to other organs affected by metastasis. Discovery by metastasis makes for a very poor prognosis. Approximately 10 percent of lung cancer victims survive five years. Symptoms related to the lung tumor are dyspnea, coughing, and hemoptysis. Diagnosis is made by X-ray and tissue biopsy.

**TREATMENT** Treatment includes chemotherapy, surgery, and radiation. If the tumor is discovered early, surgical removal may mean cure, but this is rarely the case.

## Diseases of the Pleura and Chest

Diseases of the pleura and chest may be caused by infection, trauma, or other diseases. Pain and shortness of breath are the common symptoms. The severity of the disorders can range from mild to severe, depending on the cause, the individual's age, medical history, and other complicating factors.

**Pleurisy (Pleuritis).** Pleurisy is the inflammation of the membranes covering the lung (visceral pleura) and lining the chest cavity (parietal pleura).

**ETIOLOGY** Pleurisy may be due to bacterial infection of the pleura. Secondary pleurisy often follows trauma, pneumonia, tuberculosis, and neoplasm.

**SYMPTOMS** The main symptom of pleurisy is a sharp chest area pain that increases with inspiration and coughing. Pain may be so severe that it limits movement in the affected area. Diagnosis is made by completion of a history and physical examination. Auscultation of the lungs may produce a squeaky, rubbing sound during inspiration.

**TREATMENT** Treatment is aimed at the cause and also includes symptomatic treatment with analgesics, heat application, and taping the chest to restrict movement and thus decrease pain.

**Pneumothorax.** Pneumothorax is a collection of air in the pleural cavity, often resulting in partial or complete collapse of the lung on the affected side (Figure 9–13). Spontaneous pneumothorax occurs when air is leaked into the pleural space from within or from the lung.

**ETIOLOGY** Common causes include pulmonary disease, tumor, or pulmonary tissue tear. Traumatic pneumothorax occurs when air enters the pleural cavity from outside the chest. Causes include gunshot wound, stabbing, or crushing of the chest. A rib fracture often causes a traumatic pneumothorax.

**SYMPTOMS** No matter the cause of the pneumothorax, symptoms are related to the degree of lung

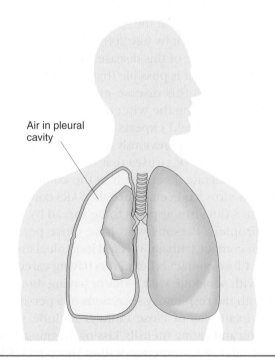

Air in pleural cavity

**FIGURE 9–13** Pneumothorax.

## The Harmful Effects of Smoking

Smoking tobacco products is the main cause of preventable death in the United States. Some of the other harmful effects of smoking include:

- its link to cancer, particularly cancer of the lung, larynx, esophagus, pancreas, bladder, kidney, and mouth. Thirty percent of cancer deaths are linked to smoking.
- heart and cardiovascular disease, especially stroke
- increased heart rate
- chronic bronchitis and emphysema
- decreased rate of lung tissue growth
- impaired level of lung function
- shortness of breath, especially with exercise, and increased phlegm production
- heartburn and peptic ulcers
- premature birth and low birth weight if used during pregnancy
- shortened life span with increased risk of morbidity
- addiction to nicotine

---

collapse. Complete lung collapse causes a sudden, severe chest pain, followed by severe dyspnea and symptoms of shock. Respirations are weak and shallow. Sucking breath sounds may be heard at the site of a traumatic wound. Increased air pressure on the affected side may cause a shift of the mediastinum toward the unaffected side. The condition of mediastinal shift is a medical emergency. Emergency treatment includes placing an occlusive dressing, clean hand, or plastic material over the sucking chest wound to prevent additional air from entering the chest.

Diagnosis is made by completion of a history and physical examination and chest X-ray.

**TREATMENT** Further treatment may include performance of a **thoracentesis** (THOR-rah-sen-**TEE**-sis; thora = chest, centesis = puncture) to insert a chest tube. The chest tube is used to withdraw air and assist in reexpanding the lung. Oxygen therapy and analgesics may also be prescribed.

**Hemothorax.** Hemothorax is the collection of blood in the chest cavity. Cause, symptoms, diagnosis, and treatments are the same as for a pneumothorax. Blood pressure and blood loss are monitored and treated as necessary.

**Pleural Effusion (Hydrothorax).** Pleural effusion or hydrothorax is a collection of fluid in the chest cavity.

**ETIOLOGY** Causes of hydrothorax may include congestive heart failure, tuberculosis, or pneumonia.

**SYMPTOMS** The affected individual may be asymptomatic, or may exhibit signs of dyspnea and chest or pleuritic pain. Diagnosis may be confirmed by X-ray.

**TREATMENT** Treatment may include thoracentesis to remove the excess fluid. Correction of the condition causing hydrothorax is needed to prevent reoccurrence.

**Empyema.** Empyema is the collection of pus (py = pus) in the chest cavity.

**ETIOLOGY** It may be the result of a ruptured lung abscess or an ulcerated tumor. Empyema is not as common as it was prior to the development of antibiotics.

**SYMPTOMS** Symptoms include coughing, dyspnea, and chest pain on the affected side. Diagnosis is by X-ray and thoracentesis.

**TREATMENT** Microbiologic cultures may be performed on the fluid to identify the infective organism. Antibiotic therapy is a common treatment for bacterial infections.

# Diseases of the Cardiovascular and Respiratory Systems

The cardiovascular and respiratory systems are so closely related that many diseases affect both systems. The degree to which each system is affected is often so close that it becomes difficult to classify the disease by one system over the other. For this reason, these diseases need further consideration.

**Pulmonary Embolism (PE).** Pulmonary embolism is a sudden blockage of an artery in the pulmonary system by an embolism (Figure 9–14).

**ETIOLOGY** Chapter 8 discussed the pathology of an embolism. Remember that the floating material may be a blood clot, fat globule, or piece of tissue. Commonly, a blood clot or thrombus develops in the veins of the lower legs, thighs, and pelvis. This clot then breaks loose, floats in the vascular system, and sticks in a pulmonary artery, resulting in a pulmonary embolism.

**SYMPTOMS** Symptoms of a PE vary greatly, depending on the size of the clot and the size of the area affected. Dyspnea, cough, chest pain, and apprehension are common symptoms. If the PE is severe, cyanosis, shock, and death may occur.

Factors that contribute to the development of an embolism are prolonged bed rest, obesity, and trauma or fractures of the legs or pelvis. Diagnosis is confirmed by X-ray examination, and lung scans.

**TREATMENT** Treatment is aimed at maintaining cardiopulmonary function by administering oxygen and anticoagulation medications. Prevention includes ambulation, antiembolic stockings, and leg exercises.

**Pulmonary Edema.** Pulmonary edema, if severe, may be a life-threatening medical emergency. This edema affects the tissue and air spaces of the lungs by filling them with fluid. The fluid leaks out of the vascular system due to increased vascular pressure.

**ETIOLOGY** Pulmonary edema is commonly seen as a result of congestive heart failure and resulting fluid buildup. Any disease that affects blood pressure, heart function, and blood fluid levels may lead to pulmonary edema. These diseases include hypertension, pulmonary embolism, and renal failure.

**SYMPTOMS** Pulmonary edema is characterized by dyspnea, orthopnea (ortho = straight, pnea = breath), or difficulty breathing when lying down, and a blood-tinged frothy sputum. It is diagnosed by utilizing arterial blood gases and chest X-ray. ABGs will show an increased carbon dioxide level, and chest X-rays will exhibit increased opacity or whiteness.

**TREATMENT** Treatment is aimed at reducing pressure and blood volume. Diuretics to increase urine output, cardiogenics to increase the contraction of the heart, and morphine to bring about venous dilatation may be prescribed. Mechanical respiratory ventilation may also be needed (Figure 9–15).

**Cor Pulmonale.** Cor pulmonale was discussed in Chapter 8. Remember that it is a right-sided heart fail-

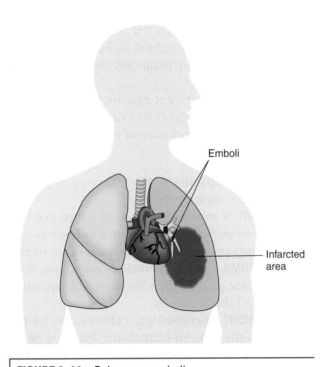

Emboli

Infarcted area

**FIGURE 9–14** Pulmonary emboli.

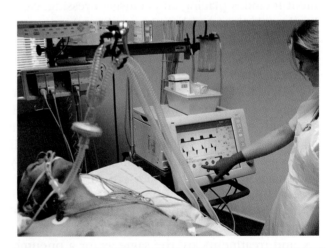

**FIGURE 9–15** Respiratory ventilator. *(Courtesy Draeger Medical, Inc., Telford, PA.)*

ure related to acute or chronic pulmonary disease. Increased pulmonary blood pressure causes enlargement of the right ventricle and decreased pumping ability. Polycythemia (poly = many, cyt = cell- red cell, emia = blood) develops as the body tries to compensate for hypoxemia (hypo = not enough, ox = oxygen, emia = blood), leading to a thickening of the blood and further increasing workload on the heart.

## TRAUMA

### Pneumothorax and Hemothorax

Pneumothorax and hemothorax often occur due to some type of trauma. Examples of trauma that often cause these conditions are fractured ribs, gun shot wounds, stabbings, and crushing chest injuries. Collapse of the lung, shock, and death are potential outcomes.

### Suffocation

Suffocation is the condition of not breathing to the point that the individual loses consciousness and eventually dies. Death is due to the lack of oxygen and the high level of carbon dioxide in the body tissues. The brain and heart are immediately affected.

**ETIOLOGY** Accidental suffocation often occurs with infants and small children playing with plastic bags. Criminal suffocation of homicide victims may be a common finding in forensic pathology. Suffocation may also be caused in a variety of other ways.

- Aspiration—aspiration of food that occludes or blocks the airway is common. As a matter of fact, this type of suffocation leads to the death of approximately one person a day in the United States!

  **TREATMENT** Treatment of food aspiration is immediate attention and may include the performance of an *abdominal thrust*, previously known as the Heimlich maneuver.

- Strangulation—accidental, suicidal, or criminal strangulation may occur in the forms of hanging or squeezing the neck with the hands, rope, wire, or a variety of other objects.

- Drowning—drowning is a common cause of accidental death, especially in children and adoles-

cent males. Drownings may be classified as wet or dry. Wet drownings are the most common (approximately 90 percent) and are characterized by water entering the airways and lungs, preventing the entry of oxygen into the system. Dry drownings are less common, and are characterized by a reflex laryngospasm that closes the glottis and does not allow water or air to enter.

**TREATMENT** Treatment of either type of drowning is immediate resuscitation and transport to an emergency department.

## RARE DISEASES

### Pneumoconiosis

Pneumoconiosis refers to a group of environmentally induced diseases that cause progressive, chronic inflammation and infection. This condition is caused by frequently inhaling the small dust particles of the offending agent for extended periods of time. Pneumoconiosis may occur within a few years, or it may take 20 or 30 years to develop. Types of pneumoconiosis, cause, and related occupations include:

- Asbestosis—asbestos, the most frequently occurring form of the disease, related to insulating and fireproofing

- Anthracosis—carbon and coal, often called "coal miner's disease" and "black lung"

- Silicosis—silicone, affects glass cutters, sand blasters, and stone masons

### Fungal Diseases

Fungal diseases affecting the lungs are caused by inhaling an airborne fungus. The lung lesions caused by fungal diseases form granulomatous inflammations like tuberculosis, but they do not cavitate or cause cavities in the lung tissue. The fungus may spread through the lung tissue and cause acute illness with symptoms of dyspnea and fever. Treatment consists of rest and antifungal medications. Two forms include:

1. Histoplasmosis—occurs primarily in the midwestern United States. This fungus is harbored in bird droppings such as those found in chicken houses, bat caves, and pigeon roosts.

## HEALTHY HIGHLIGHT

### Abdominal Thrust or Heimlich Maneuver

The abdominal thrust, previously known as the Heimlich maneuver, is a technique used to remove foreign material—usually food—from the respiratory tract of a choking victim. The procedure may be performed with the victim in a standing, sitting, or lying position. If the victim is able to talk or has wheezing breath sounds, this maneuver should not be performed. The abdominal thrust is performed on individuals who are unable to breathe.

To perform the abdominal thrust on a victim in a sitting or standing position, the rescuer assumes a position behind the victim. The rescuer wraps his or her arms around the victim's waist, allowing the victim's head, arms, and upper body to fall forward. The rescuer makes a fist with one hand and holds it in place with the other hand. The fist should be placed against the victim's abdomen at a point slightly above the umbilicus and below the rib cage. The maneuver calls for the rescuer to forcefully perform an upward thrust to this area. This maneuver may be repeated until the airway is cleared.

If the victim is or becomes unconscious, the rescuer should position the victim on his or her back with the head turned to the side. The rescuer kneels beside the victim's hips and places both hands on the abdomen slightly above the umbilicus and below the rib cage. One hand should be on top of the other. Pressure is then applied with an upward thrust. The maneuver may be repeated until the airway is cleared.

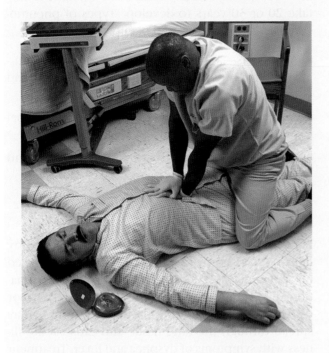
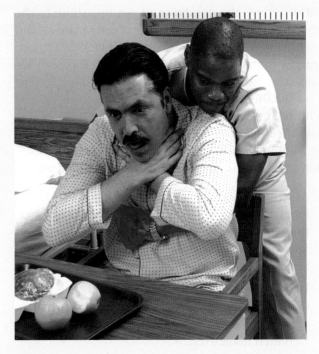

Abdominal thrust or Heimlich maneuver.

2. Coccidioidomycosis—occurs primarily in the southwestern United States. This fungus grows in hot, dry areas and produces spores that become windborne. Also known as "desert fever" and "valley fever."

## Legionnaires' Disease

Legionnaires' disease is a bacterial pulmonary infection so named as the result of an outbreak in 1976 at a convention of the American Legion held in Philadelphia. The causative bacterium is *Legionella pneumophilia*. This bacteria lives in water storage tanks and cooling systems. Legionnaires' disease may also be called Legionnaires' pneumonia because it produces typical pneumonia symptoms. It differs from other types of pneumonia in that it does not respond to the usual treatment and it may cause permanent lung damage. Legionnaires' disease is not limited to the pulmonary system like typical pneumonia. It may cause complications such as liver damage and renal dysfunction. Severe cases may need mechanical ventilation and may have a fatal outcome.

## EFFECTS OF AGING ON THE SYSTEM

The effects of aging on the respiratory system increase the risk for the older adult to develop respiratory disease. Over time, the respiratory system loses some of its elasticity, becomes less efficient, and has less reserve. Weakened respiratory muscles contribute to the ineffectiveness of the system. It can also be adversely affected by changes in posture occurring with aging, by the long-term effects of chronic diseases such as COPD, and by the changes occurring in other systems. The older adult usually has a lower tolerance for exercise due to the increased need for oxygen during exercise and the inability of the body to meet that demand.

Changes in the immune responses that occur with aging put the older adult at increased risk for acute respiratory infections. Influenza and pneumonia are common but very serious diseases affecting older adults. Pneumonia is the leading cause of death due to infections in the older population. Another respiratory disease that older people are at increased risk of developing is tuberculosis. Their reduced immunity contributes to the high incidence of TB among older adults.

Chronic respiratory diseases are particularly difficult for older people. The nature of the disease, symptoms, effects, and treatments may all contribute to the increased respiratory dysfunction, and thus, the debilitation of the individual. Many older individuals have been heavy smokers for years. The effects of smoking may have already severely damaged respiratory function and will continue to inhibit effective breathing if the individual continues to smoke. Smoking is the major cause of the high incidence of cancer of the lung in older people. Cancer of the lung is the second leading cause of death in the older adult.

## SUMMARY

The respiratory system is responsible for the intake of oxygen for the body and the removal of carbon dioxide. Decreased respiratory function greatly limits the ability of other systems because oxygen is necessary at the cellular level for all activities to occur. Diagnostic tests for respiratory diseases include physical examination, chest X-rays, arterial blood gases, and pulmonary function tests.

Respiratory diseases are a major cause of disability and death in the United States. Acute respiratory diseases such as the common cold and pneumonia occur in all age groups. Most chronic respiratory diseases are found in the older adult. Smoking is the greatest contributor to chronic respiratory disease, especially cancer of the lung.

## REVIEW QUESTIONS

### Short Answer

**1.** What are the functions of the respiratory system?

**2.** Which signs and symptoms are associated with common respiratory system disorders?

**3.** Which diagnostic tests are most commonly used to determine the type and/or cause of respiratory system disorders?

**4.** What is the most effective preventive technique for the common cold?

**5.** What behavior puts an individual at highest risk for pulmonary disease?

### Matching

**6.** Match the term on the left with the correct descriptive clause on the right.

| | |
|---|---|
| _____ asthma | **a.** Inflammation of the mucous membranes of the sinuses |
| _____ pneumothorax | **b.** High risk behavior for developing respiratory disease |
| _____ COPD | **c.** Best preventive behavior for preventing respiratory infections |
| _____ hemothorax | **d.** Hypersensitivity reaction causing constriction of the bronchi |
| _____ tuberculosis | **e.** Bacterial infection causing a primary lesion in the lung |
| _____ sinusitis | **f.** Collapse of a part of the lung with blood in the space |
| _____ cor pulmonale | **g.** Group of chronic pulmonary diseases |
| _____ hand washing | **h.** Right-sided heart failure |
| _____ smoking | **i.** Collection of air in the pleural cavity |

## CASE STUDY

**Mr. Loftin** is a 78-year-old gentleman who has been diagnosed with severe emphysema. He has been a heavy smoker since age 12 and continues to smoke. He complains about his shortness of breath, stating he cannot do much more than walk across the room without gasping for air. He has been cautioned about the effects of his continued smoking, but he responds with statements such as, "What difference does it make if I quit now? I've smoked all my life and you can't go back and change that." How would you respond to this statement? Is it too late for him to quit and receive some benefit of that behavioral change? Is any of the damage from smoking reversible? How can you explain this to Mr. Loftin?

# BIBLIOGRAPHY

Burke, L. E., & Fair, J. (2003). Promoting prevention. *Journal of Cardiovascular Nursing 18*(4), 256-265.

Carlson, B. W., & Mascarella, J. J. (2003). Change in sleep patterns in COPD. *American Journal of Nursing 103*(12), 71-73.

Carmichael, M. (2004, January 12). Cold comfort indeed. *Newsweek 143*(2), 56-57.

Consensus document on the epidemiology of sudden acute respiratory syndrome (SARS). (2003, October 17). *Weekly Epidemiology*.

Devlieger, H. (2003). The respiratory pump: Past and present understanding. *Acta Paediatrica 92*(11), 1245-1247.

Dunavan, C. P. (2003). Can't beat that cough. *Discover 24*(11), 30-31.

Enserink, M. (2003, August 21). A sequel to SARS? *Science Now*, 1-7.

Integrated immunological response represents beacon for vaccine development. (2004, March 19). *Drug Week*, 344-345.

Krauss, C. (2003, June 11). A visitor to Toronto is stricken with SARS. *New York Times 152*(52511), A7.

Modern lifestyle may increase asthma, allergy; second-hand smoke worsens it. (2003, September 1). *Biotech Week*, 98-99.

Pappas, G., Bosilkovski, M., Akritidis, N., Mastora, M., Krteva, L., & Tsianos, E. (2003). Brucellosis and the respiratory system. *Clinical Infectious Diseases 37*(7), 95-99.

Peck, H., Bray, M. A., & Kehle, T. J. (2003). Relaxation and guided imagery: A school-based intervention for children with asthma. *Psychology in the Schools 40*(6), 657-676.

Roman, M., Weinstein, A., & Macaluso, S. (2003). Primary spontaneous pneumothorax. *MEDSURG Nursing 12*(3), 161-169.

SARS—sudden acute respiratory syndrome. (2003, July). www.who.int/csr/sars/en

Sims, J. M. (2003). Guidelines for treating asthma. *Critical Care Nursing 22*(6), 247-250.

Smyth, D. (2003). Aging, cardiovascular disease and COPD. *Journal of Palliative Nursing 9*(2), 88.

Sudden acute respiratory syndrome—Singapore, 2003. (2003, May 9). *Weekly Epidemiology*.

Sudden acute respiratory syndrome (SARS). (2003, March 21). *Weekly Epidemiology*.

What everyone should know about SARS. (2004, June 10). www.cdc.gov/ncidod/sars/factsheet.htm

Whiteman, K., & Kress, T. (2003). Help me catch my breath! *Nursing 33*(12), 32-34.

Women take heart. (2003). *American Journal of Nursing 103*(12), 18.

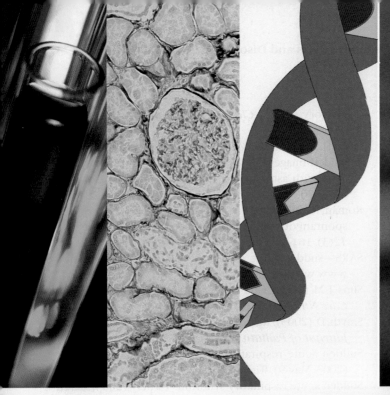
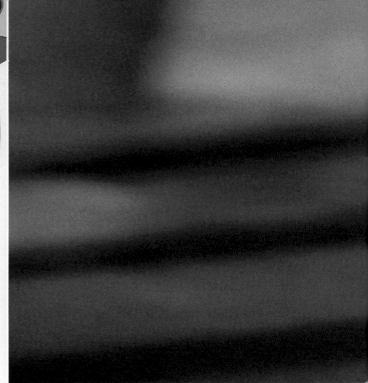

## OUTLINE

## KEY TERMS

# Lymphatic System Diseases and Disorders

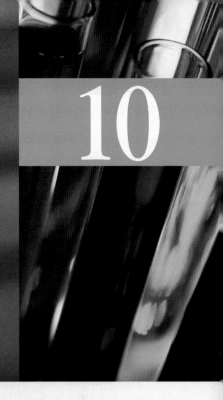

## 10

## LEARNING OBJECTIVES

*Upon completion of the chapter, the learner should be able to:*

1. Define the terminology common to the lymphatic system and the disorders of the system.

2. Discuss the basic anatomy and physiology of the lymphatic system.

3. Identify the important signs and symptoms associated with common lymphatic system disorders.

4. Describe the common diagnostics used to determine the type and/or cause of lymphatic system disorders.

5. Identify common disorders of the lymphatic system.

6. Describe the typical course and management of the common lymphatic system disorders.

7. Describe the effects of aging on the lymphatic system and the common disorders of the system.

## OVERVIEW

*T*he lymphatic system is the infection fighting system of the body. It works with the immune system to play an important role in preventing infection and maintaining one's immunity. The lymphatic system includes the lymph nodes, lymph vessels, and fluid lymph. It is a special vascular system that picks up excess tissue fluid and returns it to the blood. Disorders of the system include inflammatory conditions and neoplasms. The lymphatic system is so closely related to the immune system, the blood and blood-forming organs, and the cardiovascular system that many of the concepts and diseases of the system have already been discussed. Refer to these chapters for additional information on the lymphatic system. ■

## ANATOMY AND PHYSIOLOGY

The lymphatic system includes lymph vessels, ducts, and nodes (Figure 10–1). It is important in protecting the body from infection. It is responsible for filtering bacterial and nonbacterial products resulting from the inflammatory process. The goal of the system is to prevent these waste products from entering the general circulation. This activity may cause some inflammation of the node filtering the waste products, causing swelling and redness of the involved node.

The lymphatic system is dependent, to some extent, on the vascular system. The lymphatic system returns its fluids and other materials to the vascular system. There is diffusion of fluid between the lymphatic vessels, the interstitial spaces, and the blood capillaries.

The fluid in the lymphatic system is called **lymph**. Lymph is a clear liquid similar to plasma and contains many white cells. The conducting vessels of the lymphatic system include the capillaries, the smallest vessels, and the larger lymph vessels, which have valves much like the veins in the cardiovascular system. In the lymph vessels, the direction of flow is toward the thoracic cavity. The vessels meet in the right lymphatic duct or the left lymphatic duct, which drain into the venous system. The right lymphatic duct drains the lymph from the right half of the head, upper torso, and right arm. The rest of the lymph vessels in the body drain into the left lymphatic duct, also called the thoracic duct.

The lymph vessels have other functions besides the transportation of lymph. They also return important nutrients such as proteins and large particulate matter that have leaked out into the capillaries to the blood vessels (Figure 10–2). In the course of a day, approximately three liters of extra fluid is leaked into the tissue and not picked up by the venous system.

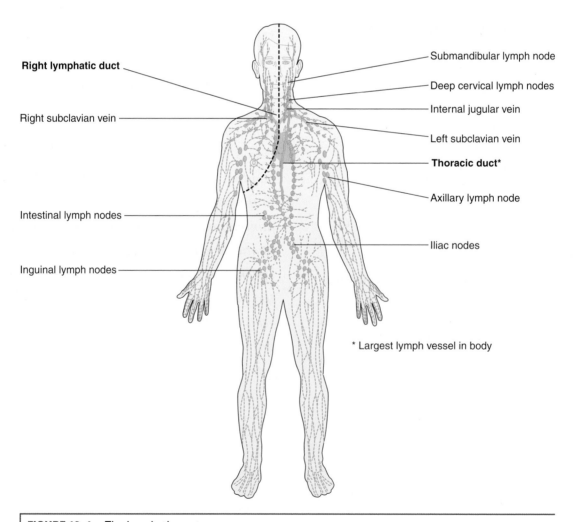

Right lymphatic duct

Right subclavian vein

Intestinal lymph nodes

Inguinal lymph nodes

Submandibular lymph node

Deep cervical lymph nodes

Internal jugular vein

Left subclavian vein

Thoracic duct*

Axillary lymph node

Iliac nodes

* Largest lymph vessel in body

**FIGURE 10–1** The lymphatic system.

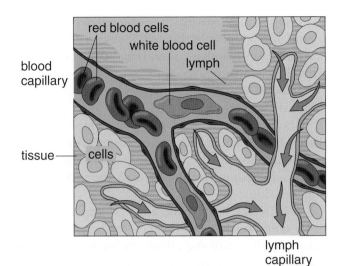

**FIGURE 10–2**  Exchange of fluids between the lymph and blood vessels.

The lymphatic system picks up this extra fluid and returns it to the blood. In addition, the lymph vessels transport toxic substances to the nodes for filtration. In the digestive process, the vessels are important in the absorption of fats. The nodes are important in the filtering process, but they also produce lymphocytes and protect the body by developing immunity to some diseases.

Organs related to the lymph system are the tonsils, thymus gland, and spleen. These organs also play a part in the body's immunity and protection system. See Chapter 5 for a discussion on immunity.

## COMMON SIGNS AND SYMPTOMS

Enlargement of the lymph glands or nodes is common, and is usually due to infection somewhere in the body. Infection stimulates activity of the nodes and glands to produce more **lymphocytes** (white cells created in the lymphatic system). Fever, fatigue, and weight loss are common with lymphatic diseases.

Most disorders of the lymphatic system are related to diseases of other systems. **Lymphocytosis** (lympho = lymph, cyto = cell, osis = increase or an abnormal increase in lymphocytes) and **lymphocytopenia** (lymphocyte = lymph cell, penia = decrease or an abnormal decrease in lymphocytes) in blood and tissue may accompany diseases of the immune system as well as the lymphatic system.

## DIAGNOSTIC TESTS

A complete blood count with white cell differential may assist in determination of inflammation or infectious diseases of the lymphatic system.

**Lymphangiography** (lim-FAN-jee-**OG**-rah-fee; lymph = lymph, angio = vessel, graphy = procedure) consists of injecting a contrast dye and taking X-rays. This procedure may be helpful in diagnosing vessel conditions. Magnetic resonance imaging and computerized tomography may also be utilized.

Biopsy of lymph glands and nodes may assist in determination of lymphoma. A special connective tissue cell called a Reed-Sternberg cell confirms a diagnosis of Hodgkin's disease.

## COMMON DISEASES OF THE LYMPHATIC SYSTEM

Diseases of the lymphatic system commonly include inflammatory conditions. Often, diseases of this system are the result of disease in another system. Disease of lymph glands may be collectively called **lymphadenopathy** (lim-FAD-eh-**NOP**-ah-thee; lymph = lymph, adeno = gland, opathy = disease). **Lymphangiopathy** (lim-FAN-jee-**OP**-ah-thee; lymph = lymph, angio = vessel, opathy = disease) is a general term to describe any disease of the lymph vessels.

### Lymphadenitis

Lymphadenitis (lim-FAD-eh-**NIGH**-tis; lymph = lymph, adeno = gland, itis = inflammation) is characterized by swelling of the lymph gland and/or nodes.

**ETIOLOGY**  Lymphadenitis is usually caused by infection somewhere in the body. Drainage of bacteria or toxic substances may cause the swelling. The location of the affected nodes may assist in determination of cause.

**SYMPTOMS**  Swelling, pain, and tenderness of the gland or node are common.

**TREATMENT**  Antibiotic treatment is helpful with bacterial infections.

### Lymphangitis

Lymphangitis (lymph = lymph, angi = vessel, itis = inflammation) is a condition of swelling of the lymph vessel due to inflammation.

**ETIOLOGY** This inflammation is commonly caused by infection with streptococcal bacteria following a trauma.

**SYMPTOMS** Lymphangitis is often characterized by a red streak at the site of bacterial entry that extends to the area lymph nodes. Other symptoms include fever, chills, and malaise. Cellulitis (inflammation of cellular or connective tissue) and leukocytosis may also be present.

**TREATMENT** Lymphangitis is commonly treated with antibiotics. Warm, moist packs and elevation of the affected area are also helpful.

## Lymphedema

Lymphedema (lymph = lymph, edema = swelling) is an abnormal collection of lymph fluid usually observed in the extremities (Figure 10-3).

**ETIOLOGY** Causes may include:

- obstruction of a lymphatic vessel
- abnormal uptake of fluid by the lymphatic capillaries due to injury
- overproduction of interstitial fluid due to increased capillary blood pressure

Lymphatic vessels may be occluded or obstructed by inflammation or by tumors. Pressure on the vessels decreases lymphatic flow. Diagnosis may be confirmed by lymphangiography.

**TREATMENT** Treatment may include antibiotics or surgical intervention, depending on cause.

Abnormal uptake of fluid by the lymphatic capillaries due to injury may be the result of surgery or radiation of tissues. Breast surgery and radiation may lead to a chronic lymphedema of the arm on the affected side.

**TREATMENT** Placing the affected arm above the heart while resting and exercise to increase lymph flow may decrease the edema. Procedures such as obtaining blood pressure and drawing blood samples should not be performed on the affected side because affected tissue is more prone to infection.

Pregnancy and constrictive clothing often cause an increase in venous pressure. This increase in venous pressure results in an increase in capillary pressure, and thus an overproduction of interstitial fluid is commonly observed in the ankles and feet. Decreasing venous pressure in these cases will relieve lymphedema.

**TREATMENT** To reduce venous pressure in the pregnant female, lying on the left side helps improve venous flow because the inferior vena cava is to the

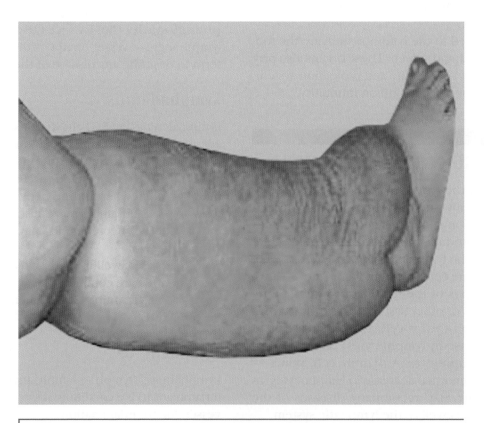

**FIGURE 10-3** Lymphedema. *(Courtesy of Mark L. Kuss.)*

right of midline. Resting with the legs above heart level will also reduce edema. Constrictive clothing should be removed or loosened when lymphedema is observed.

## Lymphoma

**ETIOLOGY** Lymphoma refers to several types of neoplasms that affect lymphoid tissue (lymph nodes, tonsils, spleen, and lymph fluid). There are many types of lymphoma but all affect normal lymphocyte production, leading to an impaired immunity.

**SYMPTOMS** Symptoms include night sweats, fever, and weight loss.

**TREATMENT** Treatment is dependent on type of lymphoma and stage of the disease. Treatment may include surgery, chemotherapy, radiation, and bone marrow transplantation. Lymphoma is discussed in more detail in Chapter 7 under the heading "Disorders of White Blood Cells."

## Mononucleosis

Mononucleosis is a viral infection that affects primarily children and young adults. It is somewhat contagious and is commonly called "kissing disease." This disease is discussed in more detail in Chapter 7 under the heading "Disorders of White Blood Cells."

## RARE DISEASES

## Kawasaki Disease

This disorder is also called mucocutaneous lymph node syndrome. It is an acute febrile disease found mostly in children and causes cervical lymphadenopathy. It resembles scarlet fever because the individual develops a rash, and some edema of the hands and feet. Other symptoms include lethargy, congestion, irritability, fever, dry skin, and reddened lips, tongue, and mucous membranes. Treatment is supportive because the disease does not respond to antibiotic therapy. This disease is rarely fatal in the acute stage, but children may die quite suddenly some years later due to coronary artery disease.

## EFFECTS OF AGING ON THE SYSTEM

As the individual ages, there is decreased ability to produce antibodies, leading to decreases in the normal immune response. This interferes with the normal ability to ward off infections. If other chronic diseases are also present, the individual may be at an even higher risk for poor healing and development of infections. In addition, as the immune response becomes less effective, the individual is more susceptible to autoimmune disorders. Many diseases of the older adult have some direct relationship to the decreased immune response. Because the lymphatic system is dependent for some of its functions on the vascular system, additional problems arise in the older person who has impaired circulation or other vascular system diseases.

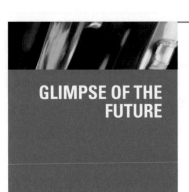

**GLIMPSE OF THE FUTURE**

## Evaluating Metastatic Lymph Nodes

Clinical trials are testing the use of Combidex (ferumoxtran-10) with MRIs in evaluating metastatic lymph nodes in patients. Combidex is a highly magnetic iron oxide preparation. Researchers have seen value in using the Combidex-enhanced MRI for more definitive diagnostic purposes. They found that using Combidex is safe and improves the ability of the physician to diagnose cancer in the nodes. In the future, this procedure may be approved for routine use in diagnosing lymph node cancers.

*Source: Muldoon, L. L. (2004).*

## SUMMARY

The lymphatic system plays an important role in the body's ability to fight infection and in immunity. The system is composed of lymph, lymph nodes, and vessels to transport the lymph. The lymphatic system also transports fluid that has leaked into the interstitial areas to the blood vessels. Diseases of the system are usually caused by infections or neoplasms, and can range from mild to severe. Treatment varies with the particular type of disease. Common symptoms include fever, fatigue, weight loss, and enlarged lymph nodes.

## REVIEW QUESTIONS

### Short Answer

1. What are the three main functions of the lymphatic system?

2. Name the four signs and symptoms associated with common lymphatic system disorders.

3. Which diagnostic tests are most commonly used to determine the type and/or cause of lymphatic system disorders?

### True or False

4.   T   F    Diseases of the lymphatic system commonly include inflammatory conditions.
5.   T   F    Lymphangiography is a biopsy of a lymph node or several nodes.
6.   T   F    Lymphadenitis is characterized by a swelling of the lymph nodes.
7.   T   F    Lymphangitis is a condition of swelling of lymph vessels due to inflammation.
8.   T   F    Lymphedema is always caused by obstruction of a lymphatic vessel.
9.   T   F    Mononucleosis is a bacterial infection that usually affects children and young adults.
10.   T   F    Lymphoma affects lymphocyte production and impairs immunity.

## CASE STUDY

**Mrs. Talik** is 78 years old and has been hospitalized frequently for repeated respiratory infections. Until the past two years, she has been relatively healthy. She has not been diagnosed with any serious chronic diseases, but does have some osteoporosis. Based on your knowledge of the aging process and the lymphatic system changes, what might be contributing to the development of these repeated respiratory infections? What can she do to decrease her risk and improve her immunity to infections?

# BIBLIOGRAPHY

A clinically useful method for evaluating lymphedema. (2004). *Clinical Journal of Oncology Nursing 8*(1), 35–38.

Data from phase III study of Combidex. (2004, October 2). *Women's Health Weekly*, 38.

Education key to managing lymphoedema. (2003). *Australian Nursing Journal 10*(8), 27.

Giguere, C. M., Bauman, N. M., & Smith, R. J. H. (2002). New treatment options for lymphangioma in infants and children. *Annals of Otology, Rhinology & Laryngology 111*(12), 1066–1075.

Hampton, S. (2003). Elvarex compression garments in the management of lymphoedema. *British Journal of Nursing 12*(15), 925–928.

Holmes, B. (2003). Stalking the enemy. *New Scientist 179*(2402), 52–55.

Lymphatic system disorders may influence anesthesia in intensive care. (2003, September 15). *Biotech Week*, 499–501.

Measles virus found in patients' tumor cells. (2001, June 7). *Blood Weekly*, 14–15.

Muldoon, L. L., Varallay, P., Kraemer, D. F., Kiwic, G., Pinkston, K., Walker-Rosenfeld, S. L., & Newelt, E. A. (2004). Trafficking of supermagnetic iron oxide particles (Combidex) from brain to lymph nodes in the rat. *Neuropathology and Applied Neurobiology 30*(1), 70–79.

October live chat to address managing lymphedema. (2003). *ONS News 18*(9), 14.

Todd, M., Welsh, J., & Moriarty, D. (2002). The experience of parents of children with primary lymphoedema. *International Journal of Palliative Nursing 8*(9), 444–451.

Witt, C., & Ottesen, E. A. (2001). Lymphatic filariasis and infection of childhood. *Tropical Medicine & International Health 6*(8), 582–606.

Woods, M. (2003). The experience of manual lymph drainage as an aspect of treatment for lymphoedema. *International Journal of Palliative Nursing 9*(8), 336–341.

Woods, M. (2003). Using reflection in the care of a patient with lymphoedema. *British Journal of Nursing 12*(14), 865–870.

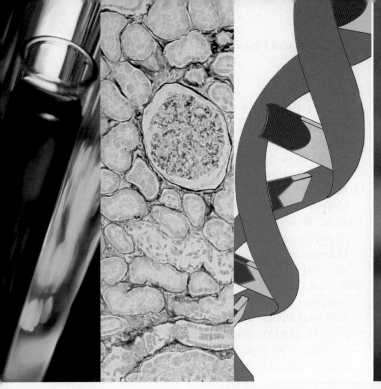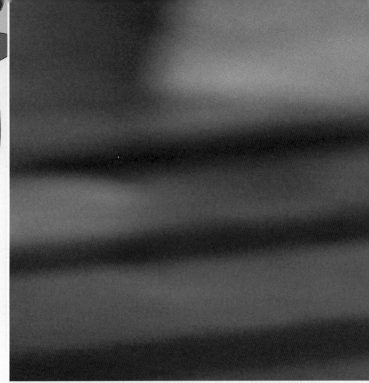

## OUTLINE

## KEY TERMS

# Digestive System Diseases and Disorders

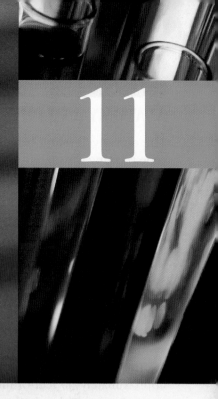

**11**

## LEARNING OBJECTIVES

*Upon completion of the chapter, the learner should be able to:*

1. Define the terminology common to the upper and lower digestive system and the disorders of the system.

2. Discuss the basic anatomy and physiology of the digestive system.

3. Identify the important signs and symptoms associated with common digestive system disorders.

4. Describe the common diagnostics used to determine type and/or cause of digestive system disorders.

5. Identify the common disorders of the digestive system.

6. Describe the typical course and management of the common digestive system disorders.

7. Describe the effects of aging on the digestive system and the common disorders of the system.

## OVERVIEW

*T*he digestive system provides nutrients for the body through the processes of ingestion, digestion, and absorption, and eliminates waste products from the system. Diseases or disorders of the digestive system are some of the most common medical problems. Because there are many differences in eating patterns, lifestyle behaviors, and inherited traits, digestive system problems vary considerably among individuals. Some digestive system problems are caused by poor nutritional habits, whereas others may be due to structural problems or a particular disease process. ■

## ANATOMY AND PHYSIOLOGY

The digestive system has been described as a long tube running through the body. It has two main purposes: (1) changing the food we eat into simpler substances so they can be absorbed into the blood and carried to all cells of the body, and (2) eliminating waste products from the body. The two major parts of the digestive system are the alimentary canal and the accessory organs, including the tongue, teeth, salivary glands, gallbladder, pancreas, and liver.

The alimentary canal (Figure 11–1) is a continuous tube running from the mouth to the anus. The term gastrointestinal (GI) tract technically refers only to the stomach and intestines, but is often used as a synonym for the alimentary canal. The alimentary canal is approximately 30 feet or nine meters in length, but most of it is coiled up in the abdomen surrounded by the peritoneum. The peritoneum is a large, serous membrane, covering the organs in the abdomen and lining the walls of the abdominal cavity. It secretes fluid to prevent friction between organs in the abdomen as they move during the process of digestion. The alimentary canal starts at the mouth where ingested food begins to be broken down to supply the body with needed nourishment. The teeth begin the process by breaking the food into smaller parts. The tongue, the organ of taste, assists the process by helping move the food in the mouth. The salivary glands, located outside the mouth with ducts leading from the glands to the mouth, secrete about 1,500 milliliters of saliva per day. The saliva continues the process of breaking down food and moistening it to make it easier to swallow. At the back of the mouth lies the pharynx, the channel for food to pass from the mouth to the esophagus.

The esophagus is a tube (about nine inches in length) that extends from the pharynx to the stomach. The walls of the esophagus are very muscular. Movement of these muscles is called peristaltic contraction. These contractions, the process called **peristalsis**, move the food from the pharynx to the stomach.

The stomach is a sac-type receptacle that lies just under the diaphragm in the upper abdomen. The

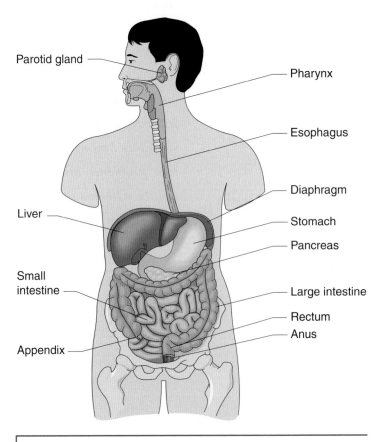

Parotid gland

Pharynx

Esophagus

Diaphragm

Liver

Stomach

Pancreas

Small intestine

Large intestine

Rectum

Anus

Appendix

**FIGURE 11–1**   The digestive system.

esophagus connects to the stomach at the cardiac orifice (opening). A thick ring of smooth muscle called the cardiac or gastroesophageal sphincter surrounds this opening. The upper portion of the stomach, at the cardiac orifice end, is called the fundus, and the middle portion of the stomach is called the body. Food is broken down in the stomach by a process of chemical changes from the action of pepsin—an enzyme—and hydrochloric acid secreted by cells in the stomach. Food is mixed with these chemicals by the contractions of the stomach. The lining of the stomach also secretes a substance called the **intrinsic factor**, which is necessary for the absorption of vitamin $B_{12}$. At the lower portion of the stomach, called the pyloric region, the stomach is connected to the first part of the small intestine called the duodenum. The opening at this end of the stomach is the pyloric orifice, which is surrounded by the pyloric sphincter. The sphincter muscles control the cardiac and pyloric openings.

The small intestine extends from the pyloric orifice to the ileocecal valve at the beginning of the large intestine. It is divided into three sections. The first section, the duodenum, is about 10 inches or 25 centimeters in length. It is the shortest of the three sections. The duodenum receives bile from the liver and pancreatic juices from the pancreas, which aid in the digestive process. The duodenum connects the stomach to the jejunum on the left side of the upper abdomen. The jejunum is the second section of the small intestine. The jejunum extends from the duodenum to the ileum. It is about seven and one-half feet or two meters in length, and is coiled throughout the abdomen. The ileum is the third section of the small intestine, attaching to the jejunum at its beginning and ending at the ileocecal valve, the beginning of the large intestine.

The major function of the small intestine is digestion and absorption of food and fluids. Material is moved through the small intestine by muscular action (peristalsis). Most of digestion takes place in the small intestine. Finger-like projections called villi are located on the inside surface of the intestine. These projections contain lymph vessels and blood capillaries. Additional extensions called microvilli cover the villi, forming a velvety surface, which greatly increases the surface area of the small intestine. As a result of this increased surface area, nutrient absorption is greatly increased. Nutrients pass into the vascular capillaries for delivery to the body cells.

The large intestine connects to the small intestine at the ileocecal valve in the right lower portion of the abdomen. The first section of the colon is called the cecum. The appendix is attached to the cecum near the ileocecal valve. The large intestine, also called the colon, is about five feet or one and one-half meters in length. Each section of the colon is named according to its anatomical position. The colon begins in the lower right quadrant of the abdomen (cecum), rises to the mid-level (ascending colon), crosses the abdomen at the umbilicus level (transverse colon), and descends on the left side (descending colon), into the pelvic cavity where it is called the sigmoid colon. The sigmoid colon forms an S-shaped tube that extends into the lower pelvic region, ending at the rectum and anus. The process of digestion and absorption continues in the large intestine. The most important function of the large intestine is the absorption of water and electrolytes, and the elimination of **feces**, the material not absorbed by the intestines.

## COMMON SIGNS AND SYMPTOMS

Diseases of this system usually result in signs and symptoms related to hemorrhage, **perforation**, and altered **motility** (movement) in the system. Hemorrhage may be mild or severe, and may originate at any site along the system. Terms identifying bleeding are **hematemesis** (HEM-ah-**TEM**-eh-sis; hemat = blood, emesis = vomiting), **hematochezia** (HEM-at-toe-**KEE**-zee-ah, bright red blood in the feces), and **melena** (meh-LEE-nah, dark tarry **stool**), due to the presence of blood.

Perforation in any area of the tract can be life threatening due to the contaminating contents of the tract and the ease of spread in the abdominal cavity. Perforation in the stomach or intestines allows spillage of contents into the abdominal cavity causing **peritonitis** (PER-ih-toe-**NIGH**-tis; an inflammation of the peritoneum). Pain is a common symptom of peritonitis. Gastric contents that are spilled are high in gastric acid and are corrosive to abdominal organs. Intestinal contents have a normally high bacterial count. Spilling of intestinal contents into the abdominal cavity causes infection, which may lead to **septicemia** (SEP-tih-**SEE**-me-ah; septic = dirty, emia = blood or bacteria in the bloodstream). Causes of perforation may include peptic ulcer, injury from gunshot or stab wounds, and untreated appendicitis.

Alteration in motility or movement of food along the tract commonly leads to a variety of signs and symptoms including nausea, vomiting, diarrhea, or constipation. Diarrhea is a disorder characterized by frequent, watery stools. Irritability of the intestinal lining causes hyperactivity of muscle contractions (peristalsis), causing a rushing of the watery contents in the small intestine through the large intestine. This rushing does not allow the large intestine the time needed to reabsorb the water. The primary concern with diarrhea, especially in young children and older people, is loss of fluids, leading to dehydration. Causes of diarrhea include a sudden increase in stress or nervous condition, bacterial or viral infection, or food poisoning.

Constipation is the opposite of diarrhea. The stool in the colon remains for an extended period of time, too much water is reabsorbed, and the stool becomes hard, dry, and difficult to pass. Constipation is commonly caused by poor dietary and elimination habits. Avoiding the urge to **defecate** (have a bowel movement) increases the amount of time the stool remains in the colon and thus increases constipation.

## DIAGNOSTIC TESTS

Diagnostic tests for the digestive system commonly include radiologic (X-ray) examinations and endoscopic (looking into the cavity with a lighted scope) examinations. An Upper GI Series, also called a Barium Swallow, allows visualization of the esophagus, stomach, and upper portion of the small intestine. In preparation for the examination, the individual must be N.P.O. (non per os or nothing by mouth) for a minimum of eight hours. Prior to the examination, the individual drinks a barium solution. This solution coats the inside of the upper tract, allowing visualization by X-ray. The physician may view a "series" or several X-rays to detect problems of the upper tract (Figure 11–2).

A lower GI series, also called a barium enema, provides visualization of the large intestine. In preparation for this radiologic examination, the individual is given an enema or laxatives the day before the examination to rid the colon of fecal material. The

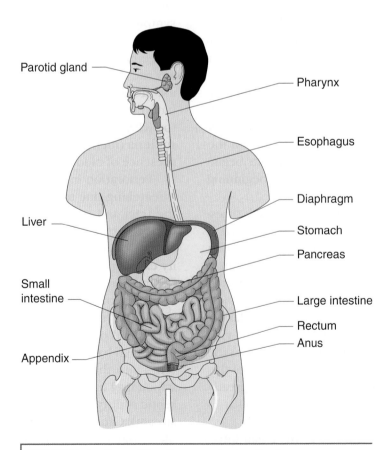

**FIGURE 11–2**  Upper GI; yellow area is visualized.

## HEALTHY HIGHLIGHT

### Good Elimination Habits

To avoid constipation, defecation should be allowed to occur when reflexes are the strongest, usually early morning following breakfast. Normal elimination habits differ from individual to individual. Some people may have bowel movements after every meal; others will have a bowel movement daily or every two to three days. Other good elimination habits include a diet high in fiber (fruits, vegetables, grains, and cereals), daily exercise, and adequate intake of fluids. Laxatives and enemas should be avoided because these artificially stimulate the bowel and may alter its normal elimination pattern. Regular use of laxatives produces dependence on them for bowel elimination.

diet is restricted to clear liquids. The day of the examination, an enema of barium solution is given to the individual to coat the lower tract and allow X-ray visualization of the large intestine (Figure 11-3).

Endoscopic examination allows the physician to look directly into the digestive organs by use of a lighted scope (Figure 11-4). The name of each procedure is identified by naming the organ that is being scoped. Examples of this include stomach (gastroscopy), colon (colonoscopy), sigmoid colon (sigmoidoscopy), and entire upper GI area (esophagogastroduodenoscopy, EGD). During an endoscopic

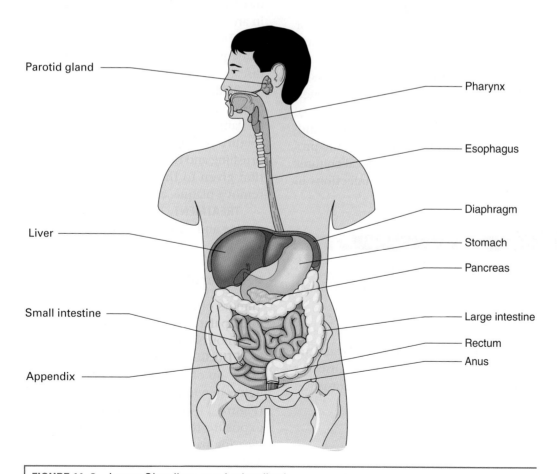

**FIGURE 11-3**   Lower GI; yellow area is visualized.

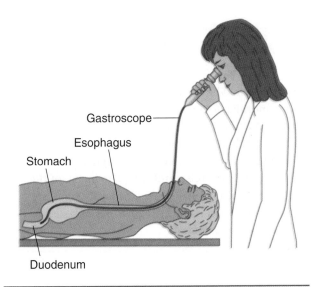

Gastroscope
Esophagus
Stomach
Duodenum

**FIGURE 11-4** Esophagogastroduodenoscopy (EGD).

examination, a physician may obtain a biopsy (small piece of tissue for examination) to determine the presence of a neoplasm or other disease processes.

Several laboratory tests may be performed to assist in the diagnosing of digestive system diseases. One of these is the Hemoccult that tests stool for **occult** (hidden) **blood**. A positive Hemoccult may be indicative of colon cancer.

Another laboratory test is an **Ova and Parasite (O&P)**. This is an examination of a stool specimen for the presence of adult parasites or their eggs (ova). Parasites identified by an O&P may include roundworms, tapeworms, pinworms, hookworms, and protozoa such as *Giardia lamblia*. Stool or fecal cultures may be utilized to determine bacterial infections in the colon.

# COMMON DISEASES OF THE DIGESTIVE SYSTEM

## Diseases of the Mouth

The primary function of the mouth is to begin the breakdown of food into smaller particles. Diseases of the mouth include those related to inflammation and tumors.

### ■ Dental Caries

Caries is a disease of the teeth.

**ETIOLOGY** Microorganisms in the mouth attack the teeth, thus producing dental cavities. Dental caries primarily affects children and young adults. The cause of caries is twofold. Bacteria are essential elements, along with a diet high in carbohydrates (sugars).

**SYMPTOMS** The bacteria stick to the tooth surface in a tough, sticky material called **dental plaque**. Acids produced by the bacteria erode the tooth surface. Prevention is based on frequently removing the plaque by brushing and flossing the teeth. A decrease in carbohydrate (sugar) intake is also helpful. The use of fluoride in drinking water and toothpaste also reduces the incidence of caries.

**TREATMENT** Treatment may range from simple dental fillings to oral surgery, depending on the extent of the caries.

### ■ Periodontal Disease

Periodontal disease affects the supporting structures of the teeth such as the gums. It is a disease that affects adults and has an increased incidence with aging. Most adults have some degree of periodontal disease. This disease is the main reason for tooth loss in an adult.

**ETIOLOGY** Dental plaque, poor oral hygiene, and inadequate diet are common factors leading to this disease.

**SYMPTOMS** The dental plaque sticks on the tooth at the gum line, often leading to **gingivitis** (inflammation of the gums with painful bleeding) (Figure 11-5). Prevention is based on frequent brushing and flossing of the teeth with special attention given to the gum line, regular dental care to remove plaque, and an adequate diet.

**TREATMENT** Treatment involves removing the plaque and treating the inflammation.

### ■ Cancer of the Mouth

Tumors of the mouth may occur on the lip, cheek, gum, palate, or tongue. A common oral cancer is squamous cell carcinoma of the lip.

**ETIOLOGY** This tumor usually occurs on the lower lip of men and is related to exposure to sunlight, chewing tobacco, and smoking pipes or cigars (Figure 11-6). Prevention is aimed at decreasing exposure to sunlight by using SPF sunscreen and wearing hats to shade the face, and eliminating the use of tobacco products.

**TREATMENT** Treatment is usually quite effective and includes radiation therapy and surgical excision.

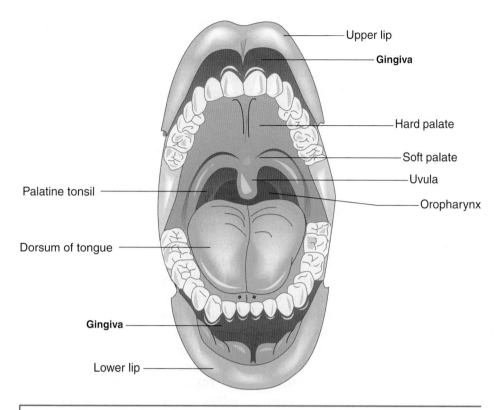

Upper lip

**Gingiva**

Hard palate

Soft palate

Uvula

Oropharynx

Palatine tonsil

Dorsum of tongue

**Gingiva**

Lower lip

**FIGURE 11–5**    Gingivitis (inflamed gingiva).

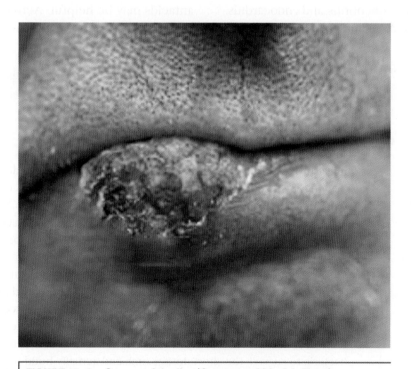

**FIGURE 11–6**    Cancer of the lip. *(Courtesy of Mark L. Kuss)*

## Diseases of the Throat and Esophagus

There are many diseases of the throat and esophagus. They range from mild to severe and acute to chronic. Infections and inflammatory conditions are some of the most common. Pharyngitis is often categorized as a respiratory problem, because the pharynx can be considered part of the respiratory system as well as part of the digestive system.

### ■ Pharyngitis

Pharyngitis is commonly called a "sore throat."

**ETIOLOGY** Pharyngitis may be caused by viral or bacterial microorganisms.

**SYMPTOMS** The most frequent and earliest symptom of pharyngitis is a sore throat. Visual examination reveals redness in the area. A common type of pharyngitis is an inflammation of the tonsils called tonsillitis. In tonsillitis, the tonsils form crypts of pus, which give the tonsils a whitish appearance.

An acute type of pharyngitis is called **strep throat**. Strep throat is caused by a **virulent** (VIR-ulent; infectious, difficult to kill) bacteria, streptococcus. This bacteria may spread into the bloodstream and produce other diseases such as scarlet fever, rheumatic fever, glomerulonephritis, and endocarditis. Diagnosis is made by examination and throat culture.

**TREATMENT** Treatment of strep throat includes identification of the organism through laboratory cultures, followed by antibiotic treatment and follow-up culture to check effectiveness of antibiotic treatment. Antibiotic treatment is quite effective if taken as prescribed.

### ■ Reflux Esophagitis

Reflux esophagitis, more recently called gastro-esophageal reflux disease (GERD), is an inflammation of tissue at the lower end of the esophagus.

**ETIOLOGY** This inflammation is caused by a reflux (backflow) of stomach acids through the cardiac sphincter upward into the esophagus.

**SYMPTOMS** The most common symptom of reflux esophagitis is heartburn, a burning sensation in the mid-chest or epigastric (epi = above, gastric = stomach) area. Long-term reflux can lead to bleeding, ulceration, and scarring of the esophagus. This scarring may cause stricture and difficulty swallowing.

**TREATMENT** Treatment is directed at reducing reflux and may include recommendations to avoid large meals, spicy foods, caffeine, and tight clothing. Medications such as stool softeners, laxatives, and antacids may be helpful. Activities that increase abdominal pressure may be restricted. Sleeping with

 **HEALTHY HIGHLIGHT**

### Tips About Strep Throat

Sore throats need to be cultured routinely to diagnose the streptococcus infection commonly called strep throat. An accurate diagnosis depends on obtaining a throat culture. Practitioners cannot determine this condition by simply viewing the throat. Even though culturing is more costly, this determination is extremely important because strep throat may lead to rheumatic heart disease and possibly heart valve deformity. Parents of children who have recurrent attacks of strep throat should also have throat cultures as they may be carriers of the strep infection. Strep throat is usually treated effectively with antibiotics.

Antibiotics should be taken as prescribed. They should always be taken until all tablets or capsules are gone. Even if the affected individual begins to feel better, the medication should be continued until completed. Discontinuing the antibiotic or saving some medicine for later may lead to bacterial resistance. If an individual does not take the prescribed number of tablets, it is possible for many bacteria to survive the short dosage time and actually build up a resistance to that antibiotic. These bacteria may then cause another attack of strep throat that cannot be treated or cured with the previously prescribed antibiotic. Taking all antibiotics as prescribed should destroy all the bacteria and eliminate the risk of bacterial resistance.

the head of the bed elevated is often helpful. Surgery on the incompetent sphincter is usually not recommended and only considered in extreme cases.

### ■ Hiatal Hernia

Hiatal hernia is a sliding of part of the stomach into the chest cavity.

**ETIOLOGY** The stomach slides upward through the natural hole in the diaphragm where the esophagus passes through to the stomach (Figure 11–7). This herniation may increase in frequency with age and the weakening of the cardiac sphincter.

**SYMPTOMS** Many hiatal hernias are **asymptomatic** (a = without, symptomatic = symptoms), but those that do cause discomfort are usually related to esophageal reflux.

**TREATMENT** Treatment is often the same as for reflux esophagitis.

### ■ Esophageal Varices

**ETIOLOGY** Unusually high pressure in the veins of the esophagus causes them to enlarge and become tortuous, resulting in esophageal varices. This increased venous pressure is due to blockage or reduced flow of blood into the liver, causing poor venous return from the esophagus. Any condition that leads to venous congestion in the liver may lead to esophageal varices. (For more detailed information on esophageal varices, see Chapter 12.) Usually, esophageal varices are related to cirrhosis of the liver. The most common cause of cirrhosis is excessive alcohol consumption. Hemorrhage of the varices can be a life-threatening condition.

**TREATMENT** The goal of treatment is to decrease venous pressure by methods such as portal vein bypass surgery and medication to lower blood pressure. Other treatments include limiting the diet to soft, non-irritating foods, and the use of stool softeners to prevent straining, which increases esophageal venous pressure. Chronic bleeding of the vessels may be treated with a sclerosing agent that hardens or destroys the vessel. Acute bleeding treatments include instillation of cold saline washings and/or the application of pressure to the site through a nasogastric tube.

## Diseases of the Stomach

Diseases of the stomach are common problems in the digestive system. Complaints of stomach pain, especially after eating, are frequently voiced to the physician. This problem increases with age due to the age-related changes in the system that are also complicated by other chronic diseases. Disorders of the stomach range from mild acute gastritis to more serious diseases such as cancer of the stomach.

### ■ Gastritis

Inflammation in the stomach is known as gastritis. Common symptoms are epigastric pain, bloating, and nausea. Acute forms of gastritis are due to irritating agents such as aspirin, alcohol, coffee, tobacco, or bacteria-laden foods. Acute gastritis usually heals rapidly and requires no treatment.

Chronic gastritis may be identified as two separate forms: fundal gastritis and *Helicobacter* gastritis. Fundal gastritis affects the proximal area of the stomach where gastric acid-producing cells are located. As people age, there is a decrease in the number of acid-producing cells, thus leading to atrophic gastritis or **achlorhydria** (AH-klor-**HIGH**-dree-ah; no hydrochloric acid) and loss of intrinsic factor (a protein produced by the gastric mucosa). Loss of this intrinsic factor leads to pernicious anemia. (See Chapter 7 for more information on anemia.) Because fundal gastritis is age-related, there is no specific treatment, although avoidance of irritating agents may be

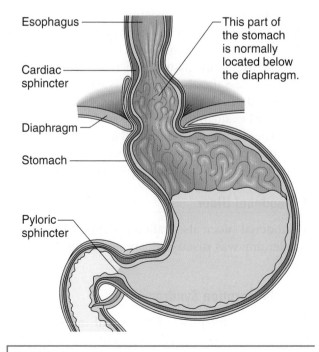

Esophagus

This part of the stomach is normally located below the diaphragm.

Cardiac sphincter

Diaphragm

Stomach

Pyloric sphincter

**FIGURE 11–7**  Hiatal hernia.

beneficial. The use of antacids may also be recommended.

*Helicobacter* gastritis is due to small bacteria commonly found in the stomach lining. The presence of the bacteria does not cause symptoms in the majority of people. Those persons affected may experience chronic gastritis. The incidence of chronic *Helicobacter* gastritis increases with age. *Helicobacter* gastritis is now thought to be a major factor in gastric ulcer formation. Diagnosis is confirmed by biopsy. A combination of medications is utilized to reduce or eliminate *Helicobacter* bacteria, and thus to reduce gastritis and ulcer formation.

### ■ Peptic Ulcer

An ulcer is an area of tissue that has eroded, leaving a crater-like appearance (Figure 11–8).

**ETIOLOGY** Development of peptic ulcers is unclear, but it is thought that contributing factors include severe stress, heavy intake of drugs (such as aspirin, steroids, and alcohol), smoking, and the presence of *Helicobacter* bacteria.

Peptic ulcers are those ulcers found in the stomach and duodenum that are caused, in part, by the action of pepsin. The stomach lining is normally protected by a thick mucous membrane lining. Pepsin is an enzyme secreted in the stomach that breaks down protein. This same enzyme, to some degree, breaks down the stomach's lining, causing ulcers.

**SYMPTOMS** Ulcer pain is caused by the hydrochloric acid in the stomach irritating the raw ulcerated area.

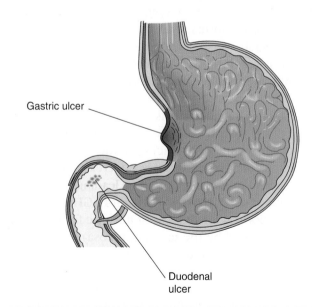

Gastric ulcer

Duodenal ulcer

**FIGURE 11–8** Peptic ulcers.

Peptic ulcers found in the stomach are called gastric ulcers and those located in the duodenum are called duodenal ulcers. Complications of peptic ulcers are massive bleeding, perforation, and obstruction.

**TREATMENT** Treatment is aimed at reducing the gastric acidity and healing of the stomach lining. Treatment includes reduction or elimination of contributory factors. Antacids to neutralize gastric acids and other gastric medications may be helpful. Antibiotics are also used to treat ulcers caused by *Helicobacter* bacteria. Surgery is warranted in severe cases that may lead to hemorrhage, perforation, obstruction, or extreme pain.

### ■ Cancer of the Stomach

Cancer of the stomach affects males in greater numbers than females.

**ETIOLOGY** Causative factors indicate some correlation to food additives and cigarette smoking. Often, this cancer goes undiagnosed until after it spreads outside the stomach and into other organs.

**SYMPTOMS** Symptoms are often vague and include loss of appetite, general stomach distress, and heartburn. Prognosis is good if the cancer is discovered early.

**TREATMENT** Treatment may include surgical resection, chemotherapy, and radiation.

## Diseases of the Small Intestine

The small intestine, consisting of the duodenum, jejunum, and ileum, secretes enzymes and absorbs nutrients for cellular functions. Disorders of the small intestine frequently manifest themselves in pain that radiates across the abdomen. This symptom alone is not enough to diagnose the specific disease process. Additional evaluation is needed such as X-ray or CT scan. The disorders of the small intestine may range from mild intestinal upset to more severe chronic problems such as ulcers or regional enteritis.

### ■ Duodenal Ulcer

A duodenal ulcer, also called a peptic ulcer of the duodenum, was discussed previously under *Peptic Ulcer.*

### ■ Malabsorption Syndrome

The primary purpose of the small intestine is to absorb nutrients. When the small intestine is unable to accomplish this function, malabsorption syndrome may be diagnosed.

## COMPLEMENTARY AND ALTERNATIVE THERAPY

### Turkey Tail Fungus for Stomach and Colorectal Cancers

The fungus known as Turkey Tail (*Trametes versicolor*) is a common forest mushroom. It has a white, tough, and fibrous flesh, usually less than 2 mm thick. The underside of its leaves contain a white to pale yellow layer of very small tubes that are vertical with three to five pores per mm. It is being used in Japan for treatment of stomach and colorectal cancers, along with traditional chemotherapy. Research has shown it to be effective for its antiviral and cholesterol lowering properties. Now, it is being used to improve the quality of life and to extend the survival rates for cancer victims. The safety of the mushroom is not well established for long-term uses or for use with other over-the-counter or prescription medications.

*Source: Hobbs, C. R. (2004).*

**ETIOLOGY** Persons with malabsorption syndrome may be unable to absorb nutrients (especially fat) and minerals. Other organ diseases such as liver disease, gallbladder obstruction, diabetes mellitus, pancreatic deficiencies, and cardiovascular disease may lead to malabsorption syndrome.

**TREATMENT** Most treatments include diet therapy for control. One of the complications of the disorder is a bleeding tendency due to the lack of vitamin K absorption.

### ■ Regional Enteritis (Crohn's Disease)

Regional enteritis is a chronic inflammatory disease most commonly affecting the small intestine, but it may also affect the large intestine. It is character-

ized by bouts of **remission** (slowing or stopping of symptoms) and **exacerbation** (x-AS-er-**BAY**-shun; flaring up of symptoms) (Figure 11–9). Regional enteritis is commonly classified as Inflammatory Bowel Disease (IBD) until complete diagnosis is made. As regional enteritis progresses, the intestinal wall becomes thickened, resulting in a narrowing of the lumen.

**ETIOLOGY** The cause of the disease has not yet been determined although genetic, immunologic, infectious and psychologic factors have been considered.

**SYMPTOMS** Symptoms include anorexia, flatulence, abdominal pain, diarrhea, and constipation. Individuals with regional enteritis tend to experience relapse or exacerbations of the condition during periods of stress or emotional upset, factors that support

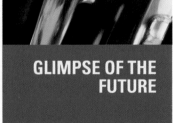

### GLIMPSE OF THE FUTURE

### Will Antioxidant Supplements Be Used to Prevent Stomach Cancers in the Future?

Antioxidant supplements may be used in the future to prevent stomach cancers. The antioxidant beta carotene has been studied alone and in combination with other vitamins such as A, C, and E, and with selenium to see if it can prevent stomach and other cancers. In this article, the researchers reviewed all the randomized trials comparing antioxidant supplement therapy with placebos for prevention of stomach cancers. The findings showed some reports of antioxidant therapy to be effective in preventing stomach cancers. Will antioxidant supplements be useful in the future to prevent these cancers? Right now, the prediction is to use caution when taking these supplements. They may be helpful, but there is not enough research at this time to tell.

*Source: Bjelakovic, G., et al. (2004).*

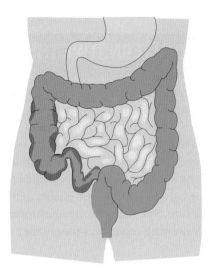

FIGURE 11–9　Regional enteritis.

the psychogenic theory. Young females are most often affected by regional enteritis.

**TREATMENT** Treatment is supportive but not likely to be curative. Approaches may involve a low-residue diet and medications to control diarrhea, inflammation, infection, and depression. Surgical resection is not curative and is performed to treat complications such as perforation and obstruction.

## ■ Gastroenteritis

Gastroenteritis (gastro = stomach, entero = intestines, itis = inflammation), as its name suggests, is inflammation of both the stomach and intestines (Figure 11-10).

**ETIOLOGY** Causes may include bacterial, viral, or parasitic invasion; ingestion of tainted food; lactose intolerance; and allergic reaction to food or drugs.

**SYMPTOMS** Gastroenteritis may have an acute and violent onset with nausea, vomiting, abdominal cramping, and diarrhea, leading to rapid fluid and electrolyte loss. Or symptoms may be less violent with stomach rumbling, malaise (ma-LAZ; general ill feeling), nausea, and mild diarrhea.

**TREATMENT** Treatment focuses on symptoms and may include antinausea medication, antidiarrhea medication, antibiotics, fluids, and nutritional support. Prognosis is generally good. Prevention of gastroenteritis includes hand washing prior to food preparation, proper refrigeration of food, and avoidance of contaminated food and water, especially in underdeveloped countries.

## ■ Inguinal Hernia

An inguinal hernia is a common problem that affects the digestive system.

**ETIOLOGY** An out-pouching of the small intestine and the peritoneum (abdominal cavity lining) into the groin area (Figure 11–11) causes this condition. Inguinal hernias are more common in males. This may be due to a congenital defect that developed as the testes descended from the abdomen into the scrotum, thus pulling part of the peritoneum into the inguinal area. Inguinal hernias also develop in both sexes due to a weakness in the abdominal wall.

The portions of the intestine that herniated may become caught and twisted, thus cutting off blood supply to the organ. If this occurs, it is called a strangulated hernia. A strangulated hernia may be life threatening and needs immediate surgical intervention.

**TREATMENT** Fortunately, inguinal hernias can be repaired surgically to prevent this potentially life-threatening situation.

Portions of the small intestine may also herniate through other openings in the body such as the femoral canal or the umbilicus. The femoral hernia, like the inguinal hernia, is more common in males. The umbilical hernia is most common in infants. Like the inguinal hernia, both are corrected surgically to prevent complications.

## Diseases of the Colon

Diseases of the colon or large intestine are common to all ages, but are found most frequently in the middle-aged and older adult with the exception of appendicitis. Common problems such as ulcerative colitis and cancer of the colon are two of the more serious conditions of the colon.

## ■ Appendicitis

The appendix is located near the junction of the small and large intestine, and although it is primarily composed of lymphoid tissues, the exact function is yet unknown.

**ETIOLOGY** Appendicitis is the inflammation of the vermiform (VER-my-form; worm-like) appendix. Infection or obstruction usually causes appendicitis. The position of the appendix near the colon allows bacteria-laden fecal contents to drop into the appendix, causing obstruction and infection. The inflamed appendix swells (see Figure 11–12), decreasing circulation and potentially leading to gangrene.

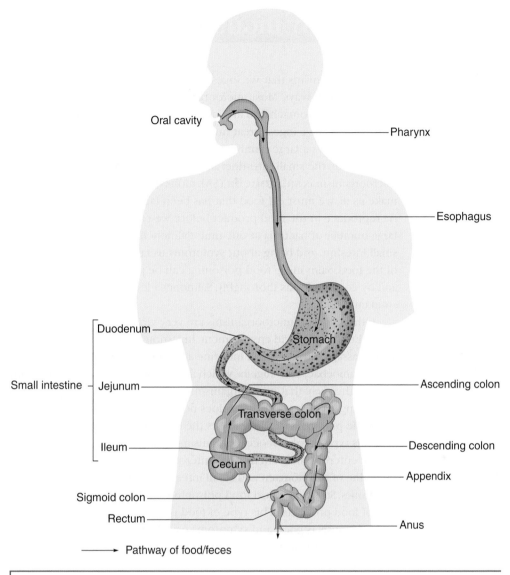

Oral cavity

Pharynx

Esophagus

Duodenum

Stomach

Small intestine

Jejunum

Ascending colon

Transverse colon

Ileum

Descending colon

Cecum

Appendix

Sigmoid colon

Rectum

Anus

→ Pathway of food/feces

**FIGURE 11–10** Gastroenteritis.

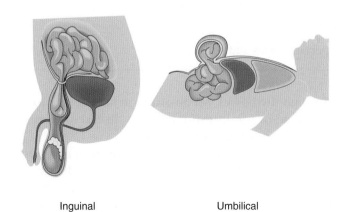

Inguinal                    Umbilical

**FIGURE 11–11** Hernias: inguinal and umbilical.

**SYMPTOMS** The pain of appendicitis usually begins with generalized abdominal pain that shifts to the lower right quadrant. Other signs and symptoms include nausea, vomiting, fever, and leukocytosis. This combination of signs and symptoms also mimics other abdominal diseases such as kidney stones, pelvic inflammatory disease, and pancreatitis, which may lead to an incorrect diagnosis.

As appendicitis progresses, the wall of the appendix thins and may rupture. Rupture of the appendix usually relieves the pain for a short time, but leads to a more severe complication of peritonitis. Before the development of antibiotics, peritonitis was usually fatal.

## HEALTHY HIGHLIGHT

### Food Poisoning

Microorganisms that we ingest (eat) may cause gastrointestinal upset in a variety of ways. Most microorganisms that we ingest are easily destroyed by the acid in the stomach and are incapacitated. Some microorganisms will only cause illness if we ingest great numbers of them at a time. Ingestion of these great numbers allows a large number of microorganisms to escape the acid environment, invade the small intestine, and cause illness. An example of this type of microorganism is **salmonella** (SAL-moh-**NEL**-ah). In order for salmonella to make us ill, we must eat food that has been tainted with salmonella. These bacteria reproduce in the food product before we eat it, thus providing ingestion of a large number of bacteria at one time. Salmonella bacteria invade the lining of the small intestine and bring about symptoms usually 24 to 48 hours after ingestion of the food. Salmonella food poisoning can be prevented by refrigerating foods and by cooking foods thoroughly. Salmonella food poisoning is determined by a stool culture.

Other types of microorganisms are very virulent and are thus able to withstand the stomach acid environment. Ingestion of even small numbers of these will allow passage into the small intestine and cause illness. These organisms include viruses, amoebae, and shigella, which are frequently spread by a fecal-oral route.

Another way that microorganisms make us ill is by producing a toxin (poisoning). The bacteria itself does not cause the harm, but the **enterotoxin** (intestine poison) it produces does the damage. Staphylococcal food poisoning is of this type. Staphylococcal organisms contaminate nonrefrigerated food and release enterotoxins. When these enterotoxins are ingested, they quickly invade the lining of the stomach and small intestine, leading to symptoms within one to four hours. Staphylococcal food poisoning can be prevented by proper refrigeration of food products. This type of food poisoning is determined by a food culture. Prognosis is good and symptoms usually resolve within 24 hours.

Following these measures can prevent most gastrointestinal upset caused by contaminated food.

- Always wash your hands before and after preparing food.
- Wash your hands before and after a meal.
- Keep eating utensils and plates clean and stored until ready for use.
- Cover and refrigerate food properly.
- Cook foods thoroughly, especially meats and seafood.

**TREATMENT** Treatment for appendicitis requires surgical removal of the appendix, preferably before rupture occurs.

### ■ Intestinal Obstruction

Intestinal obstruction may be classified as a symptom of a disease process or as a disease itself.

**ETIOLOGY** Regardless of the classification, it is identified as an inability to move intestinal contents through the bowel. An obstruction may be due to a blockage of the intestine, or to a disease or **ileus** (ILL-ee-us; absence of peristalsis).

Blockage may occur due to tumors, hernias, or **adhesions** (ad-He-zhuns) (Figure 11–13). Adhesions are areas within the colon that abnormally link together, resulting from a previous abdominal surgery or from inflammation. Blockage also may occur if the colon becomes twisted (**volvulus**; VOL-view-lus) (Figure 11–14). If the colon telescopes on itself, the

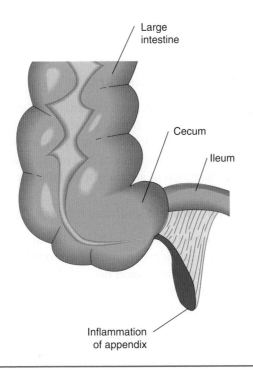

**FIGURE 11–12** Appendix.

condition may lead to a blockage called **intussusception** (IN-tus-sus-**SEP**-shun).

A decrease or absence of peristalsis that causes intestinal obstruction is classified as a **paralytic obstruction**. Colon action is paralyzed or unable to move. This type of obstruction may be a postoperative complication or may be a result of peritonitis.

**SYMPTOMS** Symptoms depend on the type and severity of the obstruction. The individual may experience mild to severe abdominal pain and distention, nausea, and vomiting.

**TREATMENT** Intestinal obstruction may be relieved by nasogastric suctioning, but more commonly, surgery is required.

## ■ Ulcerative Colitis

Ulcerative colitis is a chronic inflammation of the colon (Figure 11–15). Like regional enteritis, it is commonly called inflammatory bowel disease until diagnosis is confirmed.

**ETIOLOGY** The cause of ulcerative colitis is unknown. Exacerbations of the disease often occur during stressful times, leading one to believe that there is a psychogenic factor involved. Other causative theories include heredity and autoimmune and dietary factors. Patients with ulcerative colitis are at a high risk for developing colon cancer.

**SYMPTOMS** The colon and rectum have multiple ulcerations that lead to lower abdominal pain, blood in the stools, anemia, and diarrhea.

**TREATMENT** Treatment may include dietary limitations, stress reduction, mild sedatives, and anti-inflammatory medications. Surgery is usually considered only if conservative treatment fails. Surgical intervention often results in a colostomy (opening in the colon), either temporary or permanent (Figure

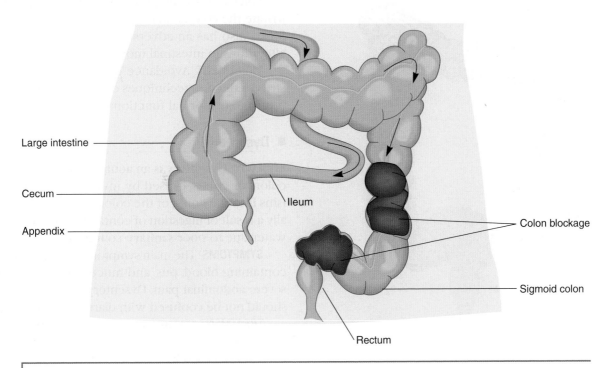

**FIGURE 11–13** Colon blockage.

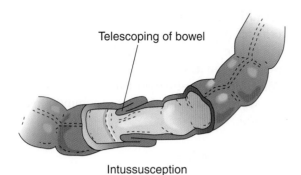

Telescoping of bowel

Intussusception

180-degree twisting of bowel

Volvulus

**FIGURE 11–14**  Volvulus and intussusception.

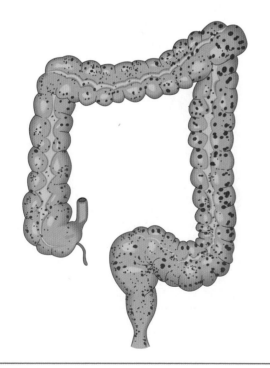

**FIGURE 11–15**  Ulcerative colitis.

11–16). If the colostomy is permanent, a portion of the colon may be removed.

## ■ Inflammatory Bowel Disease

IBD refers to both regional enteritis (Crohn's disease) and ulcerative colitis. Both diseases (as previously discussed) are chronic in nature with undetermined etiology. A general diagnosis of IBD may be used until a definite diagnosis of another bowel disorder is made.

## ■ Irritable Bowel Syndrome (Spastic Colon)

Irritable bowel syndrome (IBS) is the most common intestinal disorder. It may be commonly confused with inflammatory bowel disease (IBD), but they are not the same. Inflammatory bowel disease is an inflammation of the bowel with chronic lesions. There is neither inflammation nor lesions in irritable bowel syndrome.

**ETIOLOGY**  The cause of IBS is unknown but a strong psychogenic factor has been considered. IBS is chronic and onset usually occurs in the young adult. Frequent reoccurrence over the years is very frustrating to the affected individual and the physician.

**SYMPTOMS**  IBS is a functional disorder of motility and may cause a group of symptoms including abdominal pain and altered motility. Typically, an individual suffering from IBS has bouts of diarrhea or constipation, or both.

Spicy foods, caffeine, alcohol, and seasonings can irritate the colon and bring about symptoms of IBS. Stress also has an adverse effect and often causes alterations in intestinal motility.

**TREATMENT**  Avoidance of causative factors and stress reduction techniques often allow the colon to return to its normal functional state.

## ■ Dysentery

**ETIOLOGY**  Dysentery is an acute inflammation of the colon, or colitis, caused by invasion of microorganisms into the lining of the colon. This disease is usually a result of ingestion of contaminated food and/or water due to poor sanitary conditions.

**SYMPTOMS**  The main symptom is massive diarrhea containing blood, pus, and mucus, accompanied by severe abdominal pain. Dysentery is the disease and should not be confused with diarrhea, the symptom.

**TREATMENT**  Treatment is dependent on the cause of the disease. Antibiotics are usually effective for dysentery caused by a bacterial infection.

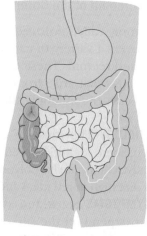

Ascending colostomy

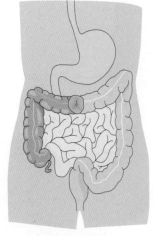

Transverse colostomy

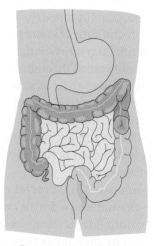

Descending colostomy

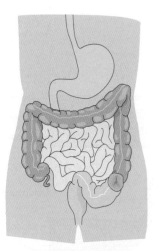

Sigmoid colostomy

**FIGURE 11–16** Colostomy locations (blue section may be surgically removed if colostomy is permanent).

## ■ Diverticulosis/Diverticulitis

Diverticulosis is a condition of having diverticula or little outpouches in the colon (Figure 11–17), especially the sigmoid colon. It may be asymptomatic (without symptoms) until the pouches become packed with fecal material and become irritated and inflamed. Once inflamed, the condition is called diverticulitis.

**ETIOLOGY** Diverticulitis increases in incidence with age, and has been associated with poor dietary habits, lack of physical activity, and poor bowel habits.

**SYMPTOMS** Low abdominal pain and cramping are indicative of diverticulitis. As this inflammatory disease progresses, it may lead to hemorrhage, per-foration, or narrowing of the lumen of the colon, and thus obstruction.

**TREATMENT** Increasing the amount of fiber in the diet is usually effective in relieving symptoms and preventing complications. Foods high in fiber include fruits, vegetables, beans, potatoes, rice, and cereals. Fiber keeps the stool soft, allowing it to move more easily through the colon. Antibiotics may be needed if acute diverticulitis develops.

## ■ Colon Polyps

A polyp (POL-ip) is an inward projection of the mucosal lining of the colon (Figure 11–18).

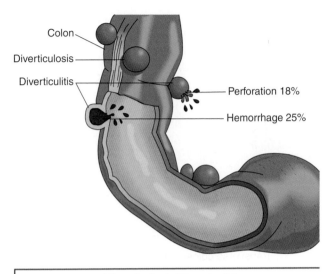

**FIGURE 11–17** Diverticulosis/Diverticulitis.

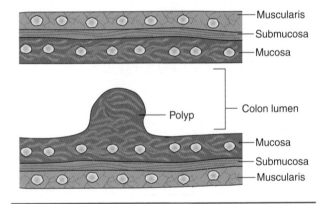

**FIGURE 11–18** Colon polyp.

**ETIOLOGY** It may be due to an inflammatory reaction, or may be caused by a benign or malignant neoplasm.

**SYMPTOMS** Polyps are commonly asymptomatic and often diagnosed during a colonoscopy (colon = colon, oscopy = procedure to look into) or sigmoidoscopy (sigmoid = sigmoid portion of the colon).

**TREATMENT** Suspicious polyps may be excisionally biopsied during these procedures. Cancerous polyps are removed by excisional biopsy or surgical resection, depending on the number and type of polyps present.

## ■ Carcinoma of the Colon and Rectum

Commonly called **colorectal** cancer, this classification covers a variety of carcinomas that arise in the colon and rectum. These tumors are usually adenocarcinomas that arise from the mucosal lining. Colorectal cancer commonly affects both sexes after the age of 40.

**ETIOLOGY** The cause of colorectal cancer is unknown. Some identified predisposing factors include ulcerative colitis, familial polyposis (many colon polyps), and a diet high in red meat and low in fiber.

**SYMPTOMS** Signs and symptoms of colorectal cancer depend on the site of the malignancy. Common symptoms may include a change in bowel habits (diarrhea or constipation), pencil sized stools, blood in the stools, anemia (due to tumor bleeding), abdominal discomfort, and obstruction.

Adenocarcinomas (the most common type found in colorectal cancer) tend to grow slowly. Eventually, the tumor may grow large enough to obstruct the lumen and spread through the colon wall. Once it has spread through the colon wall, it may gain access to the lymphatic and vascular systems, and spread throughout the body. The most common site of metastasis is the liver. Prognosis is good if the carcinoma is detected before metastasis; after metastasis, prognosis is poor.

Diagnosis of colorectal cancer may be made by stool examinations for occult blood, colonoscopy, and barium enema. Some rectal tumors also may be palpated by digital examination.

**TREATMENT** Colorectal carcinoma is one of the leading causes of death from cancer in the United States. If detected early, it is potentially curable by surgical resection.

Prevention of colorectal cancer centers around dietary changes, which include decreasing red meat and increasing fiber consumption. It is also recommended that stool examination be performed on individuals annually, beginning at age 40.

## Diseases of the Rectum

The rectum is the terminal or end part of the digestive system. The most common rectal problem is hemorrhoids. Rectal fissures and other minor problems can also occur, but cancer of the rectum is one of the most serious diseases of the rectum to be diagnosed. It is more commonly diagnosed in the older adult than at any other age.

## HEALTHY HIGHLIGHT

### Colon Cancer Prevention

Colon cancer commonly occurs after age 40. It is, therefore, recommended that everyone age 40 and over should have an annual exam, including a stool examination for occult blood. This relatively easy examination can assist with early detection of colon cancer. Prognosis for colon cancer is good if it is discovered in its early stages.

### ■ Hemorrhoids

Hemorrhoids are varicose veins in the rectum (Figure 11-19). Hemorrhoids can be internal or external. Internal hemorrhoids can be examined by a physician using a proctoscope (procto = rectum, scope = instrument used to view). Internal hemorrhoids are located on the rectal wall. External hemorrhoids are located in the lower anal canal.

External hemorrhoids are developed when internal hemorrhoids are pushed or prolapsed through the anal opening. External hemorrhoids are the ones commonly known as "hemorrhoids" and may be viewed around the anal opening. External hemorrhoids are bluish in color and may bleed with straining during bowel movements.

**ETIOLOGY** Factors that increase the risk of developing hemorrhoids include any activity that increases pressure in the anal area such as straining to have a bowel movement, frequent bouts of constipation, prolonged standing, prolonged sitting, pregnancy, and childbirth. Other causes may be related to heredity and loss of muscle tone.

Preventive measures are focused at softening the stool (which will decrease constipation and straining with bowel movements). These measures include good bowel habits (defecating when reflexes are strong), adequate fluid intake, increased fiber intake, exercise, and avoiding laxative use.

**TREATMENT** Treatment of hemorrhoids may include medications and warm sitz baths to ease the pain. Manual reduction, cryosurgery, and hemorrhoidectomy may be optional treatments, depending on the severity of the disease.

### ■ Carcinoma of the Rectum

See "Carcinoma of the Colon and Rectum."

## TRAUMA

### Trauma to the Mouth

Trauma to the mouth may be due to motor vehicle accidents, falls, abuse, burns, or any other blunt or perforating injury. The result may be broken teeth or jawbones or lesions and lacerations. Depending on the severity of the injury and the treatment needed, the individual may have difficulty eating. If the jaw is broken the individual may need to have the jaw wired closed for a period of time. This requires a special liquid nutrition program so the individual can maintain adequate intake of fluids, vitamins, and minerals. Burns and lacerations also interfere with the normal oral intake of fluid and food. The individual may need

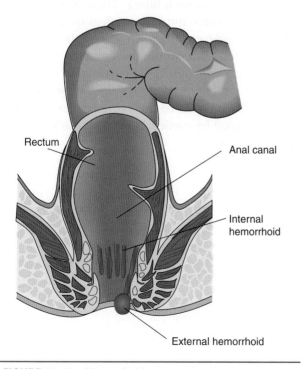

Rectum

Anal canal

Internal hemorrhoid

External hemorrhoid

**FIGURE 11–19** Hemorrhoids: internal and external.

alternate feeding methods such as parenteral (intravenous) or enteral (tube feeding) nutrition.

## Trauma to the Stomach and Intestines

Trauma to the digestive system other than the mouth is usually due to perforation (a hole through the organ). This may be the result of a stabbing, gunshot wound, or piercing by another object. This is a medical emergency because the contents of the stomach or intestines can spill out into the abdominal cavity, causing peritonitis. Commonly, the wound is surgically repaired and the individual is given antibiotics for the infection.

## RARE DISEASES

### Achalasia

Achalasia is a disorder of the esophagus that causes pain with swallowing. The peristaltic movement of the lower portion of the esophagus does not function properly. The cause of the disorder is unknown. Treatment may involve surgery and/or drug therapy.

### Gluten-Induced Enteropathy

This disease is also called celiac sprue disease or nontropical sprue disease. It is an immune problem that causes the individual to be sensitive to gluten proteins. This protein is found mainly in wheat and rye products, but also in oat and barley foods. Individuals with gluten-induced enteropathy have impaired absorption of some vitamins and proteins, fats, and carbohydrates. Gluten-induced enteropathy is treated by a dietary measure restricting all gluten-containing foods.

### Intestinal Polyps

Intestinal polyps are found along the lining of the intestine. They are benign (noncancerous) tumors. Although they usually do not cause any symptoms

for the individual, they are often surgically removed. This is a preventive treatment because polyps may increase the individual's risk of cancer.

## EFFECTS OF AGING ON THE SYSTEM

Disorders of the digestive system are common in the aging population. The incidence of problems increases with age. Some of the problems occurring in the system with age are caused by changes in the cardiovascular or neurologic system, which causes disruptions in the functioning of the digestive system. In the upper digestive system, the most common problem with aging is related to loss of teeth. Preventive dentistry has lessened teeth and gum problems in recent years, but it is still a significant factor in the older adult. The sense of taste becomes less sensitive. The motility in the esophagus decreases and may cause some distress, but it is generally asymptomatic.

Changes in the lining of the stomach and decreased secretion of hydrochloric acid increase the likelihood of digestive disorders in the older adult. Decreased circulation to the stomach increases the incidence of ulcer disease.

Lower digestive disorders are common in the older adult. The lower intestinal lining is affected much like the stomach lining. There is a decreased absorption of some nutrients such as vitamin $B_{12}$ and fats. Decreased circulation to the intestines may cause ischemia and pain in the abdomen. Decreased motility may contribute to constipation problems. The development of inflammatory disease and hemorrhoids is common to the aging process, but also may be caused by earlier problems or other predisposing factors.

## SUMMARY

The digestive system is a long, hollow tube that extends from the mouth to the anus. Its purpose is the ingestion, digestion, and absorption of fluids and nutrients, and elimination of wastes. Accessory organs of the digestive system include the liver, pancreas, and gallbladder. The most common diseases of the system are infections, ulcers, and cancer. Physiologic and lifestyle changes in older adults put them at higher risk for diseases of the digestive system.

## REVIEW QUESTIONS

### Short Answer

1. What are the functions of the digestive system?

2. Which signs and symptoms are associated with common digestive system disorders?

3. Which diagnostic tests are most commonly used to determine type and/or cause of the digestive system disorders?

### Matching

4. Match the disorders listed in the left column with the correct region of the digestive system in the right column:

| | |
|---|---|
| _____ pharyngitis | **a.** disease of the small intestine |
| _____ gastritis | **b.** disease of the mouth |
| _____ hemorrhoids | **c.** disease of the colon |
| _____ periodontal disease | **d.** disease of the throat or esophagus |
| _____ regional enteritis | **e.** disease of the rectum |
| _____ irritable bowel syndrome | **f.** disease of the stomach |

### Multiple Choice

5. Which of the following behaviors may contribute to digestive system problems?

   **a.** Eating four to six small meals per day

   **b.** Improperly cooking food

   **c.** Failure to wash hands after toileting

   **d.** Poor dietary habits

   **e.** Straining with bowel movements

   **f.** Drinking plenty of fluids daily

   **g.** Frequent use of laxatives and enemas

## True or False

**6.** T  F    The alimentary canal is a continuous tube from the mouth to the anus.

**7.** T  F    Strep throat should always be treated since it may lead to rheumatic heart disease.

**8.** T  F    The main function of the large intestine (colon) is the digestion of food.

**9.** T  F    The *Helicobacter* bacteria are contributing factors in the development of peptic ulcers.

**10.** T  F    The effects of aging put the older adult at an increased risk for digestive system problems.

## CASE STUDY

**Stacey Erin** is a 32-year-old accountant who has just been diagnosed with peptic ulcer disease. She would like some information about her disorder, what to expect in the future, and how to cope with it. What would you tell her about peptic ulcer disease? How can she prevent continued problems with her ulcer?

## BIBLIOGRAPHY

Atsushi, O. (2003). The latest advances in chemotherapy for gastrointestinal cancers. *International Journal of Clinical Oncology 8*(4), 234–238.

Birkenfeld, S. (2004). Prevalence of *Helicobacter pylori* infection in health-care personnel of primary care and gastroenterology clinics. *Journal of Clinical Gastroenterology 38*(1), 19–23.

Bjelakovic, G., Nikolova, D., Simonetti, R., & Gluud, C. (2004). Antioxidant supplements for prevention of gastrointestinal cancers: A systematic review and meta-analysis. *Lancet 364*(9441), 1219–1228.

Cooper, A. (2003). How to manage dyspepsia. *Update 67*(7), 399–401.

Crohn disease may begin with an immunodeficient condition. (2003, July 20). *Immunotherapy Weekly*, 49–50.

Diet may play a role in IBS and dyspepsia. (2003, November 3). *Health & Medicine Week*, 415–416.

Dippold, L., Lee, R., Selman, C., Monroe, S., & Henry, C. (2003). A gastroenteritis outbreak due to norovirus associated with a Colorado hotel. *Journal of Environmental Health 66*(5), 13–17.

Evans, M. R., Ribeiro, C. D., & Salmon, R. L. (2003). Hazards of healthy living: Bottled water and salad vegetables as risk factors for campylobacter infection. *Emerging Infectious Diseases 9*(10), 1219–1225.

Gallager, C., & McDowell, B. M. (2003). A guidelines-based approach for managing acute gastroenteritis in children. *Journal for Specialists in Pediatric Nursing 8*(3), 107–110.

Gastrointestinal disorder prevalent among college-age students. (2003, December 15). *Health & Medicine Week*, 212–213.

Heitkemper, M., Jarrett, M., Bond, E., & Chang, L. (2003). Impact of sex and gender on irritable bowel syndrome. *Biological Research for Nursing 5*(1), 56–65.

Henkel, J. (2003). Surgery for the severly obese. *FDA Consumer 37*(6), 41.

Hobbs, C. R. (2004). Medicinal value of turkey tail fungus Trametes versicolor (L:Fr) Pilát (Aphyllophoromycetideae). A literature review. *International Journal of Medicinal Mushrooms 6*(3), 195–218.

Home-treated water no better than plain tap in preventing GI illness. (2003, October 27). *Health & Medicine Week*, 3–5.

Horton, J. (2003). Human gastrointestinal helminth infections: Are they now neglected diseases? *Trends in Parasitology 19*(11), 527–531.

Lab tests can reveal which patients will respond to Gleevec. (2003, December 15). *Health & Medicine Week*, 343–345.

Langmead, L., & Ramptom, D. S. (2001). Review article: herbal treatments in gastrointestinal and liver disease—benefits and dangers. *Alimentary Pharmacology & Therapeutics 15*(9), 7.

Lung Lai, C., Ratziu, V., Yuen, M., & Poynard, T. (2003). Viral hepatitis B. *Lancet 362*(9401), 2089–2094.

Meineche-Schmidt, V., & Jorgensen, T. (2003). "Alarm symptoms" in dyspepsia. *Scandinavian Journal of Primary Health Care 21*(4), 224–229.

Motzer, S. A., Jarrett, M., Heitkemper, M., & Tsuji, J. (2002). Natural killer cell function and psychological distress in women with and without irritable bowel syndrome. *Biological Research for Nursing 4*(1), 31–42.

Recommendations. (2003). *Alimentary Pharmacology and Therapeutics 18*(9), 93–94.

Scientists describe germ warfare with gut bugs. (2003, August 15). *Health & Medicine Week*, 368.

The emerging role of the hedgehog signaling pathway in upper GI cancers. (2003, December 15). *Health & Medicine Week*, 337.

Uncovering gastrointestinal disorders. (2003). *Australian Nursing Journal 10*(8), 25.

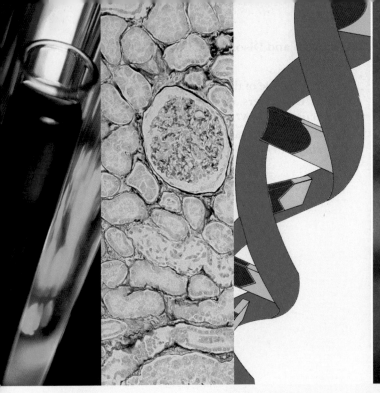
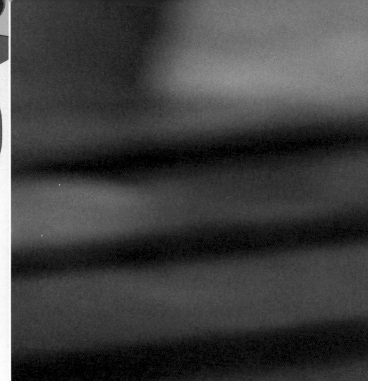

## OUTLINE

## KEY TERMS

# Liver, Gallbladder, and Pancreas Diseases and Disorders

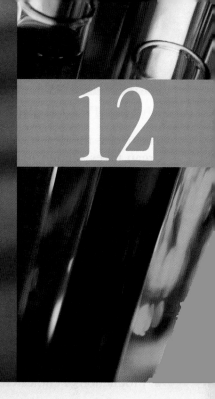

**12**

## LEARNING OBJECTIVES

*Upon completion of the chapter, the learner should be able to:*

1. Define the terminology common to the liver, gallbladder, and pancreas, and the disorders of the organs.

2. Discuss the basic anatomy and physiology of the liver, gallbladder, and pancreas.

3. Identify the important signs and symptoms associated with common liver, gallbladder, and pancreas disorders.

4. Describe the common diagnostics used to determine the type and/or cause of liver, gallbladder, or pancreas disorders.

5. Identify common disorders of the liver, gallbladder, and pancreas.

6. Describe the typical course and management of the common liver, gallbladder, and pancreas disorders.

7. Describe the effects of aging on the liver, gallbladder, and pancreas, and the common disorders of the organs.

## OVERVIEW

*The liver, gallbladder, and pancreas are the accessory organs of digestion. Although these organs are not considered part of the digestive system, they have important roles in the digestive process, as well as having many other functions in the body. Disorders of the liver, gallbladder, or pancreas can cause serious digestive problems and many other systemic disorders.* ∎

## ANATOMY AND PHYSIOLOGY

The liver is the largest solid organ of the body. This organ takes second place only to the skin as the largest organ overall (Figure 12–1). The liver has many functions, most of which are related to its chemical actions. The liver plays a role in digestion, absorption, metabolism, blood clotting, the manufacture of important chemicals, and storage of nutrients. The liver is composed of two lobes, weighs about three and a half pounds, and lies in the right upper quadrant of the abdomen. Some of the most important functions of the liver include:

- production and secretion of bile used for fat digestion
- production of cholesterol
- oxidation of fatty acids and glycerol used for body energy
- metabolism of carbohydrates, fats, and protein
- conversion of glucose to glycogen for storage and the reverse process for energy
- synthesis of amino acids
- detoxification of many drugs and other toxins
- storage of vitamins and other minerals
- production of fibrinogen and prothrombin for blood clotting

The liver receives blood from the portal system via the portal vein and the hepatic artery. About 1,450 ml of blood flows through the liver every minute. The blood returns to the circulatory system via the hepatic vein to the inferior vena cava.

Bile is continually produced in the liver. It is used to emulsify or break down lipids in the intestine. The hepatic duct connects the liver to the duodenum. When bile is not needed in the digestive process, excess bile is stored in the gallbladder.

The gallbladder is a small, pear-shaped organ lying just under the liver (see Figure 12–1). Bile is stored here until needed by the intestine in the digestive

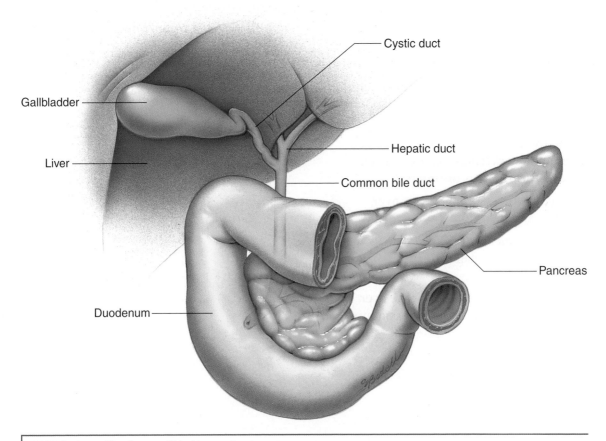

**FIGURE 12–1**  The liver, gallbladder, and pancreas.

process. Bile travels from the gallbladder to the duodenum via the cystic duct and the common bile duct.

The pancreas lies in the abdomen behind the stomach between the duodenum and the spleen (see Figure 12–1). It is both an endocrine gland (the islet cells secrete hormones) and an exocrine gland, producing and secreting most of the digestive enzymes. The pancreas secretes intestinal juices consisting of chymotrypsin and trypsin, which break down proteins; amylase, which breaks down starch; and lipase, which breaks down fats. The pancreatic juices exit the gland by way of the pancreatic duct to the duodenum.

## COMMON SIGNS AND SYMPTOMS

**Jaundice** (JAWN-dis, a yellowish discoloration of the skin) is an obvious symptom of liver disease. Jaundice also may be secondary to gallbladder disease. If a bile duct is blocked, the bile backs up into the liver and leads to jaundice.

**ETIOLOGY** Jaundice is caused by high levels of bilirubin in the blood. Bilirubin is a by-product of the breakdown of heme, the main component of hemoglobin in red blood cells. The liver filters bilirubin out of the blood and excretes it in bile. If the liver is unable to filter bilirubin and excrete it, hyperbilirubinemia (hyper = too much, bilirubin, emia = blood) or excessive bilirubin in the blood occurs.

**SYMPTOMS** Excessive bilirubin leaks into the tissues and the individual's skin, mucosa, and sclera (white part of the eye) become yellowish in color.

**TREATMENT** Bilirubin can be broken down in the skin by exposure to sunlight or direct lighting. This explains the use of "bili lights" to clear bilirubin in a jaundiced newborn infant. Excessive bilirubin is also filtered out of the blood by the kidneys, causing dark brown urine.

Pain is a common symptom of gallbladder disease, pancreatitis, and end stage pancreatic cancer. With gallbladder disease, right-sided abdominal pain commonly occurs following a meal containing fat. Acute abdominal pain occurs with pancreatitis and pancreatic cancer.

## DIAGNOSTIC TESTS

Liver function tests are blood tests to measure levels of bilirubin, albumin (blood protein), and alkaline phosphatase (enzyme). Impaired liver function will lead to elevated bilirubin and alkaline phosphatase levels, and low albumin levels.

Ultrasound is used to evaluate the liver, gallbladder, and pancreas for size, shape, and position. X-ray examinations of the gallbladder and the vessels of the gallbladder (cholecystogram and cholangiogram, respectively) utilize radiopaque dye to show the presence of gallstones, tumors, and function of the gallbladder. Ultrasonography is used more often than the above radiologic examinations.

Computer axial tomography (CAT or CT) scans may be performed to visualize the liver, gallbladder, and pancreas. Visualization of these organs aids in diagnosis of hepatic and pancreatic cancer. A liver biopsy can be performed by needle biopsy or during laparoscopic surgery. Biopsy is the most reliable test for determination of chronic hepatitis, cirrhosis, and cancer.

Blood tests to measure pancreatic function commonly include serum amylase and lipase. Amylase and lipase are digestive enzymes produced by the pancreas that break down carbohydrates and fats respectively.

## COMMON DISEASES OF THE ACCESSORY ORGANS OF DIGESTION

Diseases of the accessory organs of digestion can seriously affect the digestion and metabolism of nutrients. Symptoms of these disorders reflect an interference with the particular organ's function. Over 25 million individuals—one in ten—in the United States have been diagnosed with liver or gallbladder diseases (American Liver Foundation, 2004).

### Liver Diseases

Liver diseases can range from mild inflammation to those that destroy the liver and result in liver failure. Any disease of the liver can have serious consequences by interfering with the many functions of the liver.

#### ■ Hepatitis

**ETIOLOGY** Hepatitis is inflammation of the liver, and may be caused by the chemical action of drugs or

## COMPLEMENTARY AND ALTERNATIVE THERAPY

**Alternative Medicines for Liver Disease**

A variety of herbal medicines are used by persons with liver diseases. It is estimated that one in five individuals uses complementary or alternative therapies on a regular basis.

Specific herbals used for liver diseases include milk thistle (*Sylibum marianum*), licorice (*Glycyrrhiza glabra*), and bhuiamla (*Phyllanthus amarus*). These herbal medicines have been used in India for thousands of years to treat and prevent liver disease. Some research has shown that these are antioxidants, anti-inflammatory agents, and liver regenerating. They could be hepatotoxic in some cases and should be used with caution. Further research needs to be done to ensure their effectiveness for treatment of liver problems.

*Source: Fogden, E., & Neuberger, J. (2003).*

toxic substances. Chronic alcoholism often leads to hepatitis prior to the functional changes seen with cirrhosis. The most common cause of hepatitis is a group of viruses. This form of hepatitis is often called viral hepatitis, and is the form most commonly thought of when one considers hepatitis.

Viral hepatitis is the most prevalent liver disease in the world. It is often asymptomatic. When symptoms do occur, they may be so vague that the disease is misdiagnosed. This explains why approximately 40 percent of Americans have antibodies to hepatitis A and 10 percent have antibodies to hepatitis B, yet these individuals do not recall ever having hepatitis.

Viral hepatitis occurs in five basic types. A different virus causes each type. The types of hepatitis are A, B, C, D, and E.

1. Hepatitis A—the most benign or harmless form of hepatitis. Total recovery occurs 98 percent of the time. This virus is spread by fecal-oral route. It commonly affects children and young adults, especially in areas where there is poor sanitation and overcrowding. Symptoms are usually very vague and similar to "flu," often leading to misdiagnosis. The virus is shed in the feces and the affected individual does not become a carrier of the disease. Hepatitis A never leads to chronic hepatitis or cirrhosis. There is a vaccine available. The vaccine is recommended for those traveling or living in a high-risk area.

2. Hepatitis B—a serious form of hepatitis formerly called "serum hepatitis." It was once thought that hepatitis B was only spread by contact with blood

as occurs with blood transfusions and contaminated needles. But it is now known that saliva, urine, feces, and semen may spread the virus, which also qualifies it as a sexually transmitted disease. Hepatitis B also may be spread transplacentally (across the placenta from mother to unborn infant). This virus is a major health problem because individuals may become carriers of the virus. Approximately 125,000 new infections occur every year in the United States. This virus may be carried for years or even a lifetime. Carriers are not only a threat to others but also are at high risk for developing chronic hepatitis and cirrhosis. About one out of every 250 persons is a carrier of hepatitis B. Those at high risk for hepatitis B are drug addicts, homosexuals, blood recipients, and health care workers. A vaccine is available and is 95 percent effective in prevention of the disease.

3. Hepatitis C—similar to hepatitis B because it also is spread by blood or sexual contact. Hepatitis C differs from B in that it attacks the RNA of a cell whereas hepatitis B attacks the DNA. Once hepatitis C was distinguished from hepatitis B, it was found to be the cause of most cases of hepatitis following blood transfusion (posttransfusion hepatitis). Hepatitis C is more likely to become chronic hepatitis than form B. Approximately 50 percent of those affected with hepatitis C will develop chronic hepatitis and cirrhosis. Over 12,000 individuals die each year from hepatitis C.

4. Hepatitis D—also called the "delta virus." It requires the presence of hepatitis B to replicate. Infection

with both B and D may cause more prominent symptoms, and a greater risk of developing chronic and fulminant hepatitis.

5. Hepatitis E—similar to hepatitis A in that it is spread through fecal-oral route. It is commonly due to water contamination. Chronic hepatitis does not develop with hepatitis E, but this virus in pregnant women may be fatal.

**SYMPTOMS** Jaundice is often the first symptom that signals a liver problem, although not all individuals become yellow. Interestingly, those who become more jaundiced are more likely to have a good recovery than those who are less jaundiced. Individuals with mild jaundice are more likely to develop chronic hepatitis. Other symptoms include malaise, anorexia, myalgia (myo = muscle, algia = pain), fever, and abdominal pain. Physical examination may reveal **hepatomegaly** (HEP-ah-toh-**MEG**-ah-lee; hepato = liver, megaly = enlargement). Dark-colored urine and clay- or light-colored stools are related to the inability of the liver to form normal bile.

**TREATMENT** Treatment for viral hepatitis is symptomatic. Adequate rest and good nutrition are essential. Approximately 85 percent of affected individuals recover in six weeks. The most serious complications with hepatitis are development of chronic hepatitis and **fulminant** (FULL-ma-nant; to occur suddenly and with great intensity) hepatitis. Chronic hepatitis develops in one out of four cases and often leads to cirrhosis of the liver. Fulminant hepatitis is an acute hepatitis that causes extensive necrosis of liver tissue. Symptoms include a high fever, hemorrhages from the skin and mucous membranes, confusion, and stupor. Coma often develops and leads to death. Even with prompt and supportive care, fulminant hepatitis is 90 percent fatal.

Prevention of hepatitis involves good hygiene, and special care when handling needles and body secretions. Vaccines are available for some types of viral hepatitis.

## ■ Cirrhosis

Cirrhosis (sir-ROH-sis) of the liver is a chronic, irreversible, degenerative disease also known as end-stage liver disease. Cirrhosis is characterized by the replacement of normal liver cells with nonfunctioning fibrous scar tissue known as "hobnail liver." This change in structure and function of the liver cells leads to impaired blood flow and altered function of the liver.

**ETIOLOGY** The most common cause of cirrhosis is chronic alcoholism. Cirrhosis is more common in males than females. It also may be idiopathic, or it may be the end result of other diseases such as chronic hepatitis and congestive heart failure. The development of the disease often takes years. There are usually no symptoms until serious structural and functional changes in the liver tissue have occurred. If symptoms occur, they are usually mild and nonspecific. Symptoms may include loss of appetite, nausea, indigestion, weakness, and weight loss.

As the disease progresses, the abnormal scar tissue alters blood flow through the liver and leads to a variety of complications. Altered blood flow through the liver results in blood backing up in the hepatic portal vein. The relationship of the liver, hepatic portal system, and digestive system is as follows:

■ The purpose of the hepatic portal system is to carry venous blood from the spleen and digestive organs (esophagus, stomach, intestines) to the liver (Figure 12–2). The liver plays a major role in the digestive system by detoxifying and metabolizing nutrients before releasing them into the systemic blood in the inferior vena cava. For example, if an individual consumes a meal with an alcoholic beverage, these nutrients are absorbed into venous blood in the small intestine, and transported to

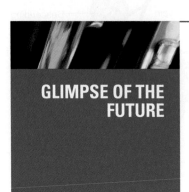

**GLIMPSE OF THE FUTURE**

### A New Treatment for Chronic Hepatitis B and Liver Disease

Using antiviral therapy for persons diagnosed with chronic hepatitis B or liver disease is now being tested. The drug lamivudine in doses of 100 mg per day has been used in trial studies to check its potential effectiveness for reducing the severity of some liver diseases. Early results are somewhat positive but further testing is indicated. In the future, this antiviral drug, as well as others, may be found to be helpful in the treatment of chronic hepatitis B and advanced stage liver disease.

*Source: Liaw, Y. et al. (2004).*

the liver to be filtered, detoxified, and stored. The liver's responsibility, in part, is to keep blood glucose levels from soaring when an individual eats a high carbohydrate meal. Nutrients are filtered, metabolized, stored, and released as needed into the systemic circulation by the liver. Toxins such as alcohol are detoxified. If alcohol consumption is too great or outpaces the liver's ability to detoxify the blood, the blood alcohol level will rise.

■ If the liver is obstructed for any reason, blood will back up in this portal system. As blood backs up, pressure increases in the portal vein and is called **portal hypertension**.

**SYMPTOMS** Complications of severe cirrhosis may include:

1. Varicosities—portal hypertension causes varicosities (varicose veins) of the veins of the digestive system

organs. Varicosities are commonly located in the esophagus (**esophageal varices**) (Figure 12–3). Esophageal varices (**VER**-ah-SEEZ) are prone to rupture, leading to massive hemorrhage, shock, and death. Other sites of varicosities include the rectum (hemorrhoids) and anterior abdominal wall. Varicosities across the front of the abdomen are often quite torturous and unsightly. This condition is called **caput medusae** (Medusa's head) because the physician who named the condition was reminded of Medusa's head when observing the varicosities. Medusa, in Greek mythology, was a woman who had snakes on her head in place of hair.

2. Splenomegaly—portal hypertension also causes increased pressure on the organs that are connected or drained by the portal system. Often, this passive congestion in the spleen leads to **splenomegaly** (SPLEE-no-**MEG**-ah-lee; spleno = spleen, megaly =

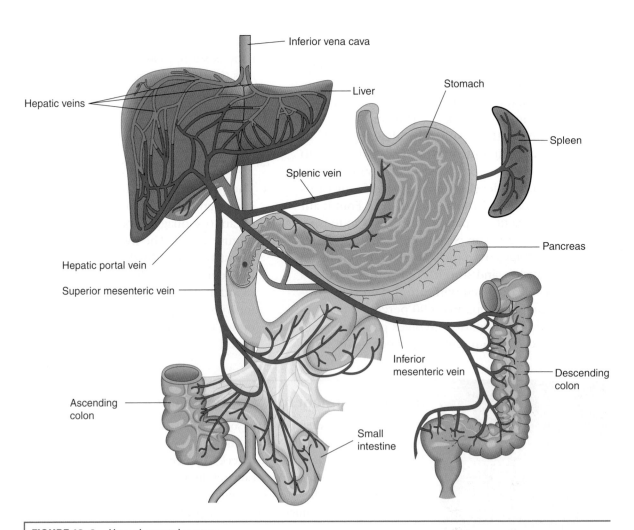

**FIGURE 12–2** Hepatic portal system.

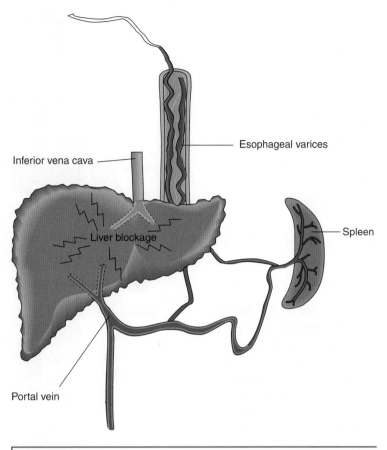

Inferior vena cava

Esophageal varices

Liver blockage

Spleen

Portal vein

**FIGURE 12–3**  Esophageal varices.

enlarged). Splenomegaly often causes increased blood cell destruction, leading to anemia, leukopenia, and thrombocytopenia.  Thrombocytopenia (thrombo = clot, cyto = cell, penia = decrease) increases the risk of bleeding.

3. Gastrointestinal hemorrhage—due to thrombocytopenia and inability of the liver to secrete blood proteins essential for clotting. **Hematemesis** (HEM-ah-**TEM**-eh-sis; hemat = blood, emesis = vomiting) is often the first symptom of severe cirrhosis.

4. **Ascites** (ah-SIGH-teez)—an accumulation of fluid in the abdominal cavity. This condition develops as a result of liver failure and portal hypertension. The increased pressure on the veins of the portal system causes leaking of serum into the abdomen. Often, this fluid enlarges the abdomen to the point of causing difficult breathing. Excessive abdominal fluid may be drained by piercing the abdominal wall with a large bore needle. This procedure is called an **abdominocentesis** (ab-

DOM-ih-no-sen-**TEE**-sis; abdomino = abdomen, centesis = puncture).

5. Edema—often develops in the ankles and feet as a result of liver failure. The normal liver produces a blood protein called **albumin** (AL-byou-men). Albumin is responsible for the osmotic pressure of blood. Osmotic pressure deals with the movement of fluid from the blood through the capillaries to the tissues and back into the blood. Without osmotic pressure, blood fluid tends to leak into the tissues and remain there. A decrease in albumin allows this to occur, leading to edema in the feet and ankles.

6. Jaundice—usually results from the obstruction of the bile ducts. This obstruction usually occurs as normal tissue is replaced by fibrous scar tissue, characteristic of cirrhosis.

7. Altered sex hormone metabolism—the normal liver inactivates small amounts of estrogen secreted by the adrenal glands in both the male and female.

As a result of normal liver activity, estrogen is inactivated and has no effect on the male. The cirrhotic liver is not capable of inactivating estrogen and thus the male has feminizing effects. These feminizing effects are evidenced by:

- **gynecomastia** (GUY-neh-koh-**MAS**-tee-ah)—an enlargement of the breasts
- **palmar erythema**—palms of the hands become reddened in color
- **spider angiomas**—small dilated blood vessels on the face and chest
- female hair distribution—absent or reduced chest and pubic hair
- testicular atrophy—decrease in testicle size

8. Hepatic encephalopathy—the liver is often unable to detoxify the blood of nitrogenous waste products such as ammonia. This waste product circulates in the blood and may affect the brain, causing mental confusion, stupor, and a characteristic shaking or tremor. This shaking, combined with hallucinations, is called **delirium tremens** (dee-LIR-ee-um TREE-mens) or DTs. Further depression of the nervous system may lead to hepatic coma and ultimately, death. The clinical features of cirrhosis of the liver in the male are shown in Figure 12–4.

Cirrhosis has an unfavorable prognosis with most individuals surviving only 10 to 15 years after diagnosis. The appearance of ascites is a prognostic indicator as a majority of individuals with cirrhosis die within five years after the onset of ascites. Individuals die of massive bleeding from esophageal varices, hepatic encephalopathy, and other metabolic disorders.

**TREATMENT** Treatment of cirrhosis is directed at the cause to attempt to prevent further liver damage. Alcohol is strictly prohibited regardless of the cause of the cirrhosis. Adequate nutrition and rest are necessary. Vitamins, minerals, and diet supplements may be needed to prevent malnutrition. Diuretics may be needed to reduce edema and ascites.

### ■ Liver Cancer

Primary and benign tumors of the liver are rare. When primary tumors do develop, they are more likely to occur in individuals with cirrhosis. Men are five times more likely to develop liver cancer than women. Secondary liver tumors are the most com-

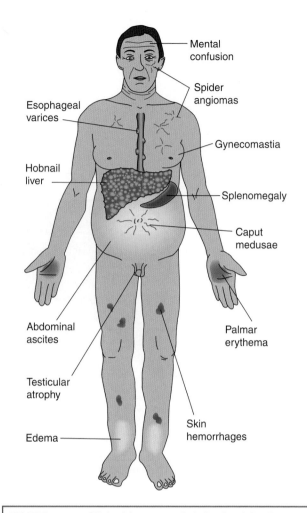

**FIGURE 12–4** Clinical features of cirrhosis of the liver in the male.

mon, and usually are the result of metastasis from cancers in the breast, digestive system, and lungs. Liver cancer is usually discovered late or end stage because symptoms of anorexia, weight loss, and abdominal discomfort are so nonspecific. Diagnosis is confirmed by biopsy. Treatment of liver cancer may involve surgery, chemotherapy, and radiation. Even with aggressive treatment, prognosis is very poor with only 10 percent of affected individuals living five years after diagnosis.

## Gallbladder Diseases

Gallbladder disorders usually cause symptoms related to indigestion when eating fatty foods. Nausea, pain, and excessive gas are the most common symptoms. Nutritional changes and a variety of surgical procedures can be used to treat the disease.

## ■ Cholecystitis

**ETIOLOGY** Cholecystitis (KOH-lee-sis-**TYE**-tis; chole = bile or gall, cyst = bladder, itis = inflammation) or inflammation of the gallbladder is usually caused by obstruction of bile flow due to a gallstone. When bile flow is obstructed, bile in the gallbladder becomes overly concentrated and irritates the lining of the gallbladder, leading to inflammation. When a fatty meal is eaten, fat in the duodenum stimulates the gallbladder to contract and release bile.

**SYMPTOMS** This contraction of the inflamed gallbladder causes mild to severe pain in the right upper quadrant of the abdomen. This pain, combined with a history of nausea and vomiting after meals, is indicative of cholecystitis. Ultrasound and cholecystogram confirm diagnosis of cholecystitis. Cholecystogram involves swallowing a dye that is absorbed by the liver and excreted into the bile. Radiographic pictures are made to confirm the presence of stones.

Complications of cholecystitis include rupture of the gallbladder, leading to peritonitis. Chronic cholecystitis may cause bile to back up into the liver, leading to liver damage and cirrhosis.

**TREATMENT** Treatment for cholecystitis is aimed at the cause. Gallstones often obstruct the gallbladder or one of its ducts. Treatment of choice for cholecystitis caused by stones is surgical removal by a procedure called **cholecystectomy** (KOH-lee-sis-**TECK**-toh-me; chole = bile or gall, cyst = bladder, ectomy=removal). Cholecystectomy may be performed using an abdominal incision or it may be removed using a laparoscope (laparo = abdomen, scope = scope). Removal of the gallbladder using a laparoscope is called laparoscopic cholecystectomy (LAP-ah-**ROW**-skop-ic KOH-lee-sis-**TECK**-toh-me). Laparoscopic cholecystectomy is performed through several small abdominal incisions. This type of procedure drastically reduces discomfort and the length of hospital stay as compared to the larger abdominal incision.

After a cholecystectomy, the bile continues to be excreted by the liver into the common bile duct and simply drips into the duodenum as it is produced. As long as the individual does not take in an excessive amount of fatty foods, the amount of bile will be sufficient to break down the consumed fat and normal digestion will occur.

## ■ Cholelithiasis

**ETIOLOGY** Cholelithiasis (KOH-lee-lih-**THIGH**-ah-sis; chole = bile or gall, lith = stone, iasis = condition) is the presence of gallstones in the gallbladder or bile ducts (Figure 12–5). Over one million people in the United States are diagnosed each year with gallstones and over 500,000 undergo surgery for removal of the stones (American Liver Foundation, 2003).

**SYMPTOMS** Gallstones are often asymptomatic. If symptoms do occur, they are usually related to blocking the outflow of the gallbladder or of its ducts. Symptoms include nausea, vomiting, and right upper quadrant pain following meals with fat. A cholecystogram and ultrasound, along with a positive history, will confirm the diagnosis.

Gallstones form from bile salts and cholesterol. The stones may vary in size, shape, number, color, and composition. The reason for stone development is not understood, but females develop stones more commonly than males. The three most important risk factors for developing gallstones include excessive body weight, increasing age, and being female. In general, individuals developing cholelithiasis have several factors in common called the five Fs of cholelithiasis. They include 1. Female 2. Fair complexion 3. Fat or obese 4. Fertile or has had children 5. Forty years of age or older.

Complications of cholelithiasis include cholecystitis and jaundice.

**TREATMENT** Extracorporeal shockwave lithotripsy (litho = stone, tripsy = destruction) (ESWL)

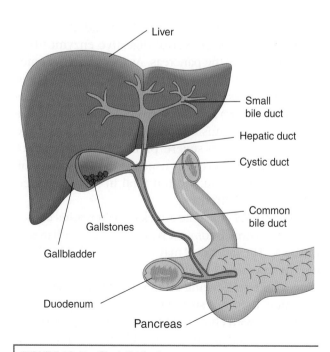

**FIGURE 12–5** Cholelithiasis.

may be performed in an effort to break up the stones so they can be passed. If this procedure is not effective or is not recommended, cholecystectomy is performed.

## Pancreas Diseases

Diseases of the pancreas are often quite advanced by the time symptoms appear. Some pancreatic disorders are associated with alcoholism. Replacement or supplements of pancreatic enzymes and insulin may be necessary when the pancreas is not functioning properly or is surgically removed.

### ■ Pancreatitis

Pancreatitis is an inflammation of the pancreas that may range from mild to fatal. With pancreatitis, the pancreas becomes inflamed, edematous, hemorrhagic, and necrotic.

**ETIOLOGY** This disease is similar to cirrhosis of the liver in that most cases of severe pancreatitis are due to alcoholism.

Pancreatitis also may be caused by blockage of pancreatic ducts by gallstones. Many cases of pancreatitis are idiopathic (of unknown cause). Diagnosis of pancreatitis is often made based on the individual's history and is confirmed by blood testing. A high blood **amylase** (pancreatic enzyme) is indicative of pancreatitis.

Pancreatitis differs from inflammation of other organs due to the powerful digestive enzymes that are produced by the pancreas. As this organ becomes diseased, these enzymes often escape the pancreatic cells and ducts, causing digestion of the pancreas (**autodigestion**) and the surrounding tissues. If this destruction extends into blood vessels, hemorrhage occurs, leading to severe pain and shock. Acute hemorrhagic pancreatitis usually follows an alcohol-drinking spree and is often fatal in spite of emergency medical attention.

**SYMPTOMS** An acute attack of pancreatitis causes sudden, severe abdominal pain that often radiates to the back. The individual may find some relief by drawing the knees up toward the abdomen. Other symptoms exhibited during an acute attack are nausea, vomiting, diaphoresis (sweating), and tachycardia. Individuals with chronic pancreatitis may complain of constant back pain and frequent bouts of mild symptoms similar to those of an acute attack. As the disease progresses, the pancreatic tissue is replaced with fibrous tissue and function is lost. As endocrine function is lost, the individual has symptoms of diabetes mellitus. Digestive disorders including malabsorption occur when exocrine function is impaired.

**TREATMENT** Treatment and prognosis of pancreatitis depends on the cause. Pancreatitis caused by gallstones is treated successfully by removing the gallbladder and the involved stones. Treatment for idiopathic and alcohol-related pancreatitis is palliative as there is no cure. Individuals must stop drinking alcohol, and are treated with analgesics and nutritional support. Prognosis for these types of pancreatitis is poor.

### ■ Pancreas Cancer

Pancreatic cancer is usually an adenocarcinoma that occurs in the head of the pancreas.

**ETIOLOGY** The cause of this tumor is unknown, but known carcinogens include cigarette smoking, drinking large amounts of coffee, chemical exposure, and consuming a high-fat diet. Diagnosis is usually confirmed by biopsy.

**SYMPTOMS** As pancreatic tissue is destroyed, the individual may experience abdominal pain, back pain, nausea, vomiting, loss of appetite, weakness, jaundice, and fatigue. Symptoms usually do not occur until late in the disease process after metastasis has already occurred.

**TREATMENT** Treatment may include surgical resection, chemotherapy, and radiation. This tumor usually responds poorly to all therapies and prognosis is very poor. Supportive care is provided, including pain management and nutritional support.

## RARE DISEASES

## Primary Biliary Cirrhosis

**ETIOLOGY** Primary biliary cirrhosis is a chronic liver disease that gradually destroys the bile ducts in the liver. The cause is unknown, but it may be related to immune system dysfunction. Destruction of bile ducts decreases bile excretion from the liver and causes a chronic inflammation, resulting in cirrhosis. The disease is much more common in middle-aged females than males.

**SYMPTOMS** Signs and symptoms of the disease include jaundice, edema, itching, and abnormal liver function studies.

**TREATMENT** Treatment is directed at relieving the symptoms. A liver transplant may be necessary.

## Gilbert's Syndrome

Gilbert's syndrome is a congenital liver disorder that usually has its onset in the teenage or young adult years. Symptoms include increased serum bilirubin and jaundice. It is more common in males. It is usually left untreated because it does not seem to adversely affect liver function.

## Hemochromatosis

Hemochromatosis is a disorder in which the body absorbs and stores excessive amounts of iron. It is the most common inherited disease affecting approximately one million people in the United States (American Liver Foundation, 2003). Eventually, damage to the liver may occur. It is diagnosed by blood tests for iron levels. Treatment requires blood (about one to two units) to be removed weekly until iron levels return to normal. This regimen must be continued every four months for life to keep the iron levels within normal limits.

## EFFECTS OF AGING ON THE SYSTEM

The older adult who develops hepatitis usually undergoes a more severe infection than a younger person does with the same disease. The mortality rate for hepatitis increases with age. Older people may be at an increased risk for developing hepatitis if any of the following factors are present:

- a depressed immune system
- increased contact with a variety of caregivers
- poor nutrition
- increased intake of medications
- poor hygiene
- multiple blood transfusions

Cirrhosis in an older person may be of unknown etiology or due to chronic alcohol intake. It is usually progressive, severe, and the prognosis is poor. Bile stones are also seen more frequently in the older adult. Surgery is usually the treatment of choice, but may not be an option due to the age of the individual and other complicating disorders. Pancreatic disease is also common in the older adult population. Replacement of pancreatic enzymes may be needed if the pancreas is not producing adequate amounts.

## SUMMARY

Diseases of the liver, gallbladder, and pancreas have serious effects on digestion and metabolism. The liver has many functions in the body, so when it is diseased, a variety of other disorders may result. If the liver fails completely, a transplant is necessary. Hepatitis is the most common liver disorder. It is usually viral in nature. Cirrhosis of the liver is a chronic, progressive disease most commonly related to alcohol ingestion. Gallbladder disease affects thousands of individuals annually. Gallstones are the most common cause of gallbladder problems. Pancreatic disorders are often not diagnosed until late in the disease process because early symptoms are often not apparent. If the pancreas is not functioning properly, pancreatic enzymes and hormones may need to be supplemented. The older adult is at increased risk for developing disorders of the liver, gallbladder, and pancreas.

## REVIEW QUESTIONS

### Short Answer

1. What are the functions of the liver, gallbladder, and pancreas?

2. Which signs and symptoms are associated with common liver, gallbladder, and pancreas disorders?

3. Which diagnostic tests are most commonly used to determine the type and/or cause of liver, gallbladder, or pancreas disorders?

## Multiple Choice

4. Which of the following is the cause of jaundice?

   a. Increased levels of amylase in the blood

   b. Decreased levels of pancreatase in the blood

   c. Increased levels of bilirubin in the blood

   d. Decreased levels of lipase in the blood

5. Impaired liver function leads to an elevation in which of the following tests?

   a. Bilirubin and alkaline phosphatase

   b. Albumin and bilirubin

   c. Alkaline phosphatase and amylase

   d. Amylase and albumin

6. Diseases of the liver, gallbladder, or pancreas generally have an adverse effect on which of the following?

   a. The immune system          c. The inflammatory process

   b. Digestion and metabolism    d. The endocrine system

7. Which of the following types of hepatitis is the most common?

   a. Hepatitis A                 c. Hepatitis C

   b. Hepatitis B                 d. Hepatitis D

8. Individuals at high risk for developing hepatitis B include which of the following?

   a. Drug addicts

   b. Blood recipients

   c. Health care workers

   d. All of the above

9. Which of the following is the best definition of cirrhosis?

   a. A chronic, degenerative disease of the pancreas

   b. An acute irreversible disease of the liver

   c. An abnormality of the liver caused by alcoholism

   d. A chronic, degenerative, irreversible disease of the liver

**10.** Ascites is an accumulation of fluid in the abdominal cavity usually due to which of the following conditions?

a. Pancreatic cancer

b. Liver failure and portal hypertension

c. Cholelithiasis

d. Cirrhosis

## True or False

**11.** T  F  Gallbladder disorders usually cause symptoms related to indigestion when eating high-fat foods.

**12.** T  F  A cholecystogram is a radiographic exam used to diagnose cholecystitis.

**13.** T  F  Gallstones are most commonly found in obese middle-aged men.

**14.** T  F  A high serum amylase is usually diagnostic for pancreatitis.

**15.** T  F  The older adult who develops hepatitis usually experiences a much milder episode of the disease than a young person.

## CASE STUDY

**Ms. Fisher** is a 68-year-old lady with the classic symptoms of gallbladder disease. She is diagnosed with gallstones and is scheduled for surgery in two weeks. She asks you about the cause of gallstones and why she would develop them. How would you respond to her? What typical factors put an individual at risk for developing gallstones?

## BIBLIOGRAPHY

American Liver Foundation. (2003). http://www. liverfoundation.org. Gall stones: A National Health Problem.

American Liver Foundation. (2003). http://www. liverfoundation.org. What is Hemochromatosis?

American Liver Foundation. (2005). http://www. liverfoundation.org. Hepatitis and Liver Disease in the United States.

Desjardins, L. A. (2002). Heptocellular carcinoma. *Clinical Journal of Oncology Nursing 6*(2), 107–108.

FDA gives orphan drug approval to REXIN-G. (2003, October 12). *Medical Letter on the CDC & FDA*, 35–36.

Fogden, E., & Neuberger, J. (2003). Alternative medicines and the liver. *Liver International, 23*(4), 213–220.

Gobel, B. H., & Baldwin, P. D. (2003). Chemical hepatitis. *Clinical Journal of Oncology Nursing 7*(1), 1–3.

Kipp, A. (2003). Daily aspirin use linked with pancreatic cancer. *Access 17*(10), 6.

Lemaigre, F. (2003). Development of the biliary tract. *Mechanisms of Development 120*(1), 81–87.

Liaw, Y., Sung, J., Chow, W., Lee, C., Yuen, H., Tanwandee, T., Tao, A., Shue, K., Keene, O., Dixon, J., Gray, D., & Sabbat, J. (2004). Lamivudine for patients with chronic hepatitis B and advanced liver disease. *New England Journal of Medicine, 351*(15), 1521–1530.

Noninfectious liver disorders: Assessment and diagnosis/adult autoimmune hepatitis. (2003). *Nurse Practitioner 28*(12), 32–33.

Obesity increases risk of pancreatic cancer. (2003, September 6). *Health and Medicine Week*, 571–572.

Rahemtullah, A., Middraji, J., & Pitman, M. (2003). Adenosquamos carcinoma of the pancreas. *Cancer: Diagnosis, Treatment, Research 99*(6), 372–378.

Strassberg, C. P., Vogel, A., & Manns, M. P. (2003). Autoimmunity and hepatitis C. *Autoimmunity Reviews 2*(6), 322–331.

Study: Link to regular aspirin use found. (2003, November 27). *Women's Health Weekly*, 97.

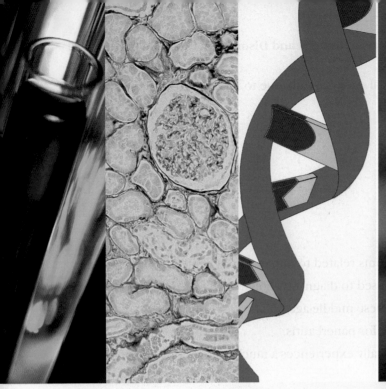
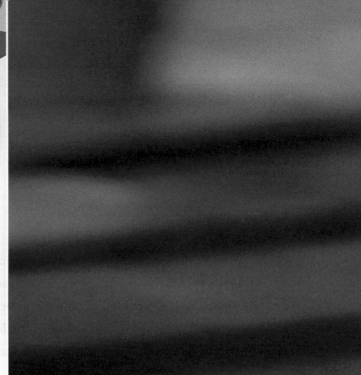

## OUTLINE

- Anatomy and Physiology
- Common Signs and Symptoms
- Diagnostic Tests
- Common Diseases of the Urinary System
  *Urinary Tract Infection (UTI)*
  *Diseases of the Kidney*
  *Diseases of the Bladder*
- Trauma
  *Straddle Injuries*
  *Neurogenic Bladder*
- Rare Diseases
  *Goodpasture Syndrome*
  *Interstitial Cystitis*
- Effects of Aging on the System
- Summary
- Review Questions
- Case Study
- Bibliography

## KEY TERMS

# Urinary System Diseases and Disorders

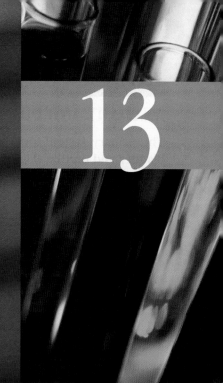

# 13

## LEARNING OBJECTIVES

*Upon completion of the chapter, the learner should be able to:*

1. Define the terminology common to the urinary system and the disorders of the system.

2. Discuss the basic anatomy and physiology of the urinary system.

3. Identify the important signs and symptoms associated with common urinary system disorders.

4. Describe the common diagnostics used to determine the type and/or cause of urinary system disorders.

5. Identify common disorders of the urinary system.

6. Describe the typical course and management of the common urinary system disorders.

7. Describe the effects of aging on the urinary system and the common disorders of the system.

## OVERVIEW

The urinary system maintains homeostasis in the body by excreting and reabsorbing important electrolytes, compounds, and water. It also excretes wastes from the body in the form of urine. Disturbances in other systems such as the circulatory or nervous systems can adversely affect the functioning of the urinary system. Urinary disorders range from mild infections to very serious diseases such as cancer of the bladder or kidneys. ■

## ANATOMY AND PHYSIOLOGY

The urinary system includes the kidneys, ureters, bladder, and urethra (Figure 13–1). The kidneys are located behind the intestines at the mid-back level. Each kidney is about the size of a man's fist and weighs about 150 grams. The kidneys are responsible for removing waste products from the bloodstream. Every minute, about one-fourth of the blood circulating in the body passes through the kidneys. Toxic wastes and unused nutrients are filtered and pass out of the body as urine. The kidneys also regulate fluid and electrolyte balance, acid-base balance, assist in the metabolism of calcium, and help regulate blood pressure. The kidneys are composed of nephrons that act as filters, selectively filtering, excreting, or reabsorbing what is needed by the body to maintain homeostasis. They monitor the amount of salts and other chemicals needed for proper body functioning. The kidneys also produce an active form of vitamin D necessary for strong bones.

The ureters are tubules that run from the kidney to the bladder (see Figure 13–1). They transport the urine from the renal pelvis to the bladder where it is stored until emptied, usually a conscious effort by the individual. The bladder, a muscular organ that holds urine, can usually store about 350–500 ml. This amount varies from individual to individual and is affected by many other factors, especially bladder tone, neurologic disease, and urologic disorders. Micturition is the process of voiding or emptying the bladder. This usually occurs in response to stimuli to the pelvic nerves.

The urethra is a hollow tube running from the bladder to the external opening (the meatus) for excretion (see Figure 13–1). The urethra is significantly longer in males than in females. The urethra serves as the passageway for urine in the female, and for both urine and semen ejaculation in the male.

Urine is normally clear, slightly yellow to gold in color, and free of sediments. Some drugs can change the color of urine. Urine has its own distinct odor but is not foul smelling unless disease is present. There are some foods that will change the odor of urine as their by-products are excreted such as asparagus. Urine has a normal specific gravity of 1.005–1.030 and a pH of about 6. Changes in these values may indicate disease.

## COMMON SIGNS AND SYMPTOMS

Common signs and symptoms of urinary tract diseases include any abnormality in urine or in the ability to urinate. Some of these include:

- **hematuria** (hem-ah-TOO-ree-ah; hema = blood, uria = urine) or blood in the urine
- **pyuria** (pye-YOU-ree-ah; py = pus, uria = urine) or pus in the urine
- **proteinuria** or protein in the urine. A specific protein, albumin, may be identified, resulting in **albuminuria**
- **dysuria** (dis-YOU-ree-ah; dys = difficult or painful, uria = urine) or difficulty or pain with urination
- **nocturia** (nock-TOO-ree-ah; noc = night, uria = urine) or increased voiding at night
- **oliguria** (OL-ih-**GOO**-ree-ah; olig = scanty or few, uria = urine) or a decrease in urine output
- **anuria** (ah-NEW-ree-ah; an = without, uria = urine) or no urine output
- **frequency** or urinating frequently
- **urgency** or the need to urinate immediately

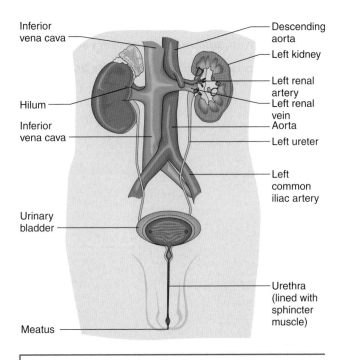

Inferior vena cava
Descending aorta
Left kidney
Left renal artery
Left renal vein
Aorta
Hilum
Inferior vena cava
Left ureter
Left common iliac artery
Urinary bladder
Urethra (lined with sphincter muscle)
Meatus

**FIGURE 13–1** The urinary system.

Varying degrees of pain in the low back or flank area also may be indicative of urinary disease. Other symptoms include nausea, vomiting, malaise, and fatigue. Urinary system diseases also may affect the cardiovascular and respiratory systems, leading to hypertension, edema, and shortness of breath.

## DIAGNOSTIC TESTS

A **urinalysis** (YOU-rih-**NAL**-ih-sis; urine analysis) is the most common test performed to diagnose urinary system diseases. This test is important because the results can confirm the presence of many different urinary tract disorders. A urinalysis uses a urine sample to test for pH, specific gravity, presence of protein, glucose or sugar, and blood. It also includes a microscopic examination to determine the presence of bacteria, crystals, and casts. The specific test, normal findings, abnormal findings, and pathologies are summarized in Table 13–1.

A **urine culture and sensitivity (C&S)** may be performed in the laboratory if the urinalysis shows an abnormal number of white cells or bacteria in the urine. If the bacteria count is greater than 100,000 bacterium per ml or cc of urine, a diagnosis of urinary tract infection is confirmed. A lesser number may be indicative of a contaminated specimen or the presence of a mild infection. A culture helps determine the type of bacteria present and a sensitivity will help determine the most effective antibiotic to prescribe for treatment. A urine specimen collected for a culture may be obtained by the clean catch method or sterile technique. The **clean catch** method involves cleaning the urethral meatus, voiding a moderate amount of urine to flush out the urethra, then catching a urine specimen in a sterile container. Catching the specimen after urinating as described above is considered a "mid-stream" catch, and is part of the proper technique of obtaining a clean catch specimen. A sterile technique involves placing a sterile urinary catheter into the bladder to obtain a sterile urine specimen.

Blood tests may be performed to determine if waste products are being filtered out adequately by the glomerulus, thus checking kidney function. The two most common nitrogenous waste products that are normally filtered from the blood are **urea** and **creatinine**. A **blood urea nitrogen (BUN)** test will determine the levels of urea nitrogen or waste product in the blood. A **creatinine clearance test** is a blood test to determine the ability of the renal glomeruli to filter creatinine out of the blood after creatinine is ingested by the subject. High levels of waste products in the blood is

**TABLE 13–1** Urinalysis Values

| Urinalysis | Normal Values | Abnormal Results |
|---|---|---|
| Color | Clear amber | Very light or very dark; cloudy |
| Odor | Pleasantly aromatic | Offensive, unpleasant |
| Albumin (protein) | Negative | Albuminuria |
| Acetone | Negative | Ketonuria |
| Red Blood Cells | 2-3/HPF | Hematuria |
| White Blood Cells | 4-5/HPF | White, cloudy urine |
| Bilirubin | Negative | Bilirubinuria |
| Glucose | Negative | Glycosuria |
| Specific Gravity | 1.005–1.030 | Higher or lower than normal |
| Bacteria | Negative | Present |
| Casts | Rare | Present-several to many |
| pH | 4.6–8.0 | Higher or lower than normal |

called **uremia** (you-REE-me-ah; ur = urine, emia = blood). Uremia is a toxic condition of the blood.

Radiologic examination of the urinary system includes **kidneys-ureter-bladder (KUB)**, **intravenous pyelogram (IVP)**, and **cystogram**. A KUB is a common X-ray of the structures of the urinary tract to determine abnormalities. An IVP is an X-ray taken after injecting dye into the individual's bloodstream. The dye accumulates in the urinary tract, improving the ability to visualize and identify obstructions, tumors, and deformities. A cystogram (cysto = bladder, gram = picture) is an X-ray taken of the bladder after a radiopaque dye is instilled into the bladder using a urinary catheter. A cystogram helps determine shape and function of the bladder.

**Cystoscopy** (sis-TOS-koh-pee; cysto = bladder, scopy = procedure to look) is an invasive procedure to look into the urethra and bladder using a lighted scope (Figure 13–2). Stones, tumors, and areas of infection and inflammation can be viewed by use of a cystoscope. Additional instruments may be used to allow the physician to obtain a tissue biopsy or crush bladder stones.

Biopsies of the kidney and bladder are often performed to determine the presence of disease. Bladder biopsies are often obtained by using a cystoscope as previously mentioned. Renal biopsies are often obtained by using X-ray technique to guide a fine needle through the flank area to remove a core of renal tissue.

**Catheterization** of the urinary bladder is a sterile procedure. A soft catheter is passed through the urethra and into the bladder for the purpose of instilling fluids or medication into the bladder and/or removing urine. Sterile technique must be maintained to prevent urinary tract infections. Urinary catheterization to remove urine may be done to relieve urinary retention, empty the bladder prior to a procedure, obtain a sterile urine specimen for testing, or as a treatment for incontinence. If the catheter is removed as soon as the urine is drained, the catheterization is temporary and is called an **in and out catheterization**. If the catheter is placed for a longer period of time, as commonly occurs for urinary incontinence, a balloon on the end of the catheter is inflated to hold the catheter in the bladder and the catheterization is called an **indwelling catheter**. If the catheter is inserted surgically through the pelvic wall, as is often done after urinary tract surgeries, it is called a **suprapubic catheter** (Figure 13–3).

# COMMON DISEASES OF THE URINARY SYSTEM

Diseases of the urinary system can affect either gender at any age. Urinary tract infections are the most common disorders of the system. Many of the diseases of the urinary system have similar symptoms in their early stages of development such as dysuria, oliguria, and frequency of urination.

## Urinary Tract Infection (UTI)

Urinary tract infection is a broad diagnosis covering any infection of the urinary tract including the urethra, bladder, and kidneys (Figure 13–4A).

**ETIOLOGY** UTIs may be caused by a virus or fungus, but by far the most common infection is due to bacteria.

Bacteria may reach the urinary tract through the blood (hematogenous infection) or by entering the tract through the urethra (ascending infection). Hematogenous infection is less common and is usually the result of septicemia. In this case, the urinary tract is a site of secondary infection. Primary infection may begin in the respiratory or gastrointestinal tract, and be carried to the urinary tract through the blood.

Ascending infection is by far the most common route of infection. With ascending infection, bacteria enter the urethra and climb or ascend upward

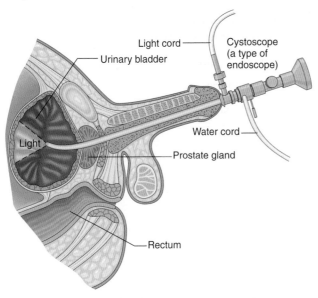

Light cord
Urinary bladder
Cystoscope (a type of endoscope)
Water cord
Prostate gland
Light
Rectum

**FIGURE 13–2** Cystoscopy.

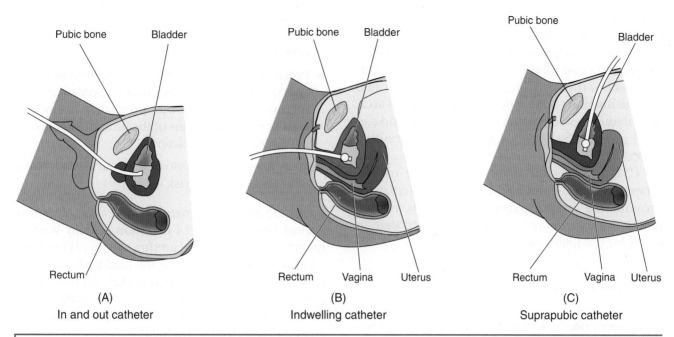

(A)
In and out catheter

(B)
Indwelling catheter

(C)
Suprapubic catheter

**FIGURE 13–3**   Types of urinary catheterizations.

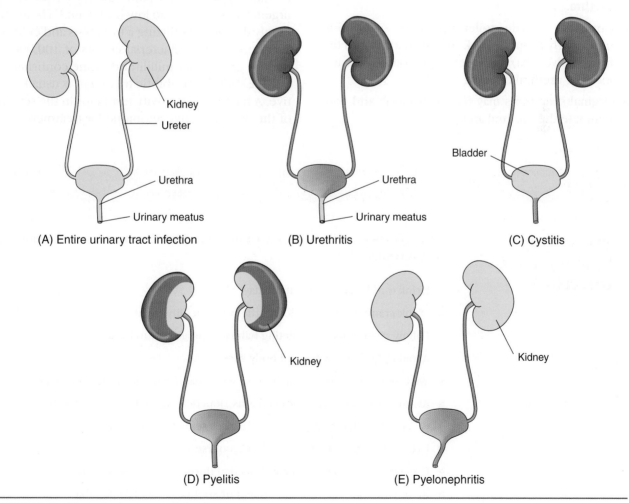

(A) Entire urinary tract infection

(B) Urethritis

(C) Cystitis

(D) Pyelitis

(E) Pyelonephritis

**FIGURE 13–4**   Sites of urinary tract infections.

toward the kidneys, infecting the various organs as they progress. Approximately 80 percent of the time, the bacteria causing ascending infection is *Escherichia coli* (*E. coli*). This bacterium is a normal flora of the intestine, and is commonly found in large numbers around the anal and perineal area. Sexual intercourse, bladder catheterization, and surgical procedures increase the risk of ascending infection.

UTIs in males are quite rare, and are usually related to obstruction of the tract by an enlarged prostate or a sexually transmitted disease. Ascending UTIs are far more common in females than in males for the following reasons:

■ Anatomically, the female urethra is shorter than the male urethra, allowing bacteria to ascend more easily.

■ Anatomically, the female urethral opening is closer to the rectal area than that of the male, allowing migration of bacteria from the rectal area to the urethra.

■ Improper female toileting habits or wiping improperly from the back (rectal area) toward the front (vulva area) pulls rectal bacteria toward and into the urethral opening.

■ Vaginal secretions may harbor bacteria and contaminate the urethral area.

■ Sexual intercourse may cause trauma to the urethra and bladder, leading to inflammation and potential infection.

■ Pregnant females are more susceptible to infection due to the pressure of the heavy uterus on the urinary tract and that pregnancy hormones tend to relax the organs of the urinary tract, allowing easier entry by bacteria.

■ Male prostatic secretions have an antibacterial effect, reducing the risk of UTI.

There are several natural preventive measures against UTIs. The act of urination actually washes most bacteria out of the urethra. A low pH (acidity) and the presence of urea in the bladder have a bactericidal effect. Also, the ureters close off during urination to prevent urine from refluxing up the ureter to the kidney. Other preventive measures are discussed in the Healthy Highlight.

**SYMPTOMS** Signs and symptoms of UTI may include dysuria, flank pain, urinary frequency and urgency, hematuria, and low back pain. UTIs are commonly diagnosed utilizing a urinalysis and culture of a urine specimen. Bacterial counts of 100,000 bacteria or greater per milliliter of urine confirms UTI.

**TREATMENT** Antibiotic treatment is usually effective. A bacterial sensitivity test helps in the selection of the most effective antibiotic for treatment.

 **HEALTHY HIGHLIGHT**

## Preventing Urinary Tract Infections

Females who suffer frequent UTIs may find the following measures helpful in preventing UTIs.

■ Drink 6 to 8 glasses of water a day

■ Drink cranberry juice to lower the pH or acidify the urine

■ Follow correct female toileting habits; wiping front to back

■ Avoid tight fitting jeans and body suits

■ Wear underwear and/or pantyhose with absorbent cotton perineal panels

■ Avoid perfumed soaps, bubble baths, douches, and feminine deodorants

■ Cleanse the genital area before and after sexual intercourse

■ Urinate before and after sexual intercourse

■ Use a water-soluble lubricant if needed during sexual intercourse

■ Remove a contraceptive diaphragm or sponge as soon as possible

As previously discussed, UTI includes infection of any of the organs of the urinary tract. Types of urinary tract infection include urethritis, cystitis, ureteritis, pyelitis, and pyelonephritis. A brief discussion of each follows.

## ■ Urethritis

Urethritis (YOU-reh-**THRIGH**-tis; urethri = urethra, itis = inflammation) is more common in males than females and is often a symptom of gonorrhea (Figure 13–4B). In females, urethritis may be the result of irritation due to tight clothing, application of soaps or powders to the genital area, or sexual intercourse. Urethritis commonly occurs in conjunction with cystitis. In males and females, it may be a symptom of herpes genitalis or chlamydia. Symptoms of urethritis may include swelling of the urethra, dysuria, and a urethral discharge.

## ■ Cystitis

Cystitis (sis-TYE-tis; cyst = bladder, itis = inflammation) is commonly called "bladder infection" (Figure 13–4C). Cystitis, occurring in females as they become sexually active, is called "honeymoon cystitis." Antibiotic treatment is usually effective. Antispasmodic medications, such as Pyridium, may be prescribed in addition to antibiotics to decrease the discomfort of bladder spasms. Individuals taking Pyridium should be warned that this medication normally stains the urine a reddish orange and this urine will permanently stain clothing. After treatment is completed, a follow-up urinalysis and culture is important to ensure complete elimination of all bacteria since recurrent infections are common.

## ■ Pyelitis

Pyelitis (PYE-eh-**LYE**-tis; pyelo = pelvis of kidney, itis = inflammation) is a fairly common disease among young female children (Figure 13–4D). Pyelitis is usually the result of an ascending infection from the bladder (cystitis) but also may be spread by blood (hematogenous infection). Rapid diagnosis and treatment must be initiated to prevent the spread of infection to adjacent tissue, which can cause pyelonephritis.

## ■ Pyelonephritis

Pyelonephritis (PYE-eh-loh-neh-**FRY**-tis; pyelo = pelvis of kidney, nephr = kidney, itis = inflammation) may be due to an ascending or a hematogenous infection, and may affect one or both kidneys (Figure 13–4E). Obstruction or blocking of urine flow in the urinary tract caused by pregnancy, prostate enlargement, stones, or tumors increases the risk of pyelonephritis. Commonly, abscesses form in the kidney and rupture, filling the kidney pelvis with pus and leading to pyuria (pyo = pus, uria = urine). Other symptoms include a sudden onset of fever and chills with flank pain and hematuria. Pyelonephritis is usually treated effectively with antibiotics, but repeated bouts of acute pyelonephritis or chronic pyelonephritis leads to scarring of the kidney. Chronic pyelonephritis may eventually lead to uremia and kidney failure.

## Diseases of the Kidney

Diseases of the kidney affect the filtering system of the body. This, in turn, affects the homeostatic balance of fluids and electrolytes. If left untreated, kidney diseases can affect all other body systems and interrupt their functioning. Symptoms of kidney disease may first appear in an affected system rather than in the urinary system. An example of this is an elevated blood pressure caused by inappropriate reabsorption of sodium and water.

## ■ Glomerulonephritis (Acute)

Acute glomerulonephritis is an inflammation of the glomerulus or filtering unit of the kidney. It is the most common disease of the kidney.

**ETIOLOGY** This disease usually affects children and young adults within one to four weeks following a strep throat infection. Other streptococcus infections such as scarlet fever and rheumatic fever also may be the cause of this problem. Glomerulonephritis with this etiology also may be called acute poststreptococcal glomerulonephritis. In addition to streptococcus bacterial infections, virus, other bacteria, and parasites also may lead to this disease.

Glomerulonephritis is nonsuppurative, or in other words, it is not associated with bacterial infection and pus formation. Inflammation in this case is the result of tissue destruction caused by the individual's immune system. Glomerulonephritis is a type of allergic or immune disease caused by an antigen–antibody reaction. The causative agent (bacteria, virus, parasites) produce antigen that stimulates the individual's immune system to produce antibodies. These antibodies, stick to the antigen, thus producing large antigen–antibody complexes. These large complexes circulate in the bloodstream until they become trapped in the tiny capillaries of the glomerulus. The trapping of these complexes blocks the glomerulus, leading to increased pressure, irritation, and the inflammatory response.

The outpouring of neutrophils and serum as a part of the inflammatory response increases pressure and decreases blood flow to the glomerulus. Ultimately, the glomerulus weakens and becomes permeable, allowing red blood cells and blood plasma proteins to leak into Bowman's capsule and appear in the urine.

**SYMPTOMS** Signs and symptoms of glomerulonephritis are flank pain, fever, loss of appetite, and malaise (general ill feeling). The eyes and ankles may appear edematous (swollen). Oliguria and hematuria are frequent signs of glomerulonephritis. A urinalysis may show albuminuria (albumin = a blood protein, uria = urine) and casts (proteins that mold to the shape of the kidney tubules).

**TREATMENT** Treatment is usually supportive. Antipyretic (anti = against, pyretic = fever) and diuretic (increase urine output) medications may be prescribed. Dietary management may include restrictions on salt, protein foods, and fluids. If a secondary bacterial infection occurs, antibiotics may be prescribed. Prevention is aimed at proper antibiotic treatment for streptococcal infections. Proper treatment of strep throat in children and young adults decreases the number of antigen-antibody complexes, thus reducing the risk of developing glomerulonephritis.

Prognosis for glomerulonephritis is generally good. Children usually recover at a slightly better rate than adults. Those who do not recover may progress into chronic glomerulonephritis.

## ■ Glomerulonephritis (Chronic)

**ETIOLOGY** Repeated bouts of acute glomerulonephritis may lead to a chronic condition. This chronic condition may extend over several years with periods of remission and exacerbation. During this time, a number of the glomeruli are destroyed, leading to an inability of the kidney to produce urine. This decrease in urine output leads to an increase in fluid volume in the blood, retention of salt, edema, and ultimately hypertension.

**SYMPTOMS** Symptoms of chronic glomerulonephritis include those mentioned in the acute disease plus hypertension. Uremia (you-REE-me-ah; ur = urine, emia = blood or urine waste in the blood) and

kidney failure may occur during late stages of the disease. Prevention of chronic glomerulonephritis is prompt treatment of the acute form.

**TREATMENT** Treatment for symptoms of uremia and renal failure may include peritoneal dialysis or hemodialysis.

## ■ Hydronephrosis

Hydronephrosis (HIGH-droh-neh-**FROH**-sis; hydro = water, nephro = kidney, osis = condition of) is a collection of urine in the renal pelvis due to some type of obstruction.

**ETIOLOGY** This accumulation of urine leads to dilation and distention of the kidney pelvis. Causes of obstruction include congenital defects in urinary tract structure, kidney stones, tumors, enlarged prostate, and urinary tract infections. If the obstruction is unrelieved, permanent damage may occur and the kidney pelvis becomes nonfunctioning.

**SYMPTOMS** One or both kidneys may be affected depending on the position of the obstruction (Figure 13–5). If one kidney is affected, the disease may go undetected as the other kidney continues to function adequately. If both kidneys are involved, anuria and uremia may develop. Diagnosis is confirmed by pyelogram.

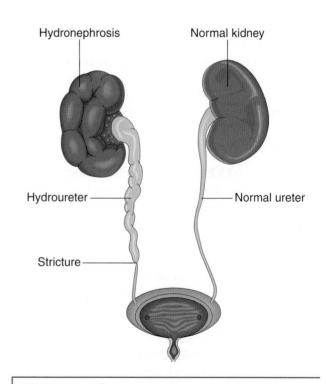

**FIGURE 13–5** Hydronephrosis.

**TREATMENT** Treatment involves immediate draining of the kidney pelvis by surgical intervention or immediate relief of the obstruction.

## ■ Renal Calculi

Renal calculi are commonly called "kidney stones." These stones are often composed of calcium salts and other substances. Size, location, and number of stones may vary (Figure 13-6).

**ETIOLOGY** Urinary stones are more common in males than females and commonly occur between ages 30 and 50. Cause of stone formation is unknown in most cases, but some precipitating factors include dehydration, chronic urinary tract infection, and immobility or prolonged bed rest, leading to release of calcium from the bones. Less commonly, stones are the result of metabolic disorders such as hyperparathyroidism, severe bone disease, and gout.

Staghorn calculi are one of the more common types of stones. These calculi form in the pelvis of the kidney and may become so large that they fill the entire kidney pelvis. Calculi commonly form in the kidney, but they also may form in the urinary bladder. Bladder stones cause difficulty with emptying the bladder, often leading to frequent or chronic bladder infections. Individuals may frequently form small kidney stones that easily pass through the urinary tract unnoticed. Stones may be present in the kidney, yet cause no problems. It is only when stones become caught in the ureters or obstruct the urinary tract that problems and symptoms arise.

**SYMPTOMS** Typical symptoms of kidney stones are hematuria and renal or urinary colic. Urinary colic is an extreme, spasmodic flank pain often described as "the worst pain I've had in my entire life." This pain is caused by the contraction of an obstructed ureter.

Diagnosis is commonly confirmed by utilizing an IVP. A KUB and renal ultrasound also may be beneficial for diagnosis.

**TREATMENT** Treatment during an acute attack of kidney stones includes administering pain medication and increasing fluid intake with the hope that the stone will pass in the urine. Urine is often strained through a filtering device in an effort to catch the stone for identification. Even though stones feel like they should be quite large to the individual passing them, the ones that are voided and filtered are usually quite small, ranging in size from a grain of salt to a small piece of rice.

If the urinary tract is totally obstructed, emergency surgery must be performed to prevent hydronephrosis and kidney damage. Surgery called a "stone basket procedure" may be performed. This procedure involves passing a retrieval instrument through the urethra, bladder, and ureter in an effort to remove the stone. Another method of removing stones is to break the stones into pieces for retrieval or in hopes that they may be passed. This breaking of the stone is called a **lithotripsy** (litho = stone, tripsy = breaking). During lithotripsy, the affected individual is placed in a tub of water and external shock waves are emitted into the water, shattering the hard stones (Figure 13-7).

Prevention of further stone development may include medications, correcting any causative metabolic conditions, and increasing water intake.

## ■ Polycystic Disease

**ETIOLOGY** Polycystic disease is an inherited disease that causes massive enlargement of both kidneys due to development of multiple grape-like cysts (Figure 13-8). These cysts may cause the kidneys to increase in weight up to 20 times the normal weight. Polycystic disease is a slow, progressive disease that affects teenagers and young adults, usually leading to renal failure by age 30 to 40. There is no cure for the disease.

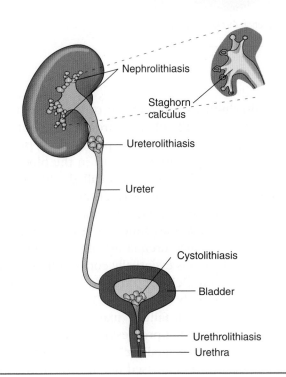

Nephrolithiasis

Staghorn calculus

Ureterolithiasis

Ureter

Cystolithiasis

Bladder

Urethrolithiasis

Urethra

**FIGURE 13–6** Types and location of renal calculi.

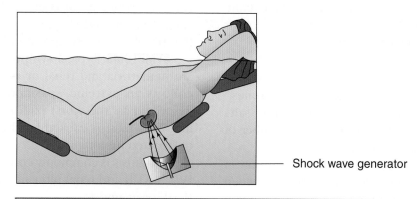

**FIGURE 13–7**  Lithotripsy.

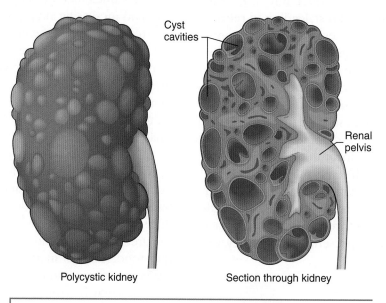

Cyst cavities

Renal pelvis

Polycystic kidney

Section through kidney

**FIGURE 13–8**  Polycystic kidney.

**SYMPTOMS**  As the disease progresses, kidney tissue is destroyed and function becomes increasingly impaired. Hypertension generally develops as the kidneys fail. Symptoms include lumbar pain, hematuria, and recurrent urinary tract infections. Diagnosis may be confirmed by family and clinical history, and an intravenous pyelogram (IVP).

**TREATMENT**  Treatment involves management of hypertension and urinary tract infections. Dialysis and kidney transplant are needed for end-stage treatment.

## ■ Renal Failure

Renal failure is the failure of the kidneys to perform the function of cleansing the blood of waste products. The primary method of cleansing the body of waste involves the liver forming urea and the kidneys filtering this product out of the blood to be excreted in urine. Blood urea nitrogen and creatinine are nitrogenous wastes, end products of protein metabolism. The amount of urea in the blood can be measured with a blood test called a blood urea nitrogen (BUN). Creatinine levels also can be measured in the blood. BUN and creatinine levels are utilized to measure kidney function. A high urea level in the blood is called uremia, literally meaning urine in the blood. Urea is eventually converted to ammonia, leading to toxicity and related symptoms in all systems of the body (Figure 13–9).

**ETIOLOGY**  Renal failure may occur suddenly (acute renal failure) or progress over a longer period of time (chronic renal failure). Acute renal failure is usually related to decreased blood flow to the kidneys due to conditions such as hemorrhagic or surgical shock, embolism, congestive heart failure, and

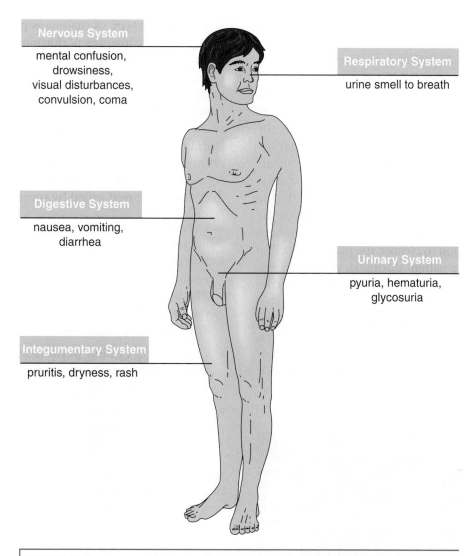

**Nervous System**

mental confusion,
drowsiness,
visual disturbances,
convulsion, coma

**Respiratory System**

urine smell to breath

**Digestive System**

nausea, vomiting,
diarrhea

**Urinary System**

pyuria, hematuria,
glycosuria

**Integumentary System**

pruritis, dryness, rash

**FIGURE 13–9**   Areas of the body affected by toxic levels of circulating ammonia.

dehydration. Blockage of urine flow, caused by tumors, stones, or enlarged prostate, also may lead to acute failure. Reversal of acute renal failure, which involves treating the cause of the failure, is usually quite successful. Dialysis may be needed temporarily to remove toxic wastes from the individual's blood until kidney function is restored. Individuals in acute renal failure are placed on a limited diet to allow the kidneys to rest and regenerate function.

Chronic renal failure occurs slowly and is usually the result of chronic kidney disease such as glomerulonephritis, pyelonephritis, renal hypertension, and polycystic disease. Long-term substance abuse, alcoholism, and diabetes also may cause chronic renal failure.

**SYMPTOMS** Symptoms of renal failure are not significant until approximately 75 percent of kidney function has been destroyed. Symptoms may include those of acute failure, plus problems of infertility, impotence, and bone weakness, leading to pain and fractures.

**TREATMENT** Treatment includes management of the related cause of the failure, limiting protein and sodium in the diet, and monitoring fluid intake and urine output. Medications may include antihypertensives, diuretics, and antibiotics as needed. Dialysis and kidney transplantation may be options for long-term treatment.

Dialysis is a procedure that cleanses the blood of waste products when the kidneys have failed or are failing to perform this function. There are two types of dialysis. Both of the types of dialysis require the same components: the patient's blood, a semipermeable membrane, and a washing or dialyzing solution. In both types of dialysis, the waste products in the individual's blood pass through the semipermeable membrane by diffusion to enter the dialyzing solution, thus cleansing the blood.

The most common type of dialysis is hemodialysis (Figure 13-10). During hemodialysis, the individual's blood is routed out of an artery (usually the brachial or radial artery) and through an artificial kidney machine, or hemodialyzer, which mechanically cleans the blood. This machine is filled with a semipermeable cellophane-like material and dialyzing solution. As blood passes through the machine, the waste products diffuse through the membrane into the dialyzing solution to cleanse the blood. The clean blood re-enters the patient through a venous access. One common problem with hemodialysis is maintaining vascular access. Commonly, an arteriovenous (AV) shunt is created by placing catheters in the needed artery and vein (Figure 13-11). These vessels are connected (shunted) with silicone rubber tubing. Common complications of AV shunts include infection and clotting.

The other type of dialysis is peritoneal dialysis. This procedure involves performing a paracentesis to instill dialyzing solution into the peritoneal cavity. This type of dialysis utilizes the membrane that lines the peritoneal cavity to act as the semipermeable membrane. The dialyzing solution is allowed to stay in the abdomen for varying amounts of time (dwell time). During this time, waste products diffuse out of the peritoneal capillaries and into the dialyzing solution. Solution is then drained and disposed of. Peritoneal dialysis may be performed by several methods.

■ Continuous ambulatory peritoneal dialysis (CAPD) is a self-dialysis that does not utilize a machine. Solution drains by gravity into and out of the peritoneal cavity by way of a permanently connected catheter. The waste solution drains into a bag worn around the individual's waist. CAPD is performed several times a day and usually once at night (Figure 13-12).

■ Continuous cycling peritoneal dialysis (CCPD) uses a cycling machine and takes place while the individual sleeps.

■ Intermittent peritoneal dialysis (IPD) is performed several times a week, usually in a medical clinic.

Hemodialysis is a much faster and more efficient process than peritoneal dialysis, but it is also much more expensive and more time-consuming. Also, access to an artificial kidney machine may be limited to large metropolitan areas.

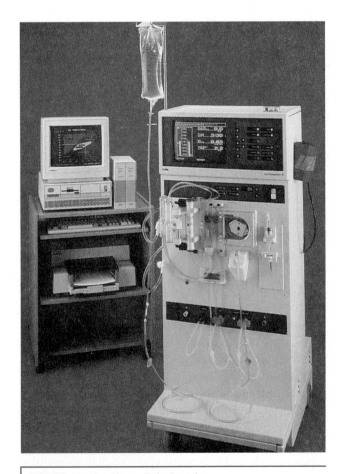

**FIGURE 13-10** Hemodialysis unit.

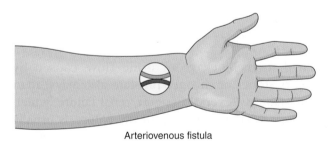
Arteriovenous fistula

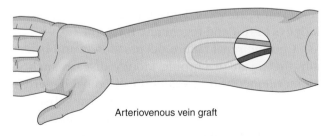
Arteriovenous vein graft

**FIGURE 13-11** Hemodialysis sites: AV Shunts.

## COMPLEMENTARY AND ALTERNATIVE THERAPY

### Women on Dialysis Need to Be Wary of Herbal Medicines

Women with end-stage renal disease who are on dialysis need to be careful using herbal preparations. The safety of many herbal medicines such as black cohosh, ginseng, and soy products, often used by women to treat menopausal symptoms, has not yet been established. Further research needs to be done to test the effects of these products and the safety of patients who are already in renal failure.

*Source: Roemheld-Hamm, B., & Dahl, N.V. (2002).*

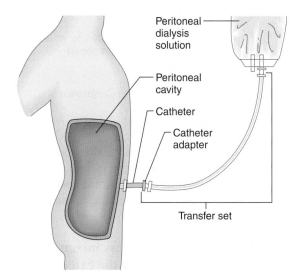

Peritoneal dialysis solution
Peritoneal cavity
Catheter
Catheter adapter
Transfer set

(A) Infusion of solution.

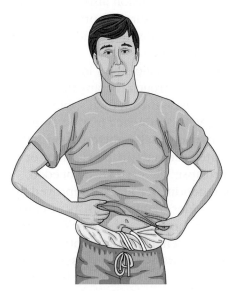

(B) Empty solution container is rolled up and hidden under clothing.

**FIGURE 13–12** Continuous ambulatory peritoneal dialysis.

Renal transplantation is a procedure to transplant a kidney of a donor into a recipient. This is a relatively simple surgical procedure performed on individuals with chronic renal failure commonly due to diabetes, hypertension, and glomerulonephritis. Best results from kidney transplants are obtained when the donor and recipient are close human leukocyte antigen (HLA) matches or are histocompatible. An identical twin provides the greatest probability of match with a fraternal twin, sibling, parent, and child the next best matches in that descending order. The greatest problems with renal transplant are obtaining a kidney that is histocompatible with the recipient, postoperative organ rejection, and complications with lifelong administration of immunosuppressant medications.

### ■ Adenocarcinoma of the Kidney

Cancer of the kidney is relatively uncommon.

**ETIOLOGY** The cause of this tumor is unknown although cigarette smoking is considered to be a risk factor. Adenocarcinoma of the kidney frequently metastasizes to the liver, brain, and bone before symptoms appear.

**SYMPTOMS** The most common initial symptom is painless hematuria. Later, as the tumor increases in size, the individual experiences flank pain and fever. A KUB, IVP, CT, and biopsy of the kidney may be utilized to confirm the diagnosis.

**TREATMENT** Treatment, whether metastasis has occurred or not, is **nephrectomy** (neh-FRECK-toh-me; nephr = kidney, ectomy = excision or removal). If metastasis has occurred, chemotherapy and radiation also may be utilized. Prognosis varies with the extent of spread. Cure may be possible if no metastasis has occurred, but with metastasis, prognosis is poor.

# Diseases of the Bladder

With the exception of incontinence, diseases of the bladder are relatively uncommon compared to the many other disorders of the urinary system. However, incontinence is very common, especially in the older adult. It can cause many physical and psychological problems for an individual.

## ▪ Urinary Incontinence

Urinary incontinence is the loss of control of urine flow. It is estimated that over 15 million people have this disorder and 85 percent of them are female. Forty percent of females age 60 and older suffer with urinary incontinence.

**ETIOLOGY** Pregnancy, childbirth, hysterectomy, and menopause may all affect female continence. Males are also affected by incontinence but not nearly as often as females. As males age, the prostate is often enlarged, leading to urinary "dribbling" or inability to control flow. Prostate surgery also may affect continence.

**SYMPTOMS** Incontinence affects all areas of an individual's life by disrupting sleep, physical activity, travel plans, and sexual activity. Often, the fear of urinary accidents drives affected individuals away from social activity and into a life of seclusion.

There are several types of incontinence. Stress incontinence is the inability to hold urine when the bladder is stressed by coughing, sneezing, or laughing. Urge incontinence occurs with a sudden uncontrollable urge to empty the bladder. Overflow incontinence is caused by the bladder not properly emptying and leaking when overfilled.

**TREATMENT** Incontinence may be managed by wearing sanitary napkins, incontinence pads, adult diapers, and/or waterproof briefs. Males also may use external appliances to catch the urine.

Stress incontinence may be improved by several different treatments, depending on the cause of the incontinence. A common noninvasive treatment employs frequently emptying the bladder, and exercising the pelvic muscles and external sphincter to strengthen these structures. Exercises of these muscles are called Kegel exercises. Kegel exercises are performed by tightening or contracting the pelvic muscles like one would do in an effort to hold or stop urine flow. Performing repetitions of 20 to 40 Kegel exercises several times a day can be quite effective in controlling some types of stress incontinence (Figure 13–13).

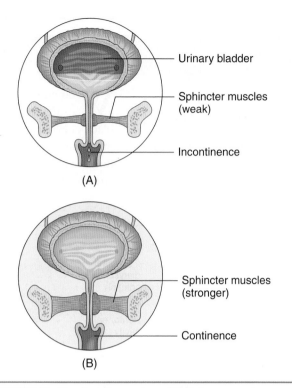

**FIGURE 13–13** Kegel exercises: (A) Before exercises, pelvic muscles are thin, the sphincter is weak, and the urethra cannot close; (B) After exercises (three months), the muscles are thicker and stronger, closing the sphincter.

Another treatment for stress incontinence involves collagen injections near the external sphincter to narrow the urethra (Figure 13–14). Laparoscopic bladder suspension also may be a treatment of choice. Another surgical procedure performed to suspend the bladder neck and urethra to correct urinary incontinence is called Marshall-Marchetti-Krantz (MMK). Female stress incontinence may be improved with estrogen therapy because low estrogen levels weaken the urethral sphincter.

Overflow incontinence may be controlled with medications and/or self-catheterization. If the bladder has herniated through the pelvic floor or if there is vaginal prolapse, surgery may be needed.

Urge incontinence may be improved by bladder training. Bladder training consists of emptying the bladder every hour for a week or so, then gradually increasing the length of time until one is toileting every three hours. Kegel exercises also may help. Surgery is usually a last alternative because it is quite expensive.

In males, urinary incontinence is common following prostate surgery. To control this incontinence, exercise is necessary. If exercise does not control the

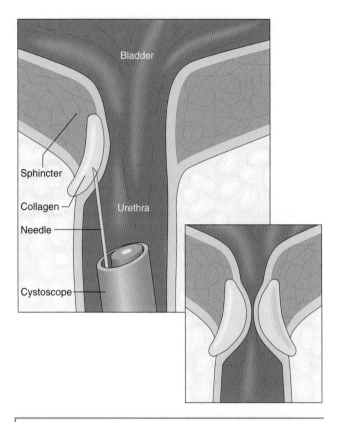

FIGURE 13–14   Collagen injection for incontinence.

incontinence, collagen injections may be needed. Another treatment option is surgical insertion of an artificial sphincter. This artificial device has a valve that an individual can activate to control urine flow.

Urinary incontinence in both sexes may be related to other diseases such as stroke and urinary tract infection. Medications to control hypertension, sleeping pills, antihistamines, and muscle relaxants also may cause urinary incontinence.

## ◼ Transitional Cell Carcinoma of the Bladder

Bladder cancer is the most common neoplasm of the urinary tract. It usually occurs in males after age 60 and is three times more common in males than females. Transitional carcinoma arises from the lining of the bladder. Bladder cancer commonly metastasizes before symptoms appear, making it highly malignant.

**ETIOLOGY**   The cause of these tumors is unknown, but the most important risk factor is cigarette smoking, which increases the chance of cancer proportionate to the number of cigarettes smoked during the life of the affected individual. Other predisposing factors include exposure to industrial chemicals and chronic cystitis.

**SYMPTOMS**   Symptoms include hematuria, dysuria, and nocturia, but as previously mentioned, these symptoms do not usually appear until late in the course of the disease. Diagnosis may be confirmed by cystoscopy and biopsy.

**TREATMENT**   Treatment depends on the stage of the tumor. **Transurethral resection (TUR)** (trans = through, urethral = urethra; resection = partial excision) may be performed to remove the tumor, or more frequently, a **radical** (radical = a treatment that seeks to cure, aggressive, not pallative or conservative) **cystectomy** (sis-TECT-toh-me, cyst = bladder, ectomy = excision or removal) is performed. If metastasis has occurred, radiation and chemotherapy also may be utilized. Prognosis depends on the stage of the tumor when discovered. Usually, discovery is late in the course of the disease and prognosis is poor. Prevention is aimed at avoiding exposure to industrial chemicals, prompt treatment of cystitis, and cessation of cigarette smoking.

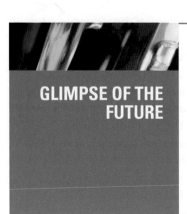

**GLIMPSE OF THE FUTURE**

### A New Drug for Bladder Cancer

Trials to test the effectiveness of the drug EOquin™ for individuals with superficial bladder cancer are underway. The initial trial was completed and the researchers reported positive findings. EOquin™ was safe and well tolerated by the subjects in the study. Most of the patients showed a complete disappearance of the bladder tumor after receiving six treatments over a six-week period. The second phase of the trial will start soon. Perhaps in the near future, EOquin™ will be routinely used to treat superficial bladder cancer.

*Source:* Health & Medicine Week. *(2004).*

# TRAUMA

## Straddle Injuries

Straddle injuries commonly cause injury to the urethra. This type of injury occurs when an individual accidentally falls in a straddling position. Straddle injuries are more common in males. Instances when straddle injuries may occur include walking a fence or roof beam or, in some cases, riding a horse or motorcycle. Treatment varies, depending on the severity of the injury.

## Neurogenic Bladder

**ETIOLOGY** Neurogenic bladder is dysfunction of the bladder due to some type of injury to the nervous system supplying the urinary tract or bladder. A common trauma that causes neurogenic bladder is a spinal cord injury such as those sustained in motor vehicle accidents or diving accidents. Other traumatic causes include cerebrovascular accidents, strokes, tumors, and herniated lumbar disks. Diabetes, dementia, and Parkinson's disease are metabolic disorders that often lead to neurogenic bladder.

**SYMPTOMS** Symptoms of neurogenic bladder vary, depending on the nerves involved. Individuals may have no feeling of the need to void or they may feel like they need to void all the time. Other symptoms are mild to severe urinary incontinence, difficulty or inability to empty the bladder, and bladder spasms. Neurogenic bladder is difficult to diagnose. A detailed history and physical, neurologic examinations, and a series of urologic studies may be needed to confirm a diagnosis.

**TREATMENT** Treatment goals are aimed at prevention of urinary tract infections and controlling incontinence. Indwelling urinary catheters may be utilized to control incontinence. Intermittent self-catheterization may be taught to individuals unable to empty the bladder to prevent hydronephrosis and possible renal failure.

The prognosis of neurogenic bladder depends on the possibility of reversing the nerve damage. Herniated lumbar disks that cause neurogenic bladder are commonly repaired and rapidly restore bladder function. If nerve damage is permanent, neurogenic bladder will also be permanent.

# RARE DISEASES

## Goodpasture Syndrome

Goodpasture syndrome is an autoimmune disorder characterized by glomerulonephritis and pulmonary hemorrhage. For some unknown reason, the body's own antibodies attack the membranes of the kidneys and lungs, leading to symptoms of hemoptysis (he-MOP-tih-sis; hemo = blood, ptysis = saliva) or coughing or spitting up blood, dyspnea (dys = difficulty, pnea = breathing), chest pain, and anemia. Goodpasture syndrome usually results in renal failure and ultimately, death.

## Interstitial Cystitis

Interstitial cystitis is a chronic "nonbacterial" cystitis due to inflammation of the inner lining of the bladder.

**ETIOLOGY** Typically, this disease affects young women and is thought to be autoimmune in nature.

**SYMPTOMS** The inflammation and swelling of the inner lining of the bladder decreases the capacity of the bladder, leading to the need to urinate frequently. Often, the lining is ulcerated, leading to hematuria. Other symptoms include pain above the pubic area and lower abdomen, bladder fullness, and urgency.

**TREATMENT** Treatment includes instillation of liquid medications into the bladder to distend the bladder and treat the disorder. Treatment may be needed for up to 12 weeks, but response to treatment is generally good.

# EFFECTS OF AGING ON THE SYSTEM

The most common problem of the urinary system in the older adult is urinary incontinence. It is frequently due to changes in other body systems in the aging process rather than the urinary system. Because the urinary elimination process is primarily controlled by the nervous system, changes with aging or diseases of this system may affect the individual's ability to control urine flow. Individuals with Alzheimer's disease, brain tumor, or other disorders of the nervous system may not be aware of the urge to urinate or be able to communicate the need to urinate.

In older males, benign prostatic hypertrophy is a common disorder that often causes urinary frequency, dribbling, pain or burning with urination, and difficulty starting the urine flow. In older females, the changes in estrogen levels may cause a decrease in vaginal muscle tone, and along with the changes in structure, may cause increased frequency and some urine incontinence. Changes in lower abdomen muscle tone, usually the result of multiple pregnancies or obesity, also contribute to some urinary incontinence in the older adult female. (See Chapter 17 for more information on changes in the female and male reproductive systems.)

Older individuals with other common system disorders such as stroke or severe circulatory impairment may not feel the urge to urinate, and thus have urinary incontinence. Chronic urinary tract infections also may affect bladder function so that the result over time is urinary incontinence.

Urinary problems in the older adult may not be due to the aging process at all, but to many other events occurring in the individual's life. Fecal impactions that are common in the institutionalized older individual also can cause urinary incontinence.

Some medications can cause changes in the ability of the bladder to empty thoroughly, causing overflow incontinence. Many older adults take medications such as antidepressants, narcotic pain relievers, or cardiac drugs that may cause some urinary retention, eventually resulting in incontinence.

Older adults who have mobility problems frequently have urinary incontinence. Individuals who have some difficulty rising from a chair or bed, or who walk slowly often have periods of incontinence simply because they cannot get to the restroom in time. Lack of mobility causes the individual to be dependent on others for toileting and this frequently leads to urinary incontinence problems. This is extremely common in the institutionalized older adult.

## SUMMARY

The urinary system includes the kidneys, ureters, bladder, and urethra. It maintains homeostasis in the body by excreting and reabsorbing important electrolytes, compounds, and water. Urinary disorders range from mild infections to very serious diseases such as cancer. The most common signs and symptoms of urinary dysfunction include an abnormality in the urine or in the individual's ability to urinate. The most common disorders of the urinary system include infections and incontinence. Some diseases are diagnosed by urinalysis or urine culture and sensitivity. However, radiologic examinations are also used. A cystoscopy may be performed for diagnostic or treatment purposes. In the older adult, urinary incontinence is the most frequent problem of the system. Urinary disorders may be the result of urinary system pathology, or the result of disease or malfunction of other body systems.

## REVIEW QUESTIONS

### Short Answer

1. What are the functions of the urinary system?

2. Which signs and symptoms are associated with common urinary system disorders?

**3.** Which diagnostic tests are most commonly used to determine the type and/or cause of urinary system disorders?

**4.** What is the most common urinary problem in the older adult population?

## Matching

**5.** Match the disorders listed in the left column with the correct definition in the right column.

| | |
|---|---|
| _____ urethritis | **a.** most commonly used diagnostic test for urinary system disorders |
| _____ pyuria | **b.** pus in the urine |
| _____ oliguria | **c.** an inflammation of the filtering components of the kidney |
| _____ anuria | **d.** difficulty urinating |
| _____ nocturia | **e.** excision of the kidney |
| _____ cystectomy | **f.** inflammation of the urethra |
| _____ dysuria | **g.** frequent urination at night |
| _____ nephrectomy | **h.** surgical removal of the bladder |
| _____ urinalysis | **i.** scanty urine output |
| _____ pyelonephritis | **j.** absence of urine output |
| _____ glomerulonephritis | **k.** inflammation of the kidney pelvis |

## CASE STUDY

**Ms. Hayden,** age 55, has been noticing a small amount of urine leakage at intervals when she participates in her low-impact aerobics class. She has noticed this problem for about a year now, but thinks it is nothing to worry about. She tells you that this occurs every time she does aerobics now and asks what you think the cause might be. She is also embarrassed to ask her physician about it. How would you respond to Ms. Hayden? Do you think this is a problem for concern? Should she seek medical advice?

## BIBLIOGRAPHY

Clinical data presented from EOquin™ trial in superficial bladder cancer. (2004, July 19). *Health & Medicine Week*, 107–108.

Color doppler sonography is a standard method renal artery stenosis screening. (2004, January 6). *Cancer Weekly*, 172–173.

Few bladder cancer markers exist, new tissue analysis methods may help ID more. (2004, January 2). *Drug Week*, 77–78.

Folkert, V. W. (2003). Intravenous iron therapy in chronic kidney disease and peritoneal dialysis patients. *Nephrology Nursing Journal 30*(5), 571–577.

Hanson, K. (2002). BCG installations for bladder cancer and latent tuberculosis infection. *Urologic Nursing 22*(2), 132–133.

HIV/AIDS and HIV nephropathy. (2003). *Nephrology Nursing Journal 30*(1), 64–68.

Interstitial cystitis. (2003). *Postgraduate Medicine 114*(6), 59–60.

Kaplow, R., & Barry, R. (2002). Continuous renal replacement therapies. *American Journal of Nursing 102*(11), 26–34.

Kunin, C. M. (2003). Definition of acute pyelonephritis vs. The urosepsis syndrome. *Archives of Internal Medicine 163*(19), 2393.

Newer methods and drugs offer opportunities to treat renal cell carcinoma. (2003, December 12). *Drug Week*, 300–301.

Overactive bladder treatment study results confirm efficacy and tolerability. (2003, November 7). *Drug Week*, 295–296.

Research shows cancer can be diagnosed in urine. (2004, January 6). *Cancer Weekly*, 102–103.

Researcher's pinpoint possible cause of chronic bladder cancer. (2003, December 4). *Women's Health Weekly*, 5–7.

Roemheld-Hamm, B., & Dahl, N. V. (2002). Herbs, menopause, and dialysis. *Seminars in Dialysis 15*(1), 53–59.

Sofer, D. (2003). Chronic kidney disease: The emerging epidemic. *American Journal of Nursing 103*(12), 23.

Stein, A. (2003). Aging is more than skin deep. *Nursing 33*(2), 32–33.

Szromba, C. (2003). Smoking in chronic kidney disease. *Nephrology Nursing Journal 30*(5), 578–579.

The von Hippel-Lindau gene, kidney cancer, and oxygen sensing. (2003, December 12). *Drug Week*, 251–252.

Urologist studies herbal remedies for prostate and urinary diseases. (2004, January 2). *Drug Week*, 198–199.

Wareing, M. (2003). Urinary retention: Issues of management and care. *Emergency Nurse 11*(8), 24–27.

Wilson, P. (2004). Polycystic kidney disease. *New England Journal of Medicine 350*(2), 151–164.

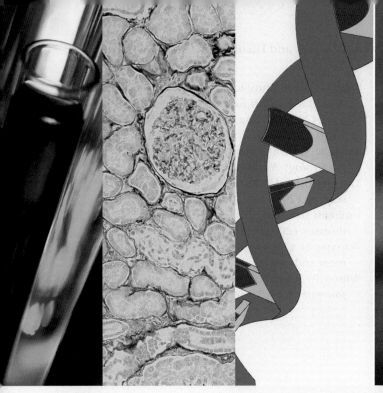
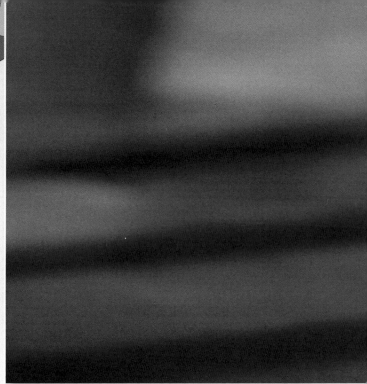

## OUTLINE

## KEY TERMS

# Endocrine System Diseases and Disorders

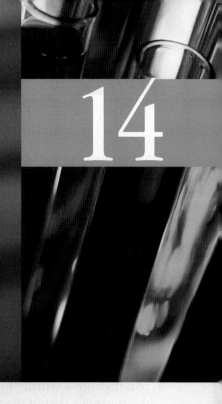

**14**

## LEARNING OBJECTIVES

*Upon completion of the chapter, the learner should be able to:*

1. Define the terminology common to the endocrine system and the disorders of the system.

2. Discuss the basic anatomy and physiology of the endocrine system.

3. Identify the important signs and symptoms associated with common endocrine system disorders.

4. Describe the common diagnostics used to determine the type and/or cause of endocrine system disorders.

5. Identify common disorders of the endocrine system.

6. Describe the typical course and management of the common endocrine system disorders.

7. Describe the effects of aging on the endocrine system and the common disorders of the system.

## OVERVIEW

*The endocrine system is a highly complex system of glands that secrete important hormones for a variety of body functions. The glands of the system work in harmony, discharging the hormones into the bloodstream as needed. The disorders of the system may be caused by problems in the primary gland or from problems in another gland whose secretions control the primary gland. Disorders of the endocrine system may be related to oversecretion of the gland's hormones or undersecretion of its hormones. ∎*

## ANATOMY AND PHYSIOLOGY

The endocrine system consists of many glands located throughout the body (Figure 14–1). It includes the following glands:

1. hypothalamus—located beneath the thalamus in the area of the third ventricle of the brain

2. pituitary or hypophysis—located at the base of the brain

3. pineal—located behind the midbrain

4. thymus—located in the mediastinal cavity under the sternum, near the heart

5. thyroid—located in the neck on each side of the trachea

6. parathyroids—usually four glands, imbedded in the posterior part of the thyroid

7. adrenals—two glands, one on top of each kidney

8. pancreatic islets—imbedded in the pancreas

9. ovaries (female) and testes (male)—one ovary on each side of the uterus or one testis in each side of the scrotal sac

Each of these glands has a unique function and delivers its secretion as needed into the bloodstream. Table 14–1 lists the glands, their hormones, and the functions of each hormone. The mechanism known as "negative feedback" controls the amount of hormones secreted into the bloodstream. Although the hypothalamus monitors the hormone secretions, negative feedback regulates the amount secreted. In the negative feedback system, levels of the particular hormone in the bloodstream trigger the release of the hormone as needed. If the concentration of the hormone in the blood is low, the sequence of events stimulates the gland to secrete more hormones. In like manner, if the concentration of the hormone in the blood is higher than normal, the feedback mechanism triggers the gland to suppress the release of more hormones.

The hypothalamus, located in the third ventricle area of the brain, contains neurosecretory cells that secrete hypothalamic hormones. These hormones regulate the function of the anterior pituitary gland. The hypothalamus also produces the two hormones stored in the neurohypophysis or posterior pituitary gland.

The pituitary gland, also known as the hypophysis gland, is divided into two distinct parts. The ade-

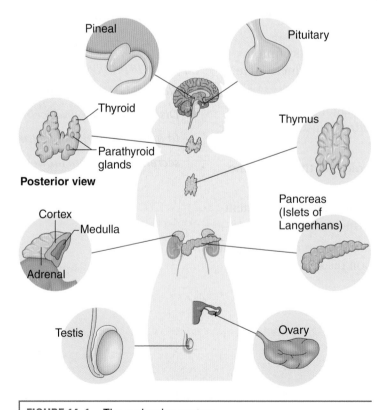

**FIGURE 14–1**   The endocrine system.

nohypophysis, or anterior part of the gland, produces several hormones that affect other endocrine glands. These include adenocorticotropin hormone (ACTH), thyrotropin hormone (TSH), somatotropin hormone (STH), melanocyte stimulating hormone (MSH), lactogenic hormone (prolactin), follicle-stimulating hormone (FSH), and luteinizing hormone (LH; also called interstitial cell-stimulating hormone, ICSH).

The posterior pituitary, also called the neurohypophysis, stores two hormones that are secreted by the hypothalamus. Oxytocin (pitocin) helps the progress of labor in the pregnant female and causes uterine contractions after childbirth. It also affects the cells in the breasts, causing a release of milk during lactation. The antidiuretic hormone ADH, also known as **vasopressin**, is also released from the neurohypophysis. It affects the reabsorption of water from the renal tubules.

The pineal gland, located behind the mid-brain, secretes melatonin. It may also secrete other hormones that interact with the hypothalamus and the pituitary gland to cause the secretion of hormones from other glands.

The thymus gland, located just below the clavicle behind the sternum, secretes thymopoietin, a hormone that stimulates the development of lymphocytes. Lymphocytes are important for immunity development and prevention of infections.

The thyroid gland, located in the neck on either side of the trachea, secretes thyroxine ($T_4$), triiodothyronine ($T_3$), and calcitonin. These hormones are released as needed in response to the thyroid-stimulating hormone secreted by the pituitary gland. Thyroxine and triiodothyronine increase metabolic activity. Calcitonin affects the regulation of calcium and works in opposition to the hormone secreted by the parathyroid gland.

Imbedded in the posterior part of the thyroid gland are the parathyroid glands. There are usually four parathyroid glands, but there can be more. The parathyroid glands secrete parathormone, important in the regulation of calcium and phosphorus in the body.

The adrenal glands, located on top of each kidney, have two distinct parts. The cortex, the outer part, secretes **mineralocorticoids**, **glucocorticoids**,

**TABLE 14–1**　The Endocrine Glands: Their Hormones and Hormone Functions

| Endocrine Gland | Hormone | Hormone Function |
|---|---|---|
| Hypothalamus | Inhibiting hormones and Releasing hormones | Inhibits or releases hormones from the anterior pituitary |
| Hypophysis (Pituitary) | Adenocorticotropin hormone (ACTH) | Stimulates release of adrenal cortex hormones |
| Adenohypophysis (Anterior Pituitary) | Thyrotropin hormone (TSH) Somatotropin hormone (STH) Melanocyte stimulating hormone (MSH) Lactogenic hormone (prolactin) Follicle-stimulating hormone (FSH) Luteinizing hormone (LH; also called interstitial cell-stimulating hormone, ICSH). | Stimulates release of thyroid gland hormones Stimulates growth Stimulates melanin production Stimulates mammary gland and lactation Stimulates estrogen secretion Induces ovulation in females and testosterone secretion in males |
| Neurohypophysis (Posterior Pituitary) | Antidiuretic hormone (ADH) Oxytocin | Increases reabsorption of water in the distal tubules of the kidneys Stimulates uterine contraction and the initiation of breast milk flow in females and increases the ejection of sperm into the seminal fluid in males |
| Pineal | Melatonin | Affects circadian rhythms |

*(continued)*

**TABLE 14–1** **The Endocrine Glands: Their Hormones and Hormone Functions (Continued)**

| Endocrine Gland | Hormone | Hormone Function |
|---|---|---|
| Thymus | Thymopoietin | Causes immune response development in the newborn and maintains it in the adult |
| Thyroid | Triiodothyronine ($T_3$) Thyroxine ($T_4$) Calcitonin | Stimulates growth and development and regulates metabolism Increases calcium deposits into the bones |
| Parathyroid | Parathormone (PTH) | Regulates calcium and phosphate levels and increases reabsorption of calcium from the bones |
| Adrenals Adrenal Cortex | Glucocorticoids Mineralocorticoids Sex hormones | Affects stress reactions; promotes protein and fat use to raise blood sugar Affects sodium and water reabsorption Promotes sodium and water reabsorption Develops secondary sex characteristics |
| Adrenal Medulla | Epinephrine Norepinephrine | Fight or flight response Increases blood pressure and metabolism Causes vasoconstriction and increases blood pressure |
| Pancreas Islets Alpha Cells | Glucagon | Increases blood glucose levels and is counterregulatory to insulin |
| Beta Cells | Insulin | Regulates protein, carbohydrate, and fat metabolism |
| Delta Cells | Somatostatin | Counterregulatory to insulin, glucagon, and somatotropin (STH) |
| Ovaries | Estrogen Progesterone | Regulates development, maturation, secondary sex characteristics and the reproductive cycle in females |
| Testes | Testosterone | Regulates growth and development, maturation, secondary sex characteristics and the reproductive system in males |

and **androgens**. The mineralocorticoids promote sodium retention. The glucocorticoids affect the metabolism of protein, glucose, and fats. **Cortisol** is the main glucocorticoid and is important for metabolism of carbohydrates. The androgens enhance masculinization. The most common androgen hormone is testosterone. The adrenal medulla or middle section secretes epinephrine and norepinephrine.

The beta cells located in the pancreas secrete **insulin**, another important hormone. Insulin is most important in the metabolism of glucose, but it also promotes fatty acid synthesis and promotes amino acid entry into cells. Insulin secretion is regulated by the feedback mechanism and by counterregulatory hormones such as **glucagon**, cortisol, epinephrine, and the growth hormone.

The ovaries and testes secrete the sex hormones, as they are commonly known. The ovaries secrete **estrogen** and **progesterone**, important for development and maturation, and maintaining the functions of the reproductive system. The testes secrete testosterone, important for growth and development, secondary sex characteristics, and maintaining the reproductive system functions. See Chapter 17 for more information about the reproductive system.

## COMMON SIGNS AND SYMPTOMS

Most endocrine disorders are due to hypo- or hyper-secretion by a gland. Diagnosis is dependent on matching the signs and symptoms with the hormone dysfunction. The difficulty in diagnosing endocrine disorders is related to tracking the problem to the correct source. A pituitary dysfunction can easily lead to signs and symptoms of multiple gland disorders. For example, a decreased secretion of thyroid-stimulating hormone from the pituitary may initially lead one to believe that the thyroid gland itself is dysfunctional. Some common signs and symptoms of endocrine system disorders include mental abnormalities, lethargy or fatigue, and tissue atrophy.

## DIAGNOSTIC TESTS

The only endocrine glands that can be physically examined are the thyroid glands and testes. Enlargement or atrophy of these glands can be felt. Severe enlargement also can be seen. Assessment of proper function of the endocrine organs can be accomplished with blood or urine testing for the hormones they produce. Computerized tomography (CT) and magnetic resonance imaging (MRI) may be utilized to check for presence of tumors or alteration in organ size.

## COMMON DISEASES OF THE ENDOCRINE SYSTEM

Endocrine diseases are the result of abnormally high or low hormone secretion by endocrine glands. Abnormal secretion may be due to the size of the gland. Abnormally large or hypertrophied glands tend to produce abnormally high hormone levels, whereas abnormally small or atrophied glands tend to produce abnormally low levels. Abnormal gland size may be the result of injury to the gland by surgery, trauma, infection, or radiation. Abnormal

function of endocrine glands leads to many different physical and mental abnormalities. Abnormalities vary with the amount of hormone secreted (hypersecretion or hyposecretion) by the gland and the age of the individual involved.

## Pituitary Gland Diseases

The anterior pituitary gland produces tropic hormones. Tropic means going toward or changing. These tropic hormones go toward or stimulate target organs to grow or produce specific hormones. Growth hormone (GH or somatotropin) promotes growth and development of all body tissues. Other target organs are the thyroid, adrenal gland, testes, and ovaries.

### ■ Hyperpituitarism

**ETIOLOGY** Hyperpituitarism is an abnormal increase in the activity of the pituitary gland. This oversecretion especially affects growth hormone (GH) production, leading to excessive growth of bones and tissues.

**SYMPTOMS** If hyperpituitarism occurs before puberty, **giantism** occurs (Figure 14–2). Children

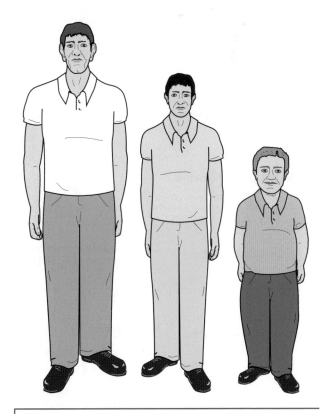

**FIGURE 14–2**  Giantism and dwarfism. (Right) A dwarf. (Left) A giant. A normal sized individual is in the center.

affected with hyperpituitarism may grow as much as six inches in a year. Sexual development is usually slowed. Mental development may be normal or retarded. Giantism is usually the result of a tumor on the pituitary gland.

**SYMPTOMS** If hyperpituitarism occurs in an adult, **acromegaly** (ACK-roh-**MEG**-ah-lee; acro = extremity, megaly = enlargement) occurs. In the adult, the long bones are unable to grow in length, but the small bones of the hands, feet, and face enlarge. Facial features become coarse, the nose and lips enlarge, and the skin and tongue thicken, leading to slurred speech. Acromegaly is a chronic, disfiguring disease that usually shortens life expectancy and often leads to congestive heart failure and respiratory and cerebrovascular diseases.

**TREATMENT** In children, surgical removal, radiation, and drug therapy may be utilized in an attempt to decrease the secretion of GH and slow the growing process. Prognosis for giantism is usually good. In adults, surgical removal of pituitary tumors often leads to hypopituitarism and these tumors tend to recur.

## ■ Hypopituitarism

**ETIOLOGY** Hypopituitarism is an abnormal decrease in the activity of the pituitary gland, leading to a deficiency or absence of any of the tropic hormones.

**SYMPTOMS** Because the pituitary gland is the master gland, hypopituitarism may lead to a variety of problems involving the function of all target organs (Figure 14–3). Growth hormone and gonadotropin are the most common deficiencies in hypopituitarism. The degree of hypopituitarism may range from mild to severe. A decrease in growth hormone leads to impaired growth of all body tissues with the most severe decreases causing **dwarfism** (see Figure 14–2). Children affected with dwarfism are proportionately small, underdeveloped sexually, and may or may not suffer from mental challenges. Gonadotropin deficiency may lead to abnormal development or absence of secondary sexual characteristics. In adult women, this deficiency may cause amenorrhea and infertility. Adult men may have a lowered testosterone level, decreased libido (la-BE-doe; sex drive), and abnormal loss of facial and body hair. A decrease in ACTH and TSH may lead to metabolic disorders. If the pituitary gland is destroyed or nonfunctional, a condition called **panhypopituitarism** (pan = all) exists. Panhypopituitarism may lead to all the preceding disorders and result in fatal complications.

Diagnosis may be confirmed by clinical history and blood testing. A blood test may be utilized to help determine the area of dysfunction. The dysfunction could be the pituitary, involve the individual target organ, or it may involve both. Specific blood hormone

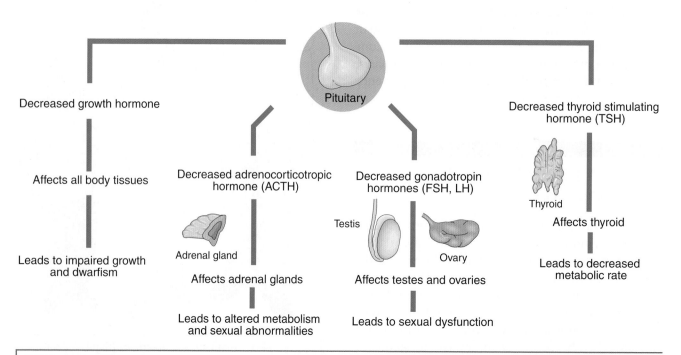

Decreased growth hormone

Affects all body tissues

Leads to impaired growth and dwarfism

Decreased adrenocorticotropic hormone (ACTH)

Adrenal gland

Affects adrenal glands

Leads to altered metabolism and sexual abnormalities

Pituitary

Decreased gonadotropin hormones (FSH, LH)

Testis

Ovary

Affects testes and ovaries

Leads to sexual dysfunction

Decreased thyroid stimulating hormone (TSH)

Thyroid

Affects thyroid

Leads to decreased metabolic rate

**FIGURE 14–3** Effects of hypopituitarism.

tests to determine pituitary function may include each tropic hormone (GH, TSH, FSH, LH, ACTH). Target organ function may be assessed by testing blood levels of each individual organ hormone ($T_3$, $T_4$, estrogen, progesterone, testosterone, cortisol).

**TREATMENT** Treatment of hypopituitarism involves hormone replacement of needed hormones. Constant monitoring and adjusting of hormone levels is needed for optimum results.

### ■ Diabetes Insipidus

Diabetes is a general term meaning "passing through," and is used to describe a variety of disorders characterized by **polyuria** (POL-ee-**YOU**-ree-ah; poly = many, uria = urine) or excessive urination. There are several types of diabetes. Diabetes mellitus, a disorder of the pancreas, is the disease most often thought of as diabetes. Diabetes mellitus and gestational diabetes will be discussed later in the chapter.

**ETIOLOGY** Diabetes insipidus is caused by a decrease in the release of vasopressin, or antidiuretic hormone (ADH), by the posterior portion of the pituitary gland.

**SYMPTOMS** Without antidiuretic (anti = against, di = run through, uri = urine) hormone, the individual has excessive polyuria and may urinate between two and 15 gallons of urine in 24 hours. The urine quality is colorless and dilute. The individual experiences excessive **polydipsia** (POL-ee-DIP-see-ah; poly = many, dipsia = thirst or drinking) in an effort to overcome dehydration. Other symptoms include hypotension, dizziness, and constipation.

Testing for diabetes insipidus includes a urinalysis and a water restriction test. The urinalysis of an affected individual will show colorless urine with a very low specific gravity. The water restriction test includes limiting the suspected individual's water intake for several hours while measuring the urine output, blood pressure, and urine concentration. After several hours, the individual is given vasopressin medication. If the medication decreases urine output and increases urine concentration, the diagnosis of diabetes insipidus is confirmed.

**TREATMENT** Treatment of diabetes insipidus is administration of vasopressin medication. Prognosis is generally good.

## Thyroid Gland Diseases

The activity of the thyroid gland affects the entire body. The hormone released by the thyroid gland (thyroxine) regulates metabolism, or the rate that calories are used. In this way, thyroxine also regulates body heat, ensuring that the body is kept warm, even in a cold environment. Thyroxine also stimulates the gastrointestinal system by increasing gastric secretions and peristalsis. To make thyroxine, the thyroid gland uses iodine. Without iodine, thyroxine cannot be produced. Diseases of the thyroid gland are primarily those of hypersecretion and hyposecretion.

### ■ Hyperthyroidism

**ETIOLOGY** Hyperthyroidism occurs when the thyroid gland secretes excessive thyroxine. This condition is due to an **adenoma** (AD-eh-**NO**-ma; adeno = gland, oma = tumor) on the thyroid.

**SYMPTOMS** This growth on the thyroid produces a characteristic **goiter** (GOI-ter) or noticeable protrusion of the thyroid gland (Figure 14–4). Overproduction of thyroxine increases metabolism, leading to symptoms of tachycardia, nervousness, hyperactivity, and excessive excitability. The individual has a tremendous appetite but loses weight to the point of extreme thinness. Diarrhea is common because thyroxine speeds up peristalsis of the gastrointestinal tract. High metabolic rate causes high heat production, leading to excessive sweating and an intolerance to heat. The skin is always moist and the individual has extreme thirst due to this water loss.

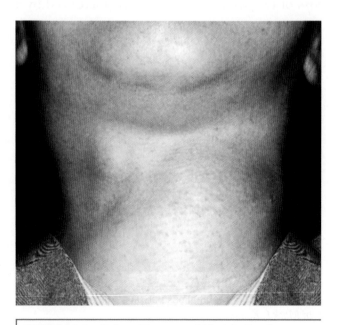

**FIGURE 14–4**  Goiter. *(Courtesy of Mark L. Kuss)*

**TREATMENT** Medications to reduce thyroxine production are often effective. In some cases, surgery may be needed to reduce the size of the thyroid and decrease thyroxine production.

**ETIOLOGY** Hyperthyroidism caused by an autoimmune condition is called Graves' disease. Antibodies stimulate the thyroid, leading to glandular hypertrophy. Graves' disease commonly affects young women.

**SYMPTOMS** Symptoms include those previously discussed. One very distinguishing characteristic of Graves' disease is a stare in the eyes due to **exophthalmos** (ECK-sof-**THAL**-mos; abnormal protrusion of the eyeballs) (Figure 14–5). This protrusion of the eyeballs is due to edema in the tissues behind the eyes. Exophthalmos may be so severe that the eyelids will not close. Unfortunately, this condition does not resolve when the hyperthyroidism is corrected.

**TREATMENT** Graves' disease may be treated with medication, radiation of the thyroid, or surgical removal of all or part of the gland. If the entire gland receives radiation or is removed, hormonal supplement will be needed for the life of the individual.

A sudden, life-threatening exacerbation of all symptoms of hyperthyroidism is called **thyroid storm**. This condition may occur in an individual with severe hyperthyroidism or during the immediate postoperative period following a thyroidectomy (ectomy = excision or removal of). Symptoms of thyroid storm include severe tachycardia with heart rates reaching 200 beats per minute, tachypnea, and loss of temperature regulation characterized by a

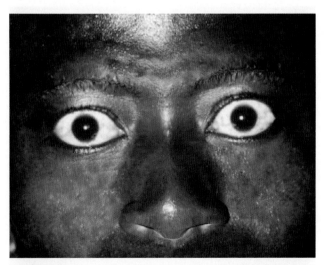

**FIGURE 14–5** Exaphthalmos in Graves' disease. *(Courtesy of Mark L. Kuss)*

rapid and steady increase in body temperature. Emergency medical intervention must be initiated in order to save the individual's life.

## ■ Simple Goiter

**ETIOLOGY** Simple goiter is an enlargement of the thyroid gland generally due to inadequate dietary iodine. The thyroid gland enlarges as it attempts to produce thyroxine without adequate iodine supply.

**SYMPTOMS** This condition usually affects females and may be asymptomatic until the thyroid gland enlarges to the point that it forms a noticeable mass at the front of the neck. If the gland is extremely enlarged, it may cause pressure on the trachea and esophagus, and cause dyspnea and dysphagia (dys = difficulty, phagia = swallowing). Simple goiter also may occur due to ingestion of large amounts of **goitrogenic** (goiter-producing) foods or drugs such as turnips, cabbage, and lithium.

**TREATMENT** Treatment includes administration of potassium iodide initially, followed by increasing iodine in the diet by adding iodized salt. If the cause is related to goitrogenic foods or drugs, avoidance of these often leads to cure. If the goiter is unresponsive to treatment, surgery may be needed to reduce the size of the gland. Treatment is aimed at stopping the enlargement of the gland, but it will not reduce the current size of the gland. Surgery also may be needed to improve physical appearance, and decrease difficulty with breathing and swallowing.

## ■ Hypothyroidism

**ETIOLOGY** Hypothyroidism is the decrease in normal thyroxine production. This condition occurs more frequently in women and is usually due to thyroid gland dysfunction rather than pituitary dysfunction. Hypothyroidism may be the result of surgical or radiation treatments to cure hyperthyroidism.

**SYMPTOMS** Symptoms of hypothyroidism are the opposite of those for hyperthyroidism. The affected individual is fatigued, drowsy, sensitive to cold temperature, has thin nails, brittle hair, and gains excessive weight. The individual becomes sluggish, mentally and physically. Diagnosis is confirmed by clinical history and blood hormone tests.

**TREATMENT** Treatment with thyroid hormone replacement is usually rapid and effective. Regardless of the cause, the symptoms, diagnosis, and treatment plan for hypothyroidism are quite similar.

The most common natural cause of hypothyroidism is an autoimmune disorder called Hashimoto's disease. It is believed that lymphocytes react with thyroid tissue, leading to atrophy and destruction of the thyroid gland tissue.

Advanced hypothyroidism in an adult is called **myxedema** (MICK-seh-**DEE**-mah). Myxedema commonly occurs in middle-aged women.

**SYMPTOMS** Symptoms of myxedema include those previously mentioned for hypothyroidism, plus a characteristic swelling or bloating of the facial tissue, thickened tongue, and puffy eyelids.

**TREATMENT** This condition responds well to treatment with thyroxine hormone replacement. Symptoms usually disappear after a few months of treatment.

Hypothyroidism in infants can be quite devastating, leading to mental and physical growth challenges. Congenital hypothyroidism is called **cretinism**.

**SYMPTOMS** If not corrected, the child is dwarfed with a short, stocky body build, and a protruding tongue and abdomen. The face is abnormal with a broad nose, puffy eyelids, and small eyes. Sexual organs fail to develop (Figure 14–6). Muscle growth

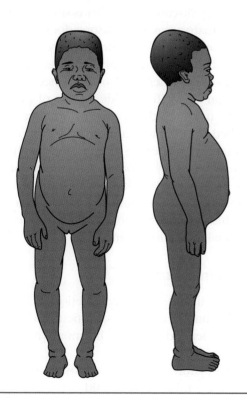

**FIGURE 14–6** Cretinism.

is retarded to the point that the child is unable to stand or walk. The earlier this condition is discovered, the better the prognosis. For this reason, many states mandate a thyroid blood test on newborns.

## Parathyroid Gland Diseases

Parathyroid glands function in the regulation of blood calcium levels. Most of the body's calcium (approximately 99 percent) is stored in the bones, but the remaining one percent circulates in the blood. Blood calcium plays a vital role in blood clotting and muscle contraction, thus affecting heart function. If blood calcium levels drop, parathyroid hormone (parathormone, PTH) acts to increase the level by increasing calcium absorption in the digestive tract, releasing calcium from bone stores, and saving calcium excretion in urine. When blood calcium levels are restored to normal, parathormone is no longer released. Like other endocrine glands, most endocrine diseases of the parathyroid are related to hypersecretion or hyposecretion.

### ■ Hyperparathyroidism

Hyperparathyroidism is a condition of overproduction of parathormone by one or more of the four parathyroid glands.

**ETIOLOGY** Oversecretion is usually due to a glandular tumor or idiopathic hyperplasia of the gland. Excessive parathormone production causes excessive blood calcium levels called hypercalcemia (hyper = excessive, calc = calcium, emia = blood).

**SYMPTOMS** As previously discussed, this calcium is pulled from the bones, leading to bone weakness and spontaneous fractures. Hypercalcemia also leads to kidney stones because the urinary system—under the influence of parathormone—retains calcium, further increasing blood calcium levels. The digestive system increases absorption of calcium, leading to abdominal pain, vomiting, and constipation. Hypercalcemia also leads to hyperactivity of cardiac muscle, thus causing arrhythmias. Blood tests for parathormone levels assist with diagnosis.

**TREATMENT** Treatment of hyperparathyroidism is directed at the cause. Removal of a tumor or removal of the parathyroid glands may be necessary. Only one-half of one parathyroid is necessary to maintain normal parathormone levels. Other treatments include diuretics to increase urine output, thus forcing excretion of calcium, and limiting dietary intake of calcium. Prognosis is generally good with adequate treatment, although cardiac arrest may occur with severe hyperparathyroidism.

## ■ Hypoparathyroidism

Hypoparathyroidism is a decrease in the normal amount of parathormone secreted, which leads to abnormally low blood calcium levels.

**ETIOLOGY** This condition is usually the result of surgical removal of all parathyroid glands in an effort to treat hyperparathyroidism or following a thyroidectomy.

**SYMPTOMS** Low blood calcium levels (hypocalcemia) causes irritability to muscles called **tetany**. Tetany should not be confused with the infectious disease tetanus (lockjaw). The tetany associated with hypoparathyroidism affects primarily the face and hands, causing uncontrolled contraction of these muscles. Testing for hypocalcemia and hypoparathyroidism involves checking for Chvostek's (VOHS-tecks) and Trousseau's (true-SOHs) signs (Figure 14–7).

**TREATMENT** Treatment with calcium and vitamin D, which controls absorption of calcium from the gastrointestinal tract, will cure the problem.

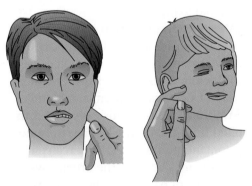

(A) Positive Chvostek's (VOHS-tecks) Sign. Tapping over facial nerve causes facial muscle spasm.

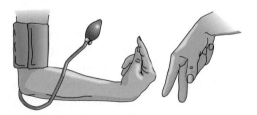

(B) Positive Trousseau's (True-SOHS) Sign. Pressure to nerves and vessels of upper arm causes muscle spasm.

**FIGURE 14–7** Tetany of the hand and face: (A) Chvostek's sign. (B) Trousseau's sign.

## Adrenal Gland Diseases

The adrenal glands, also called the suprarenals because they sit atop the kidneys, have two distinct parts that function quite differently. The inner part, called the medulla, releases two hormones, epinephrine (adrenaline) and norepinephrine, when stimulated by the nervous system. These hormones have a direct effect on the vascular system and are known as *fight or flight* hormones. The cortex, or outer part of the adrenal gland, is controlled by the pituitary gland's release of adrenocorticotropic hormone (ACTH). The adrenal cortex secretes several hormones.

1. Mineralocorticoids—the primary hormone is **aldosterone**, and regulates salt balance.

2. Glucocorticoids—the primary hormone is cortisol (**cortisone**) or **hydrocortisone**, which regulate carbohydrate metabolism.

3. Sex hormones—the primary ones are androgens and estrogens and provide male and female characteristics, respectively. Males and females have both of these androgenic sex hormones.

Cortisone is a hormone frequently used to treat inflammatory diseases like arthritis since it acts as an anti-inflammatory agent. Cortisone does not cure the inflammatory condition; it only relieves the inflammation and the associated pain. Prolonged use of cortisone is avoided whenever possible since it has some detrimental side effects. Side effects of prolonged cortisone use include hypertension, ulcers, puffy face called "moon face," and drowsiness. The anti-inflammatory properties of cortisone reduce the body's inflammatory response. This alteration in the immune system may mask the symptoms of an infection, allowing it to go unnoticed until it is in advanced stages. This side effect of prolonged cortisone use can be potentially life threatening.

## ■ Hyperadrenalism

Hyperadrenalism is the oversecretion of hormones by the adrenal cortex. The specific forms of hyperadrenalism depend on which hormones are secreted in excess.

Conn's syndrome is due to an overproduction of aldosterone, a mineralocorticoid.

**ETIOLOGY** This form of hyperadrenalism is most often due to an adrenal cortex tumor.

**SYMPTOMS** Conn's syndrome causes retention of sodium, leading to hypertension, muscle weakness, polyuria, and polydipsia.

**TREATMENT** Removal of the tumor usually leads to a good prognosis.

Cushing's syndrome is due to an overproduction of the glucocorticoid cortisol.

**ETIOLOGY** Cushing's syndrome may be caused by a tumor on the pituitary gland or on the adrenal cortex. Prolonged administration of large doses of glucocorticoid steroids (cortisone) will also cause this syndrome.

**SYMPTOMS** Classic symptoms include a round "moon-shaped" face and a "buffalo hump" on the upper back. Other symptoms include fatigue, weakness, poor wound healing, a rotund abdomen with pencil thin arms and legs, hypertension, and striae (stretch marks) on the skin (Figure 14–8).

**TREATMENT** Surgical removal of the tumor or the adrenal cortex may correct the condition. Lifetime hormone therapy to replace this hormone is then needed. Cushing's syndrome may develop in individuals receiving long-term glucocorticoid steroids.

These individuals need to be carefully monitored for symptoms of Cushing's syndrome.

**ETIOLOGY** Androgenital syndrome is due to an overproduction of sex hormones by the adrenal cortex. Androgenital syndrome is also known as adrenal virilism (masculinity or feminization), depending on the excessive hormone.

**SYMPTOMS** Adrenal virilism occurs when hypersecretion of androgen leads to premature sexual development in male children, also called precocious (early development) puberty. In female children, overproduction of androgen leads to excessive hair growth on the legs, chest, and abdomen; an enlarged clitoris; a deepened voice; and amenorrhea (ah-MEN-oh-**REE**-ah; a = without, menorrhea = menses). If adrenal feminization occurs due to excessive estrogen production, female children experience premature sexual development (precocious puberty). Male children with an overproduction of estrogen experience gynecomastia (GUY-neh-koh-**MAS**-tee-ah; excessive breast development), testicular atrophy, and decreased libido. Virilism in the adult female leads to symptoms of hirsutism (HER-soot-izm), or abnormal

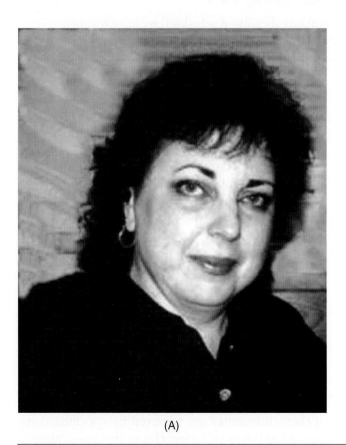

(A)

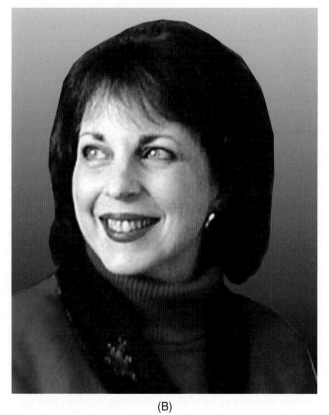

(B)

**FIGURE 14–8** Cushing's syndrome. (A) Individual affected with Cushing's. (B) Same individual after treatment. *(Courtesy of Ruth Jones)*

**HEALTHY HIGHLIGHT**

## Using Steroids Therapeutically

- Anabolic steroids are synthetic derivatives of testosterone that have anabolic (tissue-building) effects. These drugs were initially used by athletes to increase strength and endurance. Because of their potential for abuse, steroids have been placed in the Controlled Substance Act in category C-III. General uses include treatment for chronic infections, some types of anemia, extensive burns, and severe trauma.

- Use of steroids to enhance athletic performance is not recommended and has been banned in professional athletics. Serious irreversible side effects occur with long-term use of steroids and include kidney damage, increased risk of liver tumors, and increased risk of heart disease. Long-term steroid users have increased irritability and aggressive behavior. In women, masculinization occurs as evidenced by a deepening of the voice, hirsutism, menstrual difficulties, and male patterned baldness. Males experience a decrease in testosterone production, leading to testicular atrophy, decrease in sperm production, and impotence. Individuals taking steroids need to follow these recommended guidelines.

  - A well-balanced diet, including adequate proteins and carbohydrates, should be followed during steroid therapy.

  - Never share steroid medications with others.

  - Do not stop these medications abruptly. A scheduled weaning regimen should be determined and monitored by a qualified physician.

---

hair on the face and body, decreased breast size, and amenorrhea. Feminization in the adult male leads to gynecomastia, testicular atrophy, and decreased libido.

**TREATMENT** Treatment of adrenal cortex tumors usually involves surgical removal of the tumor.

### ■ Hypoadrenalism

Hypoadrenalism is an uncommon undersecretion of hormones by the adrenal cortex called Addison's disease.

**ETIOLOGY** Causes of Addison's disease include an autoimmune disorder, tumor of the pituitary gland, tuberculosis, and prolonged steroid hormone therapy. As much as 90 percent of the adrenal cortex may be destroyed before hyposecretion occurs.

**SYMPTOMS** Symptoms of Addison's disease may be mild to life threatening. Lack of mineralocorticoids allows depletion of sodium, leading to diarrhea and dehydration. Deficiency in glucocorticoids affects blood sugar levels, leading to **hypoglycemia** (HIGH-poh-gly-**SEE**-me-ah; hypo = decreased, glyc = glucose, emia = blood). Increased ACTH levels by the

pituitary lead to a hyperpigmentation or increased skin coloring, ranging from yellow to dark brown. This increased skin color affects the palms, elbows, scars, skin folds, and the areola of the nipples. Hormone blood levels can be measured to confirm the diagnosis.

**TREATMENT** Treatment includes corticosteroid therapy.

## Pancreatic Islets of Langerhans Diseases

The pancreas is both an exocrine and endocrine gland. As an exocrine gland, it secretes digestive juices by way of ducts into the digestive system. As an endocrine gland, it secretes two hormones—insulin and glucagon—directly into the blood. Both of these hormones are secreted by specialized tissue called **islets of Langerhans** that are scattered throughout the pancreas. Insulin and glucagon have an antagonistic relationship. Insulin lowers blood sugar while glucagon raises it. The overall effect of these hormones is maintaining a normal blood sugar level (80–120 mg/dl).

When blood sugar levels rise, for instance, after a meal, insulin is secreted. Insulin assists in moving sugar out of the blood and into the tissues, thus decreasing the blood sugar level (Figure 14–9). Without adequate insulin, the blood sugar level rises and the tissues are depleted of sugar.

Sugar, or glucose, is the primary source of energy for all tissue cells. Without glucose, cells must burn fats and proteins for energy. When tissue cells burn fats and proteins, they produce a waste product called **ketones**. Ketones are picked up by the blood to be filtered and excreted by the kidneys. Acetone, a part of this ketone waste, is excreted by the respiratory system, giving the affected individual a "fruity" or sweet smelling breath. This condition of having ketones in the blood, breath, and urine is called ketosis. Chemically, a large part of ketones is acidic in nature, which leads to metabolic acidosis or a low pH in the body tissues. For this reason, ketosis is often called **ketoacidosis**.

When carbohydrates or sugars are eaten, the extra sugar, the amount not needed for immediate energy, is stored primarily in the liver as **glycogen**. If blood sugar levels drop, for instance, during exercise, the pancreas secretes glucagon. Glucagon circulates in the blood and stimulates the liver to release glycogen in the form of glucose, thus raising the blood sugar to normal.

## ■ Diabetes Mellitus

**ETIOLOGY** Diabetes mellitus is a chronic disease affecting carbohydrate or sugar utilization due to inadequate production of insulin by the pancreatic islets of Langerhans. This is the most common and major disease of the endocrine pancreas and is commonly known simply as diabetes.

**SYMPTOMS** Diabetes is characterized by symptoms of polyuria (excessive urination), polydipsia (excessive thirst), and polyphagia (excessive eating). **Glycosuria** (GLYE-koh-**SOO**-ree-ah; glyco = glycogen or sugar, uria = urine) or the "spilling of sugar in the urine" is also a common symptom. The excessive sugar in the blood, known as **hyperglycemia** (hyper = excessive, glyc = glycogen or glucose, emia = blood), causes the kidney to filter out part of the excess, resulting in glycosuria. Hyperglycemia indicates that sugar is not being pulled into the tissues, and cells are using fat for energy, resulting in the formation of ketones (the waste product of fat metabolism). Ketones can be found in the blood and urine, and smelled on the breath.

There are two types of diabetes mellitus:

1. Type 1, formerly known as insulin-dependent diabetes mellitus (IDDM) or juvenile onset diabetes. This form of diabetes is the most serious. It usually occurs quite suddenly, and affects children and young adults before age 25. This form of diabetes requires daily injections of insulin. Insulin must be

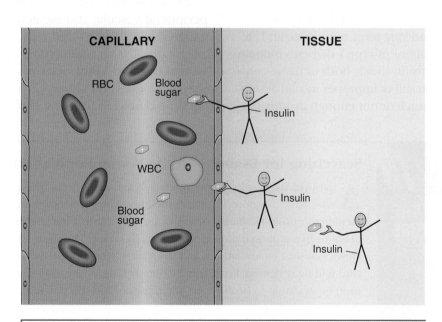

**FIGURE 14–9** Effect of insulin on blood sugar. Insulin assists in moving sugar out of the blood and into the tissues, thus decreasing blood sugar levels. Think of insulin as "offering a hand" in pulling blood sugar levels down.

injected because digestive juices would destroy oral forms. Type 1 is thought to be caused by an autoimmune disorder. It is thought that affected individuals inherit a genetic tendency for the disease. The immune system, when triggered by a virus or some other stressor, develops antibodies and begins war against the islets of Langerhans, thereby destroying the insulin-secreting cells. Affected individuals generally do not secrete any insulin, making regulation of blood glucose levels quite difficult. Individuals with Type 1 must follow a strict diet, monitor blood sugar levels on a regular basis, and administer the needed amounts of insulin. Exercise and stress can alter insulin needs and must be considered as part of the treatment plan.

2. Type 2, formerly known as non-insulin-dependent diabetes mellitus (NIDDM) or adult onset diabetes. This is the more common form of diabetes mellitus. It usually has a gradual onset and occurs most often in obese females over age 40. This form of diabetes is thought to be due to a "wearing out" of the pancreatic islets of Langerhans. It is believed that excessive carbohydrate consumption over the life of the individual places such a heavy demand on the pancreas to produce the needed insulin, this increased demand literally "wears out" the pancreatic cells leading to Type 2. Insulin injections are rarely needed because Type 2 is usually controlled with diet, exercise, and oral medications that stimulate insulin secretion.

Complications of diabetes mellitus may be classified as immediate and long term. Immediate and life-threatening complications of Type 1 diabetes include diabetic coma and insulin shock. Both of these complications occur as a result of improper insulin administration: either too much or not enough insulin. Diabetic coma may occur as a result of not administering enough insulin or taking in too many carbohydrates in the diet. Symptoms of diabetic coma are those related to hyperglycemia and include polyuria, polydipsia, dehydration, and ketoacidosis. Diabetic coma usually progresses rather slowly. The affected individual becomes lethargic and, if untreated, slips into a coma. The individual in a coma will have a slow deep-breathing pattern and fruity or sweet smelling breath. Individuals in diabetic coma require emergency medical treatment with insulin and intravenous fluids.

Insulin shock occurs quite rapidly and is the result of taking too much insulin, not eating enough food, or participating in excessive exercise. The affected individual becomes hypoglycemic with symptoms of diaphoresis (sweating), light-headedness, and trembling. Without treatment, the affected individual progresses quite rapidly into a state of confusion, followed by coma. Individuals in insulin shock need immediate emergency medical treatment with intravenous glucose to raise blood sugar levels (Table 14–2).

Long-term complications of diabetes usually appear gradually after many years. With improper carbohydrate metabolism, **lipids** or fats are pulled into the bloodstream to be utilized for cellular energy. This increase in lipids in the vascular system leads to atherosclerosis. Atherosclerosis leads to a variety of complications including myocardial infarction, cerebrovascular accidents or strokes, and peripheral vascular disease. The poor circulation caused by peripheral vascular disease is the cause of diabetic gangrene in the feet and legs, which may lead to amputation. Poor circulation also leads to poor wound healing. Atherosclerosis also affects the vessels of the eyes and kidneys. The retinas of the eyes become damaged, causing **diabetic retinopathy**

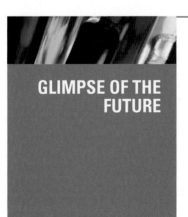

**GLIMPSE OF THE FUTURE**

### Searching for Diabetes in the Young Population

A national study is being conducted that focuses on individuals under age 20 who have diagnosed diabetes mellitus. The study is looking at age, gender, incidence, ethnicity, socioeconomics, development, and classification of diabetes in about five million children in the United States. The data will come from interviews, physical examinations, and laboratory studies. Risk factors and types of care will be reviewed. From this extremely large study, important information will soon be available to health care practitioners and the public about diabetes in the young population.

*Source:* Controlled Clinical Trials *(2004).*

| TABLE 14–2 | Emergency Treatment of Diabetic Coma or Insulin Shock |

**Step 1—Determine a Need for Intervention**

Unfortunately, it is usually difficult to determine if an affected individual is suffering from diabetic coma or insulin shock, especially if found in a comatose state. The best rule to follow in this case is "when in doubt—sugar." Raising an already elevated glucose level is not as life threatening as allowing the blood sugar level to remain low or to drop even farther.

**Step 2—Administer Glucose**

If the individual is still alert, drinking fruit juice with sugar added can be effective in raising blood sugar level. If juice is not available, candy of any type will help. If the individual is unconscious and emergency medical assistance is not available, turn the individual on his or her side and place table sugar or hard candy in the lower cheek of the mouth to help raise blood sugar. Emergency medical assistance should be sought immediately.

**Additional Important Information**

Diabetics should wear a diabetic alert tag and should carry some type of carbohydrate treat with them at all times to be used during a hypoglycemic reaction. If an incident occurs, the tag alerts the medical responder or other individuals aiding the person that he or she is diabetic and, thus, could be having a hypoglycemic or hyperglycemic reaction. This saves time between assessing the victim for probable cause of the problem and treating the person. The diabetic alert tag also helps those who are assisting the individual to recognize the "fruity breath" of a hyperglycemic diabetic as ketone breath rather than mistaking it as alcohol breath. Allowing a hyperglycemic individual to "sleep it off" could be a fatal mistake.

(retino = retina, opathy = disease) and leading to blindness. Damage to the kidney leads to kidney failure, a frequent cause of death in individuals affected with diabetes.

Diagnosis is confirmed by a positive history of symptoms along with blood glucose testing.

**TREATMENT** Diabetes cannot be cured. Management of the disease is dependent on education and a lifetime commitment to following the treatment regimen of diet, medication, and exercise. The long-term goal is to prevent the development of complications.

■ **Gestational Diabetes**

**ETIOLOGY** Gestational diabetes occurs during pregnancy.

**SYMPTOMS** The condition may be either asymptomatic or present the same symptoms of diabetes mellitus. This type of diabetes is usually discovered with routine urine testing during prenatal visits.

## COMPLEMENTARY AND ALTERNATIVE THERAPY

**Alternative Therapy Use in Diabetic Neuropathy**

Complementary and alternative therapies are frequently used by individuals with chronic neuropathies, especially those with diabetes. According to a recent study, patients with diabetic neuropathy use vitamins, acupuncture, manipulation, magnets, and other herbal drugs to relieve chronic pain. Most of these patients reported that they did not confer with their physician before trying alternative therapies. The patients stated they were not getting relief from traditional medicine and chose a variety of alternative therapies for the pain relief.

*Source: Brunelli, B., & Gorson, K. C. (2004).*

Destruction of insulin by the placenta, and blocking of insulin action by elevated levels of estrogen and progesterone lead to gestational diabetes. It is important that this condition be discovered because it may lead to fetal or neonatal mortality.

**TREATMENT** Gestational diabetes is treated like diabetes mellitus with exercise, dietary control of carbohydrate intake, and medications. Injectable insulin may be needed to control blood sugar levels. Oral hypoglycemic medications are contraindicated as these pass across the placenta and may lead to fetal birth defects or hypoglycemia. Gestational diabetes usually disappears after delivery. If this condition does not disappear with delivery, the affected individual will need to continue diabetic management. Women affected with gestational diabetes are often affected later in life by adult onset diabetes.

## ■ Hypoglycemia

Hypoglycemia (HIGH-poh-gly-**SEE**-me-ah; hypo = decreased, glyc = glucose, emia = blood) is an abnormally low blood sugar. Hypoglycemia occurs any time the blood glucose level drops below 60 mg/dl, although individuals may become symptomatic at different blood glucose levels. Some individuals tolerate unusually low blood glucose levels whereas others do not.

**ETIOLOGY** Some common causes of hypoglycemia are fasting, skipping meals, and excessive exercise. Hypoglycemia is also caused by administration of too much insulin, as previously discussed. Other causes of hypoglycemia include pancreatic adenoma, gastrointestinal disorders, and some hereditary disorders.

**SYMPTOMS** Symptoms are the same as previously discussed for diabetes, and include lightheadedness, diaphoresis, and trembling. If untreated, symptoms may progress to include mental confusion and coma. Most individuals have had an episode of hypoglycemia at one time or another. Diagnosis is confirmed by a positive clinical history and blood glucose testing. Acute hypoglycemia needs immediate emergency treatment with intravenous glucose administration.

**TREATMENT** Treatment of hypoglycemia is dependent on cause. Diabetics should carry glucose tablets or candy to take at the first sign of hypoglycemia.

## Reproductive Gland Diseases

Sexual development can be affected by the release of androgens from the adrenal cortex, as previously discussed, by the pituitary and by the sex organ (**gonad**). The male gonad is the testis and the female gonad is the ovary. Gonads function as endocrine glands in the production of hormones. The pituitary controls the function of the gonads by releasing gonadotropin. Gonadotropin stimulates the testes to produce the male hormone testosterone and the ovaries to produce the female hormone estrogen. Dysfunction of the pituitary or the gonad can lead to endocrine disorders.

## ■ Hypergonadism

**ETIOLOGY** Hypergonadism is the condition of increased hormone production before puberty, which produces precocious sexual development in both sexes. Diagnosis of hypergonadism is confirmed by positive clinical history and blood testing for evidence of elevated sex hormones.

**TREATMENT** Treatment for both sexes involves removal or radiation of tumors and administration of hormones to suppress or counteract the sex hormone.

*In the male*, onset of puberty usually occurs around age 13; with hypergonadism, this development occurs before age 10.

**ETIOLOGY** Causes of hypergonadism include unknown causes, testicular tumors, and pituitary tumors.

**SYMPTOMS** Signs of precocious sexual development include the growth of a beard and pubic hair and enlargement of the penis and testes. Spermatogenesis occurs, rendering the individual fertile. Rapid growth of muscle and bone leads to early uniting of the epiphyses and a premature stoppage of growth in the long bones.

*In the female*, onset of puberty usually occurs around age 10; with hypergonadism, this development occurs before age 8.

**ETIOLOGY** Hypergonadism in females is primarily due to idiopathic causes. Uncommon causes include ovarian and adrenal tumors.

**SYMPTOMS** Signs of precocious sexual development include onset of menarche, appearance of pubic and underarm hair, and breast enlargement. Ovarian development renders the individual fertile, making pregnancy possible.

## ■ Hypogonadism

Hypogonadism is the condition of decreased sex hormone production by the age of normal puberty.

**ETIOLOGY** *In the male*, causes of hypogonadism include dysfunctional testes, undescended testes, or loss of the testes due to castration. Testes also may fail to develop due to a pituitary disorder, resulting in the lack of gonadotropin.

**SYMPTOMS** Loss of the male gonads before puberty causes eunuchism, or the lack of development of sex characteristics, because male characteristics are brought about by testosterone. Castration in the adult male will lead to a decrease in libido, but masculinity is maintained.

**TREATMENT** Administration of testosterone is quite effective in treating hypogonadism in the male.

**ETIOLOGY** *In the female*, causes of hypogonadism include missing or dysfunctional ovaries.

**SYMPTOMS** Without estrogen, female sex characteristics do not develop. Female children become abnormally tall because the long bones do not fuse normally without estrogen.

**TREATMENT** Administration of testosterone and estrogen is quite effective in treating hypogonadism in male and the female respectively.

## TRAUMA

Head injury can result in multiple organ dysfunction if the pituitary is involved. Hypersecretion and hyposecretion may occur with injury to any of the individual organs. Organ destruction and failure can be life threatening when the pituitary, pancreas, and adrenal glands are involved.

## RARE DISEASES

Most diseases of the endocrine system discussed above are relatively uncommon with the exception of thyroid problems and diabetes mellitus. Other extremely rare endocrine disorders may be found in children or young adults. Cancer of most of the glands of the endocrine is also somewhat rare. The thyroid, ovaries, and testes are the most common sites for cancer development.

## EFFECTS OF AGING ON THE SYSTEM

As the individual ages, there are changes that occur in the endocrine glands. Decreases in the secretions from the glands alter the body's ability to respond to stressors, diseases, and other changes that occur from aging. The older adult is at high risk for hypoglycemic reactions and excessive fluid loss due to reduced levels of glucocorticoids and aldosterone. Digestive and metabolism problems are common due to reduced secretions of pancreatic and thyroid hormones. The secretions from the gonads are reduced, resulting in changes in secondary sex characteristics. Because glucose tolerance lessens with age, the serum glucose levels tend to be higher in the older adult. Diabetes mellitus is common in the older population but usually can be regulated by dietary adjustments. With all the other changes that occur during the aging process, diabetes becomes a very serious condition, adversely affecting many systems.

## SUMMARY

The endocrine system is a very complex system of many glands located throughout the body. Each of the glands has a unique function and delivers its hormones into the bloodstream. The hormones help the body's growth, regulation, and metabolism. Overproduction or underproduction of any one gland can cause dysfunction in other systems. If the gland malfunctions in childhood, the result is a different disorder than if the gland malfunctions in adulthood. The most common endocrine disorder overall is diabetes mellitus. The older adult with an endocrine disorder is at risk for other systemic problems. Secretions from the endocrine glands decrease slowly with age.

## REVIEW QUESTIONS

### Short answer

1. What are the functions of the endocrine system?

2. Which signs and symptoms are associated with common endocrine system disorders?

3. Which diagnostic tests are most commonly used to determine the type and/or cause of endocrine system disorders?

### Multiple Choice

4. Which of the following is not an endocrine gland?

   a. Pituitary                  c. Liver
   b. Adrenal                    d. Ovaries

5. What function does the somatotropin hormone perform?

   a. Promotes absorption of calcium in the bones
   b. Stimulates the thyroid to produce its hormones
   c. Stimulates growth
   d. Promotes development of sex characteristics

6. Acromegaly is defined as which of the following?

   a. An overgrowth of the long bones of the body
   b. An abnormal decrease in the activity of the pituitary gland
   c. A tumor located in the anterior pituitary
   d. A chronic disorder characterized by large feet, hands, and facial bones

7. Cretinism is defined as which of the following?

   a. Congenital hypothyroidism
   b. Congenital hypopituitarism
   c. Severe chronic lack of growth hormone
   d. An impaired growth of all body parts

8. Hypoadrenalism is also known as which of the following disorders?

   a. Acromegaly                 c. Cushing's syndrome
   b. Myxedema                   d. Addison's disease

9. In Type 1 diabetes mellitus, the individual needs replacement of which of the following?

   a. Steroids                   c. Insulin
   b. Antidiuretic hormone       d. Estrogen

**10.** The individual affected by Type 2 diabetes mellitus can usually control the disorder by:

**a.** Insulin injections      **c.** Replacement hormones

**b.** Diet and oral medications      **d.** Steroid therapy

## Matching

**11.** Match the hormone in the left column with its gland in the right column. Some glands may be used more than once.

| | |
|---|---|
| _____ ACTH | **a.** anterior pituitary |
| _____ triiodothyronine | **b.** posterior pituitary |
| _____ oxytocin | **c.** pineal |
| _____ mineralocorticoids | **d.** thyroid |
| _____ melatonin | **e.** adrenals |
| _____ estrogen | **f.** testes or ovaries |
| _____ insulin | **g.** pancreatic islets |
| _____ norepinephrine | |
| _____ ADH | |
| _____ calcitonin | |

## CASE STUDY

**Mrs. Webb** is 78 years old and has been hospitalized frequently for repeated respiratory infections. Until the past two years, she has been relatively healthy. She has not been diagnosed with any serious chronic diseases but does have some osteoporosis. Based on your knowledge of the aging process and the endocrine system changes, what might be contributing to the development of these repeated respiratory infections? What can she do to decrease her risk and improve her immunity to infections?

## BIBLIOGRAPHY

Brown, V. (2003). Disrupting a delicate balance. *Health Perspectives 111*(12), 1590–1597.

Brunelli, B., & Gorson, K. C. (2004). The use of complementary and alternative medicines by patients with peripheral neuropathy. *Journal of the Neurological Sciences 218*(1/2), 59–66.

Col, N. F., Surks, M. I., & Gilbert, H. (2003). Subclinical thyroid disease: Clinical applications. *Journal of the American Medical Association 291*(2), 239–242.

Diabetic foot ulcers. (2003). *Nursing Supplement 33*(27), 27.

Griffin, C. (2003). Using A1C to gauge blood glucose control. *Nursing 33*(12), 72.

Hall, G. (2003). Diabetes. *Practice Nurse 25*(11), 38–42.

Lamendola, C. (2003). Early and more vigorous detection of diabetes. *Journal of Cardiovascular Nursing 18*(2), 103–107.

McConnell, E. A. (2003). About diabetes insipidus. *Nursing 33*(6), 84.

Olohan, K., & Zappitelli, D. (2003). The insulin pump. *American Journal of Nursing 103*(4), 48–56.

SEARCH for diabetes in youth: A multicenter study of the prevalence, incidence and classification of diabetes mellitus in youth. (2004). *Controlled Clinical Trials, 25*(5), 458–471.

The natural history of thyroid disorder changes during pregnancy. (2003, November 17). *Health & Medicine Week*, 263–264.

Without Addison disease management in pregnancy, fetal, mother risk is serious. (2003, December 12). *Biotech Week*, 451–452.

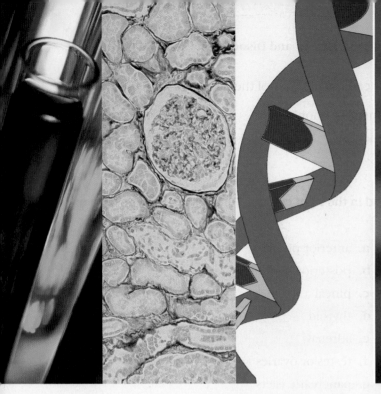
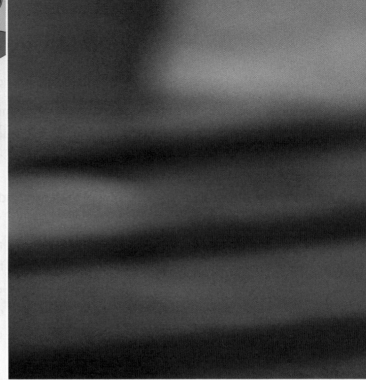

## OUTLINE

## KEY TERMS

# Nervous System Diseases and Disorders

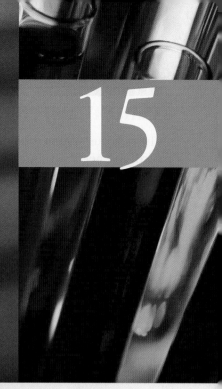

**15**

## LEARNING OBJECTIVES

*Upon completion of the chapter, the learner should be able to:*

1. Define the terminology common to the nervous system and the disorders of the system.

2. Discuss the basic anatomy and physiology of the nervous system.

3. Identify the important signs and symptoms associated with common nervous system disorders.

4. Describe the common diagnostics used to determine the type and/or cause of nervous system disorders.

5. Identify common disorders of the nervous system.

6. Describe the typical course and management of the common nervous system disorders.

7. Describe the effects of aging on the nervous system and the common disorders of the system.

## OVERVIEW

*The nervous system is a complex system that provides communication from the brain to the rest of the body and from the body back to the brain. It is responsible for the individual's ability to reason, interact with other individuals, understand complex ideas, and to respond both intellectually and physically. Disorders of the system can affect any or all other normal functioning in the individual. Because brain and spinal cord injury often causes irreversible damage, the individual with a nervous system disorder may become a victim of severe, permanent, neurological deficits.* ■

## ANATOMY AND PHYSIOLOGY

The nervous system is composed of the brain, spinal cord, and nerves (Figure 15-1). It is divided into the central nervous system (CNS) and the peripheral nervous system (PNS). The CNS includes the brain and the spinal cord. The PNS includes the autonomic nervous system (ANS), the cranial nerves, and the spinal nerves. The central nervous system communicates with organs and other body systems via the peripheral nervous system.

### The Central Nervous System (CNS)

The brain is a complex structure located within the protective covering of the skull. It is divided into the cerebrum, cerebellum, and brain stem. The cerebrum is divided into two hemispheres that can be further subdivided into lobes. Each of these lobes has a specialized function (Figure 15-2). The basal ganglia structure is also part of the cerebrum. It is called the gray matter and is located deep in the hemispheres. Another part of the cerebrum is called the diencephalon. It is where the hypothalamus and thalamus are located. They are active in controlling the body's sleep/wake pattern and are involved in the actions of the pituitary gland (see Chapter 14 for more information).

The cerebellum is located in the lower back part of the brain. It is important in coordination and fine motor movements.

The brainstem makes up the last part of the brain. It is subdivided into the mid-brain, pons, and

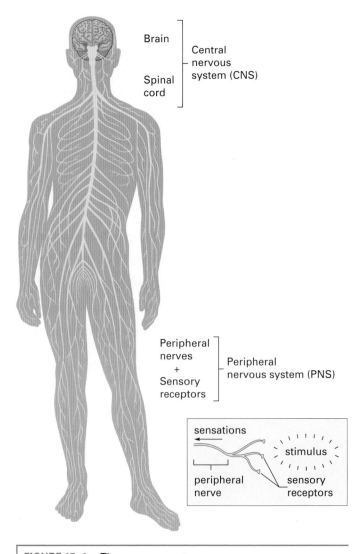

**FIGURE 15–1** The nervous system.

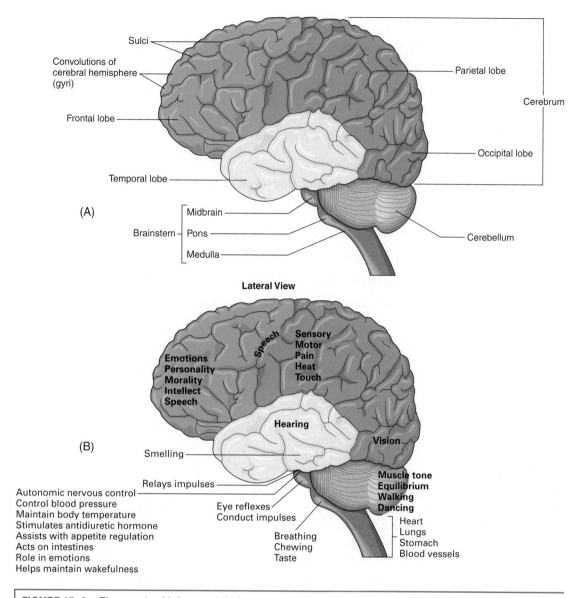

Sulci

Convolutions of
cerebral hemisphere
(gyri)

Frontal lobe

Temporal lobe

Parietal lobe

Cerebrum

Occipital lobe

(A)

Midbrain

Brainstem — Pons

Medulla

Cerebellum

**Lateral View**

**Emotions
Personality
Morality
Intellect
Speech**

Speech

**Sensory
Motor
Pain
Heat
Touch**

**Hearing**

**Vision**

(B)

Smelling

Relays impulses

Autonomic nervous control
Control blood pressure
Maintain body temperature
Stimulates antidiuretic hormone
Assists with appetite regulation
Acts on intestines
Role in emotions
Helps maintain wakefulness

Eye reflexes
Conduct impulses

Breathing
Chewing
Taste

**Muscle tone
Equilibrium
Walking
Dancing**

Heart
Lungs
Stomach
Blood vessels

**FIGURE 15–2**   The cerebral lobes and their specialized functions.

medulla. It contains some nerves and is responsible for transmitting impulses that control respiration, swallowing, wakefulness, and other activities.

The spinal cord is a continuous structure running through the vertebral column from the medulla to the tailbone. The spinal cord is composed of both white and gray matter. It has ascending and descending pathways that transmit impulses. Sensory impulses (pain, temperature, and touch) travel from the spinal cord to the brain. Motor impulses (for movement of muscles) travel from the brain to the spinal cord.

The meninges are membranes that cover the brain and spinal cord. The meninges are divided into three layers: the dura mater (outer cover), the arachnoid (middle layer), and the pia mater (inner layer). They provide both protection and support for the system.

## The Peripheral Nervous System (PNS)

The autonomic nervous system controls the functions of the body's organs, and innervates smooth muscle and cardiac muscle. It is divided into the parasympathetic and sympathetic systems. The parasympathetic system controls the changes in the body needed to relax and restore function such as returning blood pressure to normal after it has increased in response to some need. The sympathetic system controls the changes in the body needed to respond to stressors

**TABLE 15–1** The Cranial Nerves

| Cranial Nerve | Function |
|---|---|
| I. Olfactory | Smell |
| II. Optic | Sight |
| III. Oculomotor | Movement of the eyeball, pupil, and eyelid |
| IV. Trochlear | Movement of the eyeball |
| V. Trigeminal | Chewing; pain, temperature, and touch of face and mouth |
| VI. Abducens | Movement of the eyeball |
| VII. Facial | Movement of the face and secretion of saliva; taste |
| VIII. Auditory | Hearing and balance |
| IX. Glossopharyngeal | Swallowing and secretion of saliva; taste and sensation in the mouth and pharynx |
| X. Vagus | Sensation and movement in the pharynx, larynx, thorax, and gastrointestinal system |
| XI. Accessory | Movement of the head and shoulders |
| XII. Hypoglossal | Movement of the tongue |

such as increasing the heart rate or blood pressure. This is often called the "fight or flight" response.

There are 12 pairs of cranial nerves that control sensation and movement in the area of the head and neck (Table 15-1). The 31 pairs of spinal nerves are divided into eight cervical, 12 thoracic, five lumbar, five sacral, and one coccygeal. Each spinal nerve innervates a designated area of the skin. These areas are called dermatomes (Figure 15-3). Each of the spinal nerves sends sensory impulses from the body organs and surfaces to the spinal cord for transmission to the brain, and returns motor impulses from the brain to the spinal cord and then to the muscles.

## COMMON SIGNS AND SYMPTOMS

Common signs and symptoms of nervous system disorders include headache, nausea, vomiting, weakness, mood swings, and fever. Symptoms specific to the nervous system include the following.

▪ Disturbance in motor function (or ability to move) including:

**1.** stiffness in the neck, back, or extremities

**2.** inability to move any part of the body

**3.** seizures or convulsions

**4.** paralysis

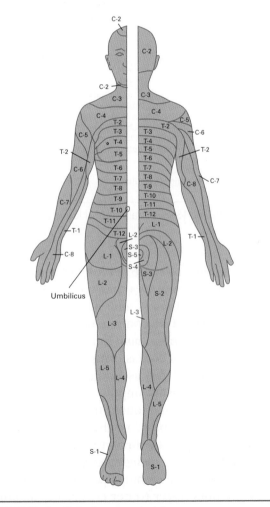

**FIGURE 15–3** Spinal nerves and dermatomes.

- Disturbance in sensory function (or ability to sense or feel) including:
  1. visual difficulties
  2. inability to speak
  3. paralysis
- Alteration in mental alertness or cognitive function including:
  1. extreme or prolonged drowsiness
  2. stupor, unconsciousness/coma
  3. amnesia or extreme forgetfulness

## DIAGNOSTIC TESTS

A neurologic examination includes testing motor, sensory, and mental function. This examination is often performed on any individual presenting with an injury to the head, neck, or spinal column, or exhibiting neurologic symptoms. Motor testing includes checking reflexes, gait, and posture. Sensory testing includes checking the ability to feel using pinprick or application of heat, cold, or vibration. Ability to see and smell also may be part of sensory testing. Testing of mental or cognitive function includes asking simple questions related to name, occupation, and location. Further testing may include simple math problems or questions about current events.

The most important laboratory test utilized in neurologic examination is the analysis of cerebrospinal fluid (CSF). The fluid is examined under a microscope to determine the presence of bacteria, leukocytes, red blood cells, neoplastic cells, and other microorganisms. To obtain this fluid, a lumbar puncture must be performed. This procedure consists of positioning the affected individual in a knee/chest position to widen the vertebral disk space, inserting a spinal needle into the meningeal space around the spinal cord, and withdrawing CSF. During the procedure, a special manometer may be connected to the spinal needle so intracranial pressure (ICP) can be measured. Because the skull is a rigid structure, any increase in the size of the brain tissue by swelling, tumor, infection, or hematoma will cause an increase in intracranial pressure. If pressure becomes too high, the brain will herniate or move downward through the foramen magnum, the only opening available. When this occurs, coma and rapid death may occur as this places pressure on vital centers in the brain stem.

Radiologic examinations include X-rays of the skull and vertebral column for fractures and other abnormalities. A myelogram, or picture of the spinal cord, may be utilized for diagnosis of a herniated nucleus pulposus (HNP) or herniated disk, tumor, or nerve root compression. Angiograms may help in determining vessel occlusion and hematomas in individuals exhibiting symptoms of cerebrovascular accident or stroke.

Electroencephalography (EEG) is a procedure to evaluate electrical brain activity. A damaged area of the brain may exhibit abnormal electrical activity as may occur with cerebrovascular accident and epilepsy. EEG is also used to determine brain death.

CT and MRI are both valuable tools to assess the anatomy of the brain and spinal cord.

## COMMON DISEASES OF THE NERVOUS SYSTEM

The diseases of the nervous system can range from mild to severe, depending on the particular condition. Age-related factors may influence the severity of the disease but many nervous system disorders can affect the individual at any age.

## Infectious Diseases

Infections of the nervous system are more common in the young but can be found in older adults as well. Early diagnosis and treatment is essential to reduce the permanent neurologic deficits that may result from the infection.

### ■ Encephalitis

Encephalitis is an inflammation of the brain tissue.

**ETIOLOGY** It is caused by a variety of microorganisms including bacteria and viruses, or as a complication of measles, chickenpox, or mumps. Viruses may be spread by mosquitoes and carried from animal to man or man to man.

**SYMPTOMS** Symptoms include headache, elevated temperature, and a stiff neck and back, but may progress to lethargy, mental confusion, and even coma. Encephalitis is usually diagnosed by finding the causative agent in spinal fluid obtained by lumbar puncture.

**TREATMENT** Treatment is supportive. Antiviral medication may be effective in some types of encephalitis. Prognosis is guarded because some forms of encephalitis have a high mortality rate. Severe encephalitis may leave the individual with permanent neurologic impairment.

## ■ Meningitis

Meningitis is inflammation of the meninges, the covering of the brain and spinal cord.

**ETIOLOGY** Meningitis may be caused by anything that causes an inflammatory response including bacteria, virus, fungus, and toxins such as lead and arsenic. Some forms of meningitis are more contagious and more lethal than other forms of the disease. The most common cause of meningitis is bacterial invasion by *Neisseria meningitides*. Bacteria and virus usually reach the meninges after invading and infecting other parts of the body such as the middle ear, sinuses, and upper respiratory tract; or they may be carried to the meninges in the blood as in septicemia.

**SYMPTOMS** Symptoms of meningitis often include a sudden onset of high fever, severe headache, photophobia (fear of light), and a stiffness in the neck that resists bending the neck forward or sideways (**nuchal rigidity**). As the disease progresses, drowsiness, stupor, seizures, and coma may occur. Diagnosis is usually confirmed by finding the causative agent in the spinal fluid obtained by lumbar puncture.

**TREATMENT** Antibiotic treatment of bacterial meningitis is usually quite effective. Other treatments include antipyretics, anticonvulsive medications, and a quiet, dark environment. If untreated, meningitis can be fatal, especially in infants, children, and older individuals. Meningitis may cause permanent neurologic damage in children, leading to hearing loss, learning challenges and development, and epilepsy. Good hand washing practices can help prevent the spread of the disease.

## ■ Poliomyelitis

**ETIOLOGY** Poliomyelitis is a viral infection affecting the brain and spinal cord. Polio was a major crippling and life-threatening disease affecting children prior to the development of a vaccine in the 1960s. Immunization programs since that time have virtually eliminated the disease in the United States. The poliomyelitis virus enters the body through the mouth and nose. It crosses the gastrointestinal tract into the blood, then travels to the brain and spinal cord. The virus is spread by oropharyngeal secretions and by infected feces.

**SYMPTOMS** Symptoms of polio include muscle weakness, neck stiffness, and nausea and vomiting. As the disease progresses, muscles atrophy and deteriorate. Muscles of the arms, legs, and respiratory system may become paralyzed. Diagnosis is made by clinical examination and confirmed by culturing the virus from the throat, feces, or spinal fluid.

**TREATMENT** Treatment is supportive and includes analgesics and bed rest during the acute phase. Long-term physical therapy and use of braces may be needed. If the respiratory system is involved, mechanical ventilation may be necessary.

## ■ Tetanus

**ETIOLOGY** Tetanus is a highly fatal infection of nerve tissue caused by the bacteria *Clostridium tetani*. The effect of the toxin produced by this bacterium on the central nervous system leads to voluntary or skeletal muscle contraction.

**SYMPTOMS** The first symptom is typically a stiffness of the jaw, commonly called "lockjaw," and is due to strong jaw muscle contractions. This disease affects both the musculoskeletal system and the nervous system. More detailed information about tetanus is found in Chapter 6, musculoskeletal system diseases.

## ■ Rabies

**ETIOLOGY** Rabies is an often fatal encephalomyelitis caused by a virus. It primarily affects animals such as dogs, cats, fox, raccoons, squirrels, and skunks, but can be transmitted to humans through a bite by an infected animal. Like tetanus, this virus travels slowly to the spinal cord and brain, so the location of the bite is significant. Incubation time is from one to three months. Shorter incubation times are related to the position of the bite, making bites to the face and neck more serious than those to the extremities.

**SYMPTOMS** Symptoms of rabies include fever, pain, paralysis, convulsions, and rage. In animals, a change in temperament is often noticed. Wild animals may become friendly and family pets may become aggressive. Another classic symptom is spasm and paralysis of the muscles of swallowing. The sight of water or attempting to drink water causes throat spasms leading to **hydrophobia** (hydro = water, pho-

**HEALTHY HIGHLIGHT**

## Polio Vaccine Precautions

There are three distinct polioviruses designated as types 1, 2, and 3. Dr. Jonas Salk developed an injectable vaccine against only one form of polio called a monovalent vaccine. This vaccine used dead virus to stimulate the production of antibodies against polio. Dr. Albert Sabin later developed an oral vaccine against all three forms of virus called a trivalent vaccine (TOPV—Trivalent Oral Polio Vaccine). This is a live vaccine using weakened virus to stimulate antibody production.

Immunosuppressed individuals must follow precautions with polio vaccines. Immunosuppressed individuals include those who are:

- Affected with chronic disease
- Taking chemotherapy
- Receiving radiation treatments
- Taking immunosuppressive medications for organ transplants
- On long-term steroid treatment

Precautions for immunosuppressed individuals include the following:

- Do not take the live trivalent vaccine since this may lead to contracting polio
- Do not change diapers or come in contact with feces of children recently treated with TOPV
- Do not come in contact with nasal secretions or vomitus of children recently treated with TOPV

---

bia = fear). Inability to swallow also causes a drooling of frothy saliva, an identifying symptom in animals.

**TREATMENT** Treatment of rabies includes immediate washing of the area with soap and water, followed by medical attention. A series of antirabies injections needs to be given before the virus has time to reach the brain. Any animal bite needs to be immediately investigated. The biting animal should be confined and placed under observation for symptoms of rabies, and viral cultures should be obtained. If the animal cannot be captured and must be killed, care should be taken not to destroy the head because the brain must be examined for presence of disease. If the animal cannot be found, the injured individual will need to take the series of injections immediately.

There is no cure for rabies. Treatment is palliative and includes strong muscle relaxants to reduce convulsions. Untreated cases end with severe convulsions and respiratory arrest. Death usually occurs within two to five days after onset of symptoms. Prevention of rabies begins with vaccination of family

pets and education of children in recognizing and avoiding animals with rabid symptoms.

## ■ Shingles

**ETIOLOGY** Shingles is an acute viral disease caused by *herpes zoster*, the same virus that causes chickenpox. The only difference between chickenpox and shingles is the level of the affected individual's immunity. Chickenpox usually appears in children with little or no immunity, and shingles occurs in adults with limited immunity. It is thought that *herpes zoster* virus is a chickenpox virus that has been dormant, usually for years, after recovery from chickenpox. This virus tends to flare up or become active during periods of stress or immunosuppression, caused by other disease processes, trauma, and aging. Approximately 50 percent of people over age 80 will have an episode of shingles.

**SYMPTOMS** Shingles is characterized by an itching, painful, red rash, and small vesicles or blisters that follow the course of a sensory nerve (Figure 15–4). The resulting neuritis or inflammation of the nerve results in a stabbing, sharp pain that usually is more severe at night. Symptoms may last for 10 days to several weeks. The pattern of rash and blisters usually appears on the body trunk and runs toward the midline. Shingles also may appear on the face, causing severe conjunctivitis. Diagnosis is made on the basis of the appearance of lesions. A viral culture or blood test for the herpes virus may be performed to confirm the diagnosis.

**TREATMENT** Treatment is symptomatic and involves administration of antiviral medication, analgesics, and antipruritics (medications to reduce itching).

# Vascular Disorders

Vascular disorders of the nervous system can be quite severe, causing long-term debility. Some vascular disorders can be prevented or reduced in severity by lifestyle changes.

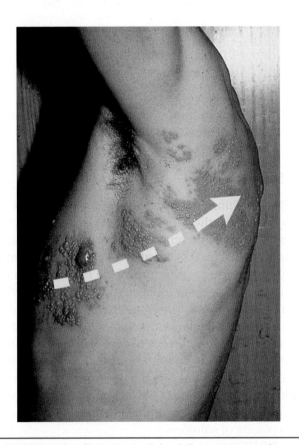

**FIGURE 15–4** Shingles: vesicles follow a nerve pathway. *(Courtesy of Robert A. Silverman, MD, Pediatric Dermatology, Georgetown University)*

## ■ Cerebrovascular Accident (CVA or Stroke)

**ETIOLOGY** Cerebrovascular accident, commonly called a stroke, is due to poor blood supply to the brain. Strokes usually occur in people over 50 years of age and are a major cause of death in this age group. A common causative factor is arteriosclerosis. A CVA is to the brain what a heart attack is to the heart. Lack of blood flow to the brain causes brain tissue death. The three common causes of poor blood supply or lack of blood flow are:

■ cerebral thrombus—a clot in a brain artery and the most common cause of vessel occlusion. Thrombus formation usually occurs in an area where the vessel is narrowed by arteriosclerosis. Symptoms usually appear gradually until blood flow is inadequate.

■ cerebral embolism—usually due to a small piece of a thrombus or arterial plaque breaking loose, and traveling in the artery until it wedges and occludes the vessel. Symptoms usually appear quite suddenly.

■ cerebral hemorrhage—the rupture of an artery filling the surrounding brain tissue with blood. Cerebral hemorrhage is usually due to hypertension and arteriosclerosis (see Arteriosclerosis in Chapter 8). Hypertension and arteriosclerosis cause the vessel to tear and hemorrhage. Another cause of cerebral hemorrhage is a weakened artery due to an aneurysm. Symptoms are very sudden with hemorrhage.

**SYMPTOMS** When an area of the brain loses blood supply, the individual suddenly loses consciousness, and may die or have permanent neurologic disability. About one-third of individuals with a CVA will die. An equal number will live with and without disability (Figure 15–5). The symptoms of CVA are numerous, depending on the area of the brain affected, and the severity of the occlusion or hemorrhage. Common symptoms include **dysphasia** (dis-FAY-zee-ah; dys = difficulty, phasia = speaking), **dysphagia** (dis-FAY-jee-ah; dys = difficulty, phagia = swallowing), **hemiparesis** (HEM-ee-**PAR**-ee-sis; hemi = one half, paresis = paralysis), confusion, and poor coordination.

Diagnosis of CVA is made and confirmed by physical examination, EEG, CT scan, and/or MRI. One indicator of the location of brain damage is shown by the pattern of hemiparesis, if present. Hemiparesis affecting the left side is indicative of right-sided brain injury whereas hemiparesis affecting the right side is

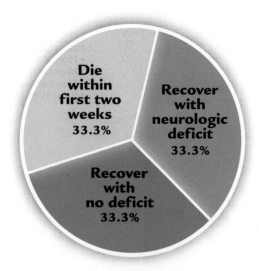

**FIGURE 15–5**   CVA: prognosis for individuals affected by CVA/stroke.

indicative of left-sided brain injury. Symptoms of right- and left-side brain damage vary to some degree (Figure 15–6).

**TREATMENT**   Treatment of CVA depends on the severity of the stroke and the symptoms. Anticoagulant and hypertensive medications may be given to control the formation of clots and to lower blood pressure. For those individuals with physical disability, a rehabilitation program, including the needed services of physical therapy and speech therapy, must be set up early and continued until the individual has gained maximum potential.

Prevention of stroke is directed toward avoiding risk factors that include:

1. smoking
2. high-fat diet
3. obesity
4. lack of exercise

These factors also play a role in arteriosclerosis, a main cause of CVA. Surgical intervention includes removal of plaque in the carotid arteries to improve blood flow and reduce the risk of a thrombus. This surgical procedure is called a **carotid endarterectomy**.

### ■ Transient Ischemic Attack (TIA)

Transient ischemic attacks are sudden, mild "mini strokes."

**ETIOLOGY**   They are due to insufficient blood supply to the brain. They may serve as a warning of an impending stroke and are often due to artery narrowing by arteriosclerotic plaque.

**SYMPTOMS**   Symptoms, like those of CVA, depend on the area of the brain that is affected. Some common symptoms are weakness of an arm and/or leg, dizziness, slurred speech, and a mild loss of consciousness. Total loss of consciousness usually does not occur. Symptoms usually subside within a few minutes to an hour.

**TREATMENT**   Diagnosis and treatment are similar to CVA. Arteriograms may be utilized to locate vessel occlusion. Surgery may be attempted in some instances to improve blood flow.

## Functional Disorders

Functional disorders of the nervous system include degenerative disk disease, headache, epilepsy, and Bell's palsy. These conditions, although varying in severity, are some of the most common problems of the system. The cause of the disorder may be found, but in many cases, it is unknown. Treatment of structural disorders is directed toward the relief of symptoms and assisting the individual in maintaining maximum function in activities of daily living.

### ■ Degenerative Disk Disease

**ETIOLOGY**   Degenerative disk disease is actually a degeneration or wearing away of the intervertebral disk of the musculoskeletal system, but the results so severely affect the neurologic system that it will be considered in this chapter. The wearing away of the disk between the vertebrae of the back allows the vertebrae to bump or rub against each other. As these vertebrae move closer together, the opening for the spine and nerve roots becomes smaller, causing pressure on the nerves. The condition of narrowing of nerve root openings in the spinal column is called **spinal stenosis** (stenosis = narrowing).

**SYMPTOMS**   Common symptoms include difficulty walking, radiating pain in the back and in one or both legs. This pain often follows the nerve path and may be **intractable** (difficult to stop or control). Degenerative disk disease usually affects older individuals, but may be related to trauma or congenital defects in younger individuals. Diagnosis is made on the basis of clinical history, X-ray, myelography, CT, or MRI.

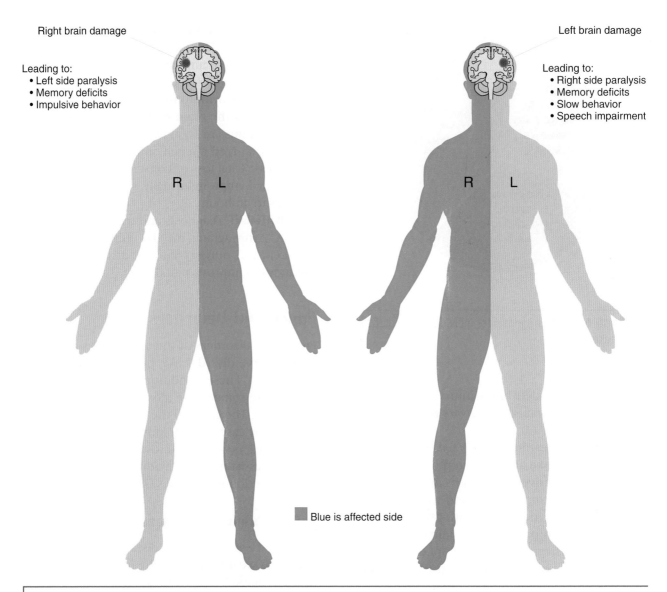

Right brain damage

Leading to:
• Left side paralysis
• Memory deficits
• Impulsive behavior

R    L

Left brain damage

Leading to:
• Right side paralysis
• Memory deficits
• Slow behavior
• Speech impairment

R    L

Blue is affected side

**FIGURE 15–6** Symptoms of right and left CVA vary to some degree.

**TREATMENT** Treatment initially involves resting the back and legs. A back brace may be of some help. Long-term treatment involves analgesics, anti-inflammatory medications, and exercise to ease the pain. A laminectomy, surgery to remove part of the vertebrae and widen the nerve root opening, may be the treatment of choice. In severe cases, surgery to fuse the vertebrae and free the nerve root may be performed. Often, older individuals affected with degenerative disk disease and spinal stenosis are not medically stable enough to endure surgery.

## ■ Headache

Headache, or **cephalalgia** (SEF-ah-**LAL**-jee-ah; cephal = head, algia = pain), is one of the most common disorders of humans. It is usually a symptom of another disease rather than a disorder in and of itself. Disorders that typically have headaches as a symptom may include sinusitis, meningitis, encephalitis, hypertension, anemia, constipation, premenstrual tension, and tumors to name only a few. Most headaches are not related to disease but are basically caused by two mechanisms:

1. tension on the facial, neck, and scalp muscles

2. vascular changes in arterial size (dilation or constriction) of the vessels inside the head

**ETIOLOGY** Many factors produce headaches including stress, noise, toxic fumes, lack of sleep, and alcohol consumption.

**SYMPTOMS** Headaches may be acute or chronic, and may affect different areas of the head. The pain may range from mild to unbearable and incapacitating. Pain may be constant or intermittent, and may be described as pressure, throbbing, or stabbing. Interestingly, brain tissue does not contain sensory nerves, so the sense of pain must come from the pain receptors in the meninges, facial tissue, or scalp. Some of the more common types of headaches include:

- Tension—caused by stress, strain, and tension on the facial, neck, and scalp muscles. Pain is typically in the occipital area.

- Cluster—may be caused by stress, emotional trauma, or unknown reasons. These headaches occur at night after falling asleep. The pain is generally a severe, throbbing pain behind the nose and one eye. The skin in this area becomes reddened, and the nose and eye water. The pain generally subsides after one or two hours, but may recur several times during the night.

- Postlumbar puncture—a severe headache affecting up to 40 percent of individuals following a lumbar puncture. It is thought to be due to leakage of spinal fluid through the needle puncture site. This type of headache is often prevented by positioning the individual flat in bed without a pillow for two or three hours following this procedure.

- Migraine—a severe, incapacitating headache commonly accompanied by nausea, vomiting, and visual disturbances. Individuals affected by migraines may experience a visual **aura** or a sensation that precedes the event including flashing light, dim vision, or photophobia. This type of headache may begin in adolescence, and diminish in intensity and frequency with age. Migraine headaches occur twice as often in women than men. The cause is still unknown although they tend to run in families, suggesting some type of inheritance pattern. Some foods that trigger migraines are chocolate, wine, and cheese. It is also thought that these are vascular headaches caused by altered arterial blood flow.

Diagnosis of the cause of headache is dependent on individual history and physical examination. Testing may include X-ray, EEG, MRI, and CT scans.

**TREATMENT** Treatment is dependent on cause. Treatment with analgesics and bed rest in a quiet, dark room is usually effective for most tension-type headaches. Muscle relaxants, muscle massage, warm baths, and biofeedback also may be effective. Vascular headaches may be relieved by the use of vasoconstrictor medication.

### ■ Epilepsy

Epilepsy is a chronic disease of the brain. It is characterized by intermittent episodes of abnormal electrical activity in the brain. This activity may be compared to an arrhythmia of the heart.

**ETIOLOGY** The cause of epilepsy may be due to brain tumors, neurologic disease, or scar tissue in the brain due to trauma or stroke. More commonly, the

---

## COMPLEMENTARY AND ALTERNATIVE THERAPY

**Feverfew for Migraine Headaches**

Feverfew (*Tanacetum parthenium*) has had the reputation of relieving headaches since the 1700s. In recent years, scientific research has been done to determine if the plant actually can affect migraine headaches. It appears to alleviate migraines by reducing the spasms and vessel swelling that cause the problems. The plant is a small bush covered with a daisy-like flower in the summer months. The leaves of the plant, and sometimes the flowers, are used to produce the tablets or tincture of feverfew. The leaves are also eaten directly but may cause sores in the mouth. The taste is quite bitter, so it is difficult to swallow in its natural state. The potential dangers of feverfew have not been established, so caution should be used by anyone taking the herb, especially pregnant women and children.

*Source: Kelville, K. (2000).*

cause cannot be determined during the individual's life or even on autopsy.

**SYMPTOMS** The most noted symptom of epilepsy is a convulsive seizure. A **convulsion** is an abnormal muscle contraction. A **seizure** is actually a sudden attack, but it is commonly used to indicate a convulsive seizure. Not all seizures are characterized by convulsions and not all convulsions are due to epilepsy. Convulsions may occur in a nonepileptic individual due to conditions such as excessive temperature (hyperpyrexia), hypoglycemia, hypocalcemia, and drug or alcohol toxicity.

The most common types of seizures are:

■ **Petit mal** seizures are also called absence seizures. These commonly occur in children and are often outgrown during puberty, but they may last a lifetime. These seizures consist of a brief change in the level of consciousness without convulsions. The involved individual may show symptoms of blank staring, blinking, and/or twitching of the eyes or mouth. The individual may remain seated or standing with loss of awareness of surroundings. Often, the individual seated only appears to have a loss of attention or absentmindedness. Episodes often last only a few seconds but may occur multiple times during the day.

■ **Grand mal** seizures are the type most often thought of as epilepsy. These seizures are characterized by convulsions, loss of consciousness, urinary and fecal incontinence, and tongue biting. Epileptic individuals often have an aura with grand mal seizures, allowing the individual time to lie down or call for support. Auras may include tingling of the fingers, ringing in the ears, and visual disturbances. Grand mal seizures often begin with a crying out as the contraction of the respiratory muscles forces exhalation. This is followed by generalized rhythmic contractions of the skeletal muscles of the body, arms, and legs. Contractions may last one to two minutes, but consciousness will return more slowly. The involved individual is often weak, drowsy, confused, and has no memory of the seizure event.

A life-threatening event is a state of continued convulsive seizure with no recovery of consciousness called **status epilepticus**. This is a medical emergency because treatment is needed to prevent cerebral anoxia and possible death.

 **HEALTHY HIGHLIGHT**

**First Aid for Seizures**

A seizure is a sign of a malfunction of some part of the brain's electrical system. Most seizures in individuals diagnosed with epilepsy are not emergencies, but they could be in others. It is always wise to call for assistance (medical personnel) when unsure.

In the event of a seizure, complete the following steps:

■ Look for a medical ID
■ Loosen tight clothing
■ Protect the individual from harm or nearby hazards
■ Protect the head by placing a cushion/padding under it
■ Do not attempt to place a tongue blade, any hard object, or your fingers in the individual's mouth
■ Turn the individual to a side-lying position
■ Avoid tightly restraining the individual
■ Stay with the individual until other assistive personnel arrive
■ Reassure the individual and offer assistance as consciousness returns

Diagnosis of epilepsy is made on the basis of EEG, CT, and cerebral angiograms. EEG may reveal altered brain activity, CT may indicate alteration in brain structure including tumors, and cerebral angiograms may reveal alteration in blood flow. Blood tests may be performed to indicate disorders of hypoglycemia and drug or alcohol toxicity.

Anticonvulsive medications are the treatment of choice for epilepsy. Close monitoring and adjusting of medications are needed to get the best effect. Medications are effective in preventing or reducing seizures 80 percent of the time. Education and emotional support of the affected individual and family members are needed because this disease is often feared due to lack of education. Goals for epileptic individuals should be aimed at maintenance of a normal lifestyle.

### ■ Bell's Palsy

**ETIOLOGY** Bell's palsy is a disease affecting the facial nerve (seventh cranial nerve), causing unilateral (one-sided) paralysis of the face. It commonly occurs in individuals 20 to 60 years of age. This disease is idiopathic, but possible causes include autoimmune problems and viral disease.

**SYMPTOMS** Symptoms include a drooping weakness of the eye and mouth, with inability to close the affected eye and drooling of saliva. The affected individual is unable to whistle or smile, and has a distorted facial appearance (Figure 15–7). Diagnosis is made on the basis of clinical history and symptoms.

**TREATMENT** Treatment includes analgesics and anti-inflammatory medications. If the individual is unable to close the affected eye, protection of the eye with a patch and artificial tear medication may be needed. Warm, moist heat, electrical nerve stimulation, and massage may be prescribed to prevent facial muscle atrophy. Prognosis for Bell's palsy is good with most cases resolving spontaneously in two to eight weeks. Plastic surgery may be prescribed to correct the facial deformities caused by chronic disease.

## Dementias

Dementia (dee-MEN-she-ah) is a loss of mental ability due to the loss of neurons or brain cells. Dementia may be caused in several ways. One of the most common dementias is senile (old) dementia and is related to degeneration of cells with aging. The most common cause of senile dementia is Alzheimer's disease. For this reason, Alzheimer's and senile dementia are

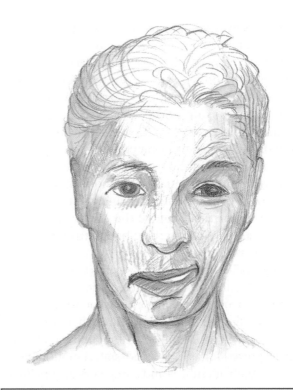

**FIGURE 15–7** Facial appearance of Bell's palsy.

often used synonymously, but in reality, an individual may have senile dementia without Alzheimer's. Vascular dementia also may be considered a form of senile dementia since it tends to occur in older individuals.

### ■ Alzheimer's Disease

**ETIOLOGY** Alzheimer's (ALTZ-high-merz) disease is a form of dementia characterized by the death of neurons and replacement of these neurons by microscopic plaques. It is the most common cause of dementia among older people. The disease usually affects individuals 70 years and older. The number of cases increases with age with an estimated 50 percent of individuals over age 85 affected. The cause of Alzheimer's disease is unknown, but factors being considered are heredity, viral infection, autoimmunity, and aluminum toxicity. Research also shows a higher rate of Alzheimer's in individuals with a history of head trauma.

**SYMPTOMS** Symptoms of the disease begin with mild mental impairment characterized by loss of short-term memory, inability to concentrate, and slight changes in personality. As the disease progresses, the affected individual struggles with communication skills, uses meaningless words, and cannot form sentences. Increased forgetfulness, along with the difficulties in communication, lead to irritability and agitation. In the final stages, which may take five to 10 years to develop, the affected individual's mental and physical capabilities are severely affected. The affected individual becomes restless, disoriented, incontinent, hostile, and combative, and is totally dependent on a caregiver. Death is usually due to a secondary cause such as infection.

Diagnosis cannot be positively made until after death with autopsy. Initially, a diagnosis may be made on the basis of symptoms after ruling out other brain diseases. In the final stage of the disease, CT or MRI may reveal the characteristic brain atrophy and microscopic plaques.

**TREATMENT** Treatment is supportive as there is no known cure for Alzheimer's disease. As the individual's capabilities decline, care is focused on safety and maintaining adequate nutrition, hydration, and personal hygiene. Mobility and mental capabilities are supported for as long as possible. Emotional support of family members and caregivers is of primary concern.

### ■ Vascular Dementia

**ETIOLOGY** Vascular dementia is caused by atrophy and death of brain cells due to decreased blood flow. Atherosclerotic plaque is the common cause of decreased blood flow and is common with aging.

**SYMPTOMS** Because the atherosclerotic plaques develop slowly, so do symptoms. Symptoms progress so slowly that they often go unnoticed by family members until they become quite severe. Symptoms include changes in memory, personality, and judgment. Irritability, depression, and sleeplessness also may occur. Personal hygiene is lacking and is often the sign that alerts family members to the condition. The affected individual may become disoriented and become lost in familiar surroundings. Diagnosis is made on the basis of a history and physical, and blood flow testing. Arteriograms of the carotid and cerebral arteries will reveal narrowing of vessels, stenosis, and arteriosclerotic plaques.

**TREATMENT** Treatment is aimed at increasing blood flow to the brain. If the cerebral arteries are involved or narrowed, medications may help improve blood flow. Carotid artery plaques can be surgically cleaned by a carotid endarterectomy (END-ar-ter-**ECK**-toh-me; endo = inside, arter = artery, ectomy = excision of). Prognosis depends on the effectiveness of treatment and the amount of brain cell death. If treatment is not possible or effective, or if a large amount of brain tissue has been lost, the affected individual will become progressively more demented and may need institutionalization for care.

### ■ Head Trauma Dementia

**ETIOLOGY** Head trauma dementia is due to death of brain cells related to head trauma. A type of head trauma dementia is Boxer's dementia, and is caused by repeated blows to the head as in the sport of boxing. Other types of trauma may be those sustained in accidents, especially motor vehicle accidents, and sports-related activities. The death of brain cells may be caused by the injury itself or due to edema and increased intracranial pressure. This increase in pressure decreases or halts blood flow to brain cells, leading to cell death.

**SYMPTOMS** Symptoms of head trauma dementia include a decrease in mental intellect and cognitive function. The affected individual may be unable to perform activities that were easily completed prior to the injury. Diagnosis is made on the basis of history, cranial X-rays, MRI, and CT.

**TREATMENT** Treatment is aimed at correcting the damage if possible, preventing further damage, and maintaining the existing healthy tissue. Dead brain cells cannot be replaced so damage is permanent. Therapy and rehabilitation is needed to regain as much function as possible. Individuals suffering severe head trauma may need institutionalization for long-term care.

### ■ Substance-Induced Dementia

**ETIOLOGY** Substance-induced dementia is due to brain cell death caused by toxicity of drugs and toxins. This type of dementia may be caused by repeated exposure to, or use, or abuse of, certain substances. Commonly, those substances include alcohol, cocaine, heroine, lead, mercury, and fumes of paints, paint thinners, and insecticides to name only a few. Brain cell death often persists long after the exposure to the substance ends.

**SYMPTOMS** Symptoms of mental impairment and decreased cognitive ability are permanent, and often worsen over a period of time.

## Sleep Disorders

Sleep may be described as a needed state of unconsciousness. It is thought that sleep is a period of time that the body is actively restoring and repairing itself as an increased amount of growth hormone is released during sleep. Sleep also provides a time of recuperation of mental activities. It is believed that there is an increase in metabolic rate in the brain during sleep that allows it to be more alert and efficient during waking hours. Sleep deprivation of just one night can lead to changes in personality, lack of muscle coordination, and decreased coping ability. There is a great variability in sleep requirements among individuals and different ages. Infants need 16 to 20 hours of sleep every 24 hours. This need for sleep decreases into adulthood with adults generally requiring between 6 to 9 hours of sleep, and older adults requiring even less sleep. Sleep disorders may be due to a variety of causes. Sleep disorders are tested by polysomnography, a procedure measuring a variety of physical variables related to sleep.

## ■ Insomnia

Insomnia is the inability to fall or stay asleep. The affected individual arises physically and mentally tired, irritable, and anxious.

**ETIOLOGY** The cause of insomnia may be related to stress, pain, fear, depression, and cardiovascular or thyroid disorders. Drugs such as caffeine, alcohol, nicotine, and bronchodilators also may cause insomnia. Eventually, the fear of being unable to fall asleep may become a cause. Insomnia is more common in females and occurs increasingly with age. The diagnostic definition of insomnia is sleeplessness for more than one month that is interfering with the individual's social or work habits.

**TREATMENT** Treatment consists of identifying and removing the cause. One may develop a sleep routine with a scheduled bedtime and awakening time. Counseling may be needed to assist the individual in managing or reducing stress and anxiety.

## ■ Sleep Apnea

Sleep apnea (ap-NEE-ah; a = without, pnea = breathing) is a sleep disorder characterized by periods of apnea or breathlessness.

**ETIOLOGY** This condition occurs more frequently in men and may be related to obesity, hypertension, and airway obstruction. Alcohol ingestion and smoking also may be causative factors.

**SYMPTOMS** The diagnostic definition of sleep apnea is more than five periods of apnea lasting for at least 10 seconds each per hour of sleep. These breathless periods are followed by sudden gasps or snorts for air. Other symptoms may include (1) excessive daytime sleepiness to the point that the individ-

ual may fall asleep during driving, work, or in the middle of a conversation; (2) extreme snoring that may not awaken the affected individual but easily awakens family members; and (3) personality changes, depression, and impotence. Sleep apnea can be divided into three categories:

1. Obstructive apnea, caused by nasal obstruction
2. Central apnea, caused by a disorder in the brain's respiratory control center
3. Mixed apnea, a combination of both obstructive and central apnea

Diagnosis is confirmed by monitoring the affected individual during sleep for apnea and low blood oxygen levels.

**TREATMENT** Treatment is based on cause. Obstructive types and mixed types are treated with weight-loss therapy, and if needed, surgery to correct nasal obstruction. Individuals affected by obstructive apnea also may benefit from oxygen administration during sleep. Central apnea is more difficult to control and may be treated with medications to stimulate breathing.

## Tumors

Brain tumors may be classified as primary or secondary.

**ETIOLOGY** Primary tumors start in the brain tissue, whereas secondary tumors occur in other areas and metastasize to the brain. The ratio of primary versus secondary tumor is about 50:50. Common sites of primary tumor that metastasize to the brain include breast and lung. Tumors also may be classified as benign and malignant (see Chapter 3). Benign tumors of the brain often become malignant if surgical removal is not possible. The growth of benign tumors in the confined space of the skull places pressure on the brain tissue and blood vessels, leading to loss of function and death of normal tissue. Tumors may occur in any area of the brain.

**SYMPTOMS** Symptoms are varied, depending on the area involved, and include headache, vomiting, seizures, mood and personality changes, visual disturbances, and loss of memory. Diagnosis is made on the basis of clinical history, symptoms, X-ray examinations, CT, MRI, and biopsy. A biopsy is the most definitive study to determine the type of tumor, and to assist with treatment and prognosis. Further studies may be needed to determine the primary location of metastatic brain tumors.

**TREATMENT** Treatment may include surgery, radiation, and chemotherapy. Treatment and prognosis are dependent on the type and location of the tumor.

# TRAUMA

Injuries to the brain, neck, and spinal cord are a main cause of disability and death nationwide. Trauma to the head can cause edema, increased intracranial pressure, hemorrhage, and infection, resulting in brain damage. Injury to the neck and spinal cord may lead to temporary or permanent paralysis.

## Concussions and Contusions

**ETIOLOGY** A blow to the head by an object, fall, or other trauma such as an automobile accident may cause a concussion or contusion.

**SYMPTOMS** Both conditions cause a disruption of normal electrical activity in the brain, which, in turn, causes immediate unconsciousness, often described as being "knocked out." This state of unconsciousness may last a few seconds to several hours. The affected individual often awakens with **amnesia** or loss of memory. Other symptoms are headache, blurred vision, and irritability. The involved individual may suddenly draw up the knees and begin vomiting.

A concussion is the less serious of the two conditions and does not involve injury to the brain. A contusion, on the other hand, is a physical bruising of the brain tissue. This physical bruising may lead to the development of a hematoma, increased intracranial pressure, and permanent brain damage. If the bruised tissue is in the area of the impact, it is referred to as a *coup* lesion. *Coup* lesions often occur with direct injury such as an injury obtained in a direct blow to the head. If the injury occurs on the opposite side of the brain, it is called a *contracoup* lesion. *Contracoup* contusions often occur when the head is in motion and is stopped suddenly, causing a rebound effect to the opposite side (Figure 15-8) as is often found in automobile accidents. *Contracoup* injuries are commonly accompanied by a *coup* injury at the point of impact. Brain contusions are often accompanied by skull fractures.

Diagnosis of both conditions is made on the basis of a history of the injury, neurologic examination, cranial X-ray, CT, or MRI.

**TREATMENT** Treatment of a concussion consists of bed rest in a quiet area under direct observation. The affected individual should be awakened every two to four hours and observed for changes in consciousness, eye pupil size, mood, and behavior. An individual suffering with a contusion should be hospitalized for continuous monitoring. Analgesic, sedative, and stimulant medications should not be given to individuals with head injuries as these medications may mask symptoms and make assessment difficult.

## Skull Fractures

The greatest danger of a skull fracture is the resulting brain tissue damage (Figure 15-9). Bony fragments may cut into the brain tissue, severing a vessel and causing a hematoma. Brain damage may cause temporary or permanent damage.

**SYMPTOMS** The position of the fracture will cause a variety of symptoms. A fracture near the base of the skull may injure the respiratory center of the brain, causing the individual to stop breathing. Fractures in other areas may lead to hemiparesis and seizures.

Another potential problem is infection of the brain tissue through the fracture site. Diagnosis is made on the basis of clinical history, physical examination, cranial X-rays, and CT scan.

**TREATMENT** Treatment is dependent on the type and position of the fracture. A craniotomy (cranio =

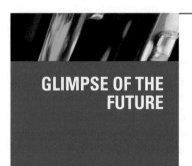

**GLIMPSE OF THE FUTURE**

### Gene Therapy Treatment for Brain Cancer

Combination immunogene therapy (CIT) is being tested for use as a treatment for brain cancer. This therapy uses two genes to strengthen the body's immune system. The combination of genes also destroys cancer cells. So far, it has been effective in the first trial in brain cancer patients. In the future, CIT may be the commonly used treatment for brain cancer.

*Source:* Gene Therapy Weekly *(2004).*

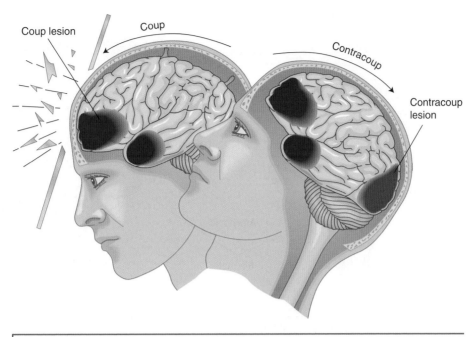

**FIGURE 15–8**  Coup and contracoup lesions.

skull, otomy = incision) may be performed to relieve intracranial pressure due to swelling. Surgical repair of the fracture may be performed if the fractured bone is pressing on the brain tissue. Protective headgear may be needed until the fracture site is healed.

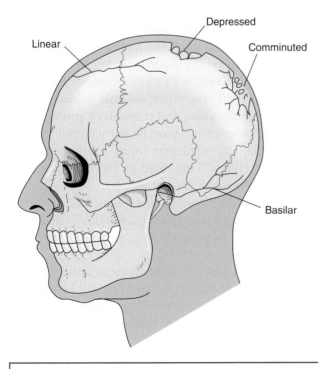

**FIGURE 15–9**  Common sites and types of skull fractures.

## Epidural and Subdural Hematomas

**ETIOLOGY**  A blow to the head is the common cause of an **epidural** (EP-ih-**DOO**-ral; epi = above, dural = dura, outer meninges) hematoma. Such a blow may be obtained in a fight or accident. Blood vessels are ruptured, and hemorrhage or seep blood between the bony skull and the first or outer meninges, the dura mater (Figure 15–10). Blood usually collects rapidly over a period of hours, pushing the dura away from the inner bony skull.

A **subdural** (SUB-**DOO**-ral) hematoma is usually the result of the head hitting a stationary object. This injury is often seen with falls, characterized by striking the head on the floor or a solid object. Subdural hematomas are characterized by blood collecting between the outer (dura mater) layer and the middle (arachnoid) layer. Subdural hematomas generally develop more slowly over a period of days.

**SYMPTOMS**  Symptoms of an epidural hematoma occur within a few hours after injury and may include headache, dilated pupils, nausea, vomiting, and dizziness. As the hematoma grows, the individual may lose consciousness and develop an increase in intracranial pressure.

**SYMPTOMS**  Symptoms of a subdural hematoma are due to increased intracranial pressure. Symptoms may include hemiparesis, nausea, vomiting, dizziness, convulsions, and loss of consciousness.

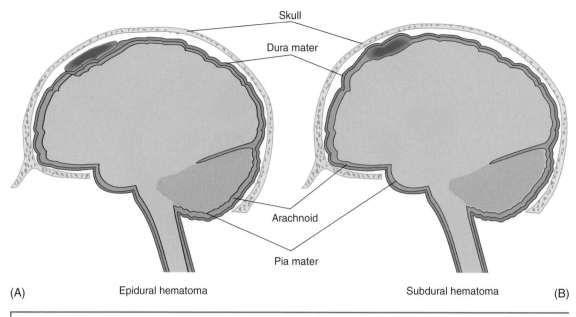

**FIGURE 15–10**  (A) Epidural and (B) subdural hematomas.

Diagnosis of a cerebral hematoma is made on the basis of clinical history, cranial X-ray, CT, or MRI. Hematomas, generally, are accompanied by a skull fracture.

**TREATMENT** Treatment of epidural and subdural hematomas is aimed at decreasing intracranial pressure. Pressure may be relieved by a special craniotomy called "bur holes" to drain the blood and **cauterization** (KAW-ter-eye-**ZAY**-shun; electrical burning of tissue) to stop the bleeding. If intracranial pressure is treated promptly, prognosis is good. Untreated, increased intracranial pressure can be fatal.

## Spinal Cord Injury—Quadriplegia and Paraplegia

The spinal cord is protected by the bony vertebral column.

**ETIOLOGY** When this column is fractured or injured, the spinal cord also may suffer injury. The spinal cord may be injured at any level, but the mobility of the neck causes this area to be the most vulnerable. The site of the injury, the type of trauma, and the degree of injury will all play a role in determining whether paralysis will occur and whether it will be temporary or permanent.

**SYMPTOMS** Injury to the spinal cord may result in varying degrees of loss of movement and feeling below the area of injury. Refer to Figure 15–11 while reading the following material for a better understanding of spinal cord injuries and preventive measures.

Injury to the neck is common in automobile accidents and sports accidents. Automobile accidents commonly lead to injury in the form of whiplash.

Injury to the highest level of the cervical spine (C1–C3) is usually fatal. Injuries to the cervical spine or neck area (C1–C4) may lead to **quadriplegia** (KWAD-rih-**PLEE**-jee-ah; quadri = four, plegia = paralysis). Quadriplegia is the loss of movement and feeling in the trunk and all four extremities with the accompanying loss of bowel, bladder, and sexual function. Other life-threatening symptoms include hypotension, **hypothermia** (hypo = low, thermia = heat or temperature), bradycardia, and respiratory problems. In some cases, respirations must be permanently assisted with mechanical ventilation. Injury to the lower cervical spine (C5–C7) may lead to varying degrees of paralysis of the arms and shoulders.

Injury to the thoracic or lumbar section of the spinal cord may lead to **paraplegia** (PARA-ah-**PLEE**-jee-ah; para = beyond or two like parts, plegia = paralysis).

Paraplegia is a loss of movement and feeling in the trunk and both legs. Loss of bladder, bowel, and sexual function are common. Paraplegia is often the result of a fall or an injury resulting in compression to the lower spine.

**TREATMENT** Treatment of suspected spinal cord injury victims includes seeking emergency medical treatment immediately, and not moving the victim

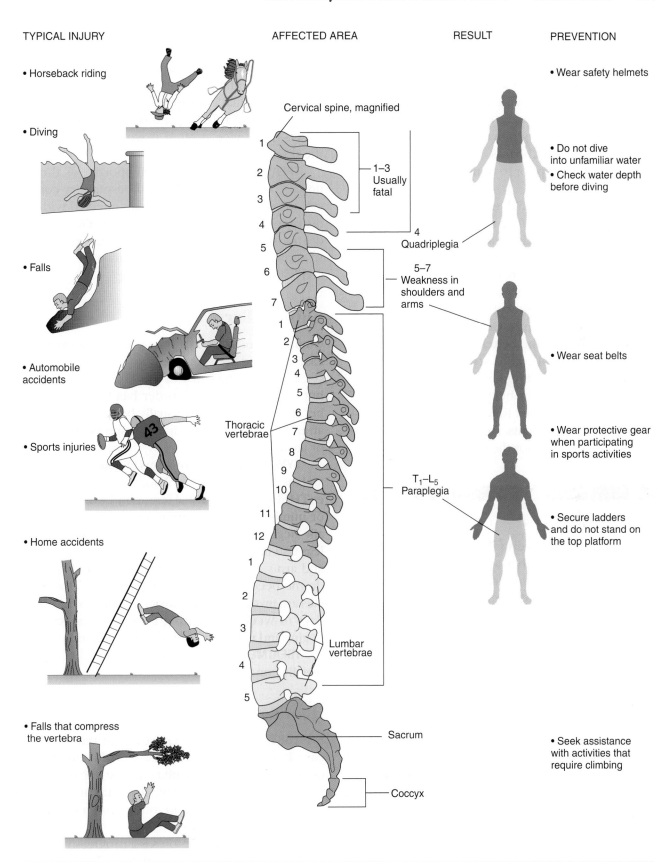

TYPICAL INJURY

- Horseback riding
- Diving
- Falls
- Automobile accidents
- Sports injuries
- Home accidents
- Falls that compress the vertebra

AFFECTED AREA

Cervical spine, magnified

1
2
3
4
5
6
7

1–3 Usually fatal

4 Quadriplegia

5–7 Weakness in shoulders and arms

Thoracic vertebrae

1
2
3
4
5
6
7
8
9
10
11
12

$T_1$–$L_5$ Paraplegia

Lumbar vertebrae

1
2
3
4
5

Sacrum

Coccyx

RESULT

PREVENTION

- Wear safety helmets
- Do not dive into unfamiliar water
- Check water depth before diving
- Wear seat belts
- Wear protective gear when participating in sports activities
- Secure ladders and do not stand on the top platform
- Seek assistance with activities that require climbing

FIGURE 15–11    Spinal cord injuries.

unless the surroundings are unsafe or life threatening as in the case of fire or flood. The head and neck should only be moved in life-threatening situations such as choking or respiratory arrest. Movement at this time should be very cautious. Emergency medical treatment is aimed at maintaining the position of the spine by limiting movement with use of special collars and backboards. The head, neck, and spine are stabilized prior to transporting in an emergency vehicle.

Diagnosis is made on the basis of history of injury, neurologic examination, spinal X-rays, MRI, and CT scan. Treatment includes realignment and stabilization of the bony spinal column, and **decompression** or release of pressure on the spinal cord. Treatment may include surgery and special medications. Much of the early treatment is aimed at preventing further spinal cord injury. Generally, the earlier the treatment is begun, the better the prognosis. If the damage to the spinal cord is severe, there is little or no hope of regaining movement and feeling. Paralysis, initially, results in the inability to move the extremities; but with time, reflex functions may return, leading to spastic movements. Early and intensive rehabilitation is necessary for the best prognosis.

# RARE DISEASES

Although some of the disorders discussed here are familiar to the public, they are actually rare diseases of the nervous system, considering all the various disorders that affect this system. Many of them have had exposure in the media due to their intensive solicitations for research. Generally, they are considered to be rare degenerative and debilitating disorders.

## Amyotrophic Lateral Sclerosis (ALS)

Amyotrophic lateral sclerosis, also known as Lou Gehrig's disease, is a destructive disease of the motor or movement neurons.

**ETIOLOGY** The cause of ALS is unknown, although genetic and viral-immune factors have been suggested.

**SYMPTOMS** ALS is characterized by atrophy of the muscles, leading to a progressive loss of movement of the hands, arms, and legs. As the disease progresses, loss of muscle function in the face and chest area leads to difficulty talking, chewing, swallowing, and breathing. Eventually, the loss of motor function

causes quadriplegia. One distinguishing factor of ALS is that there is not a loss of sensory neurons. The individual can feel the extremities but movement is impaired. Mental function is unaffected, so the affected individual is aware of the condition and may take an active role in planning care. ALS usually affects men twice as often as women, with onset of the disease after age 50.

**TREATMENT** Treatment is supportive as there is no cure for ALS. Management of respiratory complications is vital as most individuals affected with ALS die of respiratory failure. ALS is eventually fatal, with death usually occurring four to six years after onset. In some cases, affected individuals have remained active for 10 to 20 years after onset.

## Guillain-Barré Syndrome

Guillain-Barré syndrome is an acute, progressive disease affecting the spinal nerves.

**ETIOLOGY** The cause of this disease is unknown, but an autoimmune disorder has been suggested because the symptoms usually begin 10 to 21 days after a febrile illness such as a respiratory infection or gastroenteritis.

**SYMPTOMS** Early symptoms include nausea, fever, and malaise. Within 24 to 72 hours, **paresthesia** (PAR-es-**THEE**-see-ah; abnormal sensation, burning, tingling, or numbness), muscle weakness, and paralysis usually begin. These symptoms generally begin in the legs and move upward, but may also start in the face and arms and move downward. Guillain-Barré syndrome becomes life threatening if respiratory muscles are involved. Symptoms may progress for several days to weeks. Once progression ceases, recovery begins and may require three to 12 months.

**TREATMENT** Treatment is supportive. Recovery is usually complete.

## Huntington's Chorea

**ETIOLOGY** Huntington's chorea is an inherited disease. It is a dominant gene disorder affecting 50 percent of all children in families where one parent has Huntington's. This disorder does not appear until middle age, so children are often grown before the parent shows symptoms.

**SYMPTOMS** Huntington's is a progressive degeneration of the brain, characterized by loss of muscle control, and **chorea** is a constant, jerky, uncontrollable movement. The disease also leads to mental deterioration with symptoms of personality change, moody behavior, and loss of memory. Over a period of years, dementia (dee-MEN-she-ah; total mental incapacitation) occurs.

**TREATMENT** There is no cure for Huntington's chorea. Treatment is supportive and protective with institutionalization often necessary to provide the needed care. Genetic counseling is needed in families with this inheritance pattern.

## Multiple Sclerosis (MS)

Multiple sclerosis is a disease that causes demyelination of the nerves of the central nervous system. Myelin, as one will recall, acts as an "insulator" around nerves much like the insulation around an electric cord. Demyelination allows information to "leak" from the nerve pathway, leading to poor or absent nerve transmission.

**ETIOLOGY** The cause of MS is not clear. It is thought that a genetic predisposition plays some part, because it is 15 times more likely to occur in first degree relatives of affected persons. It is also believed that the immune system and viral infection play a part.

**SYMPTOMS** Symptoms caused by demyelinating lesions are muscle weakness, lack of coordination, paresthesia, speech difficulty, loss of bladder function, and visual disturbance, especially diplopia (double vision). Symptoms are varied, depending on the location of the lesions, making diagnosis difficult.

MS usually affects young adults between the ages of 20 to 40 years. It is characterized by periods of remission and exacerbation, usually over a period of several years.

**TREATMENT** Physical therapy and muscle relaxants may be helpful to maintain muscle tone and reduce spastic movement. The severity of the disease varies from individual to individual, but generally speaking, most affected individuals live a normal life span.

## Parkinson's Disease

Parkinson's disease is a slow, progressive brain degeneration, usually developing in individuals in their late 50s and 60s. Parkinson's affects men more often than women.

**ETIOLOGY** The cause is unknown, but individuals with Parkinson's have been found to have a defi-

ciency of the neurotransmitter dopamine in the brain.

**SYMPTOMS** Classic symptoms include the following:

- Rigidity and immobility of the hands, and a very slow speech pattern

- A fine tremor in the hands described as a "pill rolling" motion of the fingers

- An expressionless facial appearance with a fixed stare and infrequent blinking called Parkinson's facies

- An abnormal "bent forward" posture that includes a bowed head and flexed arms (Figure 15–12)

- A peculiar gait of short, fast-running steps due to the abnormal posture that makes the individual tend to stumble forward and leading to frequent falls

**TREATMENT** Treatment of Parkinson's is symptomatic. Dopamine replacement medications may be utilized. These medications do not stop the progression of the disease, but they may help with symptoms. Physical therapy for muscle soreness and psychological support are also helpful.

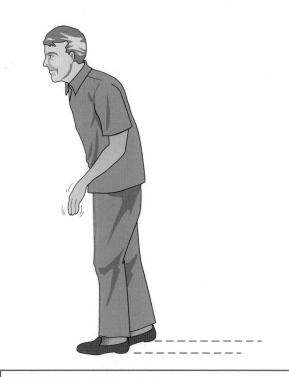

**FIGURE 15–12** Parkinson's disease.

## EFFECTS OF AGING ON THE SYSTEM

The effects of aging on the nervous system are some of the most noticeable to the older adult. Along with aging, there is a decrease in nervous system activity in the brain and spinal cord. This is due to a loss of neurons and the shrinking of the hypothalamus. Research has shown that continued active use of the brain decreases this process to some extent, but some changes still occur. With these changes in the brain and spinal cord come many changes in the individual's functioning. As the individual ages, there is a loss in short-term memory but not in long-term memory. There is also a slower general reaction time. The older person also may have difficulty completing fine

motor skills. General touch perception is somewhat diminished, too, so the individual may have difficulty distinguishing temperature changes and pain stimuli.

Vision ability is one of the first changes the individual often notices. There is a loss of visual acuity and a decrease in peripheral vision. Some individuals also become intolerant to very bright light, and have difficulty adapting to changes in light from dark to bright. Some hearing loss is a subtle process that occurs at different levels in individuals. Taste sensation also may diminish over time.

Sleep patterns are usually affected in the aging process. Generally, the older adult does not sleep as well at night, but makes up for this deficit by taking short naps throughout the day or in the early evening.

## SUMMARY

The nervous system is a highly complex system responsible for the individual's ability to reason, interact with other individuals, understand complex ideas, and to respond both intellectually and physically. Disorders of the system usually result in symptoms involving many other systems.

Injuries to the brain, neck, and spinal cord are a main cause of disability and death nationwide. Permanent neurologic deficits are common in brain and spinal cord injuries.

Changes in the nervous system with aging result in some of the most commonly seen symptoms. Losses in the senses are the most noticeable problems seen in the older adult. Changes in vision and hearing are some of the earliest symptoms realized by the middle-aged individual. Alzheimer's disease is one of the most common disorders of the nervous system diagnosed today.

## REVIEW QUESTIONS

### Short Answer

1. What are the functions of the nervous system?

2. Which signs and symptoms are associated with common nervous system disorders?

3. Which diagnostic tests are most commonly used to determine the type and/or cause of nervous system disorders?

### Matching

4. Match the disorders listed in the left column with the correct description in the right column:

_____ encephalitis      **a.** inflammation of the covering of the brain/spinal cord

_____ tetanus

_____ meningitis

_____ transcient ischemic attack

_____ cephalalgia

_____ concussion

_____ contusion

_____ subdural hematoma

_____ Alzheimer's disease

_____ Amyotrophic lateral sclerosis

_____ Multiple sclerosis

_____ Bell's palsy

**b.** a disorder affecting the seventh cranial nerve

**c.** disruption in the electrical activity of the brain, causing unconsciousness

**d.** blood collection between the dura mater and arachnoid layer of the brain

**e.** physical bruising of the brain

**f.** infection of nerve tissue

**g.** disease characterized by the demyelination of nerves of the CNS

**h.** inflammation of brain tissue

**i.** headache

**j.** a neurodegenerative disease characterized by cognitive dysfunction

**k.** destructive disease of the motor neurons

**l.** mild stroke

## CASE STUDY

**Mr. Speed** is a 57-year-old gentleman who has been recently diagnosed with Alzheimer's disease. He is in the early stage of the disease at this point in time. Mrs. Speed is quite concerned about the progression of the disease, whether Mr. Speed can still be employed, if he can be left alone for several hours at a time, and what medications he will be required to take. How would you respond to her concerns? Is there other information that would be helpful to the Speeds? Where can they find more information about Alzheimer's disease?

## BIBLIOGRAPHY

Acello, B. (2003). Handling an unwelcome comeback: Postpolio syndrome. *Nursing 33*(11), 32–34.

Age-related outcomes in patients with brain tumors linked to thymic cells. (2003, December 10). *Immunotherapy Weekly*, 26–27.

Brain tumor growth requires abnormal cellular neighbors. (2004, January 2). *Drug Week*, 85–86.

Coffman, S. (2003). Bicycle injuries and safety helmets in children. *Orthopaedic Nursing 22*(1), 9–15.

Epidural hematoma. (2003). *Nursing 33*(8), 96.

Experimental drugs show promise in halting brain tumors. (2003, December 12). *Drug Week*, 72–73.

Gene therapy may be useful in cancer treatments. (2004, July 1). *Gene Therapy Weekly*, 40–41.

Gordon, B. M., & Meyers, J. S. (2003). Leptomeningeal metastases. *Clinical Journal of Oncology Nursing 7*(2), 151–155.

Kelville, K. (2000). Earth medicine. *Better Nutrition, 62*(8), 20.

Lae, E., Mangarin, E., & Kelvin, J. F. (2003). Nursing management of patients receiving sterotactic radiosurgery. *Clinical Journal of Oncology Nursing 7*(4), 387–392.

Lyme disease: New guidelines. (2003). *American Journal of Nursing 120*(10), 17.

Many brain tumors may be associated with unknown heritable conditions. (2004, January 28). *Biotech Week*, 168–169.

Marrs, J., & Newton, S. (2003). Updating your peripheral neuropathy "know-how". *Clinical Journal of Oncology Nursing 7*(3), 299–303.

Mason, D. J. (2003). It's all in my head. *American Journal of Nursing 103*(7), 61.

New head injury guidelines. (2003). *British Journal of Nursing 12*(17), 1002.

Norrving, B. (2003). An enigmatic encephalopathy. *Practical Neurology 3*(4), 248–250.

Price, A. M., Collins, T., & Gallagher, A. (2003). Nursing care of the acute head injury: A review of the evidence. *Nursing in Critical Care 8*(3), 126–133.

Sterotactic radiosurgery for metastatic brain tumors benefits selected patients. (2004, January 28). *Biotech Week*, 437–438.

Yamamoto, L., & Magalong, E. (2003). Outcome measures in stroke. *Critical Care Nursing Quarterly 26*(4), 283–295.

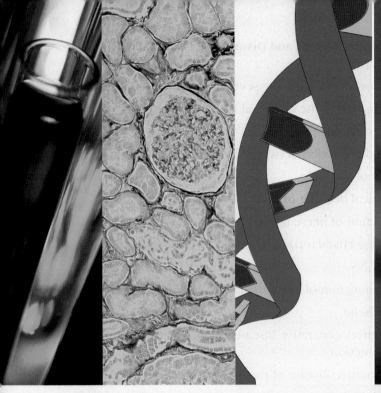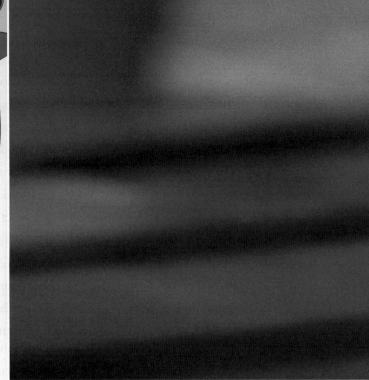

## OUTLINE

## KEY TERMS

# Eye and Ear Diseases and Disorders

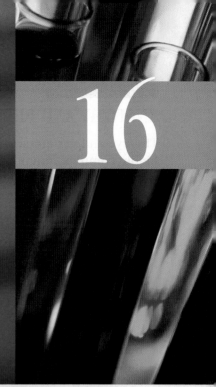

## 16

## LEARNING OBJECTIVES

*Upon completion of the chapter, the learner should be able to:*

1. Define the terminology common to the eye and ear.

2. Discuss the basic anatomy and physiology of the eye and ear.

3. Identify the important signs and symptoms associated with common eye and ear disorders.

4. Describe the common diagnostics used to determine the type and/or cause of eye and ear disorders.

5. Identify common disorders of the eye and ear.

6. Describe the typical course and management of the common eye and ear disorders.

7. Describe the effects of aging on the eye and ear, and the common disorders of these organs.

## OVERVIEW

*The eyes and ears are the major sensory organs of the body. They are extremely important to most individuals to maintain the quality of life and ease of functioning. However, although sensory deficits affect many people adversely, a high quality lifestyle is still possible after sensory losses. Individuals with visual and hearing impairment learn to function extremely well in activities of daily living. Disorders of the sensory organs are frequently the result of other system problems. Early detection of vision or hearing impairment may prevent permanent loss of these senses.* ■

## ANATOMY AND PHYSIOLOGY

The eye and ear are sensory organs that perform highly complex functions in the individual. They each are unique in their structure and function.

## Eye

The eyeball is the sensory organ of sight located in the bony orbit of the skull. It is about one inch in diameter. The eyeball consists of extraocular and intraocular structures (Figure 16-1). The extraocular structures include the following:

- muscles that hold the eyeball in place and allow movement of the eyeball
  - superior and inferior rectus—move eye up and down
  - medial and lateral rectus—move eye toward the nose and toward the temple
  - superior and inferior oblique—move the eye to the right and left vertically
- cranial nerves that innervate the eye and its structures
  - optic (II)
  - oculomotor (III)
  - trochlear (IV)
  - trigeminal (V)
  - abducens (VI)
  - facial (VII)
- eyelids that cover the anterior portion of the eyeball, regulate light entering the eye, protect the eye, and lubricate the eye
- conjunctivae (clear transparent membranes) protect the eye from foreign objects
- lacrimal glands (tear glands) clean and moisten the eye

The intraocular structures consist of some parts of the eye visible externally and parts visible only through an ophthalmoscope. The intraocular structures include the following:

- sclera—white area covering the outside of the eye except over the pupil and iris
- cornea—clear tissue covering the pupil and iris
- iris—round disk of smooth and radial muscles giving the eye its color
- pupil—round opening in the iris that changes size as the iris reacts to light and dark
- anterior chamber—space between the cornea and iris/pupil that is filled with clear fluid called aqueous humor
- posterior chamber—space between the iris and lens that is filled with aqueous humor
- lens—clear fibers enclosed in a membrane that refract and focus light to the retina

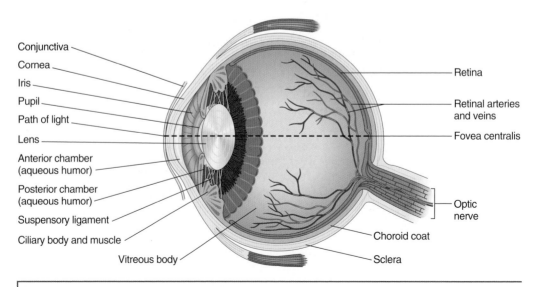

Conjunctiva
Cornea
Iris
Pupil
Path of light
Lens
Anterior chamber (aqueous humor)
Posterior chamber (aqueous humor)
Suspensory ligament
Ciliary body and muscle
Vitreous body

Retina
Retinal arteries and veins
Fovea centralis
Optic nerve
Choroid coat
Sclera

**FIGURE 16–1**   The eyeball: cross-section view.

- posterior cavity—the space in the posterior part of the eyeball filled with a thick, gelatinous material called vitreous humor

- posterior sclera—white opaque layer covering the posterior part of the eyeball

- choroid layer—the layer between the sclera and retina containing blood vessels

- retina—the inside layer of the posterior part of the eye that receives the light rays (visual stimuli)

The mechanism of vision occurs after impulses leave the retinae and travel through the optic nerves to the brain. At the optic chiasm, the nerve fibers cross and continue to the thalamus. These fibers synapse with other neurons that send the impulses to the right and left visual area of the occipital lobe of the brain. Because the tracts cross at the optic chiasm, the stimuli coming from the right visual fields are translated in the visual area of the left occipital area, and the stimuli coming from the left visual fields are translated in the visual area of the right occipital lobe (Figure 16-2).

## Ear

The structures of hearing and equilibrium are divided into the external ear, the middle ear, and the inner ear (Figure 16-3). The external ear includes the pinna (auricle) and the external auditory canal. The pinna is mostly cartilaginous tissue with a small amount of

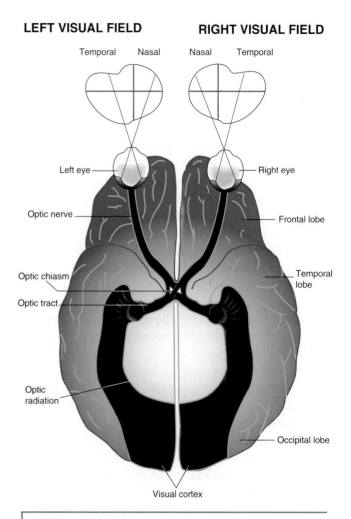

**FIGURE 16–2**  The visual pathways of the eye.

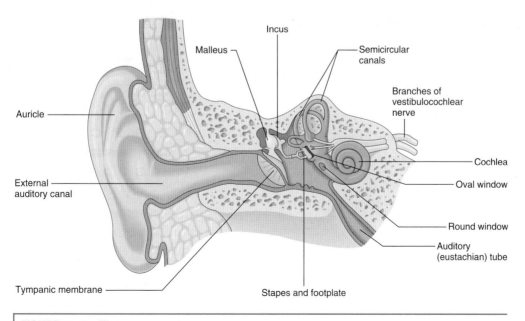

**FIGURE 16–3**  The ear.

adipose tissue in the earlobe. The external auditory canal is about one inch in length, and contains hair and wax (**cerumen**, se-ROO-men) producing glands. The external ear and middle ear are separated by the tympanic membrane (eardrum).

The middle ear, also called the tympanic cavity, is a small space containing three bones: the malleus (hammer), incus (anvil), and stapes (stirrup). Next to the stapes is the oval window that leads to the inner ear.

The inner ear is the most sophisticated part of the ear. It is responsible for both hearing and equilibrium (balance). The inner ear consists of a fluid-filled space housing the vestibule, the semicircular canals, the round window, and the cochlea. The structures in the vestibule are responsible for maintaining equilibrium during movement of the head. The semicircular canals assist the body in adjusting to changes in direction. The movement of fluid in this area can cause symptoms of dizziness. The cochlea is the organ of hearing.

The outer ear (pinna) picks up sound waves that are sent through the external auditory canal to the tympanic membrane. The membrane vibrates in reaction to the sound waves striking it. These vibrations pass through the three tiny middle ear bones, through the oval window, and into the fluid in the cochlea. Receptor cells respond and transfer the sounds into electrical impulses that travel to the brain via the acoustic nerve. The receiving area of the brain for auditory impulses is in the temporal lobe.

## COMMON SIGNS AND SYMPTOMS

Common signs and symptoms of eye disease that need medical attention include:

■ pain or burning in or around the eye

■ decreased visual acuity or ability to see

■ any visual disorder such as seeing flashes of light

■ eye redness

Common signs and symptoms of ear disease that need medical attention include:

■ otalgia (oh-TAL-gee-ah; oto = ear, algia = pain; ear pain)

■ deafness

■ vertigo (VER-tih-go; dizziness)

■ tinnitus (tin-EYE-tus; ringing in the ears)

## DIAGNOSTIC TESTS

### Diagnostic Tests of the Eye

An **ophthalmoscope** (aft-THAL-moh-skope; ophthalm = eye, scope = instrument used to look) is the instrument used for a basic examination of the eye. During an ophthalmoscopy (ophthalm = eye, oscopy = procedure to look), the fundus or interior aspect of the eye is examined. The retina, vessels, and optic disk of the eye can be visualized easily.

Visual acuity is measured by the use of a Snellen chart (Figure 16–4). The chart contains lines of letters in varying sizes with predetermined numbers at the end of each line. The predetermined numbers indicate the distance from which an individual with normal vision can see that particular line of letters. Normal vision is expressed as 20/20 and is considered normal vision for an individual viewing a particular

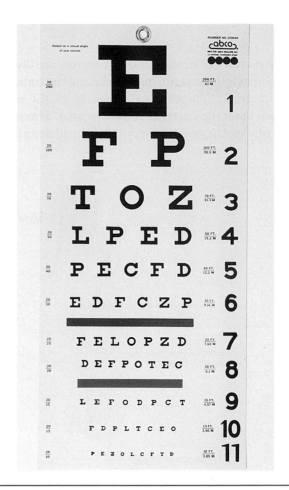

**FIGURE 16–4** The Snellen chart.

line of the chart from 20 feet away. For testing, the individual is positioned 20 feet from the chart or this distance may be simulated with the use of reflective mirrors. During the testing, one eye is covered, allowing measurement of each eye separately. The smallest line of letters the individual can read is noted and the predetermined numbers at the end of that line are recorded in a fraction. The first number, 20, expresses the fact that the individual is tested from 20 feet, and the second number expresses the distance an individual with normal vision could view those same images. For example 20/220 means that the tested individual can see at 20 feet what most people can see at 220 feet.

Diagnostic testing includes tonometry, slit-lamp examination, and retinal angiography. **Tonometry** (toh-NOM-eh-tree; tono = tone or pressure, metry = measurement) is a procedure to measure the pressure inside the eye. Tonometry is useful in determining the presence of glaucoma. A slit-lamp examination utilizes a microscope to magnify the surface of the eye. A beam of light, narrowed to a slit, is directed at the cornea. A slit-lamp examination is helpful in determining corneal abrasions, keratitis, and cataracts. Fluorescein dye may be used to improve visualization of eye disorders. **Angiography** (AN-jee-**OG**-rah-fee; angio = vessel, graphy = procedure to record) is used to discover vessel disease and problems with blood flow to the eye. Fluorescein dye is injected into a vein, usually in the arm. After the dye fills the vessels of the eye, X-rays are made showing the vessels. Vascular disorders such as those caused by diabetic retinopathy can be visualized.

## Diagnostic Tests of the Ear

An **otoscope** (OH-toh-skope; oto = ear, scope = instrument to look) is the instrument used to examine the ear. During an otoscopy (oto = ear, scopy = procedure to look) or otoscopic examination (Figure 16–5), the external canal and tympanic membrane can be visualized easily. Otitis externa and a ruptured tympanic membrane can be diagnosed using the otoscope.

The basic test for hearing is called **audiometry** (AW-dee-**OM**-eh-tree; audio = sound, metry = measure). During the test, sound is delivered in varying levels or decibles through a headset. Each ear is tested separately. The greater the amount of sound needed for the individual to hear or recognize it, the greater the amount of deafness or hearing loss.

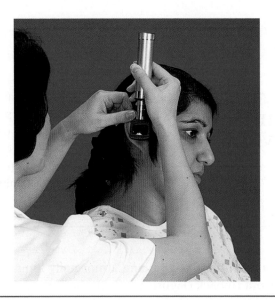

**FIGURE 16–5**  Otoscopy.

## COMMON DISEASES OF THE EYE

The most common problem of the eyes is a decrease in visual acuity or the inability to see clearly. The most common cause of poor visual acuity is refractive errors. Other common problems include those related to inflammation or infection. Infection usually affects the outer eye because of its contact with the environment. Other eye disorders are clouding of the lens (cataract), increased inner eye pressure (glaucoma), altered eye movement (nystagmus, strabismus), degenerative disorders (macular degeneration), secondary disease (diabetic retinopathy), and hereditary disorders (color blindness).

## Refractive Errors

Refractive errors are those caused by the eye's inability to correctly focus images on the retina. Approximately one-third of the population is affected by refractive errors.

**ETIOLOGY**  The cause of refractive errors is unknown although some run in families, suggesting an inheritance pattern. While these disorders affect individuals of all ages, incidence increases with age. There are four common types of refractive errors:

1. Myopia (my-OH-pee-ah) is commonly called nearsightedness or shortsightedness. Individuals with myopia can see objects that are near but have difficulty seeing distant objects. Light entering the eye of a myopic individual falls short of the retina

**Vitamins Can Help Your Vision**

Age-related macular degeneration (AMD) is a leading cause of vision loss and blindness, especially in older adults. Until recent research demonstrated the beneficial effects of vitamins on reducing or slowing the progress of the disease, there was no effective treatment for AMD. Now, recommendations are to eat a diet rich in leafy green vegetables. Individuals with intermediate or advanced AMD should take vitamin antioxidants and a zinc supplement.

*Source:* Better Nutrition, *(2004).*

---

due to the eyeball being abnormally long from front to back (Figure 16–6). **Radial keratotomy** (KER-ah-**TOT**-oh-me; kerato = cornea, otomy = incision) is a relatively new surgical procedure to correct myopia. Incisions are made in a radial fashion in the cornea in order to flatten the cornea, shortening the length of the eyeball and correcting the refractive error (Figure 16–7). Approximately two out of three individuals undergoing this procedure are able to see without the use of corrective lenses.

2. Hyperopia (HIGH-per-**OH**-pee-ah) is commonly called farsightedness. Individuals with hyperopia can see objects that are far away but have difficulty seeing close objects. Light entering the eye of a hyperoptic individual falls too far past the retina due to the eyeball being abnormally short from front to back (Figure 16–6).

3. Presbyopia (PRES-bee-**OH**-pee-ah) is a type of hyperopia that is age (presby = old age) related. Presbyopia is not due to the shape of the eyeball, but is related to the inability of the aging lens to properly focus light rays. When the eye focuses on a distant object, the muscles of the eye pull the lens into a flatter shape. As the eye focuses on nearby objects, the muscles relax, allowing the lens to return to a more spherical shape. In presbyopia, the lens does not return to the normal shape, causing light rays to fall beyond the retina (Figure 16–6). Presbyopia usually affects individuals aged 40 or older. Presbyopia may be corrected by the use of reading glasses or bifocals.

4. Astigmatism (ah-STIG-mah-tizm) is an irregularity in the surface of the cornea, causing light rays to spread over the retina rather than focusing properly on a part of the retina (see Figure 16–6). This

refractive error may lead to blurred or fuzzy vision, often described as seeing "halos" around objects.

**SYMPTOMS** Common symptoms of refractive errors include squinting, blurred vision, headaches, and rubbing of eyes. Tests for visual acuity include reading a Snellen chart and an ophthalmoscopic examination to look inside the eye.

**TREATMENT** Refractive errors are commonly corrected by use of prescriptive eyeglasses or contact lenses. There are no preventive measures for refractive errors.

## Inflammation and Infection

Inflammation of the eye and related structures is commonly caused by infectious microorganisms. Internal infections, or infection affecting the inside of the eye, are rare and are usually related to trauma. More common are inflammation or infections of the surface of the eye and its related structures. Eye infections are commonly caused by viruses and bacteria, and may be secondary to allergies, trauma, and upper respiratory infections. Microorganisms may reach the eye from the individual's hands, and contaminated washcloths and towels. Good hand washing and cleanliness are preventive measures.

### ■ Conjunctivitis

Conjunctivitis is an inflammation of the conjunctiva, the pink membrane lining the inner eyelids (Figure 16–8).

**ETIOLOGY** Conjunctivitis may be caused by excessive exposure to wind, sun, heat, and cold. The eyelids become red and swollen.

**SYMPTOMS** Affected individuals may complain of excessive tearing, itching, burning, and pain. An acute, contagious bacterial infection of the conjunc-

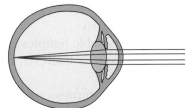

Normal eye
Light rays focus on the retina

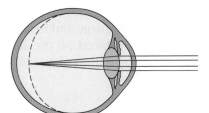

Myopia (nearsightedness)
Light rays focus in front
of the retina

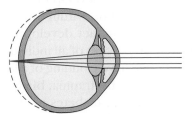

Hyperopia (farsightedness)
Light rays focus beyond
the retina

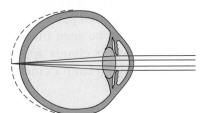

Presbyopia
Light rays focus
behind the retina

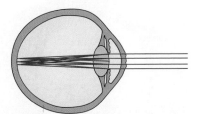

Astigmatism
Light rays focus on multiple
areas of the retina

**FIGURE 16–6** Normal eye vision, myopia, hyperopia, presbyopia, and astigmatism.

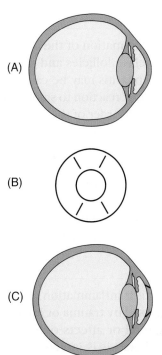

(A)

(B)

(C)

**FIGURE 16–7** Radial keratotomy. (A) Cross-section of the eye prior to surgery. (B) Small incisions are made in the cornea from the middle outward. (C) This causes the cornea to become flatter, thereby improving vision.

tiva is called pinkeye. Pinkeye may become epidemic among school-aged children.

**TREATMENT** Treatment includes warm compresses, anti-inflammatory medications, and analgesics to relieve pain. If infection occurs, cultures to identify the microorganisms, followed by antibiotic ointment or drops, may be needed.

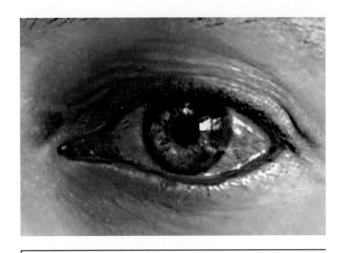

**FIGURE 16–8** Conjunctivitis. *(Courtesy of Mark L. Kuss)*

## ■ Blepharitis

Blepharitis is inflammation of the edge of the eyelid including the eyelash follicles and glands.

**ETIOLOGY** Blepharitis may be caused by bacterial infection, and allergic reaction to smoke, dust, or chemicals. Seborrhea, a disorder of the sebaceous gland or oil-secreting gland, also may cause blepharitis.

**SYMPTOMS** Affected individuals may complain of itching, burning, and a feeling of "something in the eye." The eyelids appear red, swollen, and crusted.

**TREATMENT** Treatment is directed toward removal of the cause, and may include antibiotics, allergy medication, or treatment of seborrhea.

## ■ Keratitis

**ETIOLOGY** Keratitis is inflammation of the cornea, and is frequently caused by trauma or infection. Keratitis is usually unilateral or affects only one eye. A frequent cause of keratitis is infection by herpes simplex virus secondary to an upper respiratory infection involving cold sores (herpes simplex).

**SYMPTOMS** Symptoms may include pain, **photophobia** (photo = light, phobia = fear), and excessive tearing. A slit-lamp examination of the surface of the cornea will confirm the diagnosis.

**TREATMENT** Treatment may include antibiotic ointment or drops to treat or prevent infection, and an eye patch to treat photophobia.

## ■ Stye (Hordeolum)

A stye or hordeolum (hor-DEE-oh-lum) is an inflammatory infection of a sebaceous (oil-secreting) gland of the eyelid (Figure 16–9). This gland is at the base of a hair follicle or eyelash.

**ETIOLOGY** Styes resemble pimples, are commonly caused by staphylococcus bacteria, and are often seen in blepharitis.

**SYMPTOMS** Warm compresses may relieve pain, help localize the infection, and promote drainage. Styes usually form a soft spot, open, and drain and heal without further treatment.

**TREATMENT** In some cases, styes may need to be incised to promote drainage and healing. In chronic conditions, **topical** (placed on the skin) antibiotic or systemic (taken by mouth or injection) antibiotic may be needed.

## Cataract

A cataract is a clouding of the lens of the eye (Figure 16–10).

**ETIOLOGY** Cataracts develop due to a change in metabolism and nutrition within the lens. The most common cause of cataract development is aging. Approximately 60 percent of all individuals 70 years of age or older will have clouding of a lens. Cataracts also may be caused by trauma, birth defects, and other diseases such as diabetes mellitus. Cataracts usually develop very slowly in one or both eyes.

**SYMPTOMS** The main symptom is a decrease in visual acuity or a complaint about not being able to see clearly. Other symptoms include blurred vision, glare, and a decrease in color perception. In advanced cases, the cataract can be seen through the pupil, giving the pupil a white, cloudy appearance. Diagnosis is confirmed by slit-lamp examination.

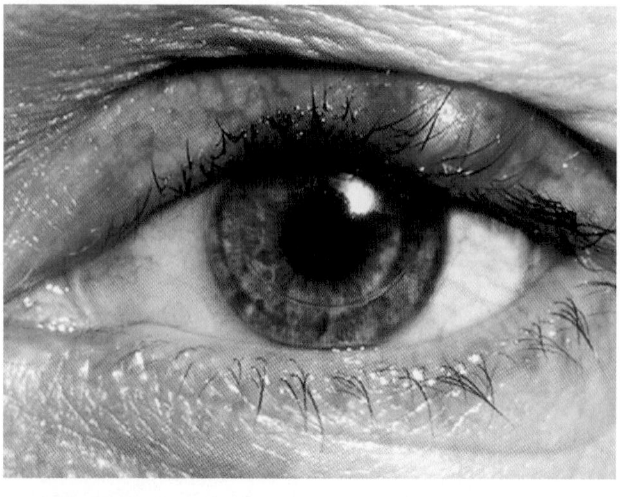

**FIGURE 16–9** Stye (hordeolum). *(Courtesy of Mark L. Kuss)*

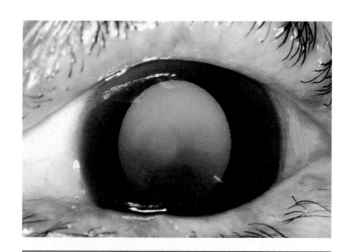

**FIGURE 16–10** Cataract. *(Courtesy of Mark L. Kuss)*

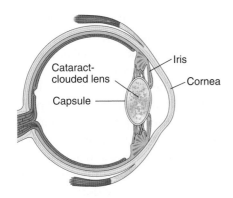

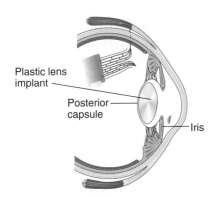

**FIGURE 16–11** Cataract extraction with placement of intraocular lens.

**TREATMENT** Cataracts are commonly treated with surgery. Cataract surgery involves removing the cloudy lens and replacing it with a clear artificial lens (Figure 16-11). This surgery, commonly called "cataract extraction with placement of intraocular lens," is routinely performed as outpatient surgery. Postoperative prognosis is good and there are no known preventive measures.

## Glaucoma

Glaucoma is a common condition characterized by excessive pressure inside the eye. The fluid inside the eye, known as aqueous humor, is produced constantly by blood. It circulates through the eye and is reabsorbed into the bloodstream.

**ETIOLOGY** Excessive pressure inside the eye occurs if too much fluid is produced or does not drain properly. There are several forms of glaucoma.

**SYMPTOMS** Generally speaking, glaucoma progresses slowly, may or may not be symptomatic, and rarely affects individuals under age 40. Increased pressure inside the eye for a continued period of time may lead to damage of the optic nerve and blindness. Permanent damage is often done before symptoms occur. For this reason, intraocular pressure should be checked on an annual basis. Diagnosis is made on the basis of an ophthalmic examination and tonometry revealing an increase in intraocular pressure.

**TREATMENT** Early treatment is essential to prevent permanent blindness. Depending on the form of glaucoma, treatment may include use of eye drops or surgery. Both are directed toward either reducing the amount of aqueous humor produced or improving the drainage.

## Nystagmus

Nystagmus (nis-TAG-mus) is a constant, involuntary movement of the eyes. Movement may be unnoticed by the affected individual. Movement may be vertical, horizontal, circular, or a combination of these. One or both eyes may be affected.

**ETIOLOGY** Nystagmus may be the result of brain tumors, disease, alcohol abuse, and congenital defects.

## COMPLEMENTARY AND ALTERNATIVE THERAPY

### Herbal Treatment for Glaucoma

Ginkgo biloba has been promoted for a variety of ailments, especially for memory enhancement. It also has been shown to assist in repairing peripheral vision that is often lost in individuals with glaucoma. In one study, subjects saw improvement in their peripheral vision after four weeks of treatment. Researchers think the herb, which is an antioxidant, increases the circulation to the eye and thus improves the vision field. Further study about the effects still needs to be done. Users of ginkgo biloba for eye problems should be cautioned to visit their ophthalmologist first.

*Source:* Vegetarian Times, *(2003).*

Diseases that cause nystagmus include Ménière's disease and multiple sclerosis.

**TREATMENT** Treatment is directed toward correction of the underlying cause. Congenital nystagmus is often untreatable and permanent.

## Strabismus

Strabismus (strah-BIZ-mus) is a disorder in which the eyes fail to look in the same direction at the same time. (Figure 16–12)

**ETIOLOGY** It is the result of muscle weakness in one or both eyes. The affected eye may deviate upward or downward, but more commonly, it looks inward (convergent strabismus) or outward (divergent strabismus). Strabismus commonly occurs in children and requires early intervention to prevent **amblyopia** (AM-blee-**OH**-pee-ah). Amblyopia is a decrease in the vision of the affected eye due to a lack of visual stimuli. The primary symptom of strabismus is **diplopia** (dih-PLOH-pee-ah) or double vision.

**TREATMENT** Treatment often consists of covering the normal eye in an effort to force the affected or "lazy eye" to function. Eye exercises and corrective lenses also may be ordered. The earlier the treatment is begun, the better. If correction is not made by the age of six or seven, the visual impairment may be permanent. Surgical intervention may be needed to correct strabismus.

## Macular Degeneration

Macular degeneration is a degeneration of the macular area of the retina. This area is important in seeing fine detail.

**ETIOLOGY** The cause of this degeneration may be due to the effects of drugs, but the most common cause is age related. Risk factors include farsightedness, light eye color, and cigarette smoking. This disease is the leading cause of visual impairment in individuals 50 years of age and older.

**SYMPTOMS** The primary symptom is a loss of central vision. Peripheral vision and color perception are unaffected. The disease generally develops slowly and painlessly, and both eyes are usually affected. As the disease progresses, reading and activities that require fine detailed vision become impossible. There may be a complete loss of central vision, but generally, blindness does not occur. Diagnosis is made on the basis of fluorescein angiography and routine examination.

**TREATMENT** Vision may be improved in some cases by laser surgery. There are some reports that individuals who eat foods high in vitamin A and zinc are at lower risk for development of macular degeneration.

## Diabetic Retinopathy

Diabetic retinopathy (RET-ih-**NOP**-ah-thee; retino = retina, opathy = disease) is the leading cause of blindness in the United States.

**ETIOLOGY** Diabetes mellitus causes vascular changes in the retina that lead to a decrease in visual acuity. These changes include capillary aneurysms (also called microaneurysms), microhemorrhages, venous dilation, and new vessel growth (Figure 16–13). The affected vessels tend to bleed easily into the retina and produce scarring.

**SYMPTOMS** Retinal scarring decreases visual acuity and may ultimately cause permanent blindness. These vascular changes tend to occur in both eyes, and are more extensive in uncontrolled diabetes or in individuals whose blood sugar is not controlled.

**TREATMENT** Laser photocoagulation treatment is usually effective, but the condition tends to recur and may need repeated treatment. Prevention is directed toward controlling blood sugar levels to reduce the retinopathy.

## Color Blindness

Normal ability to see colors diminishes with age due to the progressive yellowing of the lens. Colors become less intense, and the colors of green and blue often become more difficult to distinguish. Difficulty in distinguishing colors also may occur in young individuals affected with color blindness.

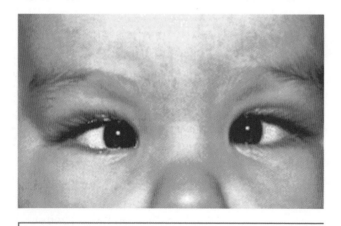

**FIGURE 16–12** Strabismus. *(Courtesy of Mark L. Kuss)*

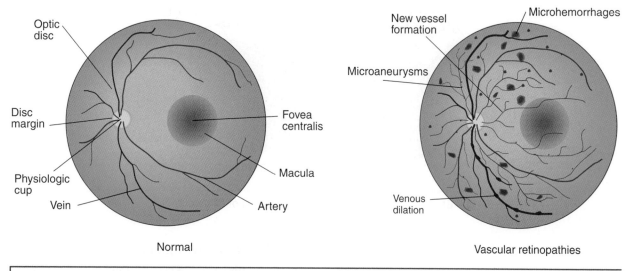

| Optic disc | | New vessel formation | Microhemorrhages |
|---|---|---|---|

**FIGURE 16–13**   Vascular changes caused by diabetic retinopathy.

**ETIOLOGY** Color blindness is an inherited, x-linked disorder that affects eight percent of the male population.

**SYMPTOMS** The most common color blindness affects the ability to distinguish between red and green.

**TREATMENT** There is no cure for color blindness. Interestingly, affected individuals may be sought to perform military duties that include the discovery of camouflage. Color blind individuals may exhibit an uncanny ability to see through camouflage, especially those utilizing shades of green.

# COMMON DISEASES OF THE EAR

The common diseases of the ear include infections and conditions of decreased hearing or total hearing loss. Gradual hearing loss may be due to a primary ear disorder such as an infection, or secondary to another disease or injury.

## Infection

The ear and related bony structures are commonly subject to infection. The middle ear is connected to the nasopharynx by way of the eustachian tube, making it easily accessible to bacteria that cause throat and respiratory infections. The external ear is open to the external environment, allowing infection from air and water. The bony mastoid process connects with the middle ear and is subject to infections affect-ing the middle ear. Ear infections are more common in infants and children.

## ■ Otitis Media

Otitis media is inflammation in the middle ear. It usually affects infants and young children, and is commonly called middle ear infection. But it may not necessarily be an infection. The middle ear is normally filled with air, but when this area fills with fluid, inflammation occurs. For this reason, otitis media is classified by the type of fluid that fills the ear. Fluid types are:

1. Serous—**ETIOLOGY** This may be due to an eustachian tube obstruction, allergy, or change in middle ear pressure, as occurs with air flight, that allows clear serous fluid to accumulate in the middle ear. This fluid accumulation causes inflammation of the middle ear but there is no infection.

   **SYMPTOMS** Symptoms are usually mild, and include a feeling of fullness in the ear and conductive hearing loss.

2. Suppurative—an infection in the middle ear.

   **ETIOLOGY** The fluid is pus due to the presence of bacteria. The **suppurative** (SUP-you-**RAY**-tive; formation of pus) form of otitis media is often due to bacteria entering the middle ear, usually from the eustachian tube during an upper respiratory infection. Blowing the nose forcefully often drives respiratory bacteria through the eustachian tube into the middle ear. Swimming in contaminated water may be another cause of suppurative infection.

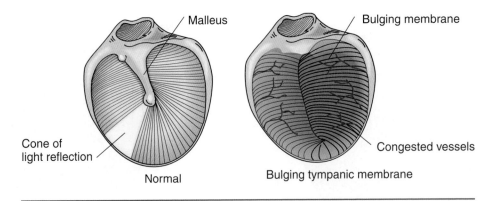

**FIGURE 16–14** Bulging tympanic membrane indicative of otitis media.

**SYMPTOMS** Symptoms include varying degrees of **otalgia** (oh-TAL-gee-ah; ot = ear, algia = pain), nausea, vomiting, fever, chills, **vertigo** (VER-tih-go; dizziness), and conductive hearing loss.

The structure and position of the eustachian tube is an important factor with either type of otitis media. If the eustachian tube is narrower, shorter, and/or more horizontally placed than normal, the individual is more prone to otitis media. Infants and young children normally have more horizontally placed and narrower eustachian tubes, thus predisposing them to otitis media. As the child grows, the tube becomes more vertical and explains why children often "outgrow" ear infections.

Diagnosis is made on the basis of otoscopy revealing a bulging tympanic membrane or eardrum (Figure 16–14). The normally pearly colored tympanic membrane is red and swollen. If the tympanic membrane is ruptured, a culture of the fluid may be performed; otherwise, cultures are not obtainable. An elevated white blood cell count, is also indicative of infection.

**TREATMENT** Treatment for both types of otitis media includes analgesics for pain and decongestants to promote drainage. Suppurative otitis media will require antibiotic therapy.

Chronic otitis media, both forms, may need surgical removal of fluid by **myringotomy** (MIR-in-**GOT**-oh-me; myringo = eardrum, tomy = incision into) to prevent rupture of the tympanic membrane, permanent hearing loss, and possible mastoiditis. To prevent further accumulation of fluid and to relieve pressure, **tympanostomy** (TIM-pan-**OSS**-toh-me; tympano = eardrum, ostomy = new opening) tubes, commonly called PE tubes or pediatric ear tubes, may be placed through the tympanic membrane during a procedure called a **tympanoplasty** (TIM-pah-no-**PLASTY**; tympano = eardrum, plasty = surgical repair) (Figure 16–15). Tubes commonly fall out after several months, but may be removed after six to 12 months. Prognosis for both types of otitis media is good if given prompt treatment. Chronic untreated otitis media may lead to severe ear damage and permanent hearing loss. Prevention of complications is

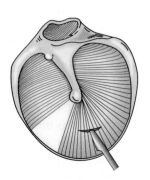
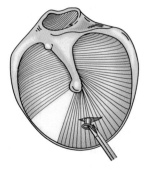
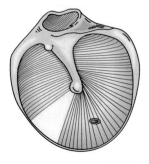

Tympanic membrane incision          Tube placement          Tympanoplasty completed

**FIGURE 16–15** Tympanoplasty.

directed toward prevention and prompt treatment of upper respiratory infections and otitis media.

### ■ Otitis Externa

Otitis externa, also called swimmer's ear or external otitis, is an inflammation of the external ear canal.

**ETIOLOGY** This disease commonly affects swimmers who spend many hours in the water. Other causes include trauma to the ear canal, that can occur when attempting to scratch or clean the ear canal, and when swimming in contaminated water. The condition often is due to bacterial or fungal infection. Wearing headphones also makes a favorable environment for the growth of microorganisms.

**SYMPTOMS** Symptoms of otitis externa include an inflamed ear canal with extreme pain, fever, **pruritis** (proo-RYE-tus; itching), and hearing loss. The ear also may drain clear or **purulent** (PYOU-roo-lent; containing pus) fluid. Diagnosis is made on the basis of an otologic examination. If an infection is suspected, a culture and sensitivity test may be needed.

**TREATMENT** Treatment includes keeping the ear canal clean and dry, analgesics for pain, and antibiotics if an infection is detected. Prevention includes wearing earplugs while showering or swimming to keep the external canal clean and dry. Decreasing the amount of time headphones are worn and keeping foreign objects out of the ears also may be helpful. Otitis externa tends to be a recurring disease that may eventually become chronic and cause hearing loss.

### ■ Mastoiditis

Mastoiditis (MAS-toy-**DYE**-tis) is inflammation of the mastoid bone or process. This bone is porous or honeycombed in appearance, and is located behind the ear.

**ETIOLOGY** Acute mastoiditis is usually the result of a middle ear infection. Infection in the mastoid bone is commonly caused by Streptococcus.

**SYMPTOMS** Symptoms include **tinnitus** (tin-EYE-tus; ringing in the ears) and otalgia (oh-TAL-gee-ah; ot = ear, algia = pain). The mastoid also may become swollen and painful. Diagnosis is made on the basis of otoscopy, (OH-**TOS**-koh-pee; oto = ear, scopy = procedure to look into), cultures, and X-ray of the mastoid bone.

**TREATMENT** Mastoiditis generally responds to antibiotic therapy. Severe or chronic mastoiditis may need surgical treatment with a **mastoidectomy**

(MAS-toy-**DECK**-toh-me; ectomy = removal or excision) to prevent complications and preserve hearing.

## Deafness

Deafness or loss of hearing is a common disease affecting more than 25 million people. There are multiple reasons for deafness, but most causes fall into two basic categories: conductive and sensory. Conductive deafness is caused by external or middle ear disorders that decrease or stop conduction of sound to the inner ear. Conductive disorders include impacted cerumen, otosclerosis, and a ruptured tympanic membrane. Sensory deafness is the result of cochlear or auditory nerve damage that impairs the ability of sound to be carried to the brain. Sensory deafness is often related to damaging noise levels and ototoxic medications.

### ■ Impacted Cerumen

Cerumen is the soft, yellow-brown secretion produced by the external ear, commonly called ear wax.

**ETIOLOGY** Impacted cerumen is a common cause of conductive hearing loss. If cerumen accumulates and becomes impacted (pressed firmly) in the ear canal, it may cause tinnitus and temporary deafness. An abnormal amount of cerumen may build up in the ear due to skin dryness, excessive hair in the ear, or a narrow ear canal. Another cause of buildup is due to excessive dust in the ear, which occurs among construction workers, farmers, and cabinetmakers, to name a few. Cerumen is normally washed out of the ear during routine showering and shampooing. An otologic examination will confirm the diagnosis.

**TREATMENT** Impacted cerumen is often removed with ear irrigations. This condition tends to recur, so routine examination should be performed.

### ■ Otosclerosis

Otosclerosis (OH-toh-skleh-**ROH**-sis; oto = ear, scler = hardening, osis = condition) is a condition characterized by bony fixation of the small bones of the middle ear. This fixation does not allow the bones to conduct vibrations from the eardrum to the inner ear, causing a conductive hearing loss. Otosclerosis occurs more commonly in females than in males. It usually affects females under the age of 35 and may be aggravated by pregnancy.

**ETIOLOGY** The cause of otosclerosis is unknown, but there is evidence of familial tendency, suggesting a hereditary cause. Diagnosis is made on the basis of physical examination, audiogram, and otoscopy.

## ◉ HEALTHY HIGHLIGHT

### Removing Impacted Cerumen

Impacted cerumen should be softened and removed gently in the following manner.

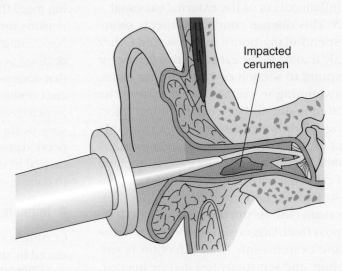

Impacted cerumen

1. Warm mineral oil or glycerin by holding it between the hands or placing the bottle in a cup of warm water.
2. Check the temperature to ensure that it is not too hot. It should be lukewarm.
3. Drop two to three drops of oil in the ear canal.
4. Gently irrigate the ear canal using a bulb syringe filled with lukewarm water.
5. Aim the water flow toward the top of the ear canal, not toward the eardrum.
6. Continue to irrigate until the impacted cerumen is removed. This may take 10 to 15 minutes.
7. Repeat steps 1–6 until the impacted cerumen is removed.

**TREATMENT** A common treatment for otosclerosis is a **stapedectomy** (STAY-peh-**DECK**-toh-me; stape = stapes, ectomy = removal or excision of). A stapedectomy involves removing the stapes bone in the middle ear and replacing it with a **prosthesis** (pros-THEE-sis; an artificial part) (Figure 16–16). Hearing is generally improved soon after surgery. If a stapedectomy is not an option for the affected individual, a hearing aid may improve hearing.

### ■ Sensorineural Deafness

Sensorineural deafness is a type of sensory deafness due to damage to the cochlea or the auditory nerve.

**ETIOLOGY** Damage to these structures is often due to exposure to loud noise. Occupational noise including heavy machinery, jackhammers, and airplane engines may lead to deafness. Teenagers and young adults are at high risk due to the popularity of playing loud music and attending music concerts that utilize large amplifiers. Diagnosis is made on the basis of audiometry.

**TREATMENT** Sensorineural deafness caused by cochlear or auditory nerve damage is often permanent. Prevention is aimed at reducing the amount of noise, and protecting the ears by using protective earphones and earplugs.

### ■ Presbycusis

**ETIOLOGY** Presbycusis (PRES-beh-**KOO**-sis; presby = old age, cusis = hearing) is a progressive sensory

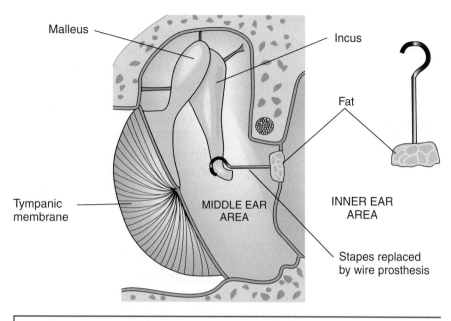

**FIGURE 16–16** Stapedectomy with wire prosthesis.

hearing loss related to aging. The cause of presbycusis is due to degenerative changes in the organs of hearing.

**SYMPTOMS** Onset of symptoms is gradual and usually begins after age 50. Initially, there is a loss of hearing of high tones, but as hearing loss progresses, lower tones become difficult to hear as well.

**TREATMENT** Use of a hearing aid may be helpful initially, but as the hearing declines, aids may become less useful.

## Motion Sickness

Motion sickness is the nauseated feeling some individuals experience when traveling by automobile, boat, or airplane.

**ETIOLOGY** The cause of motion sickness is abnormal movement of the organs of balance—the semicircular canals—that are located in the inner ear. These semicircular canals are accustomed to traveling in a horizontal plane, but movement in a vertical plane, as in a boat or bumpy airplane ride, produces an abnormal sensation in these organs, leading to motion sickness. Watching motion on a wide-screen picture also may cause motion sickness, even though the individual is not actually moving.

**SYMPTOMS** Symptoms of motion sickness include varying degrees of nausea, vomiting, diaphoresis, and vertigo. Fortunately, motion sickness usually subsides when movement stops.

**TREATMENT** To prevent this condition, antimotion sickness medication including diazepam (Valium) or scopolamine may be taken prior to a trip. Other considerations that may decrease the occurrence of motion sickness include:

■ avoidance of heavy meals prior to a trip

■ finding a seat in the most stable area of the boat or plane

■ during automobile rides, making frequent stops for short walks in the fresh air

■ not reading while traveling

■ avoiding stuffy areas, especially those with odors such as cigarette smoke

■ trying to stay cool with plenty of fresh air when possible

■ avoiding too much heat

Motion sickness may be relieved or reduced by lying down and closing the eyes.

# TRAUMA

## Corneal Abrasion

The cornea, the transparent outer layer of the eye, is subject to trauma because of its position.

**ETIOLOGY** Corneal abrasions may be caused by:

- trapping a foreign object like sand or sawdust between the eyelid and the cornea
- contact lenses that do not fit properly, are dirty or scratched, or are worn for too long a time period
- accidentally poking a finger in the eye
- extreme light, as with welding

**SYMPTOMS** Symptoms are often delayed, occurring 12 to 18 hours after the trauma, and include severe pain, tearing, and photophobia. Diagnosis is made on the basis of history and visual examination. Abrasions may be easily stained with fluorescein and viewed with a slit lamp.

**TREATMENT** Treatment includes removal of the foreign body, and antibiotic ointment or drops to prevent infection. Analgesic medications for pain may be prescribed. A pressure dressing may be applied to the eye to keep the eyelid from moving against the cornea and to reduce the pain of photophobia. Interestingly, the pain caused by corneal abrasion comes from the inside of the eyelid rubbing over the abrasion on the cornea. The cornea does not have sensory nerves. Abrasions can often be avoided by use of protective eyewear.

## Retinal Detachment

**ETIOLOGY** Retinal detachment often occurs with trauma, diabetes, and other retinopathies that cause an opening or hole in the retinal layer. This opening allows fluid from the vitreous humor to leak between the retina and choroid layer. The fluid lifts or floats the retina away from the choroid (Figure 16–17).

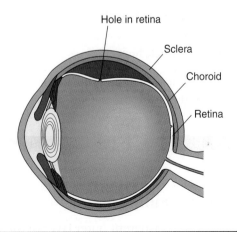

Hole in retina

Sclera

Choroid

Retina

**FIGURE 16–17** Retinal detachment.

**SYMPTOMS** As this process occurs, the individual experiences loss of vision in the detached area. Often, symptoms of retinal detachment include blurred vision, flashes of light, and floating spots. Retinal detachment is painless but needs immediate medical attention. Ophthalmoscopic examination will readily show the detachment.

**TREATMENT** Surgery is the usual treatment to seal the opening and reattach the retina to the choroid layer. This may be done using laser technology. The retina usually regains function unless extreme detachment has occurred.

## Ruptured Tympanic Membrane

**ETIOLOGY** The most common causes of a ruptured tympanic membrane are a severe middle ear infection or sticking a sharp object, such as a pencil, into the ear canal.

**SYMPTOMS** Symptoms include pain, partial loss of hearing, and usually bloody or purulent drainage. The main complication of a ruptured membrane is risk of infection. Diagnosis can be confirmed by otoscopy.

**TREATMENT** Treatment may include antibiotics to prevent infection and surgical patching of the membrane with a tissue graft. Minimal hearing loss is associated with a ruptured tympanic membrane.

# RARE DISEASES

## Retinoblastoma

Retinoblastoma is a malignant tumor of the eye.

**ETIOLOGY** It occurs during infancy and childhood, and tends to be hereditary. Often, both eyes are affected.

**SYMPTOMS** Retinoblastomas grow as intraocular masses that fill the eye and may extend into the optic nerve. The mass is usually recognized by a white light reflex seen at the pupil (cat's eye).

**TREATMENT** Untreated retinoblastoma is fatal. With treatment, 90 percent of affected children survive. Treatment includes **enucleation** (removal of the eyeball), radiation, and chemotherapy.

## Ménière's Disease

Ménière's usually affects individuals between the ages of 40 and 60.

**ETIOLOGY** The cause is unknown, although predisposing factors appear to include middle ear infections and head trauma.

**SYMPTOMS** Ménière's disease is a chronic disease of the inner ear characterized by tinnitus, vertigo, progressive hearing loss, and a feeling of fullness in the ear. Acute attacks may last from a few hours to several days with symptoms of nausea, vomiting, diaphoresis, and vertigo.

**TREATMENT** Treatment for acute attacks includes medications to control nausea and vomiting. A low-salt diet, diuretics, antihistamines, and cessation of smoking are usually effective for long-term treatment. Surgery may be performed if the disease does not respond to treatment, but a major complication of surgery is permanent deafness.

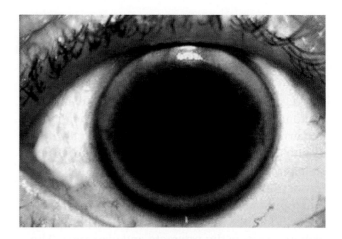

**FIGURE 16–18**  Arcus senilis. *(Courtesy of Mark L. Kuss)*

# EFFECTS OF AGING ON THE SYSTEM

The effects of aging on the sensory organs are significant. Changes in vision begin in middle age and progress through the older adult years. The change is obvious in most people, beginning with the inability to read small print or to see well in low light. These changes affect the older adult's ability to function well in society, and often cause social isolation and dependence on others.

Vision changes begin around age 40 and continue through the life span. Focusing on near objects, color perception, some sensitivity to light, and decreased visual acuity are all normal physiologic changes that occur during the aging process. Although the changes vary among individuals, most persons have about a 20/70 visual acuity by age 65. Glaucoma and cataracts are common problems of the older adult, reducing their ability to see even further. In the diabetic older person, retinopathy is a very common problem that often eventually leads to blindness. Arcus senilis is an opaque, grayish ring at the periphery of the cornea that frequently occurs in an older person. It results from fatty granule deposits in, or hyaline degeneration of, the lamellae and cells of the cornea (Figure 16–18).

Hearing changes in the older adult affect the ability to perceive what is heard, and also may affect behavior, personality, and attitudes. Many hearing problems can be corrected, but may not because of financial constraints or social concerns. The inability to hear often affects the individual's ability to communicate, and interferes with one's social life and independence. In some instances, speaking in a clear, concise manner is more beneficial than raising one's voice.

As the individual ages, the tympanic membrane becomes thinner and less flexible, reducing the conduction of sound. This is a conductive hearing loss associated with aging. If there has been damage to the eighth cranial nerve, the individual has a sensorineural loss. If both types are present, it is called a mixed hearing loss.

The slow but gradual loss of hearing called presbycusis affects more men than women. This type of hearing loss is due to degenerative changes in neurons, the bones of the middle ear, and the cochlea. High-pitched sounds become the most difficult to hear at first, but gradual loss of low-pitched sounds also occurs eventually.

Other hearing conditions seen in the older adult include otosclerosis, tinnitus, and Ménière's disease. Although some of these may begin in younger life, they are most commonly detected in later years.

## SUMMARY

The sensory organs of the body are often regarded as the most important to the individual to maintain quality of life. Visual and hearing impairments are often correctable, especially if diagnosed early in the degenerative period. Other system diseases such as diabetes often affect the sensory organs and can destroy their ability to function. Some of the most common disorders of the eyes include myopia, presbyopia, hyperopia, diabetic retinopathy, cataracts, and glaucoma. The most common diseases of the ear include tinnitus, otitis media, conduction loss, otosclerosis, and Ménière's disease. In the older adult, sensory organ disorders are common. Some losses of vision and hearing occur naturally through the aging process, whereas others are a result of other system diseases. Diagnosis and treatment of vision and hearing losses should be implemented early to prevent some of the complications of sensory dysfunction.

## REVIEW QUESTIONS

### Short Answer

1. What are some of the most common problems affecting the eyes?

2. What are some of the most common problems affecting the ears?

3. What diagnostic tests are used to diagnose or evaluate eye disorders?

4. What diagnostic tests are used to diagnose or evaluate ear disorders?

### Fill in the Blanks

5. _____ is the chronic inflammation of the eyelid.
6. The lay term for _____ is "pinkeye."
7. Extreme sensitivity to light is called _____.
8. Another term for nearsightedness is _____.
9. Farsightedness is also called _____.
10. A common eye disorder that occurs with aging is called _____.
11. The main symptom of a cataract is the gradual _____ of vision.
12. In _____, aqueous humor is produced faster than it can be drained.
13. Sudden flashes or spots before the eyes may be a sign of _____.
14. Flushing the eye with large amounts of water is the best immediate treatment for a _____ of the eye.
15. The cranial nerves that control the muscles of eye movement include _____, _____, and _____.

**16.** Within the ear, the organ of hearing is the _____.

**17.** The major symptom of ear disorders is _____.

**18.** Buzzing or ringing in the ear(s) is called _____.

**19.** Pediatric ear tubes may be placed through the tympanic membrane during a procedure called _____.

**20.** _____ is also commonly called "swimmer's ear."

**21.** The most common cause of a progressive hearing loss is _____.

**22.** The surgical treatment for progressive otosclerosis is a _____.

**23.** Vertigo is the common complaint of an individual with _____.

**24.** The slow but gradual loss of hearing common in the older adult is called _____.

**25.** Chronic otitis media may result in perforation of the _____.

## CASE STUDY

**Ms. Tesar** is a 52-year-old woman who has been doing intricate needlework for years. She has exhibited her work in many fairs and received awards for the unique self-created patterns. While having lunch with her one day, she confides that she is having difficulty seeing the eye of the needle while trying to thread it. She is also having some difficulty drawing the minute details of the patterns. She has noticed, however, that she can see a little better if she holds the needle out away from her while threading it rather than holding it close, as she was used to doing. Having just completed a unit on vision and hearing disorders in your Human Disease course, you think you can explain what is probably occurring with Ms. Tesar's eyesight. What would you tell her about this problem? How do you explain the natural changes that occur with aging? Would you recommend she make an appointment to have her eyes checked?

## BIBLIOGRAPHY

Antioxidants and eyesight. (2004). *Better Nutrition 66*(2), 24.

Brooks, Y. (2003, December 5). It's a wrap. *Times Educational Supplement, 4561,* 8–10.

Charters, L. (2004). Radial scleral ablation trial promising for presbyopia. *Ophthalmology Times, 29*(19), 68–69.

Ear, nose, & throat. (2002, July 22). *US News & World Report 133*(3), 80.

Eyes. (2003, July 28). *US News & World Report 135*(3), 120.

Ferri, R. S. (2003). Good news for "lazy eyes". *American Journal of Nursing 103*(9), 120.

Garcia, L. J., Metthe, L., Paradis, J., & Joanette, Y. (2001). Relevance is in the eye and ear of the beholder: An example from populations with a neurological impairment. *Aphasiology 15*(1), 17–38.

McGurk, V. (2003). Screening for retinopathy of prematurity. *Paediatric Nursing 15*(10), 29–32.

Quinn, L. (2002). Mechanisms in the development of type 2 diabetes mellitus. *Journal of Cardiovascular Nursing 16*(2), 1–15.

Shute, N. (2003, December 5). Seeing straight. *US News & World Report 135*(22), 58.

Sight for sore eyes. (2003). *Vegetarian Times 313,* 16.

Sulica, L., & Berhman, A. (2003). Management of benign vocal fold lesions: A survey of current opinion and practice. *Annals of Otology, Rhinology & Laryngology 112*(10), 827–833.

Zeitels, S. M., & Healy, G. (2003, August 28). Laryngology and phonosurgery. *New England Journal of Medicine 349*(9), 882–892.

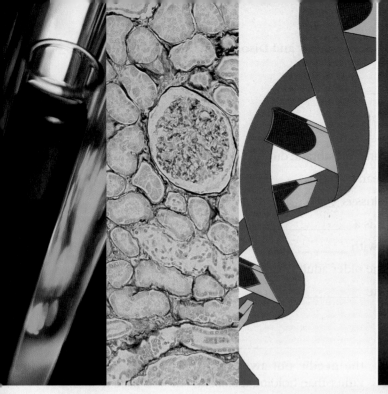
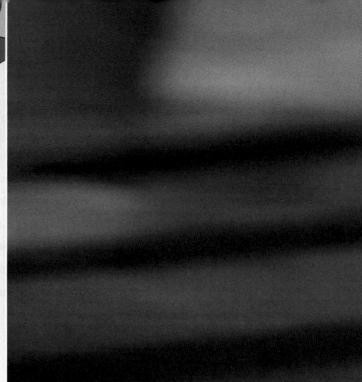

## OUTLINE

- **Anatomy and Physiology**
  *Female Anatomy and Physiology*
  *Male Anatomy and Physiology*

- **Common Signs and Symptoms**

- **Diagnostic Tests**

- **Common Diseases of the Reproductive System**
  *Female Reproductive System Diseases*
  *Diseases of the Breast*
  *Disorders of Pregnancy*
  *Male Reproductive System Diseases*
  *Sexually Transmitted Diseases (STDs)*
  *Sexual Dysfunction*

- **Trauma**
  *Rape*

- **Rare Diseases**
  *Vaginal Cancer*
  *Puerperal Sepsis*
  *Hydatidiform Mole*

- **Effects of Aging on the System**

- **Summary**

- **Review Questions**

- **Case Study**

- **Bibliography**

## KEY TERMS

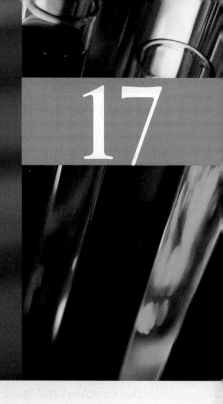

# Reproductive System Diseases and Disorders

**17**

## LEARNING OBJECTIVES

*Upon completion of the chapter, the learner should be able to:*

1. Define the terminology common to the reproductive system and the disorders of the system.

2. Discuss the basic anatomy and physiology of the reproductive system.

3. Identify the important signs and symptoms associated with common reproductive system disorders.

4. Describe the common diagnostics used to determine the type and/or cause of reproductive system disorders.

5. Identify common disorders of the reproductive system.

6. Describe the typical course and management of the common reproductive system disorders.

7. Describe the effects of aging on the reproductive system and the common disorders of the system.

## OVERVIEW

The reproductive system is a complex system of structures with a variety of physiologic functions. Some parts of the reproductive system are endocrine glands (ovaries and testes) whereas other parts are strictly involved in procreation for a time during the individual's life span. Disorders of the system are common at all ages, and may range from mild to severe, especially if not diagnosed early in the development of the disorder. Changes in the system during the aging process have both physiological and psychosocial implications. ∎

## ANATOMY AND PHYSIOLOGY

The reproductive system is quite different between the male and female. Although the anatomy and physiologic features have a few commonalities, there are enough differences to discuss them separately.

## Female Anatomy and Physiology

The female reproductive system consists of external structures and include the vulva, labia majora, labia minora, clitoris, vestibule, hymen, vaginal orifice, and vestibular glands. Internal structures include the ovaries, fallopian tubes, uterus, cervix, and vagina (Figure 17–1). The ovaries secrete the female sex hormones estrogen and progesterone. The ovaries produce ova, the reproductive cells, within the graafian follicles (microscopic sacs). After a follicle releases an ovum, it develops into a corpus luteum. This structure is created by the luteinizing hormone from the pituitary gland. The corpus luteum secretes estrogen and progesterone. The fallopian tubes are ducts that carry the ova (eggs) from the ovaries to the uterus.

The uterus is a pear-shaped muscular structure lying above the bladder in the pelvis. It is only about two inches by three inches in the nonpregnant state.

The lower part of the uterus is called the cervix (neck). The inner layer of the uterus is the endometrium. During menstruation, part of this layer is sloughed off and passed through the vagina and vaginal orifice. The vagina is the structure that receives the penis during intercourse and also becomes the birth canal during delivery of the fetus.

The hormones secreted by the ovaries are estrogens and progesterone. Secretion occurs in response to the effects of the follicle-stimulating hormone (FSH) and the luteinizing hormone (LH) produced by the anterior pituitary gland. Estrogen affects the development of secondary sex characteristics (characteristics occurring at puberty), changes in the endometrium, and growth of the uterus and vagina. Progesterone affects the development of the endometrium, assists the development of the placenta, causes enlargement of the breasts during pregnancy, prevents ova from being produced during pregnancy, and assists in the development of cells in the mammary glands.

The menstrual cycle is the process of secretion of hormones, the preparation of the endometrium for the implantation of the fertilized egg, and if the egg is not implanted, the sloughing of the layer with bleeding from torn capillaries. The cycle runs for about 28 days, but varies among individuals. The start of the menstrual flow is the first day of the

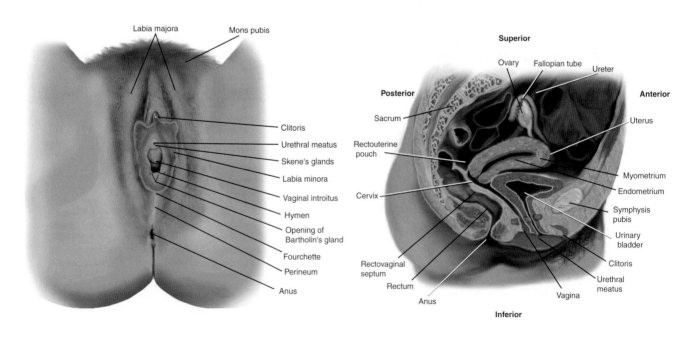

External genitalia.

Cross-section of internal structures.

**FIGURE 17–1**   The female reproductive system.

cycle and usually lasts about four to five days. After that, estrogen is secreted until the graafian follicle matures and ruptures, about halfway through the cycle. Progesterone is then secreted by the corpus luteum. As the corpus luteum ages, progesterone levels go down, causing menses and the beginning of the next cycle. Pregnancy will sustain progesterone levels maintaining the endometrium. The menstrual cycle may begin in females as young as 10 years of age, but typically begins at age 11 to 12. The ceasing of the cycle is called menopause. This usually occurs between ages 40 to 50, but varies with the individual.

The female breasts are located between the second and seventh ribs over the pectoralis major muscle of the chest. Breasts are usually almost symmetrical and may be small or very large, depending on the individual's structure, body weight, and other factors. Endocrine secretions during menstruation and pregnancy affect the breast size and composition. The breasts show little sign of development until puberty. Over a two- to three-year period, the breasts change from the flattened preadolescent stage to full breast maturity. As the female enters menopause, the breasts begin to atrophy and become more relaxed with a reduction in size.

The female breasts consist of three types of tissue: glandular, fibrous, and fat (adipose). The structure of the breast includes the nipple, areola, lactiferous ducts, lobules lined with milk-producing glands called acini, and fibrous dividers or septa. The breast also contains a network of lymph glands that drains the lymph and returns it to the circulatory system.

## Male Anatomy and Physiology

The male reproductive system includes the external organs, scrotum and penis, and the internal organs, testes, epididymis, vas deferens, urethra, seminal vesicles, bulbourethral glands, and the prostate (Figure 17–2). The penis houses the urethra, a tube that carries urine from the bladder and semen from the ejaculatory duct. At the tip of the penis is the prepuce or foreskin. The penis is composed of erectile tissue and arteries that dilate during sexual arousal. This causes the penis to become erect for the purpose of intercourse. The scrotum is a sac that hangs below the penis and holds the testes. The testes secrete testosterone (the male sex hormone) and produce sperm (the reproductive cells). Testosterone is responsible for changes occurring during puberty and secondary sex characteristics in the male.

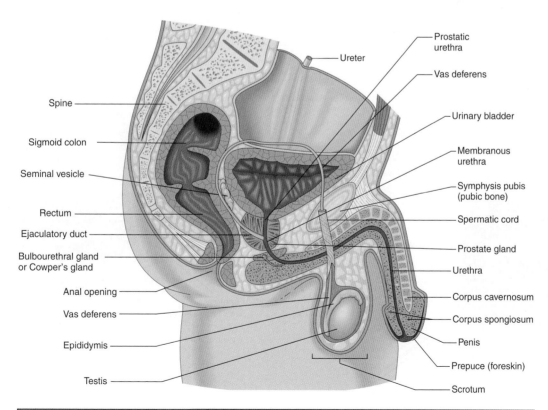

**FIGURE 17–2** The male reproductive system.

The epididymis is the duct leading from each testis to the vas deferens, the excretory duct. The vas deferens from each testis extends up into the abdomen where it connects to create the ejaculatory duct that opens into the urethra. The seminal vesicles sit behind the bladder near the neck. They secrete fluid that is part of the thick, white secretion called semen. The prostate gland and bulbourethral glands also secrete fluid that becomes part of the semen.

## COMMON SIGNS AND SYMPTOMS

Common signs and symptoms of female reproductive system diseases and disorders include:

- abdominal and pelvic pain
- fever and malaise
- abnormal vaginal drainage
- burning and/or itching of the genitals
- pain during sexual intercourse
- any change in breast tissue
- abnormal discharge from the nipple

Common signs and symptoms of male reproductive system diseases and disorders include:

- urinary disorders including frequency, dysuria, nocturia, and incontinence
- pain in the pelvis, groin, or reproductive organs
- lesions on the external genitalia
- swelling or abnormal enlargement of the reproductive organs
- abnormal penile drainage
- burning and/or itching of the genitals

## DIAGNOSTIC TESTS

Physical examination of the female reproductive system to aid in diagnosis of diseases begins with a pelvic examination. This exam includes inspection of the external genitalia, visual examination of the vagina and cervix through a speculum or instrument used to spread and hold the vaginal wall in an open position (Figure 17–3), and palpation of female internal organs by **bimanual examination**. A bimanual (two-handed) examination is so named because the

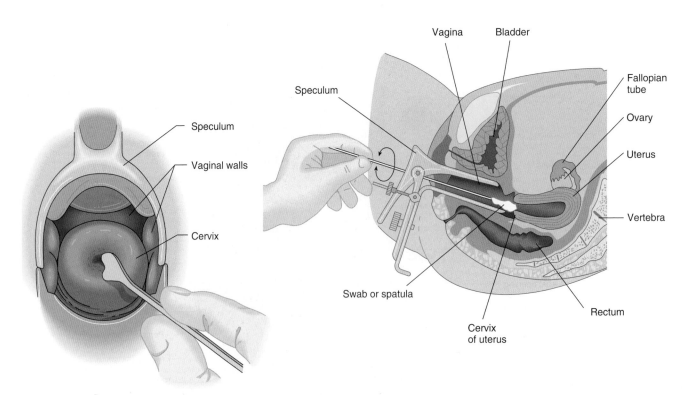

**FIGURE 17–3** Use of a speculum and obtaining a Pap smear.

physician places one hand on the abdomen and inserts fingers of the other hand into the vagina to feel the female organs between the two hands. A bimanual rectal examination allows palpation of the posterior aspect of the uterus and the rectum.

The most common test of the female reproductive system is the Papanicolaou (Pap smear) of the cervix (see Figure 17–3). Pap smears are **cytologic** (sigh-toe-LAWG-ic; cyto = cell, logic = study) examinations to discover cervical cancer. If an abnormal Pap smear is obtained, follow up may involve a cervical biopsy. A cervical biopsy entails taking a small piece of tissue from the cervix for microscopic examination. A special type of biopsy, called a cone biopsy, refers to taking a cone-shaped piece of cervical tissue including the cervical os and endocervical lining. The diagnosis of endometrial cancer is best discovered by obtaining tissue for biopsy during a **dilatation and curettage** (KYOU-reh-**TAHZH**) or **(D&C)**. This procedure involves a light surgical sedative, dilation of the cervix (dilatation), and scraping (curettage) of the uterine endometrial tissue. D&C is also commonly performed for abnormal uterine bleeding and following a spontaneous abortion.

A **laparoscopy** (LAP-ah-**ROS**-ko-pee; laparo = abdomen, scopy = scope procedure), or looking inside the abdominal cavity with a lighted scope (Figure 17–4), is commonly used to view the female organs for abnormalities, to diagnose endometrio-

sis, and perform a tubal ligation. To determine the size, position, and patency of the uterus and fallopian tubes, a **hysterosalpingogram** (hystero = uterus, salpingo = fallopian tubes, gram = picture) or X-ray of these organs may be obtained. During a hysterosalpingogram, a small tube is passed through the cervix and a radiopaque dye is injected. As the dye fills the uterus and fallopian tubes, and spills into the abdominal cavity, X-rays are taken to show patency or openness of the tubes. This procedure is commonly done as part of infertility testing.

Laboratory tests to determine reproductive diseases include microscopic examination, and culture and sensitivity of secretions or drainage from the vagina and genital lesions to determine the presence of infection. Blood tests to measure hormone levels including estrogen and progesterone are also common. Other blood testing includes **VDRL (Venereal Disease Research Laboratory)** and **RPR (Rapid Plasma Reagin)** test for syphilis.

**Mammography** (mam-OG-rah-fee; mammo = breast, ography = procedure to take a picture) is an X-ray or radiologic examination of breast tissue (Figure 17–5) to determine the presence of cysts or tumors. If an abnormal mass is discovered, further diagnostic techniques include fine needle aspiration and incisional biopsy.

Ultrasound may be performed on the pelvis to determine the presence of tumors and pregnancy, and to visualize pelvic organ position and size. Benign breast cysts may be differentiated from solid tumors by ultrasonography.

Physical examination of the male reproductive system includes visual examination of the external genitalia for tumors, lesions, or penile drainage. The testes are palpated to determine presence of tumors. A **digital rectal examination** allows the physician to feel the prostate (Figure 17–6) for abnormal enlargement (hypertrophy or hyperplasia) and tumors.

A **cystoscopy** (sis-TOS-koh-pee; cysto = bladder, oscopy = scope procedure) is performed to view the urethra and bladder with a lighted scope. This procedure allows the physician to evaluate the size of the prostate and the degree of obstruction the gland is placing on the urethra.

Biopsy of the male reproductive organs commonly involves the prostate and the testicle. Both procedures are performed to determine malignancy. To obtain a prostatic biopsy, a fine needle is guided through the rectum and into the prostate. A testicular biopsy involves the use of local anesthetic and a

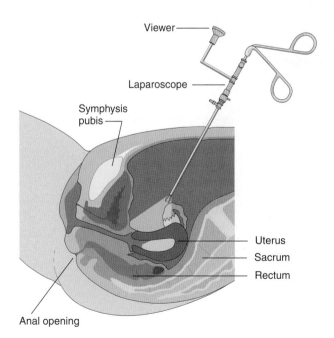

**FIGURE 17–4** Laparoscopy.

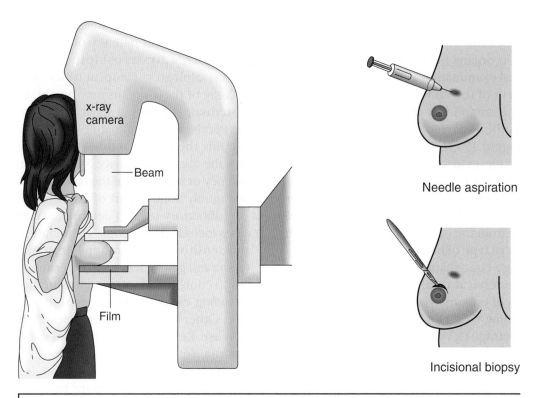

**FIGURE 17–5** Mammography, needle aspiration, and incisional biopsy.

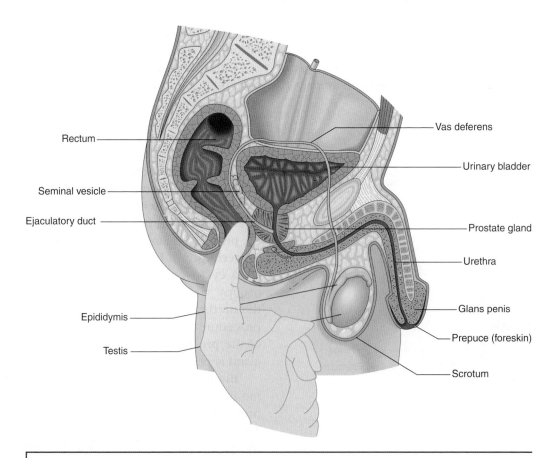

**FIGURE 17–6** Digital rectal examination.

fine needle to withdraw a small piece of tissue. Testicular biopsy also may be used to evaluate sperm production.

Laboratory tests utilized in the determination of diseases of the male reproductive system include cultures and sensitivities of penile drainage, lesions, and urine to determine the presence of infection. A blood test called a prostate specific antigen (PSA) is helpful in the detection of prostate cancer. PSA levels also assist in determining effectiveness of prostate cancer treatment. Urine estrogen levels may assist in the diagnosis of testicular cancers.

Specific laboratory tests utilized for infertility testing include microscopic examination of semen to perform a sperm count, check sperm viability or ability to survive, and look for abnormally shaped sperm. Blood tests for the hormones testosterone and LH are also utilized.

# COMMON DISEASES OF THE REPRODUCTIVE SYSTEM

Common diseases of the reproductive system involve those affecting both sexes including the pregnant female. These diseases are divided into female reproductive system diseases, diseases of the breast, disorders of pregnancy, male reproductive system diseases, sexually transmitted diseases, and sexual dysfunction.

## Female Reproductive System Diseases

The female reproductive system is affected by numerous diseases and disorders caused by inflammation, infection, tumors, cysts, and hormonal imbalances. Diseases may range from mild to life threatening. Common symptoms include pain and abnormalities in the menstrual cycle.

### ■ Premenstrual Syndrome (PMS)

Premenstrual syndrome, commonly called PMS, is a group of symptoms occurring prior to the onset of menses.

**ETIOLOGY** The cause of PMS is uncertain, but research has shown an increase in PMS with rapid hormonal changes in estrogen levels that occur during the menstrual cycle. The fact that PMS only occurs in ovulating females lends support to this cause. Other causes may be related to vitamin defi-

ciencies and psychologic disturbances. In the past, PMS was thought to be entirely due to emotional factors and stress, but it is now known to have a true physical cause.

**SYMPTOMS** Symptoms of PMS usually begin midcycle with ovulation and increase in severity until a few hours after the onset of menses. PMS symptoms can affect virtually every system of the body and include headache, nausea, and back and joint pain. There is an increase in water retention that may cause edema, bloating, weight gain, breast tenderness, and engorgement. Psychological symptoms may include irritability, mood swings, depression, and sleep disturbances. Symptoms of PMS vary significantly from one individual to another. It is unknown why some females have severe, disabling PMS whereas others are virtually unaffected.

**TREATMENT** Due to the variation in symptoms, treatment must be individualized as affected individuals have differing symptoms and respond differently to treatment. Dietary changes may be helpful and include avoidance of caffeine, chocolate, nicotine, sugar, salt, and alcohol. Developing a regular exercise program of brisk walking or swimming may be of benefit. Medications may be helpful and include the hormone progesterone, diuretics, and analgesics.

### ■ Menstrual Abnormalities

Menstrual abnormalities are a common problem in the ovulating female.

**ETIOLOGY** Causes of menstrual abnormalities vary, as does treatment. Common abnormalities include amenorrhea, dysmenorrhea, menorrhagia, and metrorrhagia. A short description of these disorders follows.

■ Amenorrhea (ah-MEN-oh-**REE**-ah; a = without, menorrhea = menstruation) is the absence of menstrual periods. If menses has not occurred by age 18, it is considered to be primary amenorrhea and may be caused by hormonal disorders, malformation or absence of female organs, pregnancy, or anorexia. Secondary amenorrhea is the absence of menses for six months or more in a female who has had regular cycles.

**ETIOLOGY** Causes include hormonal imbalance, emotional upset, depression, malnutrition, excessive fitness training, ovarian tumor, and pregnancy. Diagnosis is made on the basis of a physical examination, and hormonal blood and urine studies.

**TREATMENT** Treatment depends on cause. If no abnormalities are present, hormone administration will usually begin the menstrual cycle in primary amenorrhea. Preventive measures include adequate nutrition, exercise, and stress reduction.

■ Dysmenorrhea (DIS-men-oh-**REE**-ah; dys = difficult, menorrhea = menses) is painful or difficult menses, and is one of the most common gynecologic disorders.

**ETIOLOGY** Causes of dysmenorrhea include pelvic infections, cervical stenosis, endometriosis, and unknown causes.

**SYMPTOMS** Symptoms include dull to severe cramping pain in the pelvic area and low back pain. Pain also may radiate into the upper back, thighs, and genitalia. Pain associated with cervical stenosis and endometriosis often occurs in females prior to childbearing, and is often relieved after the birth of a child. Prognosis is good if the cause can be found and treated.

**TREATMENT** Oral contraceptives may be effective in reducing dysmenorrhea as they regulate and decrease menstrual flow. Nonsteroidal anti-inflammatory medications are helpful in reducing inflammation and pain. Application of a heating pad to the pelvic area also may be helpful.

■ Menorrhagia (MEN-oh-**RAY**-jee-ah; meno = menses, orrhagia = bursting forth, abnormal, excessive) is excessive or prolonged menstrual flow.

**ETIOLOGY** Cause may be due to uterine tumors, pelvic inflammatory disease, and hormone imbalances.

**TREATMENT** Treatment is related to cause and may include surgery to remove tumors, antibiotics to treat pelvic inflammatory disease, and hormone therapy for hormone imbalances.

■ Metrorrhagia (MET-roh-**RAY**-jee-ah; metro = uterus, orrhagia = bursting forth, abnormal, excessive) is abnormal bleeding between menstrual periods.

**ETIOLOGY** The cause is commonly due to hormonal imbalance, leading to an abnormal thickening and shedding of the endometrial tissue.

**TREATMENT** Treatment may be a D&C, returning the endometrium to normal and ending metrorrhagia.

## ■ Endometriosis

**ETIOLOGY** Endometriosis (EN-doh-ME-tree-**OH**-sis; endo = inside, metri = uterus, osis = condition of) is the abnormal growth of endometrial tissue outside the uterus. Endometrial tissue may flow retrograde during menses, and escape into the abdominopelvic cavity through the fallopian tubes, or even worse, this tissue may escape into the blood supply and be carried to sites all over the body.

The cause of retrograde flow is unknown, but use of tampons may be a causative factor. For this reason, the use of tampons is discouraged. Common sites of endometrial implantation include the ovaries, fallopian tubes, abdominal wall, and intestine. Other sites of implantation include the urinary bladder, the diaphragm, nerves and ligaments of the back, and the vulva to name only a few (Figure 17–7). This endometrial tissue continues to act under the influence of hormones, thickening and bleeding with menstrual cycles. This action causes irritation and inflammation of normal tissue surrounding the implanted endometrial tissue, thus causing the development of a special blood-filled cyst called "chocolate cyst," scar tissue, and adhesions.

**SYMPTOMS** This bleeding of endometrial tissue in the abdominopelvic cavity and other **ectopic** (eck-

---

## COMPLEMENTARY AND ALTERNATIVE THERAPY

**Using Unkei-to for Infertility**

Several Chinese herbal medicines have been used to treat ovarian dysfunction. Unkei-to is one of those products with few side effects. It has been shown to be effective in stimulating the pituitary-ovarian cycle to help correct infertility in young women. It is also used to treat menstrual disorders and abnormal uterine bleeding.

*Source: Ushiroyama, T. (2003).*

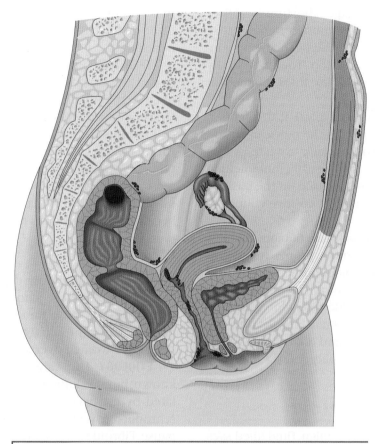

**FIGURE 17–7** Endometriosis—common sites of endometrial implants.

TOP-ick, out of normal place) areas causes **dysmenorrhea** (DIS-men-oh-**REE**-ah; dys = painful, menorrhea = menses), beginning a few days before menses and extending several days into the menstrual cycle. There may be a constant cramping pain in the low back, pelvis, and vagina. Affected individuals, usually females of childbearing age, also may have heavy menses and **dyspareunia** (DIS-pah-**ROO**-knee-ah; painful sexual intercourse).

The primary complication of endometriosis is infertility. Other complications include ectopic pregnancy and spontaneous abortion. Diagnosis is made on the basis of history and pelvic examination. A laparoscopy will confirm the diagnosis and allow visualization of the extent of the condition.

**TREATMENT** Treatment depends on affected individual's age and desire to have children. Young females wishing to have children should not delay childbearing. Treatment with various hormonal medications

may be helpful in younger individuals. Pregnancy, nursing, and menopause will not cure the condition, but do cause a remission in symptoms as the abnormal tissue shrinks when menstrual hormones are halted. In severe cases, a total or **panhysterectomy** (removal of ovaries, fallopian tubes, and uterus) may be indicated.

## ■ Pelvic Inflammatory Disease (PID)

Pelvic inflammatory disease is an inflammation of some or all of the pelvic reproductive organs. It may be mild to severe, and may involve the cervix (**cervicitis**), the inner lining of the uterus (**endometritis**), fallopian tubes (**salpingitis**), and ovaries (**oophoritis**).

**ETIOLOGY** This inflammation is commonly due to infection by bacteria that ascend from the vagina and travel upward to the pelvic cavity. Bacteria can be introduced into the female reproductive system during childbirth, miscarriage, abortion, or other gynecologic procedures. The most common cause of PID is sexually transmitted disease including gonorrhea and chlamydial infection. Young, sexually active females, and those who use IUDs, are most at risk of developing PID.

**SYMPTOMS** Symptoms are typical of an infection and include fever, chills, pain in the pelvic area, and **leukorrhea** (LOO-koh-**REE**-ah; leuk = white, orrhea = flow or discharge), a white, usually foul-smelling vaginal discharge. Diagnosis is made on the basis of a pelvic examination including a positive culture of vaginal discharge.

**TREATMENT** Treatment includes antibiotic therapy, analgesics, and bed rest. Without proper treatment, the infection may become bloodborne, **septicemia** (SEP-tih-**SEE**-me-ah; septic = dirty or contaminated, emia = blood), and may be life threatening. Inflammation of the reproductive organs may lead to the development of scar tissue and adhesions. These adhesions may cause the complications of infertility and ectopic pregnancy.

## ■ Ovarian Cyst

Ovarian cysts are commonly benign, fluid-filled sacs on or near the ovary (Figure 17–8).

**ETIOLOGY** There are two types of cysts: physiologic or those caused by a normally functioning ovary, and neoplastic, an abnormal type not related to the function of the ovary. Physiologic cysts are the most common and may become very large (grapefruit size) before producing symptoms.

**SYMPTOMS** Symptoms include low back pain, pelvic pain, and dyspareunia. Acute, extreme pain, nausea and vomiting may occur if the ovary becomes

twisted due to the weight of the cyst. Diagnosis is made on the basis of history, pelvic examination, and ultrasound.

**TREATMENT** Treatment depends on the type and size of the cyst. Small physiologic cysts usually do not need treatment and often resolve spontaneously. Oral contraceptive medication may be given for several months to help resolve physiologic tumors of various sizes. Large cysts or those of questionable type are often viewed by laparoscopy. During laparoscopy, the cyst may be removed or drained. Determination should be made as to the type of cyst because cancerous cysts need immediate treatment.

## ■ Fibroid Tumor

Leiomyomas, commonly called fibroid tumors, are benign tumors of the smooth muscle of the uterus (Figure 17–9). These tumors are the most common of the female reproductive system, occurring in one out of five women over age 35.

**ETIOLOGY** The cause of fibroid tumors is unknown, but it is known that these tumors are stimulated by estrogen, and thus tend to occur during reproductive years and regress or calcify after menopause. Fibroid tumors often appear in multiples and vary in size from small to quite large. Small fibroids are often asymptomatic.

**SYMPTOMS** Symptoms include abnormal uterine bleeding, excessive menstrual bleeding, and pain. Diagnosis is made on the basis of pelvic examination and ultrasound.

**TREATMENT** Treatment depends on the individual's age and desire for childbearing. Fibroids may be removed surgically, but in older individuals, a hysterectomy is often the treatment of choice.

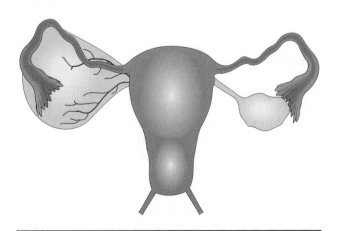

**FIGURE 17–8** Ovarian cyst.

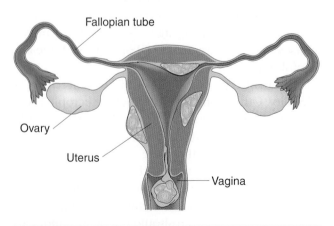

**FIGURE 17–9** Fibroid tumors.

## ■ Vaginitis

Vaginitis (VAJ-ih-**NIGH**-tis) is inflammation of the vagina.

**ETIOLOGY** It is a very common disease caused by a variety of microorganisms. Vaginitis is not dangerous but is irritating, uncomfortable, and often leads to a bladder infection.

**SYMPTOMS** Symptoms of vaginitis are burning, itching, and swelling of the vagina and external genitalia. A white "cottage cheese" appearing discharge is common with *Candida* vaginitis. Diagnosis is usually confirmed by microscopic examination of vaginal secretions, revealing the presence of the infecting organism. The most common types of vaginitis include:

1. *Candida* vaginitis—a type of fungus or yeast vaginitis. *Candida* normally cohabitates with lactobacillus bacteria in the vagina, maintaining vaginal normal flora (see Chapter 4 for more details on normal flora).

   **ETIOLOGY** If the balance between the candida and the lactobacillus is disturbed, the affected individual develops a *Candida* vaginitis. *Candida* vaginitis is the most common type of vaginitis and is commonly called a "yeast infection." To maintain a healthy vaginal normal flora, sufficient estrogen must be produced. Estrogen enhances the growth of lactobacilli, a beneficial, normal flora bacteria. Lactobacilli aids in the production of lactic acid, causing a lower vaginal pH of 4 or 4.5. This acid environment is also a deterrent to the growth of harmful microorganisms. Use of tampons, diaphragms, condoms, spermacides, vaginal douche, and deodorant sprays may easily upset the normal flora of the vagina and lead to vaginitis. Antibiotic use commonly kills lactobacilli and may lead to severe vaginitis. Candida infection is usually not spread by sexual transmission except in severe cases.

   **TREATMENT** Treatment is insertion of a miconazole tablet or cream into the vagina, or oral antifungal medication.

2. **Trichomonas** (TRICK-oh-**MOH**-nas) vaginitis— **ETIOLOGY** a parasite vaginitis that is commonly transmitted during sexual intercourse.

   **TREATMENT** In the case of *Trichomonas* vaginitis, both sexual partners must be treated with an oral antiparasitic medication to eradicate the infection.

3. Atrophic vaginitis—**ETIOLOGY** commonly occurs postmenopausal and is caused by a decrease in secretion of estrogen. Estrogen is needed to maintain the vaginal lining. Without adequate supply, the lining becomes more susceptible to infection.

   **TREATMENT** Treatment often includes estrogen therapy and the use of adequate lubrication during sexual intercourse to avoid injury to the vaginal lining.

## ■ Toxic Shock Syndrome

Toxic shock syndrome (TSS) is a severe, life-threatening illness. TSS is found almost exclusively in menstruating females using tampons.

**ETIOLOGY** It is thought to be caused by *Staphylococcus aureus*, a normal flora bacterium of the skin. This bacterium produces an increased amount of toxin when in contact with the synthetic fibers found in tampons.

**SYMPTOMS** Symptoms include the sudden onset of high fever, vomiting, diarrhea, and a dropping blood pressure. Diagnosis is made on the basis of history of tampon use and symptoms.

**TREATMENT** Treatment includes intravenous fluids to counteract shock and antibiotics to treat the infection. Untreated or delayed treatment may be fatal. Prevention is good hand washing prior to tampon insertion to decrease the number of bacteria on the individual's hands. Tampons should be changed frequently (every two to three hours) to prevent infection.

## ■ Menopause

Menopause is the natural halting of menstruation.

**ETIOLOGY** It is not a disease but rather a normal physical change related to aging. Many women consider menopause a disorder because they commonly have physical and psychological symptoms. Menopause usually takes place between the ages of 45 and 55 years. As a female ages, the ovaries produce less estrogen, causing cessation of ovulation and menstruation. This process can be surgically induced by removal of both ovaries (bilateral oophorectomy).

**SYMPTOMS** Common physical symptoms of menopause include hot flashes, night sweats, and vaginal dryness. Some women also experience psychological symptoms of depression, sleep disorders, and decreased libido or sex drive. Hormonal changes brought about by menopause increase a woman's risk of cardiac disease and osteoporosis.

**TREATMENT** Hormone replacement therapy has been the treatment of choice for more than 60 years for prevention of hot flashes and vaginal dryness in menopausal women. In the mid-1980s, estrogen also was approved as preventive treatment of heart disease and osteoporosis.

More recently, in 2002, a federally funded Women's Health Initiative (WHI) prematurely halted a hormone study finding that hormone therapy did not protect against heart disease, and actually led to a slight increase in risk of heart attacks, breast cancer, strokes, and blood clots. This same study reported benefits of reduced risk of bone fractures and colon cancer in women using hormone replacement.

Since the release of the above study, there continues to be many unanswered questions and much confusion about hormone therapy. Benefits of hormone replacement include relief or prevention of hot flashes and vaginal dryness, and decreased risk of bone fractures and colon cancer. The question is whether these benefits outweigh the risk of heart attack, breast cancer, stroke, and blood clots. Each individual has different risk levels depending on a variety of factors including family history, individual health history, the amount of hormone medication prescribed, and the length of time this medication is taken.

As with all medications, the decision to use hormone therapy is an individual one, based on review of the individual woman's health needs. The decision should be made only after detailed discussion with the physician regarding the risks and benefits of therapy. For more information, search www.hormone.org.

### ◼ Uterine Prolapse

Uterine prolapse occurs when the uterus drops or protrudes downward into the vagina. There are varying degrees of prolapse (Figure 17–10).

**ETIOLOGY** Prolapse is commonly due to aging and childbirth as these weaken the pelvic floor muscles.

**SYMPTOMS** Symptoms include heaviness in the pelvic area, urinary stress incontinence or dysuria, and low back pain. With a complete prolapse, one can easily see the uterus bulging out of the vaginal opening. Although quite uncomfortable, this condition is not an emergency or even a health risk unless there is bleeding or an inability to urinate. Diagnosis is made on the basis of a pelvic examination.

**TREATMENT** A hysterectomy is often the surgical treatment of choice, depending on the woman's age and desire to bear children.

### ◼ Cystocele

Cystocele (SIS-toh-seel; cysto = urinary bladder, cele = hernia) is the herniation or protrusion of the urinary bladder through the anterior vaginal wall (Figure 17–11).

**ETIOLOGY** This condition is often due to weakening of or trauma to the pelvic muscles related to aging and childbirth.

**SYMPTOMS** Symptoms include pelvic pressure, urinary urgency, frequency, and incontinence. Diagnosis is made on the basis of a pelvic examination.

**TREATMENT** Treatment depends on the degree of herniation. Strengthening the pelvic floor muscles with exercise may be of benefit. The specific exercise (Kegel exercise) is performed by contracting the pelvic floor muscles (this group of muscles is tightened to cut off urine flow) and releasing the muscles several times a day. If the cystocele is large or exercise is ineffective, surgery (anterior colporrhaphy) may be necessary.

### ◼ Rectocele

Rectocele is the herniation or protrusion of the rectum through the posterior vaginal wall (see Figure 17–11).

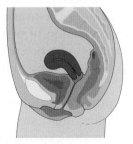 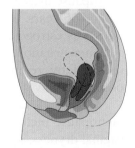 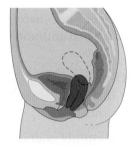 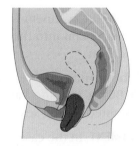

| Normal uterus | First degree prolapse | Second degree prolapse | Third degree prolapse |

**FIGURE 17–10** Uterine prolapse—varying degrees.

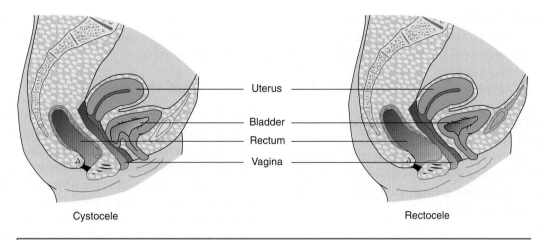

Uterus
Bladder
Rectum
Vagina

Cystocele

Rectocele

**FIGURE 17–11** Cystocele and rectocele.

**ETIOLOGY** This condition, like a cystocele, is due to trauma to this area during childbirth.

**SYMPTOMS** Symptoms include discomfort, constipation, and fecal incontinence. Diagnosis is made on the basis of a physical examination.

**TREATMENT** Treatment is commonly surgical repair (posterior colpoplasty). Often, the affected individual needs both a cystocele repair and a rectocele repair. This surgery is called an anterior-posterior or A&P repair.

## ■ Cervical Cancer

Cervical cancer is the fifth leading cause of cancer-related death in females. This cancer usually begins with **carcinoma in situ** or neoplastic cells that "sit" on the basement membrane, and have not invaded into deeper tissue. As the cancer progresses, ulceration and cervical bleeding occur.

**ETIOLOGY** Human papillomavirus (HPV) has been determined to be the cause of essentially all cervical cancer. There are over 60 types of HPV. Some types cause warts on the hands and feet of children whereas other types cause genital warts. Several types of HPV do not cause warts but cause changes to the cells in the cervix, leading to cervical cancer.

HPV is generally obtained through sexual contact. Condoms cannot prevent the spread of HPV because it is found on all genital tissues of the infected individual. Males and females are usually asymptomatic with HPV infection. Discovery of HPV is usually made when cervical changes are found with a Pap smear. It is very difficult to trace exposure to the virus because it can lay dormant on the cervix for 20 years before it causes changes to the

cells of the cervix. Activities that increase risk of HPV infection include:

■ Beginning sexual intercourse at an early age. This activity generally results in an increase in the number of sex partners over the individual's lifetime.

■ Having multiple sexual partners. Studies show that approximately 40 percent of young sexually active females carry HPV in their vaginas. Presumably, a similar percentage of males are infected.

One fact in support of these identified risk factors is that females who abstain from sexual intercourse throughout life do not get cervical cancer.

HPV infection does not cause cervical cancer in all females. Most women who have evidence of HPV on their cervix never get cervical cancer. Studies suggest that whether a female will develop cervical cancer depends on a variety of factors acting together with HPV infection. These factors include:

■ decreased resistance to infection

■ smoking—women who smoke concentrate nicotine into their cervix, which harms the cells

■ sexual intercourse with males who smoke—men also concentrate nicotine into their genital secretions, and can bathe the cervix with these chemicals during intercourse

■ marriage to a male whose previous spouse was diagnosed with cervical cancer—females married to men whose former spouse was diagnosed with cervical cancer are at greater risk of also developing cervical cancer

■ obesity

■ excessive alcohol consumption

**SYMPTOMS** Development of cervical cancer is usually slow and symptoms of abnormal cervical bleeding are easily noticed, leading to early detection of this form of cancer.

Diagnosis of cervical cancer is made on the basis of a Pap smear.

**TREATMENT** Treatment is usually surgical removal of the tumor. If metastasis has occurred, surgery is often followed by radiation therapy. If the tumor has spread into adjacent tissues, a complete hysterectomy may be performed. Untreated, the tumor becomes inoperable and fatal.

### ■ Uterine Cancer

Uterine cancer develops in the inner lining of the uterus, the endometrium, and spreads into the uterine wall. Uterine cancer also may be called endometrial cancer.

**ETIOLOGY** This type of cancer usually occurs in postmenopausal females who have never had children. Increased risk factors include infertility, obesity, and prolonged estrogen stimulation as occurs with hormone replacement therapy.

**SYMPTOMS** The symptoms of uterine cancer include abnormal bleeding, which is quite noticeable in postmenopausal females, and usually leads to early detection of this form of cancer. Diagnosis is made on the basis of visual examination and endometrial biopsy.

**TREATMENT** Treatment is very successful if the cancer is discovered in its early stages, and includes surgical removal of the ovaries and uterus, combined with radiation therapy.

### ■ Ovarian Cancer

Ovarian cancer is quite common and often fatal.

**ETIOLOGY** The cause of ovarian cancer is unknown. The ovaries' position deep in the pelvis make discovery of this tumor difficult. Often, extensive metastasis will occur before there are noticeable symptoms.

**SYMPTOMS** Symptoms include a feeling of pressure on the bladder, low abdominal or pelvic pain, and a general feeling of ill health. Diagnosis is made on the basis of physical examination and visualization of the mass during an exploratory laparoscopy.

**TREATMENT** Treatment depends on the stage of the cancer and often includes a complete hysterectomy, radiation, and chemotherapy. Prognosis is good with early detection, but as stated earlier, this is not the usual case. If metastasis has occurred, this can-

cer may be fatal in one to two years. The only preventive measure is early detection through annual gynecologic exams.

## Diseases of the Breast

Diseases of the breast are quite common and range from mild to life threatening. Breast cancer affects one in nine women in the United States. Breast self-examination and mammography are important methods of screening for cancer. Although women are most often affected with breast diseases, men also may be affected. Any change from normal in tissue shape or appearance in males or females should be called to the attention of a physician.

### ■ Fibrocystic Disease

Fibrocystic disease of the breast is the most common breast disorder of premenopausal females between the ages of 30 and 55.

**ETIOLOGY** It is thought that the development of cysts is linked to estrogen levels.

**SYMPTOMS** This disorder is characterized by:

- single or multiple fluid-filled cysts in one or both breasts
- breast tenderness and feeling of fullness prior to menstruation
- a tendency to run in families
- cysts that recede after the onset of menopause

Fibrocystic disease causes an increased risk of cancer approximately one and one-half that of the normal population. Multiple cysts also make detection of neoplasm more difficult. For these reasons, affected females need to routinely perform monthly breast self-examinations and have routine mammograms. Females with severe fibrocystic disease and at high risk of breast cancer may decide to have a **prophylactic** (preventive) mastectomy.

**TREATMENT** Measures to decrease breast pain due to fibrocystic disease include elimination of caffeine in the diet, reduction of salt intake, the use of a mild diuretic the week prior to menstruation, and the use of mild analgesics. For severe cases, hormonal therapy with synthetic androgen may be helpful.

### ■ Mastitis

Mastitis (mas-TYE-tis; mast = breast, itis = inflammation) is inflammation of the breast tissue and is a broad term covering a variety of diseases or disorders. The type of mastitis commonly thought of is **puerperal** (pyou-ER-pier-al; childbirth) mastitis.

**ETIOLOGY** Puerperal mastitis occurs when bacteria from the nursing baby's mouth or mother's hands enter the breast tissue through the nipple and cause infection.

**SYMPTOMS** Symptoms include redness, heat, swelling, pain, and often bloody discharges from the nipple. Diagnosis is made on the basis of symptoms.

**TREATMENT** Treatment includes antibiotics, application of heat, analgesics, and a firm-support brassiere to decrease discomfort.

## ■ Breast Cancer

Breast cancer is an adenocarcinoma (adeno = gland, carcinoma = cancer) of the breast ducts. It is the most common neoplasm affecting breast tissue and occurs in one out of nine females. It is second only to lung cancer as the leading cause of cancer-related deaths in females in the United States. Monthly breast self-examinations and routine mammograms are a must for early detection of breast cancer.

**ETIOLOGY** The cause of breast cancer is unknown but identified risk factors include:

- age 40 and over
- family member affected with breast cancer
- onset of menses before age 13
- menses continuing after age 50
- nullipara (nuh-LIP-ah-rah; nulli = none or no, para = births)
- first child after age 30
- obesity
- chronic breast disease

**SYMPTOMS** Symptoms of breast cancer include a nontender lump of varying size. These occur most often in the upper outer quadrant of the breast, near the axillary area. The lump may cause a dimpling of the skin or the nipple may be retracted. Often, there are no visual symptoms. Diagnosis is made on the basis of the presence of the lump, mammogram, and biopsy. A biopsy is the definitive test, and may be performed by aspiration or surgery. Prognosis is good if the lump is found early. Metastasis is common and usually affects the lungs, liver, brain, and bone. If metastasis has occurred, the prognosis may be poor.

**TREATMENT** Treatment is usually surgical removal of the mass or the breast (**mastectomy**: mas-TECK-

toh-me; mast = breast, ectomy = excision), followed by chemotherapy and/or radiation therapy. Carcinoma spread through the lymphatic system so removal of the lymph nodes and lymph vessels is a common procedure. There are several types of surgical procedures performed for breast cancer, depending on the location, size, and metastasis of the tumor. Commonly, these types of surgery include:

- lumpectomy involving removal of the lump only
- simple or total mastectomy involving removal of the breast and nipple
- modified radical mastectomy involving removal of the breast, nipple, and lymph nodes
- radical mastectomy involving removal of the breast, nipple, lymph nodes, and underlying chest (pectoral) muscles (Figure 17–12)

Mastectomy surgery not only causes an alteration in the physical image but also may lead to a variety of psychological disorders for a female. For this reason, many women decide to have reconstructive surgery (mammoplasty) performed along with the mastectomy in an effort to reduce the physical and psychological trauma. **Mammoplasty** (**MAM**-oh-PLAS-tee; mammo = breast, plasty = surgical repair or restructuring) involves reconstruction of the breast with plastic surgery and prosthetic breast implants.

## Disorders of Pregnancy

Pregnancy is a normal condition of developing a fetus in the female body. Disorders of pregnancy range from mild to life threatening. The lives of the mother and the fetus are sometimes at risk. For this reason, the importance of prenatal care cannot be stressed enough.

### ■ Ectopic Pregnancy

**ETIOLOGY** Ectopic (eck-TOP-ick; displaced) pregnancy occurs when a fertilized ovum attaches to tissue outside the uterus, most commonly in the fallopian tubes. Strictures, adhesions, and scarring of the fallopian tubes due to PID (pelvic inflammatory disease), inflammation, infection, and structural defects may cause the tube to be narrowed. Microscopic-sized sperm may travel up the tube and fertilize the ovum, but the larger ovum is unable to travel down the tube and implant normally in the uterus. Other

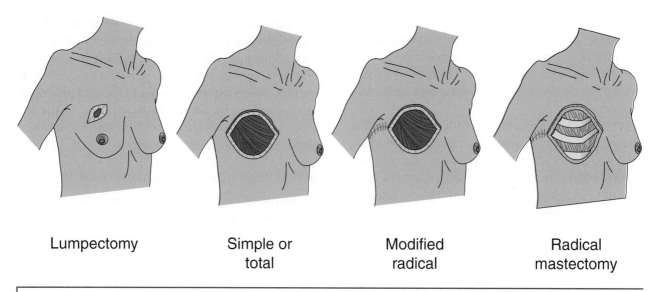

| Lumpectomy | Simple or total | Modified radical | Radical mastectomy |

**FIGURE 17–12**   Types of mastectomy.

ectopic sites include the ovary, intestine, and outside wall of the uterus (Figure 17–13).

**SYMPTOMS** Symptoms of ectopic pregnancy include acute pelvic pain, vaginal bleeding, and a positive pregnancy test. If large blood vessels are ruptured, bleeding may be heavy and the affected female may show symptoms of shock. Diagnosis is made on the basis of symptoms, a pelvic examination, and ultrasound.

**TREATMENT** Treatment is prompt surgery to terminate the pregnancy and decrease the possibility of shock, which can be life threatening. Blood replacement also may be needed. If the female wants to bear children, every effort is made to preserve the affected ovary and tube.

### ◼ Spontaneous Abortion (Miscarriage)

Spontaneous abortion is the natural termination of pregnancy before the fetus is able to live on its own. This type of abortion is commonly called miscarriage.

**ETIOLOGY** The cause of spontaneous abortion is unknown. It is believed that it may be due to abnormal fetal development, infection, drug use by the pregnant mother, and/or an incompetent cervix (one that dilates prematurely). Approximately one in every six pregnancies ends with spontaneous abortion, and 75 percent of these occur in the first 12 weeks. The risk is higher during first pregnancies.

**SYMPTOMS** Symptoms of miscarriage include vaginal bleeding, cramping, and pelvic pain, usually

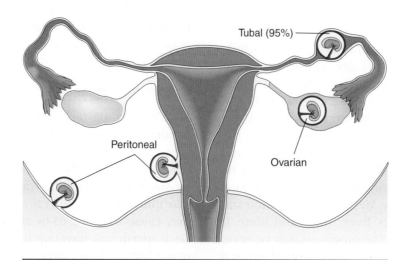

**FIGURE 17–13**   Sites of ectopic pregnancy.

in the first trimester of pregnancy. If bleeding is severe, shock is of major concern.

Diagnosis is made on the basis of symptoms and pelvic ultrasound.

**TREATMENT** Bed rest is the treatment of choice if bleeding is not severe. Bed rest is continued until spotting stops. If the individual is hemorrhaging and showing signs of shock, hospitalization may be needed to control hemorrhage and give blood replacement. Once spontaneous abortion begins, its progression is difficult to stop. A surgical D&C may be performed to remove any tissue remaining in the uterus after the abortion.

### ■ Morning Sickness

**ETIOLOGY** The cause of morining sickness is unknown but it is thought to be due to hormonal changes related to pregnancy. It is also believed that hunger may play some part in the cause. Morning sickness is diagnosed by symptoms in a pregnant female.

**SYMPTOMS** Morning sickness is the nausea and vomiting associated with pregnancy, usually occurring in the first trimester of pregnancy. Morning sickness, as its name implies, usually occurs in the morning, but it also may occur later in the day. Approximately 50 percent of pregnant females experience varying degrees of morning sickness.

**TREATMENT** Treatment is not necessary unless there is excessive vomiting, which can lead to dehydration and weight loss. This condition is then termed hyperemesis gravidarum. No antiemetic (anti = against, emetic = vomiting) medication has been approved by the Food and Drug Administration (FDA) for morning sickness, and taking medications at this time in pregnancy may lead to fetal abnormalities. Activities that may help reduce morning sickness include:

- eating something light like soda crackers before getting out of bed in the morning
- eating dry foods before drinking liquids
- eating several small meals during the day instead of three large ones
- avoiding fatty foods such as fried foods, butter, and margarine
- resting after meals

### ■ Hyperemesis Gravidarum

Hyperemesis (hyper = excessive, emesis = vomiting) gravidarum is excessive vomiting during pregnancy, leading to dehydration, weight loss, and possible electrolyte imbalances in the mother and baby. This condition is not usually life threatening, but prompt medical attention is needed to preserve the health of the mother and baby.

**ETIOLOGY** The cause is unknown but is thought to be due to an increased production of chorionic gonadotropin by the fetus. This thought is supported by the fact that hyperemesis gravidarum occurs more often in pregnancies with multiple fetuses. Diagnosis is made on the basis of symptoms.

**TREATMENT** Severe cases may be treated with intravenous fluids, and withholding all foods and oral fluids. Most cases subside by the second trimester of pregnancy.

### ■ Toxemia

Toxemia is a condition usually appearing in the third trimester of pregnancy. The name of this condition is misleading as there is no toxin in the blood, but it was once thought that the fetus produced a toxin that led to toxemia.

**ETIOLOGY** The cause of toxemia is unknown but it does tend to occur more frequently in:

- individuals with poor prenatal care
- **primigravid** (PRE-mih-**GRAV**-id; primi = first, gravid = pregnancy) females younger than 20 years of age and older than 30
- individuals with poor nutritional intake
- those who are hypertensive prior to becoming pregnant
- **multiparity** (mul-TIP-ah-rah-tee; multiple births), especially in individuals who have had five or more pregnancies

**SYMPTOMS** Toxemia is characterized by hypertension, sudden weight gain, proteinuria (protein = blood protein, urina = urine), and edema in the face, hands, and feet. It is also called **preeclampsia** (PREE-ee-**KLAMP**-see-ah). The individual with toxemia is preeclamptic before convulsions occur. Toxemia or preeclampsia, if untreated or unresolved, may progress into **eclampsia** (eh-KLAMP-see-ah). Eclampsia is a condition characterized by all the symptoms of toxemia or preeclampsia, plus the symptoms of convulsions. Eclampsia may lead to abruptio placentae, and become life threatening to the mother and baby. Diagnosis is made on the basis of symptoms.

**TREATMENT** Treatment includes frequent monitoring of blood pressure, weight, and urine protein as part of prenatal care. If symptoms of toxemia occur, a low-salt diet and antihypertensive medications may be recommended. If toxemia becomes severe, hospitalization in a quiet environment, with frequent monitoring and administration of antihypertensive medications, is the usual therapy in an effort to prevent convulsions. Prognosis is good since delivery of the baby or termination of the pregnancy resolves the problem. Good prenatal care and good nutrition greatly reduce the risk of toxemia.

### ■ Abruptio Placentae

Abruptio placentae is the sudden separation of the placenta from the uterus prior to or during labor (Figure 17–14).

**ETIOLOGY** Often, the cause is unknown but convulsions, trauma, multiple births, and chronic hypertension are known causes.

**SYMPTOMS** The degree of separation determines the symptoms. A partial separation during labor may be asymptomatic, whereas a complete separation prior to labor may be life threatening to the mother and baby. Symptoms of a complete separation may include severe abdominal pain with large amounts of vaginal bleeding (hemorrhage), shock, a decrease in fetal heart tones, and a decrease in fetal activity. Complete separations are a medical emergency, because these may lead to maternal death due to hemorrhage and death of the baby due to a lack of needed oxygen and nutrition. Diagnosis is usually made on the basis of clinical history as there is not time for other testing.

**TREATMENT** Treatment is prompt delivery, either vaginally or by surgical cesarean section (C-section). Blood replacement also may be needed.

### ■ Placenta Previa

Placenta previa is the abnormal positioning of the placenta in the lower uterus, often near or over the cervical os or opening (Figure 17–14). If the placenta is totally over the os, it is a complete placenta previa, and partial covering is a partial placenta previa.

**ETIOLOGY** The cause of this condition is unknown but risk factors include multiparity, maternal age over 35, and previous uterine surgery.

**SYMPTOMS** The affected individual has symptoms of painless, bright red vaginal bleeding during the third trimester of pregnancy. Vital signs may be indicative of shock if the bleeding is severe. Placenta previa may be life threatening to the mother due to hemorrhaging and to the baby due to anoxia. Diagnosis is made by pelvic ultrasound.

**TREATMENT** Vaginal delivery may be possible if the mother is asymptomatic or if bleeding is not severe. Severe maternal bleeding or fetal anoxia is reason to perform an emergency cesarean section.

## Male Reproductive System Diseases

The most common diseases affecting the male reproductive system include infection and diseases affecting the prostate. The positional relationship of the male urinary bladder and the prostate cause the male to experience urinary symptoms when the prostate is affected with disease.

### ■ Prostatitis

Prostatitis (PROS-tah-**TYE**-tis; prost = prostate, itis = inflammation) is inflammation of the prostate gland. This condition is more common in men over 50 years of age.

**ETIOLOGY** Cause may be unknown, or it may be the result of a urinary tract infection or infection by gonorrhea.

**SYMPTOMS** Symptoms include **dysuria** (dis-YOU-ree-ah; dys-painful, uria = urination), **pyuria** (pye-YOU-ree-ah; py = pus, uria = urine), fever, and low back pain. Diagnosis is made on the basis of a urinalysis, urine culture, and digital rectal examination.

**TREATMENT** Treatment is dependent on cause but often includes antibiotic therapy with penicillin. Warm sitz baths, increased fluid intake, and analgesics also may be prescribed. Prognosis is good as prostatitis usually responds well to treatment.

### ■ Benign Prostatic Hyperplasia (BPH)

Benign prostatic hyperplasia is also called benign prostatic hypertrophy, and is the enlargement of the prostate due to normal cells overgrowing and enlarging (Figure 17–15). BPH is common in men over the age of 60. Approximately 50 percent of males over age 65 have some degree of prostate enlargement.

**ETIOLOGY** The cause of BPH is unknown, but it is thought to be due to hormonal changes including alterations in testosterone, estrogen, and androgen levels associated with aging.

**SYMPTOMS** The enlargement of the prostate places pressure on the bladder and prostatic urethra, causing urinary obstruction and a variety of urinary

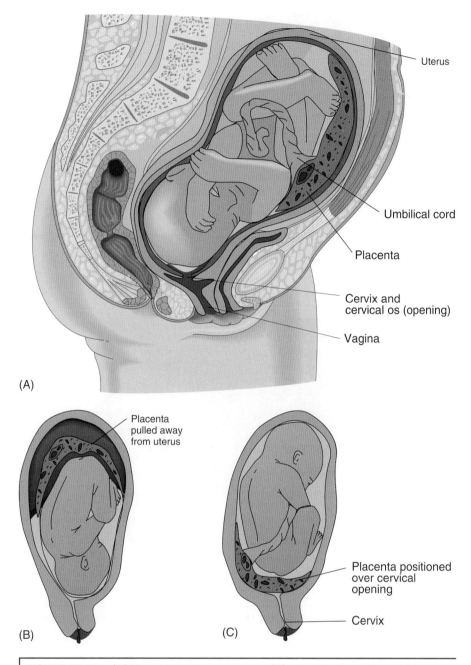

**FIGURE 17–14** (A) Normal uterine pregnancy, (B) abruptio placentae, and (C) placenta previa.

symptoms. The primary symptoms of BPH are **nocturia** (nock-TOO-ree-ah; noc = night, uria = urination) or frequently getting up at night to void, inability to start urination, a weak urinary stream, and inability to empty the bladder. The inability to empty the bladder often causes the excess urine to fill the ureters, leading to hydroureter, hydronephrosis, and frequent urinary tract infections. Diagnosis is made on the basis of symptoms and digital rectal examination revealing an enlarged prostate.

**TREATMENT** Treatment is symptomatic and may include prostatic massage, sitz baths, and catheterizations. Regular sexual intercourse may be helpful in reducing prostatic congestion. Surgery to resect or decrease the size of the prostate is a common treatment, and is called a transurethral (trans = through, urethral = urethra) resection of the prostate (TURP). This procedure is performed, as the name indicates, through the urethra. No surgical incision is needed. During a TURP, the surgeon uses a cystoscope to

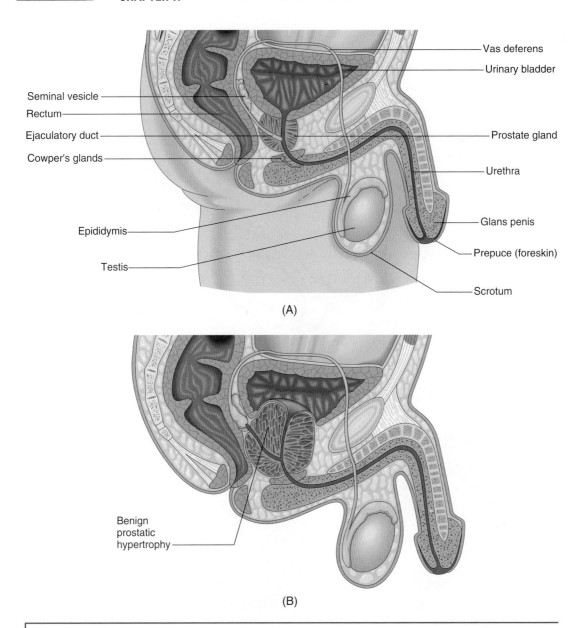

Vas deferens
Urinary bladder
Seminal vesicle
Rectum
Ejaculatory duct
Cowper's glands
Prostate gland
Urethra
Epididymis
Glans penis
Prepuce (foreskin)
Testis
Scrotum

(A)

Benign prostatic hypertrophy

(B)

**FIGURE 17–15**   Normal and enlarged prostate. (A) normal, (B) benign prostatic hypertrophy or hyperplasia (enlarged).

chisel away the excess prostate tissue causing the urinary obstruction (Figure 17–16). There are no known preventive measures for BPH. An annual prostate exam is recommended for males after age 40.

### ■ Prostatic Carcinoma

Prostatic carcinoma is a neoplasm of the prostate gland that commonly affects men after age 50. It is the second most common cause of cancer-related death in men (lung cancer is first).

**ETIOLOGY**  The cause of this cancer is unknown although some believe that testosterone levels are involved. A puzzling fact with this theory is the great racial inequity in incidence of prostatic cancer. Caucasian men are affected with prostatic cancer 10 times more often than oriental men. This fact leads to the belief that there are environmental and lifestyle factors involved. It is known that incidence does increase with age.

This adenocarcinoma grows in the outer layer of the prostate and often does not cause symptoms until it has metastasized. Common sites of metastasis include the bones of the spine and pelvis.

**SYMPTOMS**  Symptoms, when present, are similar to BPH as the urethra becomes obstructed. Digital rectal examination will reveal a hard abnormal mass.

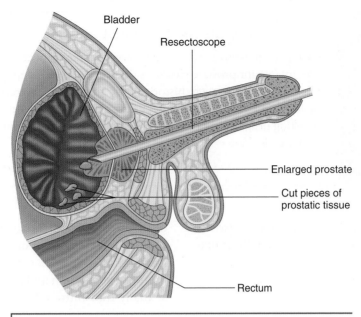

Bladder

Resectoscope

Enlarged prostate

Cut pieces of prostatic tissue

Rectum

**FIGURE 17–16** Transurethral resection of prostate (TURP).

A blood test measuring prostatic-specific antigen, also called PSA, will be elevated with prostatic cancer. Biopsy is the definitive test.

**TREATMENT** Treatment depends on the age and physical condition of the affected individual, and the degree of metastasis. If the tumor has not metastasized, complete removal and cure may be accomplished with a prostatectomy. If metastasis has occurred, treatment may involve hormone therapy to slow the growth of the neoplasm. Hormone therapy may include:

- administration of estrogen to counteract testosterone

- surgical **orchiectomy** (OR-kee-**ECK**-toh-me; orchi = testicle, ectomy = removal) or removal of the testicles to halt testosterone production

- a combination of both treatments

Much controversy exists over the benefits of hormone therapy. Many urologists do not believe an orchiectomy improves the survival rate of the affected individual. Chemotherapy and radiation treatments also may be beneficial treatments. The prognosis of prostatic carcinoma varies, depending on the age of the affected individual and the degree of spread. If the individual is older than 60 years of age, he will probably outlive the cancer and die of some other disease process. Younger individuals and those with extensive metastasis do not have as positive a prognosis. Overall, 50 to 75 percent of affected individuals live five years or more. Annual prostate examinations are recommended for early detection.

## ■ Epididymitis

Epididymitis (EP-ih-did-ih-**MY**-tis; epididym = epididymis, itis = inflammation) is inflammation of the epididymis.

**ETIOLOGY** Common causes include prostatitis, urinary tract infection, mumps, and sexually transmitted disease such as chlamydia, syphilis, and gonorrhea. Epididymitis is one of the most common diseases of the male reproductive tract and usually affects only one epididymis (unilateral).

**SYMPTOMS** Symptoms include a swollen, hard, and painful epididymis, often accompanied by severe scrotal pain and swelling. Scrotal discomfort makes walking difficult and the affected individual may walk straddle-legged to protect the scrotum.

Diagnosis is made on the basis of symptoms, urinalyis, and urine culture.

**TREATMENT** Prompt, appropriate antibiotic therapy is usually very effective. A delay in treatment may lead to complications of scarring and **sterility** (inability to impregnate a female related to sperm quality or quantity). Other treatment includes bed rest, analgesics, use of a scrotal support, and avoidance of alcohol, spicy foods, and sexual stimulation. Prevention is aimed at cause, and includes prompt treatment of causative infections, sexual abstinence,

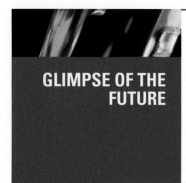

### New Treatments for Prostate Cancer

There are many new treatments for prostate cancer being studied. The mortality rate for prostate cancer is decreasing, and treatments are much more effective than they were historically. Some of the new treatments on the horizon include gene therapy, a variety of new chemotherapeutic agents, and immune-boosting drugs. Vaccines are also being studied that help the body's T-cells destroy tumor cells.

*Source: Langreth, R. (2004).*

or use of condoms during sexual intercourse to decrease the risk of infection with sexually transmitted diseases.

## ■ Orchitis

**ETIOLOGY** Orchitis (or-KYE-tis, orch = testis, itis = inflammation) is inflammation of one or both testes usually due to bacterial or viral infection or trauma. Viral mumps is the most common cause of orchitis in the adult male. Commonly, orchitis occurs in conjunction with or as a complication of epididymitis.

**SYMPTOMS** Symptoms include swelling, pain and tenderness of one or both testes, fever, and malaise. Diagnosis is made on the basis of symptoms, blood testing, and urinalysis.

**TREATMENT** Treatment is dependent on cause. If the cause is bacterial, antibiotic therapy is usually effective. Orchitis caused by mumps is treated symptomatically and includes bed rest, and analgesic and antipyretic medications. The use of a scrotal support may be helpful. Prognosis is good although atrophy of the involved testicle does occur 50 percent of the time. If both testes are involved, sterility may occur. Prevention is aimed at causative factors, and includes mumps vaccination and prevention of infection with sexually transmitted diseases.

## ■ Testicular Tumors

Testicular tumors commonly affect young males age 20 to 35, and are the most common type of cancer for this age group. Testicular tumors rarely occur in males over age 40.

**ETIOLOGY** The cause of this cancer is unknown, but predisposing factors include individuals who have been affected by **cryptorchidism** (krip-TOR-kih-dizm; crypt = hidden, orchid = testicle, ism = condition) or undescended testicle and an inguinal hernia as a child.

**SYMPTOMS** The primary symptom of a testicular tumor is a painless mass felt in the testicle. Diagnosis is made on the basis of palpation of a testicular mass and confirmed by biopsy.

## COMPLEMENTARY AND ALTERNATIVE THERAPY

### Herb Therapy for Prostate Cancer

The use of complementary and alternative therapies for prostate cancer is increasing. There is not much scientific research on these therapies but they are still being widely utilized by patients with prostate cancer, especially those in late stages. Essiac formulas are some of the most popular treatments. The formulas contain varying amounts of burdock, sheep's sorrel, turkey rhubarb root, and slippery elm. Some of the ingredients have been shown to have antimutagenic properties and also may stimulate the immune system. Although the research has not proven that essiac products reduce prostate cancer growth, there does not seem to be serious side effects from its use.

*Source: Smith, M., & Mills, E. J. (2001).*

**TREATMENT** Treatment commonly includes surgery (orchiectomy), followed by chemotherapy and radiation. Because there is no direct lymphatic connection between the testes, testicular tumors do not usually spread from one testicle to the other. Surgical removal of the affected testis is often the treatment of choice. This procedure leaves the unaffected testis, and the male is not rendered sterile or **impotent** (inability to achieve or maintain a penile erection). Metastatic testicular cancers may be treated with radical surgery involving removal of both testes and adjacent lymph nodes. This surgery may or may not affect impotency, but it will cause sterility. Males wishing to father children may elect to bank sperm prior to surgery in order to father children at a later date by means of artificial insemination. If discovered early, prognosis of testicular tumor is good with an approximate 90 percent cure rate. If metastasis has occurred, the prognosis is poor. To discover testicular tumors prior to metastasis, it is recommended that males perform regular testicular examinations.

## ■ Cryptorchidism

Cryptorchidism is a condition commonly called an undescended testicle. As the unborn male fetus develops, the testes appear first in the abdominal cavity. As the fetus grows and develops, the testes move downward through the inguinal canal and into the scrotum. If this process does not occur properly, the testes may become lodged in any position in the abdominal cavity (Figure 17–17).

**ETIOLOGY** Premature birth is a common cause of cryptorchidism and is usually time limited. The failure of both testes to descend is uncommon.

**TREATMENT** If a testis remains undescended into childhood, surgical intervention is necessary to move and secure the testis in the scrotum. This surgery is usually performed during infancy or prior to the age of five. If the testis is left in the abdominal cavity it will not function properly, but this will not affect potency or sterility as one testis can maintain adequate male hormone levels. If both testes are undescended, the male will be sterile.

## Sexually Transmitted Diseases (STDs)

Sexually transmitted diseases (STDs), formerly called venereal diseases, include a group of many diseases that are spread by intimate or sexual contact. The spread of STD is at an epidemic level in the United States. These infections are transmitted from one person to another by contact with infected skin, blood, semen, and vaginal secretions during vaginal, anal, and oral sex. Prevention is best achieved by avoiding intimate contact with infected individuals. Other precautions include use of a condom during sexual intercourse, avoiding multiple sex partners, avoiding sex with someone with an unknown sexual history, and avoiding the use of alcohol that may impair judgment concerning a sexual encounter. Treatment of STDs commonly consist of identifying sex partners, and treating the infected individuals concurrently to avoid reinfection or a "ping-pong" effect of passing the infection back and forth between involved individuals. Follow-up testing is needed after treatment to ensure the disease has been eradicated in all infected individuals.

## ■ Acquired Immunodeficiency Syndrome (AIDS)

Acquired immunodeficiency syndrome (AIDS) is a bloodborne infection commonly transmitted sexually. AIDS is the most dreaded disease of modern society and has reached global epidemic proportion. Currently, there is no cure for this immunodeficiency disease that predisposes the affected individual to a multitude of opportunistic diseases. Prevention is imperative, and must include health and AIDS education. For more details about AIDS, see Chapter 5.

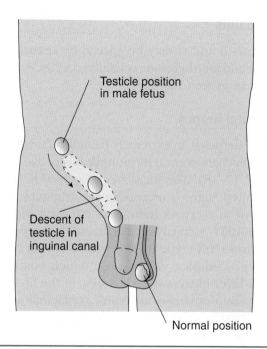

Testicle position in male fetus

Descent of testicle in inguinal canal

Normal position

**FIGURE 17–17** Cryptorchidism—pathway and common sites of hidden testis.

## ■ Hepatitis

Hepatitis B and C may be spread by sexual intercourse and are, therefore, considered STDs. For more information see Chapter 12.

## ■ Genital Herpes

Genital herpes is an extremely painful, recurring viral infection characterized by multiple blister-like lesions (Figure 17–18). The incidence of genital herpes in the United States is increasing at a frightening rate with one in every six individuals currently infected.

**ETIOLOGY** Genital herpes is caused by herpes simplex virus (HSV) type II. This virus is closely related to herpes simplex virus type I, which commonly causes fever blisters or cold sores on the lips. Both herpes simplex viruses are highly contagious and are transmitted by intimate contact between two mucous membrane surfaces. HSV I may be spread by kissing an infected individual during the active phase of the disease. HSV II is commonly spread by sexual intercourse. HSV I may be spread to the genital area by oral-genital exposure and HSV II may be spread to the lips in the same manner. Self-infection with the hands is also possible. Touching an infected area, followed by touching of the lips, genitals, or eyes, may cause self-infection. Extreme care should be taken to avoid infection of the mucous membranes of the eyes.

Herpes disease cannot be cured. The virus remains dormant in the tissues until activated by stress or lowered immunity. Sunlight, fever, emotional stress, and menses are common activators of the herpes virus.

**SYMPTOMS** Once activated, the virus produces blisters that enlarge, rupture, and ulcerate. The lesions are extremely painful, especially during sexual intercourse. Severe itching and painful urination (dysuria)

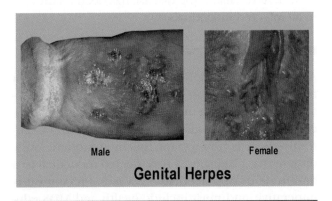

Male      Female

**Genital Herpes**

**FIGURE 17–18** Genital herpes. *(Courtesy of Mark L. Kuss)*

are common. Genital herpes infection in the male commonly produces blisters on the glans penis, the shaft of the penis, scrotum, and inner thighs. Lesions in the female commonly appear on the vulva, vagina, inner thighs, and rectal area. Childbirth in a female with active herpes infection is fatal to the infant 50 percent of the time. If the infant survives, major neurologic and ophthalmic complications usually occur. For this reason, delivery by cesarean section is performed in mothers with active genital herpes.

Herpes lesions generally last between one to three weeks, but may recur weekly, monthly, or yearly. Diagnosis is made on the basis of presence of characteristic lesions and a positive viral culture of active lesions.

**TREATMENT** Treatment is symptomatic and involves antiviral medications to reduce symptoms. Sitz baths, ice therapy, analgesics, and keeping the lesions clean and dry may help with the discomfort. Females with genital herpes should have Pap smears every six months as they are eight times more likely to develop cervical cancer.

## ■ Gonorrhea

**ETIOLOGY** Gonorrhea, also known as "clap," is a highly contagious, sexually transmitted disease, caused by the bacteria *Neisseria gonorrhoeae*. It is one of the most common STDs in the United States. This bacterial infection causes inflammation of mucous membranes of the genital and urinary systems in both males and females.

**SYMPTOMS** Gonorrhea commonly causes urethritis in the male with symptoms of purulent discharge from the penis, dysuria, and urinary frequency. Females commonly show signs of cervicitis with purulent vaginal discharge, dysuria, urinary frequency, genital itching, and a burning pain. The transmission of gonorrhea is often difficult to control because the infected individual, either male or female, may be asymptomatic. In this case, the infected individual is a carrier of the infection and may unknowingly spread the infection. Infants born to mothers with gonorrhea run the risk of developing gonorrheal eye infection, which can lead to blindness. To prevent infant blindness, it is a common practice, and is state law in some instances, that all newborns' eyes are treated with prophylactic antibiotic at birth.

Diagnosis of gonorrhea is made on the basis of a culture of secretions.

**TREATMENT** Treatment with antibiotics including penicillin, tetracycline, and ceftriaxone is usually effective. Untreated gonorrhea may lead to life-threatening, systemic infections like meningitis and endocarditis. Arthritis and sterility are also common in both the untreated male and female.

## ■ Syphilis

**ETIOLOGY** Syphilis is a serious sexually transmitted infection caused by *Treponema pallidum* bacteria. It is spread by sexual or intimate contact with contagious lesions. As soon as exposure occurs, this bacteria rapidly penetrates the skin or mucous membrane, and gains access to the vascular system, producing a systemic infection. Diagnosis is made on the basis of blood tests, VDRL, and RPR. Syphilis has a much lower incidence than gonorrhea and is more easily treated. Antibiotic treatment with penicillin or tetracycline is very effective. As a matter of fact, syphilis may unknowingly be cured with penicillin therapy for streptococcus infection such as strep throat. Untreated syphilis has a much worse outcome than gonorrhea as it may become a chronic life-threatening disease. Untreated, syphilis progresses through three distinct stages with characteristic signs and symptoms. The stages are primary, secondary, and tertiary.

1. Primary—**SYMPTOMS** This stage is marked by the appearance of a painless, highly contagious lesion called a **chancre** (SHANG-ker) (Figure 17–19). This lesion occurs at the site of bacterial entry and usually appears several weeks after contact. It may vary in appearance from pimple-like to an ulcerated sore. In the male, the chancre usually appears on the head of the penis. In the female, the chancre commonly appears on the vulva, although it may occur inside the vaginal cavity, and thus be hidden and go unnoticed. The chancre may appear at other sites in both sexes including the lips, fingers, anus, and tongue. Even without treatment, the chancre commonly disappears in 10 to 30 days, often leading to the false conclusion that the disease is cured. Lymphadenopathy, or sore swollen lymph nodes, is common.

   **TREATMENT** The disease is highly contagious during this stage but is easily cured with antibiotic therapy.

2. Secondary—After the chancre heals, a period of rest occurs that may last from six weeks to one year.

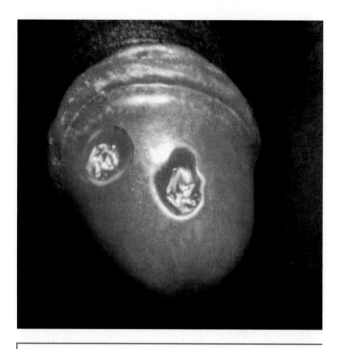

**FIGURE 17–19** Syphilis chancre. *(Courtesy of Mark L. Kuss)*

**SYMPTOMS** During this time, the bacteria rests, then rapidly grows and multiplies, causing the characteristic rash of secondary syphilis. This rash may appear in any area of the body such as the palms, soles of the feet, and mouth, or it may spread over the entire body. The rash does not itch and may be erroneously diagnosed as mumps, chickenpox, or ringworm. The individual is highly contagious during this stage. If mouth sores are present, kissing may spread the disease.

**TREATMENT** Syphilis can be easily diagnosed based on a blood test during this stage, and easily treated with antibiotics. The primary and secondary stages are often combined and called *early syphilis*.

3. Tertiary (Late or Latent)—If secondary syphilis is untreated, the bacterial organisms withdraw into single or multiple sites in the body and become dormant. The length of this dormant time ranges from one to 20 years. During this time, the infected individual may be unaware of the infection. Blood testing even may show negative results. The disease at this time is less contagious to others but is dangerous for the infected individual.

   **SYMPTOMS** Bacteria invade organs throughout the body, producing a characteristic soft gummy lesion called **gumma** (GUM-mah). Symptoms vary, depending on the organs attacked. Common problems include aortic aneurysm, heart failure, mental disorders, insanity, deafness, blindness, paralysis, and death.

**TREATMENT** Tertiary syphilis can be cured with antibiotic treatment, but the effects of the lesions are irreversible.

Syphilis in pregnant females may cause spontaneous abortion or death of the infant. Infants that survive commonly have numerous defects including physical and mental deformities, blindness, and deafness. Pregnant females should be tested for syphilis early because syphilis can be cured with antibiotic treatment during the first five months of pregnancy, thus preventing infection in the unborn child.

### ■ Chlamydial Infection

**ETIOLOGY** Chlamydial infection, due to the bacteria *Chlamydia trachomatis*, is very common in the United States and is one of the most damaging of the STDs.

**SYMPTOMS** Chlamydial infection is often called the "silent" STD because infected individuals may be asymptomatic until dangerous complications occur. Chlamydial infection is the leading cause of PID and is a major cause of female infertility. Males with chlamydial infection are usually symptomatic with drainage from the penis, burning and itching with urination due to urethritis, and epididymitis. Symptomatic females experience vaginal drainage with burning and itching of the genital area. Abdominal pain and dyspareunia may be indicative of PID. Diagnosis is made on the basis of cytologic examinations.

**TREATMENT** Treatment with antibiotic therapy is effective. Prognosis is good if treatment occurs prior to the onset of complications. Untreated females may suffer with PID and infertility. Untreated males may suffer with severe epididymitis, causing sterility.

### ■ Trichomoniasis

**ETIOLOGY** Trichomoniasis is an infection by a protozoan, *Trichomonas vaginalis*. Trichomoniasis is a fairly common STD, affecting approximately 10 percent of all sexually active individuals.

**SYMPTOMS** Most infected individuals are asymptomatic, resulting in extensive spread of the infection. If symptoms occur in the male, they commonly include urethritis, epididymitis, and prostatitis. Infected females, when symptomatic, have itching and burning of the genital area and a green, frothy vagi-

nal drainage. Diagnosis is made on the basis of microscopic examination of vaginal or penile secretions revealing the presence of the causative organism.

**TREATMENT** Treatment with an antiparasitic medication is usually very effective.

### ■ Genital Warts

**ETIOLOGY** Genital warts are due to a virus commonly spread during sexual contact (Figure 17-20).

**SYMPTOMS** Warts may be asymptomatic or may cause tenderness in the affected area. The amount of discomfort is related to the size, location, and number of warts present. These viral lesions commonly appear one to six months after exposure to an infected individual. In the male, warts are usually located on the head of the penis, but also may be found along the penile shaft and around the anus. In the female, these lesions commonly appear around the vaginal opening and may spread to the perianal area. Size of genital warts may vary from very small to three or four inches in diameter. They may appear singly or in clusters. Pregnancy tends to cause the warts to grow more rapidly. Genital warts in a pregnant female may even reach a point of occluding the vaginal canal, thus making a cesarean delivery necessary. Cervical cancer is also more common in females with genital warts. Diagnosis is made on the basis of visualization of the warts and biopsy to rule out carcinoma.

**TREATMENT** Treatment is commonly surgical or chemical removal of the infected tissue. Surgical removal does not mean cure as recurrence of genital warts is common.

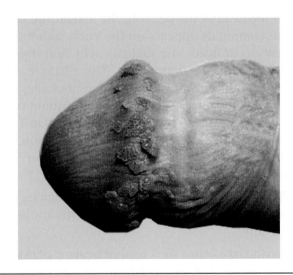

**FIGURE 17–20** Genital warts. *(Courtesy of Mark L. Kuss)*

# Sexual Dysfunction

A brief description of the most common sexual dysfunctions is provided in this section. Sexual dysfunction, whether due to physical or psychological conditions, may limit the ability of the individual to reproduce and to develop a close, nurturing sexual relationship with a significant other. The human sexual cycle progresses through stages of arousal, sexual intercourse, climax, and ends with feelings of pleasure and relaxation. Any disorder that interrupts this cycle may be considered a sexual dysfunction. Diagnosis of sexual dysfunction is dependent on general examination including a complete medical history, a sexual history including details of the dysfunction, a physical examination, and laboratory testing as indicated. Psychological disorders leading to sexual dysfunction may need treatment by psychological counselors. Success in counseling is often dependent on both partners participating and maintaining a patient and sensitive attitude toward each other.

## ■ Dyspareunia

Dyspareunia is a condition of having pain or discomfort with sexual intercourse. It may affect both males and females, although it is more common in women.

**ETIOLOGY** Dyspareunia for both sexes may be related to physical or psychological conditions. In females, common physical conditions causing dyspareunia include an intact hymen, vaginal deformity, insufficient lubrication, sensitivity to spermacide, presence of an STD, bladder infection, pelvic inflammatory disease, and endometriosis. In the male, common physical conditions causing dyspareunia include penile deformity, presence of an STD, **phimosis** (figh-MOH-sis) or an abnormally tight foreskin (Figure 17–21), prostatitis, and epididymitis. Psychological conditions in both sexes that may lead to dyspareunia include a history of past sexual abuse, fear of pregnancy, anxiety, and guilt. Diagnosis is made on the basis of general examination including a description of the type of pain and the time of occurrence.

**TREATMENT** Treatment is dependent on cause and may include instructions on extended foreplay, use of lubricating jelly, and manual stretching of the vaginal opening prior to intercourse. Infections need to be treated appropriately. Surgery may be needed to correct deformities, remove tumors, and treat endometriosis. Psychological conditions may need to be addressed with counseling.

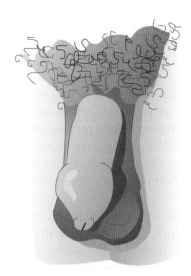

**FIGURE 17–21** Phimosis.

## ■ Female Arousal-Orgasmic Dysfunction

Female arousal-orgasmic dysfunction, also called frigidity, is the lack of sexual desire or responsiveness in a female.

**ETIOLOGY** Frigidity is seldom caused by physical conditions, but neurological disturbances such as those experienced with diabetes mellitus and multiple sclerosis may produce this condition. More commonly, frigidity is due to psychological conditions including stress, depression, fatigue, past sexual abuse, guilt, and anxiety.

**SYMPTOMS** Common signs include the inability to produce and maintain adequate vaginal lubrication and vasocongestive response, indicative of sexual arousal.

**TREATMENT** Treatment is directed at proper stimulation activities and psychological counseling.

## ■ Impotence/ED

Impotence, more recently called Erectile Dysfunction (ED), is the inability of the male to achieve or maintain an erection sufficient to complete sexual intercourse. Impotence does not affect fertility or the ability to produce offspring. Impotence is a common disorder, affecting most men at some time in their lives.

**ETIOLOGY** It is commonly the result of physical problems caused by endocrine disorders affecting testosterone levels; drug and alcohol abuse; neurologic disorders; spinal cord injury; urologic disorders; extensive pelvic surgery such as radical prostatectomy;

diabetes mellitus; arteriosclerosis, which reduces blood flow; and certain medications like diuretics, antihypertensives, and vasodilators.

Impotence is also caused by psychological factors, but these are not as common as physical problems. Psychological factors include depression, stress, guilt, sexual anxiety, sexual trauma, and disagreeable relationships. Diagnosis is made on the basis of a medical history, sexual history, and physical examination including review of medications and laboratory testing.

**TREATMENT**  Treatment is based on diagnosis and may be as simple as a change in medications, or it may be quite involved and include psychological counseling and behavior modification. Untreatable physical disorders may be treated with implantation of an inflatable penile implant. Erections also may be obtained artificially by use of external vacuum devices and injections into the penis with vasodilator medications.

## ■ Premature Ejaculation

Premature ejaculation is expulsion of seminal fluid during foreplay, prior to complete erection or immediately after the beginning of sexual intercourse. This disorder leads to the inability to satisfy the partner or impregnate a female. Premature ejaculation is fairly common, especially in young males.

**ETIOLOGY**  The cause of this disorder is usually psychologic rather than physical in nature. Common psychologic causes include, but are not limited to, guilt, anxiety, and negative feelings or dislike for the sexual partner. Physical causes are rare but may include neurologic disorders, prostatitis, and urethritis. Diagnosis is made on the basis of a medical history, sexual history, and a physical examination.

**TREATMENT**  Treatment is based on the diagnosis and may include sex therapy and instruction for both partners on techniques that help delay ejaculation. Control of male stimulation is important during lovemaking to allow the female time to reach orgasm and allow penetration into the vagina before ejaculation occurs. It is important that both partners understand that this condition is reversible with treatment.

## ■ Infertility

Infertility is the inability of a couple to achieve pregnancy after one year of unprotected sexual intercourse.

**ETIOLOGY**  Infertility may be due to male or female disorders, or a combination of both. It was once thought that female disorders were the primary cause of infertility, but currently, male, female, and combination disorders are pretty equal in occurrence. Approximately one in 10 couples experiences difficulty with infertility. Of that group, it is estimated that half will eventually be able to have a child. Common causes of infertility in the female include:

- presence of STD
- hormonal disorders
- abnormality of reproductive organs
- endometriosis
- scarring from PID; blocking of fallopian tubes
- development of vaginal antibodies that kill sperm

Diagnostic testing for the female may include a complete medical and gynecologic history and examination. Hormone levels are determined by blood testing. Ovary function and ovulation may be evaluated by recording daily basal body temperatures. The structure of the uterus and patency (openness) of the fallopian tubes may be determined by a hysterosalpingogram. Endometriosis and other pelvic conditions may be assessed by visualization during a laparoscopy.

Common causes of infertility in the male include:

- presence of STD
- chronic genitourinary infection; blocking of the tract
- structural abnormalities
- hormone imbalances

Diagnostic testing for the male may include a complete medical history and physical examination with semen analysis. Blood testing for endocrine or hormone imbalances may be beneficial. A urinalysis may assist in determination of the presence of infection.

**TREATMENT**  Treatment is based on cause with the common goal of achieving pregnancy. Treatment may include surgery to correct anatomical abnormalities or remove blockages, or medication therapy to correct endocrine or hormone imbalances and treat infection. Fertility drugs, artificial insemination with husband sperm (AIH), artificial insemination with donor semen (AID), and in vitro fertilization may be beneficial in complicated cases.

## TRAUMA

### Rape

Rape is sexual intercourse (vaginal or anal) without consent or against the will of the involved individual. Victims of rape may be any age and of either sex, but it is primarily an act violating females. The crime of rape occurs at an alarming rate, but many cases are unreported as the victim often feels embarrassed, ashamed, and guilty. Rape is a crime of violence more than of sexual passion. An acquaintance, date, spouse, or an unknown individual may carry out rape. Recent publicity has been devoted to "date rape" drugs or medication that is placed in a drink and renders the individual unconscious to the point of becoming an easy victim.

**SYMPTOMS** Signs and symptoms of rape may include, but are not limited to, torn clothing, disheveled appearance, bruises, and lacerations around the mouth, breasts, genitals, and rectum. Semen may be found on the inner thighs, in the vaginal cavity, and around the genital and rectal area if the victim has not bathed, showered, or douched after the act.

Diagnosis is made on the basis of history and physical examination. Special attention should be given to the emotional condition of the victim. Emergency guidelines are aimed at protecting the victim against disease and pregnancy, and collecting legal evidence should the victim decide to press charges against the perpetrator. Gathering of criminal evidence is best if the individual has not bathed, showered, or douched. But often, because the victim feels very "dirty and violated," these cleansing activities are performed immediately and prior to reporting the crime. Sex crime evidence gathering may involve collecting samples of clothing, hair, scrapings from under fingernails, pubic hair, semen samples, and taking pictures of areas of trauma.

**TREATMENT** Recovery from rape is difficult. Crisis intervention counselors are needed and follow-up is very important. Individuals involved with the victim need to be nonjudgmental, confirm that the individual is a victim, and assure the individual that this act of violence was not deserved.

## RARE DISEASES

### Vaginal Cancer

**ETIOLOGY** Vaginal cancer is a rare form of cancer that occurs in the daughters of mothers who used the synthetic hormone diethylstilbestrol (DES) to prevent spontaneous abortion.

**SYMPTOMS** Symptoms include leukorrhea and bloody vaginal drainage. Diagnosis is made on the basis of a Pap smear and biopsy.

**TREATMENT** Treatment usually consists of surgery, chemotherapy, and radiation.

### Puerperal Sepsis

**ETIOLOGY** Puerperal (pyou-ER-pier-al; after childbirth) sepsis is an infection of the endometrium, usually with streptococcus bacteria, following childbirth. Other names for puerperal sepsis include puerperal fever and childbed fever. In the 1800s the cause and spread of this infection was unknown. During this time, it was not uncommon for puerperal sepsis to sweep through maternity wards and kill most of the new mothers.

**SYMPTOMS** Symptoms of puerperal sepsis include chills, fever, and abdominal and pelvic pain.

**TREATMENT** The modern use of aseptic technique has made this infection uncommon in most of the world except for special instances where asepsis is not properly carried out. Without prompt and effective antibiotic treatment, this condition is often fatal.

### Hydatidiform Mole

Hydatidiform mole is the formation of grape-like cysts in the uterus that fill the uterus and give indications of pregnancy. There is no fetus although HCG levels get abnormally high.

**ETIOLOGY** The cause of hydatidiform mole may be a genetic abnormality.

**SYMPTOMS** Toward the end of the third month, the affected individual may have symptoms of bright red vaginal bleeding, nausea, and vomiting. Diagnosis is made on the basis of symptoms and no fetal heart tones.

**TREATMENT** Treatment is a surgical D&C to remove the abnormal tissue. Since individuals affected with hydatidiform mole are at higher risk for a certain type of carcinoma (choriocarcinoma), the individual should have frequent follow-up examinations.

# EFFECTS OF AGING ON THE SYSTEM

As the female ages, changes in the reproductive system may seem more distinct than in the male. The pubic hair becomes thin and gray, and the external structures become less elastic and appear more wrinkled and sagging. The internal organs shrink in size, vaginal secretions diminish, and there is less elasticity of the vagina. Although sexual stimulation is still important, as in the male, it may take increased stimulation and the aid of a vaginal lubricant to enhance sexual intercourse. Some cancers of the female reproductive system such as cancer of the uterus and ovaries are more common in the older adult. Women over age 65 should be screened regularly for these disorders.

As the female enters menopause, the breasts also begin to atrophy and become more relaxed with a reduction in size.

As the male ages, there is a decrease in testosterone production and the formation of sperm. The size of the testes also may diminish, but the functional ability of the male for sexual intercourse and reproduction continues. There is some loss of elasticity of the penis and scrotum, causing them to appear more wrinkled and sagging. There is some thinning and graying of the pubic hair. Although the male is still able to have an erection, sometimes it takes greater stimulation to achieve this. The ejaculation amount also may be diminished. The prostate slowly enlarges in most men, beginning around age 50. This prostatic hypertrophy can cause problems with urination. The prostate is also a common site for cancer development in the older male. Routine rectal examination of the prostate and laboratory levels of PSA should be completed by all adult males over age 50.

## SUMMARY

The reproductive system is a highly complex multifunction system. It has important physiologic functions, but is also very important in social relationships between individuals. Both procreation and the relationship/intercourse aspect of the system can be altered when disorders develop in the system. Common disorders of the system in the female include infections, inflammation, infertility, fibrocystic disease, pregnancy abnormalities, STDs, and cancer. In the male, common disorders include infections, STDs, impotence, and cancer. Signs and symptoms of reproductive disorders in both sexes may include pain, discharge, lesions, and abnormal enlargement of tissue. Changes occurring in the system in the older adult often affect the individual's ability to perform sexual intercourse satisfactorily. Other changes include decrease in hormone secretion, loss of elasticity of tissues, diminished lubricating secretions, and increased risk for cancer development.

## REVIEW QUESTIONS

### Short Answer

1. What are some of the common reproductive system disorders in the:

   a. Female?

   b. Male?

2. What are the common signs and symptoms of reproductive system disorders in the:

   a. Female?

   b. Male?

## True or False

**3.** T F Endometriosis is an ectopic occurrence of endometrial tissue.

**4.** T F A hernia of the bladder into the vagina is called a urethrocele.

**5.** T F Vaginal infections are very uncommon.

**6.** T F Toxic shock syndrome is characterized by high fever.

**7.** T F Intermittent painless bleeding is the most common symptom of cervical cancer.

**8.** T F Leiomyoma is a metastatic tumor of the uterus.

**9.** T F A Pap smear should be performed every two years on a female who is not high risk.

**10.** T F PMS is probably caused by a hormone imbalance.

**11.** T F Phimosis is a narrowed opening of the prepuce.

**12.** T F Epididymitis is usually caused by an infection from the bladder.

**13.** T F STDs are not common in the male reproductive system.

**14.** T F The best preventive measure for testicular cancer is the monthly self-examination.

**15.** T F One of the symptoms of benign prostatic hypertrophy is urinary retention.

**16.** T F An orchiectomy is the removal of the prostate gland.

**17.** T F Cancer of the prostate may be detected early by the PSA test.

**18.** T F The hormone testosterone is secreted by the prostate gland.

**19.** T F There is some loss of elasticity of the penis and scrotum during the aging process.

**20.** T F It may take increased stimulation and the aid of a vaginal lubricant to enhance sexual intercourse between the older adult male and female.

## CASE STUDY

**Charles Roberts** is a 63-year-old gentleman who has been having difficulty urinating. He states he tends to get up at least twice a night to void and has some difficulty getting the stream started. Is this a problem? He is basically quite healthy and does not have a family physician. He asks for your advice about this. What should you tell Mr. Roberts? Are there other questions you should ask him before giving him any information? How could you explain the effects of aging to him? Should he make an appointment with a physician?

**Janice Simmonds** is a 53-year-old first-grade school teacher. At the present time, she is single but dates on a fairly regular basis. She has been an active person all of her life. Janice has played on a tennis team for 20 years and works out at the local athletic club. She considers herself to be in great shape for her age and has never been concerned about any possible health problems. Her past laboratory history includes an average routine cholesterol level, normal blood sugar, and normal blood pressure. Her mother is still living and well but her aunt died at age 69 of breast cancer. Her father is also living and well. Janice does not consider herself at risk for any major health problems. Do you agree with her? Would you consider her at risk for breast cancer? If so, what risk factors can you identify? Is she also at risk for cervical cancer? What routine clinical examinations should she have based on her age and gender?

## BIBLIOGRAPHY

Advances in fertility technology. (2004, February 16). *Health & Medicine Week*, 774–775.

Bloom, J. R., Stewart, S. L., Subo Chang, S. L., & Banks, P. J. (2004). Then and now: Quality of life of young breast cancer survivors. *Psycho-Oncology 13*(3), 147–160.

Choices. (2004). *Better Nutrition 66*(1), 16–17.

Comparison of HRTs finds progesterone causes less bleeding. (2003, December 5). *Women's Health Weekly*, 5–6.

Epidural analgesia for labor may be linked to breast-feeding problems. (2004, March 3). *Health & Medicine Week*, 684–685.

Global strategy: Breastfeeding critical for child survival. (2004, April 15). *Women's Health Weekly*, 33–34.

Harvard heart letter urges caution on testosterone therapy. (2004, April 20). *Cancer Weekly*, 140.

Herbal treatment for PMS? (2001). *Harvard Women's Health Watch 8*(9), 7.

Kates, J. (2003). The global HIV/AIDS epidemic: Current and future challenges. Kaiser Family Foundation. www.cph. georgetown.edu.

Langreth, R. (2004). Men, cancer, & hope. *Forbes, 124*(9), 96–104.

Love, R. R., Love, S. M., & Laudico, A. V. (2004). Dilemmas in breast disease breast cancer from a public health perspective. *Breast Journal 10*(2), 136–140.

McNeil, E. (2003, June 2). Body smarts. *People 59*(21), 123–124.

New molecular-based method can assess protein expression in prostate cancer. (2004, April 12). *Health & Medicine Week*, 643–644.

Parker-Pope, T. (2003, August 25). Herbs to hormones: Women in menopause are finding relief. *Wall Street Journal–Eastern Edition 236*(39), B1.

Patients may benefit from revolutionary womb transplant surgery. (2003, August 19). *Women's Health Weekly*, 2.

Ruston, A. (2004). Risk, anxiety and defensive action: General practitioner's referral decisions for women presenting with breast problems. *Health, Risk & Society 6*(1), 25–38.

Schwartz, L. M., Woloshin, S., Fowler, F. J., Jr., & Welch, H. G. (2004, January 7). Enthusiam for cancer screening in the United States. *Journal of the American Medical Association 281*(1), 71–78.

Shedding light on the prostate. (2004, April 12). *Maclean's 117*(15/16), 80.

Smith, M., & Mills, E. J. (2001). Select complementary/alternative therapies for prostate cancer: The benefits and risks. *Cancer Practice 9*(5), 253.

Survey reveals low awareness of prostate cancer among African-American men. (2004, April 12). *Health & Medicine Week*, 643–644.

The best herb for prostate health. (2003). *Natural health 33*(6), 19.

The fetus is the father of man. (2003, August 25). *Economist 352*(8138), 95–96.

Ushiroyama, T. (2003). Endocrinological actions of Unkei-to, a herbal medicine, and its clinical usefulness in anovulatory and/or infertile women. *Reproductive Medicine & Biology 2*(2), 45–61.

What's a man to do? (2003). *Consumer Reports on Health 14*(12), 7–9.

What's new about zinc. (2004). *University of California at Berkeley Wellness Letter 20*(7), 3.

Younger survivors suffer more long-term after effects. (2004, April 8). *Women's Health Weekly*, 58–59.

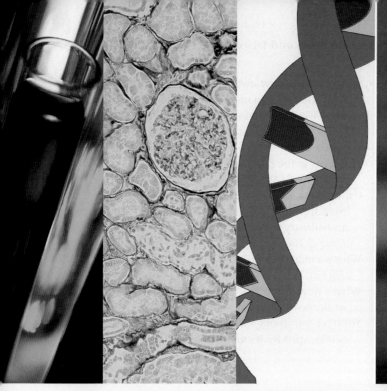
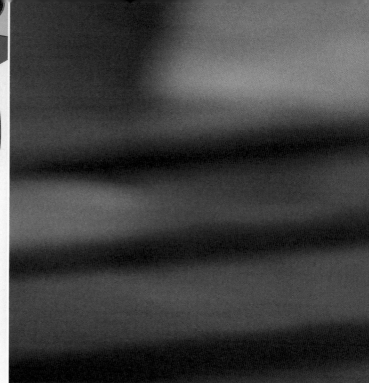

## OUTLINE

## KEY TERMS

# Integumentary System Diseases and Disorders

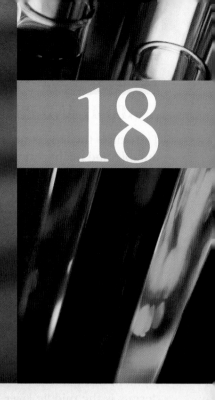

**18**

## LEARNING OBJECTIVES

*Upon completion of the chapter, the learner should be able to:*

1. Define the terminology common to the integumentary system and the disorders of the system.

2. Discuss the basic anatomy and physiology of the integumentary system.

3. Identify the important signs and symptoms associated with common integumentary system disorders.

4. Describe the common diagnostics used to determine the type and/or cause of integumentary system disorders.

5. Identify common disorders of the integumentary system.

6. Describe the typical course and management of the common integumentary system disorders.

7. Describe the effects of aging on the integumentary system and the common disorders of the system.

## OVERVIEW

*The integumentary system is composed of all the skin and its layers. The skin is also known as the largest organ of the body. It makes up about 15 percent of the total body weight. The skin is the first line of defense against disease. Many diseases of the integumentary system are the result of other body or system disorders. For instance, measles is a viral disease of the respiratory system but it is characterized by the maculopapular rash seen on the skin. Skin disorders such as psoriasis are traumatic to the individual because of the obvious lesions and the effect it has on body image. Skin disorders range from mild to severe, and acute to chronic.* ■

## ANATOMY AND PHYSIOLOGY

The skin is the largest organ of the body. It is a large, durable, and pliable organ, and is the first line of protection for the body against invading organisms. The skin also provides a sense of touch, heat and cold, and pain, and helps stabilize temperature, and fluid and electrolyte balance. The skin is composed of three layers: the epidermis, dermis, and subcutaneous level (Figure 18-1).

The epidermis or outer layer is composed of five layers: the stratum corneum, stratum lucidum, stratum granulosum, stratum spinosum, and stratum basale. The cells of the epidermis are called stratified squamous epithelial cells. Most of these are keratinocytes; the others are melanocytes that produce melanin, the pigment that darkens the skin and gives it color. The dermis is the middle layer, consisting of connective tissue and a variety of cell types. Blood vessels transverse the dermal layer to provide nutrients and oxygen, regulate heat, and remove waste products. Nerves also form a network in the dermis. They provide the sensations of heat, cold, pain, and touch.

The subcutaneous layer is composed of connective tissue containing fat cells and blood vessels. The amount of fat varies considerably with the individual. This layer protects the body against cold.

Imbedded in the dermis and extending to the epidermis are the sebaceous, apocrine, and eccrine sweat glands. The sebaceaous glands produce oil called **sebum**. The apocrine sweat glands are located in the underarms (axillae), around the nipples of the breasts, and around the umbilicus, anus, and genital areas. These glands are inactive until puberty and initiate their function with hormonal changes at that time. Their secretions are odorless, but bacteria that accumulate in these areas cause the smell referred to as body odor. Both the sebaceous glands and the apocrine glands secrete through the hair follicles. The eccrine sweat glands are found throughout the body surfaces. They secrete through the skin pores to help the body regulate heat. Some electrolytes are also lost through these sweat glands.

The hair follicles are found in the dermal layer and extend through the epidermis. The hair follicles grow in cycles, which vary with the individual, with an average growth of about 1 cm per month. Hair loss occurs continually, but is not usually obvious until a large amount is lost and not replaced. The male hormone testosterone influences hair growth, especially at puberty when hair begins to appear in the axillae and groin. It also causes the male's level of baldness later in life. Generally, soft tiny hairs cover most of the body and terminal hairs (stiffer, longer, and often darker) are found on the scalp, axillae,

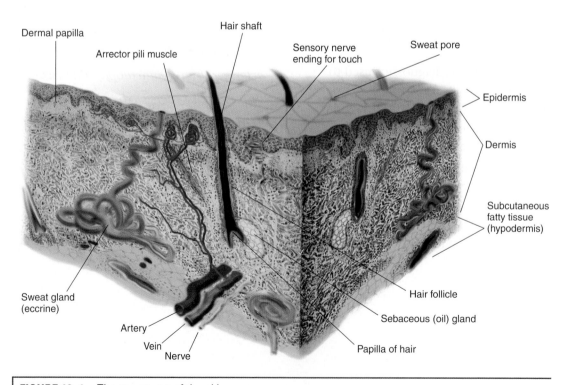

**FIGURE 18–1** The structures of the skin.

groin, eyebrows, and eyelashes of both sexes, and the face and trunk of males.

The nails are composed of **keratin** (epidermal cells in a tight web). Fingernails grow more rapidly than toenails but they are composed of the same material. The thickness and growth rate of the nail varies with the individual. Health status, nutrition, and other factors may influence nail strength and growth.

## COMMON SIGNS AND SYMPTOMS

Common signs and symptoms of integumentary diseases include the following.

- Skin **lesion** (LEE-zhun). A lesion is a very broad term meaning any discontinuity or abnormality of tissue. Lesions may be hard, soft, flat, raised, large, small, reddened, crusted, fluid filled, or pus filled to name only a few characteristics (Figure 18–2).
- Pain
- **Pruritus** (proo-RYE-tus) or itching
- Edema (swelling)
- **Erythema** (ER-oh-**THEE**-mah) or skin redness
- Inflammation

## DIAGNOSTIC TESTS

There are numerous skin diseases. Several have very characteristic lesions, leading to an easy diagnosis. But many exhibit the same or similar types of lesions and symptoms, making diagnosis difficult. Biopsy may be used in diagnosing nodules and chronic lesions. Culture and sensitivity are effective in determining the presence of bacterial infections. Blood tests are helpful, especially if there is concern about a systemic infection or metabolic disorder. Diagnosis and identification of fungal and parasitic infections may be determined by utilizing cultures and microscopic smear examinations.

## COMMON DISEASES OF THE INTEGUMENTARY SYSTEM

There are numerous diseases and disorders of the integumentary system. Diagnosis of skin disorders is often very difficult because several diseases may be characterized by the same type or similar types of lesions. Common diseases may be categorized as to cause and include infections, metabolic, hypersensitivity, idiopathic, and tumors.

## Infectious Diseases

Skin infections are quite common and usually contagious. Care must be taken to prevent spread from one area of the body to another and from one person to another. Most infections are not serious unless systemic involvement occurs. Infections of the skin may be caused by virus, bacteria, fungus, and parasites.

**Viral Diseases.** Viral skin diseases may be acute or chronic. Acute viral diseases commonly affect children and usually resolve spontaneously. Many viral infections become lifelong, with periods of remission and **exacerbation** (flaring up).

### ■ Herpes

**ETIOLOGY** Herpes is a large family of viruses.

**SYMPTOMS** It is characterized by inflammation of the skin and clusters of fluid-filled **vesicles** (VES-ih-kul).

**TREATMENT** The virus is not treatable and remains in the affected individual's body for life. Some type of balance between the host and the virus exists, with periods of viral remission and exacerbation. The virus exacerbates or flares up often during times of decreased immunity as occurs with stress. Common types of herpes virus are:

- Herpes simplex type 1—commonly called "fever blisters" and "cold sores" as febrile conditions and the common cold often bring about an exacerbation. The vesicles commonly appear around the lips and nose (Figure 18–3). Lesions appearing around the lips may be further identified as *herpes labialis* (labia = lip) and those occurring in conjunction with a fever may be further identified as *herpes febrilis*.
- Herpes genitalis, herpes simplex type 2—commonly called genital herpes. This is a highly contagious disease and is spread by direct contact. Genital herpes may be a sexually transmitted disease but transmission is not limited to sexual contact. Autoinoculation with the hands is also possible by touching the lips and then the genitals, and vice versa. Genital herpes type 2 and herpes simplex type 1 cause the same type of lesions and

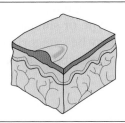

A **papule** is a small solid raised lesion that is less than 0.5 cm in diameter.

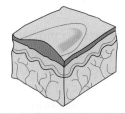

A **plaque** is a solid raised lesion that is greater than 0.5 cm in diameter.

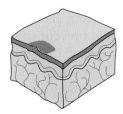

A **macule** is a flat discolored lesion that is less than 1 cm in diameter.

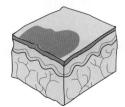

A **patch** is a flat discolored lesion that is greater than 1 cm in diameter.

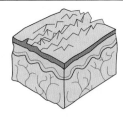

A **scale** is a flaking or dry patch made up of excess dead epidermal cells.

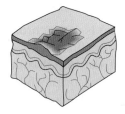

A **crust** is a collection of dried serum and cellular debris.

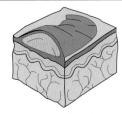

A **wheal** is a smooth, slightly elevated swollen area that is redder or paler than the surrounding skin. It is usually accompanied by itching.

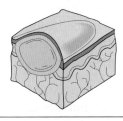

A **cyst** is a closed sack or pouch containing fluid or semisolid material.

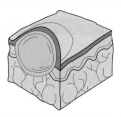

A **pustule** is a small circumscribed elevation of the skin containing pus.

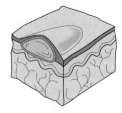

A **vesicle** is a circumscribed elevation of skin containing fluid that is less than 0.5 cm in diameter.

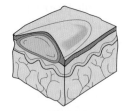

A **bulla** is a large vesicle that is more than 0.5 cm in diameter.

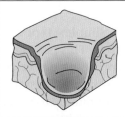

An **ulcer** is an open sore or erosion of the skin or mucous membrane resulting in tissue loss.

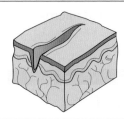

A **fissure** of the skin is a groove or crack-like sore.

**FIGURE 18–2**   Skin lesions.

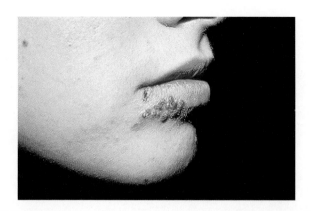

FIGURE 18–3   Herpes simplex virus 1. *(Courtesy of Robert A. Silverman, M.D., Pediatric Dermatology, Georgetown University)*

clinically cannot be separated (see Chapter 17 for more information).

- Herpes varicella—commonly called chickenpox, this is an acute, highly contagious childhood disease. Varicella is discussed in detail in Chapter 20.

- Herpes zoster—commonly called shingles. The virus that causes chickenpox in children causes zoster in adults. Shingles is characterized by painful lesions that follow the course of a spinal nerve. More detailed information may be found in Chapter 15.

### ■ Verruca (Warts)

**ETIOLOGY** Verruca, or warts, is a chronic condition caused by the *papillomavirus* affecting the keratin cells of the skin, causing cellular hypertrophy. Warts usually occur in multiples, and differ in size, shape, and appearance.

   **TREATMENT** Verruca is often resistant to treatment and recurrence is frequent. The most common types are:

1. Common warts—predominantly appear on the hands and fingers of children (Figure 18-4). These lesions are contagious, and are spread by scratching and direct contact. Although unsightly, these warts are usually painless and harmless. This type of wart often disappears spontaneously. Common warts occurring in adults should be called to the attention of a physician to ensure they are not skin cancers.

2. Plantar warts—appear on the sole of the foot. This wart usually grows inward, is smooth on the sole

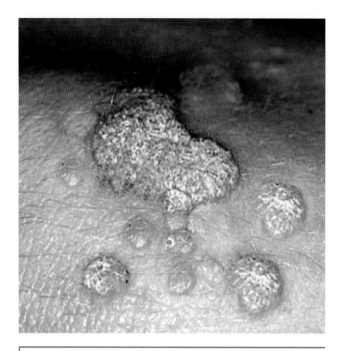

FIGURE 18–4   Verruca (warts). *(Courtesy of Mark L. Kuss)*

of the foot, and feels like a hard lump. Plantar warts contain small clotted blood vessels that appear like dark splinters inside the wart and give it a cauliflower-like appearance (Figure 18-5). This

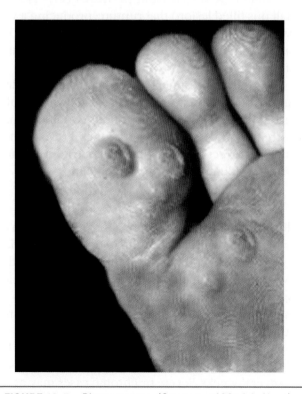

FIGURE 18–5   Plantar warts. *(Courtesy of Mark L. Kuss)*

wart commonly causes pain with walking, thus surgical removal is often the treatment of choice.

**3.** Genital warts—are a sexually transmitted disease. They are highly contagious and often need to be removed surgically. More detailed information may be found in Chapter 17.

## ■ Measles

Measles is a highly contagious childhood disease. This viral disease causes a characteristic maculopapular skin rash. For more information on measles, see Chapter 20.

**Bacterial Diseases.** Bacterial skin infections are often highly contagious, and affect individuals who are immunosuppressed or practice poor personal hygiene. These skin infections are generally caused by normal flora bacteria and are treated effectively with antibiotics.

## ■ Impetigo

**ETIOLOGY** Impetigo is a highly contagious skin disease caused by *Streptococcus* and *Staphylococcus* bacteria. The face and hands of children are most commonly affected.

**SYMPTOMS** Impetigo is characterized by the appearance of vesicles and **pustules** (PUS-tyouls; small pus-filled lesion) that rupture, producing a yellow crust over the lesions. Impetigo occurs more readily in individuals with poor hygiene, anemia, and malnutrition.

**TREATMENT** Treatment includes washing and drying the affected area several times a day, and applying antibiotic ointment. More serious conditions may also require the use of oral antibiotics. Prevention is aimed at correcting anemia and malnutrition, and following good personal hygiene guidelines.

## ■ Folliculitis

**ETIOLOGY** Folliculitis is inflammation and infection of the hair follicle, usually by *Staphylococcus* bacteria.

**SYMPTOMS** Folliculitis is characterized by the development of small pustules surrounding the hair (Figure 18–6). This condition commonly occurs in young men, and affects the thighs, buttocks, beard, and scalp.

**TREATMENT** Most cases are effectively treated by daily cleansing of the area with an antiseptic cleanser for several weeks. Severe or chronic cases may need additional treatment with oral antibiotics.

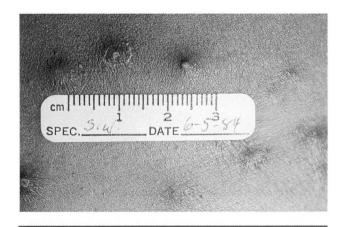

**FIGURE 18–6** Folliculitis. *(Courtesy of Robert A. Silverman, M.D., Pediatric Dermatology, Georgetown University)*

## ■ Abscess, Furuncle, Carbuncle

**ETIOLOGY** These lesions are commonly caused by the pyogenic, normal flora bacteria *Staphylococcus*.

**SYMPTOMS** Abscess, furuncle, and carbuncle are all characterized by inflammation, infection, and the formation of a capsule to wall off and prevent the spread of infection. All of these encapsulated lesions are extremely painful, usually develop a soft spot, or "come to a head," and need to be opened or surgically drained.

**TREATMENT** Antibiotic treatment is generally effective. Predisposing factors for these lesions include a lowered immunity due to the presence of other diseases and poor personal hygiene. There are some differences in these lesions. An abscess is a localized collection of pus occurring in any tissue of the body including the skin. Abscesses commonly occur around sites of trauma, embedded foreign material like splinters, and hair follicles. A small abscess occurring in the tissues of the skin is a furuncle, commonly called a boil. Furuncles generally occur around a hair follicle and may develop during an acute case of folliculitis. Boils may develop in any hairy area of the body, with common sites including the skin of the neck, back, and buttocks. Carbuncles are larger abscesses and involve several interconnected furuncles. These lesions arise in a cluster of hair follicles and have multiple drainage sites. Needless to say, carbuncles are much larger than furuncles and are less common.

## ■ Cellulitis and Erysipelas

Cellulitis is a diffuse or spreading inflammation of the skin and subcutaneous tissue.

**ETIOLOGY** The cause of cellulitis is usually the bacterium *Staphylococcus*. Cellulitis may be the extension of a wound, **ulcer**, or other skin infection.

**SYMPTOMS** The involved area is swollen, red, and painful.

**TREATMENT** Cellulitis is generally treated successfully with oral penicillin. Any cellulitis involving the face may be dangerous as this has the potential of spreading into the sinuses of the skull.

Erysipelas is a form of cellulitis commonly involving the skin of the face.

**ETIOLOGY** This infection is caused by the bacterium *Streptococcus* and may be transferred from the respiratory system to the face.

**SYMPTOMS** Fever, chills, headache, vomiting, and red, painful, edematous skin are characteristic signs and symptoms. Complications include endocarditis and septicemia.

**TREATMENT** Affected individuals are often hospitalized and treated with intravenous penicillin.

### ■ Lyme Disease

**ETIOLOGY** Lyme disease is a multisystem infection caused by bacteria transmitted to humans by the bite of a deer tick.

**SYMPTOMS** The bacteria may affect any organ, causing a variety of symptoms and possibly delaying diagnosis. Symptoms may include flu-like symptoms, arthritis, malaise, chills, and fever. A characteristic "bull's eye" skin rash is a common sign. The bull's eye is a reddened circle with a lighter center and may appear days to weeks after the infected bite. Positive blood testing for antibodies confirms the diagnosis.

**TREATMENT** Antibiotic treatment is necessary as untreated, the disease may cause arthritis and various neurologic and cardiovascular complications. Lyme disease is more prevalent in the northeast and was first discovered in 1975 in the town Lyme, Connecticut, for which it was named. Prevention of lyme disease is aimed at preventing tick bites by using insect repellant; wearing long-sleeved shirts, pants, and socks; and tucking the pants into the socks and boots when hiking or camping in grassy or wooded areas. Showering and inspecting the skin immediately after outside activities may also aid in prevention of bites. The lyme vaccine LYMErix® may be used in individuals over 15 years of age. Side effects of the vaccine include soreness and swelling at the site of injection, and some joint pain, fever, and fatigue.

**Fungal Diseases.** Fungal infections are very common and usually affect the nails and hair. Pathogenic fungi are called dermatophytes and tend to live in dead tissue. Dermatophytes often cause the skin to itch and crack, leaving it open to bacterial infections. Fungal infections are difficult to eradicate and may cause lifelong symptoms.

### ■ Tinea (Ringworm)

**ETIOLOGY** Tinea is a term used to identify any of a number of highly contagious fungal infections of the skin. Tinea infections typically affect warm, moist areas of the body, feeding on perspiration and dead skin.

**SYMPTOMS** Symptoms include itching, cracking, and weeping of the skin. Diagnosis is made on the basis of clinical appearance and microscopic examination of skin scrapings, revealing the fungi.

**TREATMENT** Treatment includes keeping the affected area clean and dry. Antifungal agents in liquid, cream, and powder forms are effective but must be used consistently over a long period of time to eradicate the fungus. Commonly, these fungal infections recur and become a chronic problem. Types of tinea include:

■ Tinea corporis—affects the smooth skin of the arms, legs, and body. It is characterized by red, ring-shaped patches with pale centers, and is commonly called ringworm although there is no worm involved. Tinea corporis is often spread from cats to humans and is common in children.

■ Tinea pedis—is the most common form of tinea infection. It is typically called athlete's foot because it is a common condition in athletes. Tinea pedis is highly contagious, and may be spread by direct contact with contaminated surfaces, such as locker room floors, showers, and towels. Athlete's foot affects the spaces between the toes, causing intense itching and burning. The affected skin peels, leaving painful cracks or fissures (Figure 18-7). Untreated athlete's foot may spread to the entire foot. Wearing cotton socks, alternating shoes to allow complete drying, and wearing sandals help to prevent and treat the fungus.

■ Tinea cruris—often occurs in conjunction with tinea pedis and is commonly called jock itch. It generally affects the scrotal and groin area of adult men. It tends to flare up during summer months, and is aggravated by physical activity, tight fitting jeans, and increased perspiration.

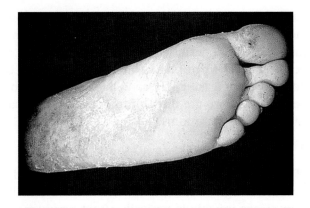

**FIGURE 18–7**   Tinea pedis. *(Courtesy of the Centers for Disease Control and Prevention)*

■ Tinea unguium—involves the fingernail or toenail, and is characterized by white patches in the nail. This tinea is difficult to treat as the fungus hides under the nail. Untreated, the fungus may destroy the entire nail, causing it to thicken, overgrow, turn white, and become brittle (Figure 18–8).

■ Tinea capitis—affects the scalp, causing areas of hair loss. This tinea occurs most often in children (see Chapter 20 for more information).

■ Tinea barbae—affects bearded areas of the neck and face, and thus is commonly called barber's itch. Shaving the affected area is helpful.

## ■ Candidiasis

**ETIOLOGY** Candidiasis (KAN-dih-**DYE**-ah-sis) is a fungal infection caused by the fungus *Candida*. This infection commonly affects individuals with chronic diseases such as diabetes mellitus, those who are on immunosuppressive medications or antibiotics, and

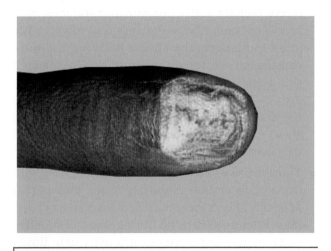

**FIGURE 18–8**   Tinea unguium. *(Courtesy of Mark L. Kuss)*

those exposed to long-term water immersion such as dishwashers, bartenders, and waitresses.

**SYMPTOMS** Candidiasis infection may produce patches of red, itchy skin with blisters and pustules. This infection commonly affects the fingernails, interdigital space or area between the fingers, mouth, and vagina. Candidiasis of the mouth is commonly called thrush. The inner cheeks and tongue are often covered with white patches of infection. Thrush is common in infants and immunosuppressed adults. Candidiasis of the vagina causes vaginitis and is discussed in detail in Chapter 17.

**TREATMENT** Antifungal medications are useful in treatment, but again, fungal infections are often difficult to eradicate and may become chronic in some cases.

**Parasitic Diseases.** Parasites are organisms that feed on a host, sometimes a human. Human parasites affecting the skin are easily spread and cause intense itching. Parasites commonly occur in crowded living conditions with inadequate bathing facilities. The two most common skin parasites are pediculosis (lice) and scabies.

## ■ Pediculosis

**ETIOLOGY** Pediculosis is infestation with lice. Lice are easily spread by direct contact with an infected individual, or may be carried by sharing of combs, brushes, towels, clothing, or bed linens. Lice are not partial to any of the socioeconomic classes, and thus affect anyone coming in contact with them.

**TREATMENT** Treatment generally includes bathing and shampooing with medicated shampoo. There are three types of lice that commonly affect humans.

1. Head lice—commonly spread among school-aged children and their families (Figure 18–9). See Chapter 20 for more information.

2. Body lice—often occur in individuals with poor hygiene practices such as transients and the homeless. Body lice can spread disease and were responsible for the spread of typhus during war times.

3. Pubic lice—are spread by sexual contact with an affected individual and are commonly called "crabs." Pubic lice infect males and females, and cause intense itching in the genital area. These lice also may spread to the eyelashes and eyebrows. Treatment includes bathing in medicated shampoo, and treating clothing and bed linens. Petroleum jelly may be applied to the eyelashes to kill lice.

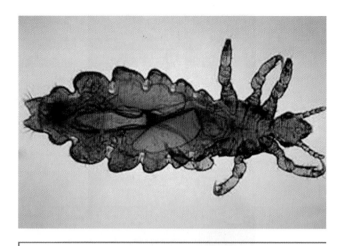

**FIGURE 18–9** Head lice. *(Courtesy of the Centers for Disease Control and Prevention)*

## ■ Scabies

**ETIOLOGY** Scabies is a condition caused by a tiny mite. The condition is commonly called the "seven year itch." Mites are transferred from one infected individual to another by direct contact.

**SYMPTOMS** Scabies commonly affect the folds of the skin such as areas beneath the breasts, under the arms, in the groin area, wrists, and between the fingers and toes (Figure 18–10). The pregnant female mite burrows into the skin and lays her eggs in a short tunnel near the surface of the skin. These burrows often appear as slightly elevated, greyish white lines. Intense itching, vesicles, and pustules develop due to hypersensitivity to the bite, the mite's feces, and the presence of the ova. The eggs hatch in three to five days; the mite matures on the surface of the skin in two to three weeks, then mates, and the cycle begins again. Diagnosis is made on the basis of microscopic

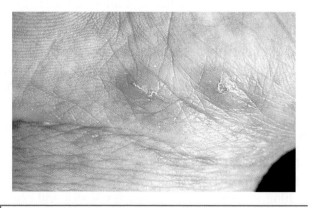

**FIGURE 18–10** Scabies. *(Courtesy of Robert A. Silverman, M.D., Pediatric Dermatology, Georgetown University)*

skin examination, often revealing the presence of mites. Female mites may be viewed at the end of the burrowed tunnel and appear as a tiny black dot.

**TREATMENT** Treatment includes application of lindane cream to the entire body, leaving the cream on for 8 to 14 hours before showering or bathing. All infected individuals must be treated to prevent reinfection. Itching may persist for three to four weeks after successful treatment.

**Metabolic Diseases.** Hyperactivity of the sebaceous gland is the cause of several different skin diseases. Inflammation and infection also may play a role in these diseases, although the primary cause is metabolic.

## ■ Acne Vulgaris

Acne is an inflammation of the sebaceous (oil secreting) glands and hair follicles of the skin, characterized by the formation of **comedones** (KOM-eh-dohs; a plugged skin pore; the open form is a blackhead; the closed form is a whitehead). Acne vulgaris is the most common form of acne, and affects a large number or crowd (vulgus = crowd) of individuals.

**ETIOLOGY** The cause of acne is unknown but it may be considered a metabolic disease because it occurs at puberty during increased production of sex hormones. An increase in these hormones, especially androgen, causes an increase in the size and activity of the sebaceous glands on the face, neck, chest, and back of males and females. Other factors contributing to the development of acne are heredity, food allergies, and endocrine disorders. Many misconceptions or misinformation exist concerning acne. Acne is not contagious, is not due to uncleanliness, lack of sleep, a lack or excess of sexual release or masturbation, venereal disease, or consumption of chocolate, colas, and fried foods.

**SYMPTOMS** Acne develops when sebaceous glands secrete excessive amounts of oil or sebum into a skin pore, eventually clogging the pore and causing the development of comedones. Sebaceous secretions at the opening of the pore may become oxidized and turn black, thus forming a blackhead. If bacteria enter the accumulated sebum and cause infection, the comedone becomes a whitehead or pimple. Acne may be mild to severe. Teens should be instructed to manage acne by:

■ cleansing the skin frequently with antibacterial soap to remove excess oil and bacteria

■ avoiding the use of heavy makeup, which contributes to clogging the skin pores

■ avoiding the temptation to squeeze comedones as this may push the collected sebum further into the skin pore causing further inflammation and infection

Comedones should be extracted gently, and pustules or pimples and cysts should be incised and drained.

**TREATMENT** Mild cases of acne are usually managed with proper cleansing and over-the-counter treatments. Severe cases need a treatment regimen prescribed by a dermatologist, and often include cleansing with prescription medications, oral antibiotic therapy (tetracycline), steroids, and retinoic acid preparations or Retin-A. Even with proper treatment, severe cases often result in permanent skin scarring. Symptoms of acne generally subside after puberty, with or without treatment.

## ■ Seborrheic Dermatitis

**ETIOLOGY** Seborrheic dematitis is a common type of dermatitis affecting the sebaceous or oil-secreting glands of the skin.

**SYMPTOMS** This disease is characterized by an increase in the production of sebum, causing inflammation in the areas of the skin with the greatest number of glands. Seborrheic dermatitis thus affects the scalp, eyebrows, eyelashes, skin behind the ears or postauricular area, the sides of the nose, and the middle of the chest. Affected skin is usually reddened and covered with greasy looking, yellowish scales. Itching may or may not be present. Seborrheic dermatitis affecting the scalp of infants is commonly called "cradle cap" (Figure 18–11). This condition usually clears by 12 months of age without treatment.

Seborrheic dermatitis affecting the scalp of adults is called "dandruff."

**ETIOLOGY** Dandruff is generally treated with special selenium-containing shampoos.

**SYMPTOMS** The eyebrows and eyelashes of an individual with seborrheic dermatitis show dry, dirty white scales. The affected nose area is generally reddened and itches. Mid-chest or sternal lesions are reddened and greasy feeling.

**TREATMENT** Treatment of these affected areas includes keeping the skin clean and dry, and using steroid creams. The cause of this type of dermatitis is unknown although heredity and stress may be factors. There is an increased occurrence in individuals

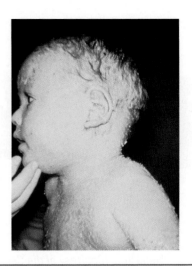

**FIGURE 18–11** Seborrheic dermatitis. *(Courtesy of the Centers for Disease Control and Prevention)*

with central nervous system disorders such as Parkinson's disease and those with impaired immunity. Individuals recovering from stressful medical conditions such as myocardial infarction or who are confined for long periods of time in nursing homes are also more prone to this condition.

## ■ Sebaceous Cyst

**ETIOLOGY** Sebaceous (seh-BAY-shus) cyst develops when a sebaceous gland becomes blocked and the sebum collects under the skin. This cyst can form anywhere on the body except in the palms of the hands and soles of the feet. Sebaceous cyst commonly develops in the scalp, neck, and groin area. A special type of sebaceous cyst is a **pilonidal cyst**. This cyst develops around a hair in the sacrococcygeal area.

**TREATMENT** Treatment of sebaceous cyst includes incising and draining the cyst although it tends to recur. Permanent treatment is surgical removal.

**Hypersensitivity or Immune Diseases.** Hypersensitivity diseases are those that are caused by an immune reaction within the body. Frequently, the cause is unknown and treatment is symptomatic.

## ■ Eczema

**ETIOLOGY** Eczema (ECK-zeh-mah) is an inflammation of the skin or type of dermatitis characterized by itching, redness, vesicles, pustules, scales, and crust, appearing alone or in combination (Figure 18–12). It is also called atopic dermatitis, as it tends to occur in

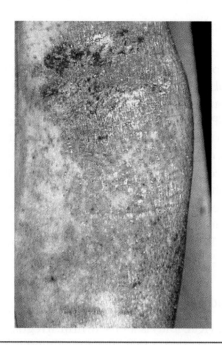

**FIGURE 18–12** Eczema. *(Courtesy of the Centers for Disease Control and Prevention)*

atopic individuals or those with a genetic predisposition to allergies. Eczema is a common allergic reaction in children, often beginning in infancy. It is believed to be due to allergies to milk, orange juice, or some other foods. Eczema in infants often disappears when the offending food is discontinued.

**SYMPTOMS** In adults, eczema often produces dry, leathery skin lesions. Stress, humidity, and severe changes in temperature are a few of the identified factors causing an exacerbation or flare-up of the condition. Diagnosis is made on the basis of clinical examination and history.

**TREATMENT** Treatment is aimed at decreasing the occurrence and severity of the condition, as there is no cure. Topical cortisone creams are often used, along with antihistamines and sedatives to treat pruritus.

### ■ Urticaria

Commonly called hives or nettle rash, this is a vascular reaction of the skin.

**ETIOLOGY** This condition is caused by contact with an external irritant such as insect bites, pollen, or plants. Urticaria also may be caused by internal irritants such as food, drugs, and contrast dye.

**SYMPTOMS** Urticaria is characterized by slightly elevated lesions that are redder or paler than the surrounding skin, and are associated with severe itching.

The elevated areas are called **wheals** (WEEL)s or hives. Scratching or rubbing the hypersensitive area may lead to formation of larger or additional wheals.

**TREATMENT** Treatment includes antihistamines and avoidance of the allergen (see Chapter 5 for more information).

### ■ Contact Dermatitis

Contact dermatitis is an acute or chronic allergic reaction affecting the skin.

**ETIOLOGY** Often, the allergen is some type of cosmetic, laundry product, plant, jewelry, paint, drug, plastic, or a variety of other agents. Often, it is difficult to determine the causative agent, and once found, complete avoidance may not be possible.

**SYMPTOMS** Allergic lesions may range from small, red, localized lesions to vesicular lesions that cover the entire body. A common example of a contact dermatitis is poison ivy (see Chapter 5 for more information).

**Idiopathic Diseases.** Idiopathic diseases of the skin have no known cause but often tend to be familial. They can range from mild to severe and are generally treated symptomatically. They tend to be chronic, with periods of remission and exacerbation of the disease process.

### ■ Psoriasis

Psoriasis (soh-RYE-uh-sis) is a chronic skin disease.

**ETIOLOGY** The cause is unknown but some hereditary basis does exist.

**SYMPTOMS** Psoriasis is characterized by red, raised lesions with distinct borders and silvery scales (Figure 18–13). These lesions generally occur on the elbows, knees, and scalp. A characteristic of the condition is the rapid replacement of epidermal cells. Normally, in a square centimeter of skin, some 25,000 cells produce 1,250 new cells with a life of 300 hours. Epidermal cells in a square centimeter of skin affected by psoriasis will number around 52,000 (twice the normal), and will produce 35,000 new cells (28 times more) with a life of only 36 hours (approximately one-eighth as long as normal). Periods of remission and exacerbation are common with psoriasis. Stress, infection, skin trauma, and sunlight tend to cause an exacerbation of the condition.

**TREATMENT** Treatment includes medications containing coal tar, ultraviolet light, and steroids.

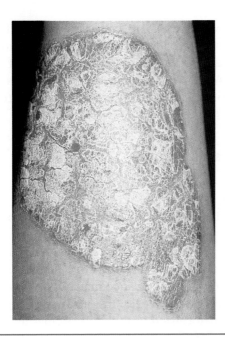

**FIGURE 18–13** Psoriasis. *(Courtesy of Robert A. Silverman, M.D., Pediatric Dermatology, Georgetown University)*

### ■ Scleroderma

Scleroderma (SKLEHR-oh-**DER**-mah; sclero = hardening, derma = skin) is a chronic autoimmune disorder characterized by hardening, thickening, and shrinking of the connective tissues of the body, including the skin. It is thought that this autoimmune reaction begins with the skin and connective tissues attracting lymph cells. These lymph cells stimulate the production of collagen, leading to the disorder. More information may be found in Chapter 5.

**Benign Tumors.** Benign tumors of the skin are relatively common. They tend to be familial and often are more common in older adults.

### ■ Seborrheic Keratosis

Seborrheic keratosis (SEB-oh-**REE**-ic KERR-ah-**TOH**-sis) is a benign overgrowth of epithelial cells.

**ETIOLOGY** This condition of unknown cause is very common among older people.

**SYMPTOMS** The lesions tend to increase in number with age, and vary in color from yellow to brown with a well-defined border. The surface of the lesion is covered with a warty scale that is soft on the trunk but harsh, dry, and rough on the hands, arms and face. These lesions are rather loose and appear to be tacked onto the skin.

**TREATMENT** They are often easily scraped off by curettage, the treatment of choice.

### ■ Keloid

A keloid (KEE-loid) is a raised, firm, irregular-shaped mass of scar tissue that develops following trauma or surgical incision.

**ETIOLOGY** It is due to an overgrowth of collagen during connective tissue repair. Keloid formation is more common in the black population. Keloids may be unsightly but are generally considered to be harmless. Surgical removal of keloids is usually not effective as it often results in the formation of another keloid. Radiation, injecting the lesion with steroids, and cryotherapy may be helpful in reducing the size of a keloid (see Chapter 4 for more information).

### ■ Hemangioma

**ETIOLOGY** Hemangioma (heh-MAN-jee-**OH**-mah; hem = blood, angio = vessel, oma = tumor) is a congenital benign tumor made up of small blood vessels forming a reddish or purplish birthmark. Common types of

---

## COMPLEMENTARY AND ALTERNATIVE THERAPY

### Alternative Therapy for Psoriasis

Historically, traditional Chinese medicines (TCM) have been used for a variety of dermatological conditions. Several research studies have shown TCM to be beneficial for psoriasis and atopic dermatitis. Perhaps practitioners of western medicine should investigate TCM for its benefits in relieving conditions such as psoriasis. The use of TCM along with conventional treatments may be the best practice in the future.

*Source: Koo, J., & Desai, R. (2003).*

hemangioma include port wine stain, strawberry, and cherry hemangioma (Figure 18–14).

- port wine stain—a dark red to purple birthmark usually appearing on the face
- strawberry hemangioma—a strawberry red, rough, protruding lesion commonly appearing on the face, neck, or trunk
- cherry hemangioma—a small, red, dome-shaped lesion

**Premalignant and Malignant Tumors.** Skin cancer is the most common type of cancer in humans, and in most cases, is due to exposure to sun. Skin cancers generally occur in multiples and appear on the face, arms, and hands of middle-aged and older individuals. The most common skin cancer is basal cell carcinoma, but the most deadly is malignant melanoma. Diagnosis is made on the basis of clinical examination and positively confirmed by biopsy. Prevention for all forms of skin cancer is aimed at avoiding overexposure to the sun and lifelong use of sunscreen with a high sun protection factor (SPF).

### ■ Actinic Keratosis

**ETIOLOGY** Actinic keratosis (ack-TIN-ick KERR-ah-TOH-sis; actinic = sun-related) is a pre-malignant condition caused by excessive exposure to the sun.

**SYMPTOMS** It is characterized by the growth of multiple wart-like lesions on sun-exposed areas of the body such as the face, arms, and legs. It is more common in fair-skinned individuals. This condition commonly occurs in middle-aged or older individuals and is also called senile or solar keratosis. Diagnosis is made on the basis of clinical examination.

**TREATMENT** Treatment is with topical medication such as Retin-A, or removal by curettage or cryotherapy.

### ■ Basal Cell Carcinoma

Basal cell carcinoma is the most common type of skin cancer. It is most common in fair-skinned, blonde hair and blue or gray eyed individuals. Basal cell carcinoma is a slow growing, locally invading tumor that does not metastasize. This is not to say that left untreated it is not dangerous. Tumors near the eyes and mouth may invade these spaces and cause much concern. Tumors on the nose, lip, and ear may lead to the loss of these tissues.

**SYMPTOMS** There is variability in the appearance of this tumor. It may appear as a raised nodule with a depressed or dented center, a smooth shiny bump that is pink to pearly white in color, or a nonhealing lesion that bleeds easily (Figure 18–15).

**TREATMENT** Treatment of basal cell carcinoma is surgical removal.

### ■ Squamous Cell Carcinoma

Squamous cell carcinoma is less common than basal cell carcinoma, but it tends to grow more rapidly and become metastatic. This tumor, like basal cell, tends to occur on sun-exposed skin. As a general rule, basal cell

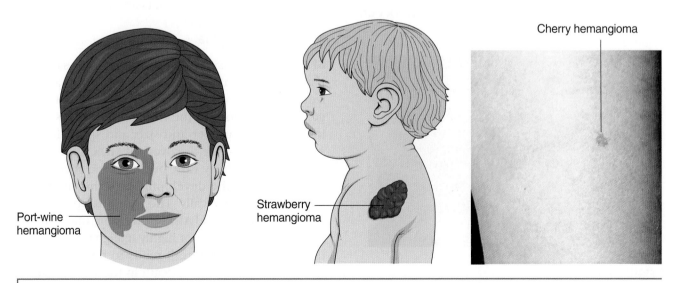

Cherry hemangioma

Port-wine hemangioma

Strawberry hemangioma

**FIGURE 18–14** Hemangiomas.

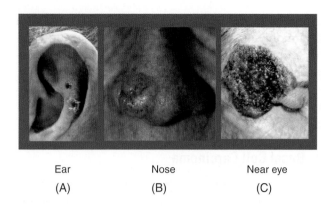

Ear          Nose          Near eye

(A)          (B)           (C)

**FIGURE 18–15**    Basal cell carcinoma: (A) ear, (B) nose, (C) near eye. *(Courtesy of Mark L. Kuss)*

carcinoma occurs on the face above the lip line and squamous cell occurs below the lip line. This tumor is often preceded by another skin lesion such as actinic keratosis, chronic ulcers, sinus tracts, or scars.

**SYMPTOM**  Squamous cell carcinoma may appear as a firm, red nodule with crusts or a slightly elevated plaque (Figure 18–16).

**TREATMENT**  Treatment is wide surgical excision with radiation treatments and follow-up for at least five years for signs of recurrence.

### ■ Malignant Melanoma

Malignant melanoma (melan = black, oma = tumor) is the most serious type of skin cancer.

**SYMPTOMS**  This tumor arises from melanocytes or skin-coloring cells, and is usually tan, brown, or dark brown in color (Figure 18–17). Often, this tumor arises in a mole, and causes a change in size and color of the mole. Malignant melanoma rarely occurs

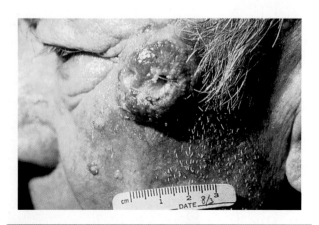

**FIGURE 18–16**    Squamous cell carcinoma. *(Courtesy of Robert A. Silverman, M.D., Pediatric Dermatology, Georgetown University)*

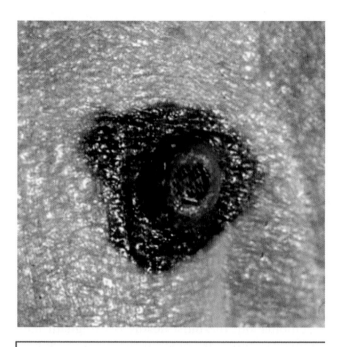

**FIGURE 18–17**    Malignant melanoma. *(Courtesy of Mark L. Kuss)*

before the age of 20 and may be related to a severe childhood sunburn. Malignant melanoma metastasizes quickly and is highly malignant. This tumor spreads into the lymph nodes and may metastasize to all organs of the body.

**TREATMENT**  Treatment depends on the degree of spread, and may include wide surgical excision, radiation, and chemotherapy. Prognosis depends on the degree of spread when discovered, but approximately 20 percent of those diagnosed with this tumor die from effects of metastasis.

### ■ Kaposi's Sarcoma

**SYMPTOMS**  Kaposi's sarcoma (KAP-oh-seez sar-KOH-mah) is a malignant vascular skin tumor characterized by bluish-red cutaneous nodules. These tumors generally develop on the toes, feet, and legs, often increasing in number and size, and spreading upward. Previous to the discovery of AIDS, Kaposi's sarcoma was relatively rare, but with the recent epidemic of AIDS, the development of this neoplasm has increased drastically. The relationship between Kaposi's sarcoma and AIDS is not fully understood. Usually, this tumor is not highly malignant except in the case of AIDS, where it tends to be widespread and is often the cause of death in these individuals.

**TREATMENT**  There is no adequate treatment for this sarcoma.

**Abnormal Pigmented Lesions.** The epidermis of normal skin contains melanocytes that produce melanin or the coloring pigment of skin. Skin color varies from light to dark, depending on the number of melanocytes present. Pigment or coloring protects the skin from burning. This explains why individuals with a fair or pale complexion burn more easily than individuals with a darker complexion. An individual's skin may contain several variations or abnormal lesions associated with pigment. These abnormal pigmented lesions include ephilis, lentigo, nevus, albinism, vitiligo, and melasma. These conditions may be unsightly but are usually harmless and easily diagnosed by a physician. Moles may cause increased concern if they undergo a change in size and shape, possible indicators of cancer. Lesions may be biopsied if cancer is suspected. A brief description of abnormal pigmented lesions follows.

- Ephilis—commonly called a freckle and is indicative of skin damage due to sunburn. The melanocytes in a freckle area are hyperreactive to sunlight, causing the darkened lesion. Freckles commonly occur in children and tend to fade in adults.

- Lentigo—a small brown spot occurring on the face, neck, and back of the hands of older adults. Commonly called liver spots, these lesions are not due to aging but to years of overexposure to the sun.

- Nevus—commonly called a mole. Nevi may be brown, black, or flesh colored, and are often due to a collection of melanocytes. These lesions may appear on any area of the body, vary in size and shape, and occur singly or in multiples. Suspicious or unsightly nevi are often removed surgically.

- Albinism—a hereditary disorder characterized by a decrease or total absence of pigment in the skin, hair, and eyes. Individuals affected with albinism have pale skin, white hair, and pale blue or pink eyes. These individuals suffer from extreme sunburn if adequate protection is not provided.

- Vitiligo (VIT-ih-**LYE**-go)—a condition characterized by destruction of melanocytes in small or large patches of skin (Figure 18–18). This condition may be due to an immune disorder.

- Melasma—characterized by dark patches of skin on the face, especially the cheeks (Figure 18–19). This condition is common in pregnant females and those taking birth control pills. It is commonly called "mask of pregnancy." Melasma usually disappears after delivery or discontinuation of birth control pills.

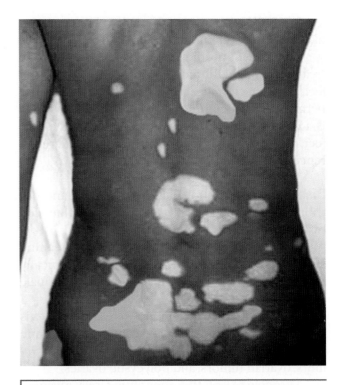

**FIGURE 18–18** Vitiligo. *(Courtesy of Mark L. Kuss)*

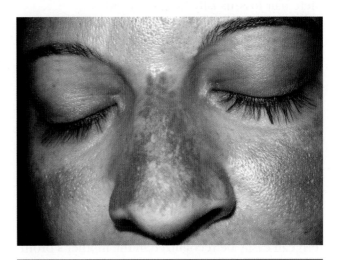

**FIGURE 18–19** Melasma. *(Courtesy of Mark L. Kuss)*

**Diseases of the Nails.** Nails act as coverings for the toes and fingers, and can be considered extensions of the skin.

**ETIOLOGY** Fungal and bacterial infections are the most common cause of nail disease. Bacterial infection of the nails is **paronychia** (PAR-oh-**NICK**-ee-ah), an infection of the skin around the nail. This condition is commonly seen in individuals whose hands are in water for long periods of time such as dishwashers, for example. This infection may cause the nail to lift away from the bed, causing acute pain.

**SYMPTOMS** Diseases of the nail may cause abnormal shape, thickening, and color changes.

**TREATMENT** Antibiotics are usually an effective treatment. Fungal infections frequently affect the feet, are often chronic in nature, and commonly cause permanent nail deformity. Tinea pedis (athlete's foot) is a common cause of fungal nail infections of the feet. Fungal infections are difficult to treat and recurrence is common.

**Diseases of the Hair.** Hair color, texture, and distribution are genetically determined and influenced by hormones.

**Hirsutism** (HER-soot-izm; in Latin meaning shaggy) is excessive growth of hair. Men typically have facial and chest hair due to stimulation by male sex hormones.

**ETIOLOGY** Hair growth in these areas in females is quite distressing, and is usually caused by hormone abnormalities due to such disorders as adrenal tumors, ovarian tumors, and polycystic ovaries.

**Alopecia** (AL-oh-**PEE**-shee-ah; in Greek meaning fox mange, which caused hair loss) is partial or complete hair loss, usually from the head.

**ETIOLOGY** Alopecia may be caused by a number of factors including aging, heredity, thyroid disease, iron deficiency, chemotherapy, radiation, and dermatitis. Alopecia may occur suddenly or over a period of time, and may be temporary or permanent. One of the most common causes of sudden, temporary alopecia is related to chemotherapy and radiation treatment. Hair growth normally returns when treatments are stopped.

A common cause of hair loss in men is an inherited trait passed to males by their mothers. The mother does not have this type of hair loss because it is influenced by male sex hormones, but the pattern can easily be recognized in the mother's brothers or the affected individual's maternal uncles. This type of alopecia is commonly called "male pattern baldness."

**SYMPTOMS** Male pattern baldness often begins around age 30 with a receding front hairline, and loss of hair on the top and back portion of the head (Figure 18–20). In some men, these areas of alopecia eventually meet, leaving hair on only the sides of the head. Alopecia in females is usually due to a hormonal or nutritional disorder.

**TREATMENT** Treatment of alopecia varies according to cause. Treatment of cause usually restores hair growth. In the case of male pattern baldness, hair

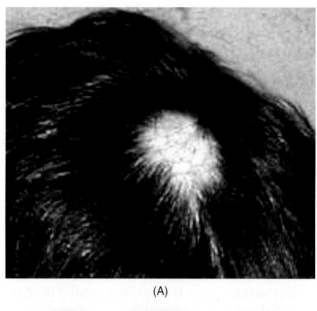

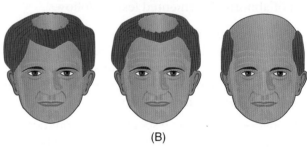

**FIGURE 18–20** (A) Alopecia. *(Courtesy of Mark L. Kuss)* (B) Male pattern baldness.

growth may be restored to some degree by certain special medications. These medications are quite expensive and loss of hair returns if treatment is discontinued. Other options include use of a wig, toupee, and hair transplantation.

# TRAUMA

The skin is the outermost organ of the human body and the body's first line of defense. The position of the skin allows it to be at high risk for receiving frequent trauma. Trauma may be the result of mechanical, thermal, electrical, radiation, or pressure injury.

## Mechanical Skin Injury

Skin is exposed to mechanical trauma in a variety of ways. Mechanical trauma may be due to blunt or sharp objects. Trauma may range from mild and insignificant to major and life threatening. Several types of mechanical skin injury include the following.

- **Abrasion**—is a common mechanical trauma caused by scraping away the skin surface. Abrasions are also called friction burns or rug burns. An abrasion is red, raw, and painful. Bleeding with an abrasion is usually minimal. A skinned knee is a typical example of an abrasion. Treatment generally consists of cleaning the area with soap and water, removing any imbedded particles such as grass or rock, applying antibiotic ointment, and covering the area with a light sterile dressing.

- **Blunt trauma**—may be caused when an individual is struck by items such as hammers and clubs, or is thrown into objects like steering wheels and walls. Falls also may be the cause of blunt trauma. Blunt trauma often causes a large bruise called a **contusion** (kon-TOO-zhun). A contusion is an accumulation of blood in the tissue without breaking the skin. The bleeding comes from injured or disrupted blood vessels.

- **Avulsion**—occurs when a portion of skin or appendage is pulled or torn away. Avulsion injuries usually occur when tissue is caught up in some type of machinery. If an appendage is completely torn away, it is termed an amputation.

- Crush trauma—occurs when tissue is caught between two hard surfaces. Crush injuries commonly involve fingers, hands, feet, and toes. The hands and fingers may be caught in doors or between objects. Crush trauma also occurs when heavy items are dropped on the fingers, hands, feet, and toes.

- Puncture injury—occurs when a sharp object such as a knife, nail, or splinter of glass or metal is forced into the tissue. Bleeding is usually minimal. A feared complication of puncture injury is tetanus as puncture injuries set up an anaerobic condition favorable to tetanus bacteria.

- **Laceration**—is a cut in the skin caused by a sharp object such as a knife, razor, glass, or metal. The edges of the laceration may be smooth, making repair easy, or the edges may be jagged, leading to a more difficult repair. A laceration with smooth even edges is commonly called an **incision**.

## Thermal Skin Injury

Thermal skin injury may be due to excessive heat or cold. Injury may be due to short-term or long-term exposure to varying temperatures. Skin injury may range from mild to severe. Untreated, severe skin injuries may become life threatening.

**Hyperthermia.** Hyperthermia (hyper = excessive, thermia = temperature) occurs when the body is overheated due to excessive exposure to the sun or a hot environment, or may be due to excessive exercise in a hot environment. There are two types of hyperthermia: heat exhaustion and heat stroke. The cause and treatment of these types of hyperthermia vary considerably.

- Heat exhaustion is sometimes called heat prostration.

  **ETIOLOGY** This type of hyperthermia commonly occurs due to excessive exercise or activity in a warm environment.

  **SYMPTOMS** The individual has profuse perspiration and loss of salt and water, leading to dehydration. The skin is cool and moist. The individual may feel weak, nauseated, and may have muscle cramps. Body temperature is usually normal.

  **TREATMENT** The affected individual should lie quietly in a cool place. Fluid and salt replacement may include drinking tomato juice or other high-sodium drinks along with water. In extreme cases, the affected individual should be transported to the hospital.

- Heat stroke is more serious than heat exhaustion.

  **ETIOLOGY** This type of hyperthermia occurs when the body's temperature-regulating mechanisms are no longer able to cope with the excessive exposure to heat.

  **SYMPTOMS** The body's core temperature rises above 105°F, and the skin is red and hot. The skin is dry with a noted absence of perspiration. The affected individual may feel nauseated, weak, and become mentally confused. In extreme cases, the confusion may progress to loss of consciousness with convulsions. Without rapid and effective treatment, brain damage and death may occur.

  **TREATMENT** Treatment is aimed at immediate and aggressive cooling of the body, by removing clothing and pouring cool water over the body, or placing the body in a cool tub or pool. The affected individual should be immediately transported to a hospital.

**Burns.** **ETIOLOGY** Burns may be caused by fire, steam, exposure to hot liquids or items, chemicals, and electricity. The degree of tissue injury is related to the intensity of the heat and duration of exposure.

Burns are classified by depth of skin injury and include first-, second- and third-degree burns.

- First-degree burns are fairly common.

    **SYMPTOMS** This burn is characterized by pain, skin redness, and swelling. First-degree burns involve only the epidermis and are often the result of sunburn. Healing generally occurs within a week, followed by peeling of the damaged epidermis.

- Second-degree burns, also called partial thickness burns, involve the epidermis and dermis.

    **SYMPTOMS** This burn is characterized by extreme pain, redness, blisters, and open wounds. Second-degree burns usually heal in two to three weeks. If the burned area becomes infected, a second-degree burn may progress into a third-degree wound.

- Third-degree burns, also called full thickness burns, involve the epidermis and entire dermis, exposing layers of fat, muscle, and bone.

    **SYMPTOMS** This burn is characterized by charred and broken tissue layers. The affected individual may exhibit signs and symptoms of shock. Tissue burned to the third degree is painless since the nerves in the dermis have been destroyed. This is not to say that individuals with third-degree burns

do not have pain; there is extreme pain, but the pain is due to the first- and second-degree burns around the area. Third-degree burns do not consist exclusively of third-degree burn areas; there is a layering of degrees of burn, with first- and second-degree areas surrounding the third-degree areas. Third-degree burns often need tissue grafting in order to heal. Scarring and deformity are common with third-degree tissue damage.

The amount of body surface burned generally correlates with the chance of survival for the affected individual. Body surface may be determined by applying the "rule of nines" (Figure 18–21). Burns exceeding nine percent of the body are serious and should be treated in large medical centers with special burn units. Generally speaking, body burns of 25 to 30 percent of the body are extremely serious, and 60 percent body burns are usually fatal. Other factors affecting the chance of survival include age, health, quality of care, and complications. Those who are older and the very young do not survive serious burns as well as other age groups. The main complications of burns are fluid loss and infection. Open tissue affected by second- and third-degree burns may leak pints to quarts of serous fluid per day, leading to dehydration

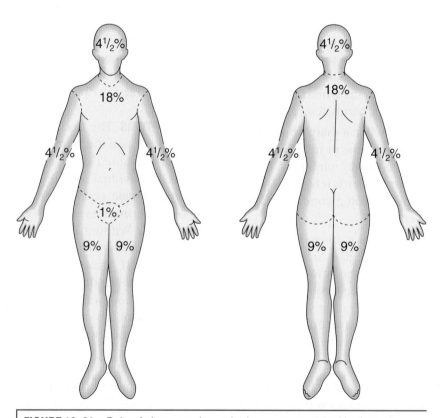

**FIGURE 18–21**　Rule of nines: used to calculate percentage of body surface burned.

and shock. Pseudomonas is the bacterium often causing infection. This bacterium is noted for its ability to spread to the blood, leading to septicemia and death.

**TREATMENT** Treatment of burns depends on the degree and type of burn. Generally, treatment will include cooling the tissue with cool water to prevent further burning. Pain is treated with analgesics ranging from over-the-counter products to narcotic analgesics, depending on the severity of pain. Antibiotics are given orally and intravenously to prevent or treat infection. Antibiotic ointments also may be applied directly to the burned area. Surgical débridement may be needed to remove charred and necrotic tissue, or this may be accomplished by whirlpool treatments. Surgery is often necessary to graft skin, remove excessive scar tissue, and reshape deformities. Surgical treatment may be needed multiple times over a period of months or years to obtain the desired results.

**Cold Injuries.**   Cold thermal injury is usually not as severe or life threatening as heat or burn injuries. Hypothermia (hypo = low, therm = temperature) occurs when the body's core temperature falls below 95°F.

**ETIOLOGY** Hypothermia occurs when the body is cold for a long period of time or is exposed to extreme cold for even short periods of time. Exposure to wind and water increase the chilling effect, and may lead to hypothermia in shorter amounts of time. Hypothermia can be fatal.

**SYMPTOMS** Symptoms of hypothermia include extreme shivering, mental confusion, blue or cyanotic extremities, and weak pulse.

**TREATMENT** Treatment includes removing wet clothing and warming the body with warm blankets, warm packs, or another person's body. Warm liquids may be given if the individual is conscious. The affected individual should be immediately transported to an emergency medical facility.

**ETIOLOGY** **Frostbite** is the freezing of tissue, usually on the face, fingers, toes, and ears. Frostbite may or may not occur with hypothermia.

**SYMPTOMS** The tissue affected by frostbite usually is painless and white in color. With warming, the skin becomes painful and turns red. Tissue affected by severe frostbite may become necrotic and need surgical débridement and amputation.

**TREATMENT** Treatment includes rapid rewarming in warm (not hot) water baths, *not* rubbing the affected tissue, and emergency treatment at a medical facility.

## Electrical Injury

Electrical tissue injury is the result of contacting unprotected or inadequately insulated electrical wiring, or coming in contact with lightning. Whatever the cause of injury, electrical tissue damage has a point of entry and an exit point. The point of entry is the area coming in contact with the electrical source and the exit point is the grounded area. Electricity travels through the body from point of entry to point of exit, causing burns and often causing deep tissue injury. A common cause of death related to electrical injury is due to respiratory and cardiac arrest. The physical jolt of electricity may cause res-

 **HEALTHY HIGHLIGHT**

**Sunburn Prevention**

Fair-skinned persons and those working in the sun—sailors, farmers, ranchers, road crew workers, and construction personnel—are at the greatest risk for development of sunburn, and ultimately, skin cancer. Prevention of sunburn includes:

- Avoiding sun exposure during the hours of 10:00 A.M. And 3:00 P.M., when the sun's rays are the strongest

- Using sunscreen with SPF of 15 or higher on all exposed skin

- Wearing a large brimmed hat to reduce sun exposure to the face, ears, and head

- Avoiding tanning beds

piratory arrest. Electrical current passing through the body may interfere with the conduction system of the heart, leading to cardiac arrest.

## Radiation Injury

Radiation injury may be caused by ionizing radiation such as X-rays and by sunlight. Of the two, sunlight injury is the most common. Exposure to sunlight for short amounts of time leads to skin redness, but prolonged exposure may cause first- and second-degree burns to the skin. Fair-skinned persons are the most easily burned due to a lower number of pigment cells in the skin. Tanning of the skin occurs as a protective mechanism. Tanned skin returns to normal color when pigmented keratocytes in the epidermis are shed. Pigmented skin cells shed approximately every 30 days. Radiation injury also may occur due to exposure to tanning beds. Tanning of the skin occurs in the same manner as with sun exposure. Tanning of the skin is a popular activity because of the cosmetically pleasant color produced. The long-term effects of tanning are not so pleasant. Prolonged exposure to sun or tanning beds causes the skin to prematurely become dry, brittle, wrinkled, and lose elasticity. These effects cause the skin to appear much older than its natural age. Another unpleasant effect of sun exposure is the development of skin cancers as discussed earlier in this chapter.

## Pressure Injury

Pressure injury is caused when placing pressure against tissue leads to a decrease in blood flow to this area. The most common type of pressure injury is a decubitus ulcer. Corns and calluses are also the result of pressure injury.

**Decubitus Ulcer.** Decubitus (dee-KYOU-bih-tus) ulcer is a pressure injury commonly called a bedsore or pressure sore. Decubitus actually means the act of lying down or the position of lying. Decubitus ulcers commonly affect the bony areas of the body such as the heels, sacrum, elbows, and head of individuals who spend prolonged amounts of time in bed. Increased pressure in these areas slows blood flow, thus leading to tissue ischemia and necrosis. Pressure sores can be avoided by frequent turning and repositioning to decrease tissue pressure and allow blood flow to the tissues. Massaging the affected area also may improve circulation.

**Corns and Calluses.** Corns and calluses are protective hyperplasias of tissue as a result of pressure. The main difference between a corn and a callus is the location. Corns are commonly found on the feet, and are due to poor or ill-fitting shoes. Corns are usually painful and the affected individual may seek to have them surgically removed. Calluses are found in the palms of the hands and are related to pressure injury to the hands, generally due to working with hand tools or performing labor. Calluses are usually not painful, and in fact, protect the hands from repeated abrasions and blisters.

## RARE DISEASES

### Elephantiasis

Elephantiasis is characterized by hypertrophy of the skin and subcutaneous tissue, giving it an elephant-like appearance. Inflammation of the lymphatic system also leads to fluid accumulation in the legs, causing them to become enlarged. Elephantiasis is caused by a parasitic worm entering the lymphatic system that causes obstruction of drainage and accumulation of fluids. This disease is most commonly seen in tropical areas like central Africa, and is spread by mosquitoes and blood-sucking flies.

## EFFECTS OF AGING ON THE SYSTEM

There are numerous changes in the integumentary system during the aging process. The epidermal layer becomes thinner and retains less water. This accounts for the easy tearing and dryness of the skin common in older adults. **Xerosis** (zee-ROE-sis; dry skin) is a major problem in older adults. They may have flaky, scaly skin and pruritus. The sweat and sebaceous glands do not function as well, further contributing to the dry skin problem. The youthful elasticity of the skin is lost, causing wrinkles and an aged appearance. If the individual has spent a great deal of time in the sun over the years, these problems will be exaggerated. The nails become thicker and may be difficult to trim. The hair becomes thinner and brittle. There may be extensive hair loss and graying.

Skin lesions are common in older people. Keratoses and skin cancers are the most common problems, especially in individuals who have been exposed

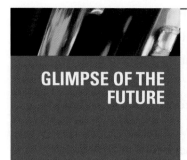

### New Treatment for Rosacea?

A new drug named Periostat® is being tested for use in rosacea treatment. In the third phase of the clinical trials, the drug has been found to be effective for reducing the inflammatory lesions common to the disease. The drug may be approved by the FDA in the future as a new prescription medication for the treatment of rosacea in adults.

*Source:* Immunotherapy Weekly *(2004, April 21).*

to sunlight for many years without using protection. Seborrheic dermatitis, rosacea, and psoriasis are frequently seen disorders. Older adults with chronic disorders such as diabetes or peripheral vascular diseases are particularly prone to develop skin problems, especially pressure injuries. Older adults are also more likely to experience burn or cold injuries since they have decreased touch sensation.

## SUMMARY

The skin is important in protecting the body from pathogens, in providing sensations of touch, heat, and cold, and in regulating body temperature. There are numerous skin conditions, some of which are manifestations of other body system diseases. Skin problems are very traumatic to the individual because they affect appearance and can cause extreme discomfort. Skin diseases range from mild to severe and from acute to chronic. Treatment for many of the skin conditions is symptomatic. Changes in the integumentary system in the older adult cause dry skin, thick, brittle nails, and graying, thinning hair. Older people are at increased risk for secondary skin disorders related to other system diseases.

## REVIEW QUESTIONS

### Short Answer

**1.** What is the main function of the integumentary system?

**2.** What are the most common symptoms of integumentary system disorders?

**3.** Which diagnostic tests are used to diagnose integumentary system disorders?

### Matching

**4.** Match the skin condition in the left column with its description in the right column.

| | |
|---|---|
| _____ herpes | **a.** a form of cellulitis commonly involving the face |
| _____ verruca | **b.** a chronic autoimmune disorder characterized by hardening |
| _____ folliculitis | and thickening of the skin and connective tissue |

_____ erysipelas

_____ tinea

_____ scabies

_____ eczema

_____ psoriasis

_____ scleroderma

**c.** a condition caused by a tiny mite that burrows into the skin

**d.** an inflammation and infection of the hair follicle

**e.** a viral disease characterized by inflammation and fluid-filled blisters

**f.** a chronic skin condition characterized by red, raised lesions with distinct borders and silvery scales

**g.** a condition caused by *papillomavirus* that affects the keratin cells, causing hypertrophy

**h.** an inflammation of the skin also known as atopic dermatitis

**i.** a group of contagious fungal diseases of the skin

## True or False

**5.**  T  F  Genital warts are a sexually transmitted disease.

**6.**  T  F  Carbuncles are most commonly caused by *Staphylococcus* bacteria.

**7.**  T  F  Pediculosis is an infestation of lice.

**8.**  T  F  Tinea capitis is also known as jock itch since it is located in the groin area.

**9.**  T  F  Comedones are plugged skin pores found in cases of acne.

**10.**  T  F  A port wine stain is a type of erythema found on the neck or trunk of the body.

**11.**  T  F  An avulsion is a traumatic crushing injury, often caused by heavy objects dropped on parts of the body such as the fingers.

**12.**  T  F  Skin cancer is the most common type of cancer diagnosed in individuals.

**13.**  T  F  Radiation injury may be caused by ionizing radiation such as X-rays and by sunlight.

**14.**  T  F  In burn injuries, the amount of body surface burned generally correlates with the chance of survival of the affected individual.

**15.**  T  F  Third-degree burns, also called partial thickness burns, involve the epidermis and dermis.

**16.**  T  F  Cold thermal injury is usually more severe or life threatening than heat or burn injuries.

**17.**  T  F  In the aging process, the elasticity of the skin is lost, causing wrinkles and an aged appearance only if the individual has had constant exposure to sunlight over the years.

## CASE STUDY

**Mrs. Moore** is a 54-year-old school teacher. She has been diagnosed with psoriasis. At the present time, she has a few patches on her arms and legs, but not an extensive amount. She asks you to give her more information about the disorder. She wants to know if it will get worse, if it will eventually heal, what she can do to relieve the symptoms, if it is contagious, if it is genetic, and what might cause it to get worse. How would you answer her questions? How much information should you give Mrs. Moore? Where might you refer her for more information? What is her long-term prognosis?

## BIBLIOGRAPHY

A common topical dental treatment also accelerates skin wound healing. (2004, April 12). *Health & Medicine Week*, 756.

Carter, K. F., Dufour, L. T., & Ballard, C. N. (2004). Identifying secondary skin lesions. *Nursing 34*(1), 68.

Coyle, B., & Polovich, M. (2004). Handling hazardous drugs. *American Journal of Nursing 104*(2), 104.

Englert, K. (2003). Stasis dermatitis in the patient with CHF. *Dermatology Nursing 15*(6), 552.

Gorgos, D. (2003). Dermatologic considerations for bioterrorism threats. *Dermatology Nursing 15*(6), 558.

Gottlieb, A. B. (2003). Psoriatric arthritis: A guide for dermatology. *Dermatology Nursing 15*(2), 107–116.

Graham, K., & Logan, J. (2004). Using the Ottawa model of research use to implement a skin care program. *Journal of Nursing Care Quality 19*(1), 18–24.

Kolve, J., & Crutchfield, C. (2003). Acne keloidalis nuchae. *Dermatology Nursing 15*(6), 551.

Koo, J., & Desai, R. (2003). Traditional Chinese medicine in dermatology. *Dermatologic Therapy 16*(2), 98–106.

Latex allergy: Separating fact from fiction. (2004). *Nursing Travel Supplement 34,* 18.

McEnroe Ayers, D. M. (2004). Melanoma. *Nursing 34*(4), 52–53.

Periostat® reduces rosacea inflammatory lesions in study patients. (2004, April 21). *Immunotherapy Weekly*, 110–111.

Pullen, R. L., Jr. (2001). Managing subacute cutaneous lupus erythematosus. *Dermatology Nursing 101*(12), 48–52.

Purnell, D., Hazlett, T., & Alexander, S. L. (2004). A new weapon against sepsis related to necrotizing faciitis. *Dimensions of Critical Care Nursing 23*(1), 18–23.

Rantz, M. J., & Zwygart-Stauffacher, M. (2004). Back to the fundamentals of care. *Journal of Nursing Care Quality 19*(2), 92.

Rudy, S. J. (2003). Overview of the evaluation and management of acne vulgaris. *Pediatric Nursing 29*(4), 287–294.

Skin assessment in neonates and children. (2004). *Pediatric Nursing 16*(3), 15–18.

Skin cancer prevention. (2004). *Dermatology Nursing 16*(1), 88.

Skin disease updates. (2004). *Dermatology Nursing 16*(1), 85.

Skin lesions afflict troops in Iraq. (2004). *Dermatology Nursing 16*(1), 83.

Study reveals that use of selenium does not prevent skin cancers. (2004). *Clinical Journal of Oncology Nursing 8*(2), 119.

Wipke-Tevis, D. D. (2004). Caring for vascular leg ulcers. *Home Healthcare Nurse 22*(4), 237–247.

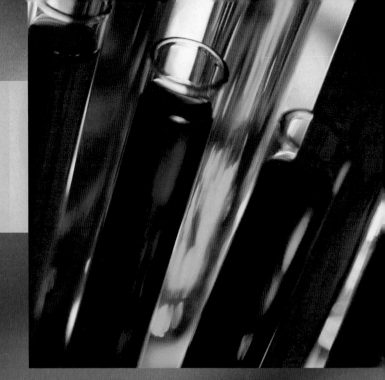

# UNIT

# III

# Genetic/Developmental, Childhood, and Mental Health Diseases and Disorders

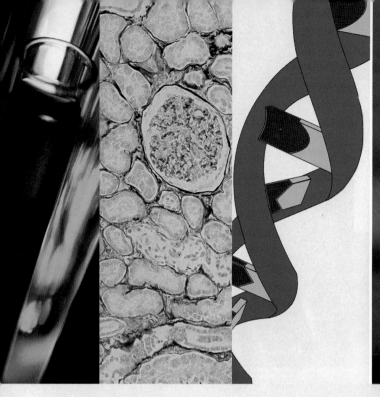
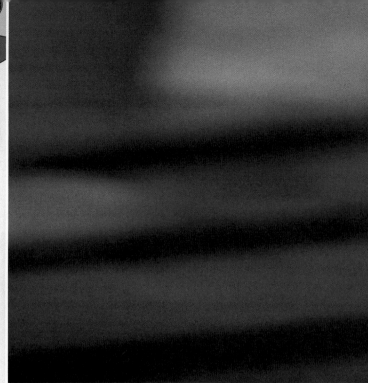

## OUTLINE

## KEY TERMS

# Genetic and Developmental Diseases and Disorders

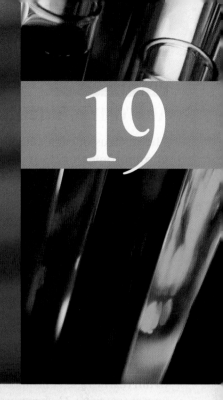

**19**

## LEARNING OBJECTIVES

*Upon completion of the chapter, the learner should be able to:*

1. Define the terminology common to genetic and developmental disorders.

2. Identify the important signs and symptoms associated with genetic and developmental disorders.

3. Describe the common diagnostics used to determine the type and/or cause of genetic or developmental disorders.

4. Identify the common genetic and developmental disorders.

5. Describe the typical course and management of the common genetic and developmental disorders.

## OVERVIEW

Genetic and developmental disorders may first appear or be diagnosed at any age throughout the lifespan. Some are readily diagnosed at birth; others do not display symptoms until childhood, adolescence, or adulthood. Although some disorders have relatively few symptoms, others are profoundly disabling and may even result in early death. In disorders such as Tay-Sachs disease, genetic testing can inform an individual if he or she is a carrier of the disease. There are many other disorders, however, in which testing is not yet available. ∎

## ANATOMY AND PHYSIOLOGY

The nucleus of each cell of the normal body has 46 chromosomes or 23 pairs of chromosomes. Most **somatic** (body) cells have the ability to reproduce in a process called **mitosis** (mi-TOE-sis). During mitosis, the 46 chromosomes duplicate and divide into two identical daughter cells, each containing 46 chromosomes (Figure 19–1). **Germ** (sex) **cells**, specifically the ova and sperm, also have 46 chromosomes, but division in these cells is different. Germ cells do not duplicate before division. This process is called **meiosis** (mi-OH-sis) and results in each cell carrying only one-half or 23 chromosomes (see Figure 19–1). Meiosis is necessary to maintain the normal 46 chromosomes in a newly formed individual. When an ovum (carrying 23 chromosomes) is fertilized with a sperm (carrying 23 chromosomes), the newly formed individual will have a combined total of the normal 46

chromosomes. One-half or 23 chromosomes will have come from each parent.

Of the 46 chromosomes each individual cell possesses, 44 chromosomes or 22 pairs determine somatic or body function, and are called **autosomes** (auto = self, somes = body). One pair (or two chromosomes) are sex chromosomes and determine the sex of the individual. Normal females have XX chromosomes as the sex chromosome and males have XY. A female germ cell or ovum undergoes meiosis and divides into two separate X chromosomes; thus, the only chromosome a female may give is an X or female chromosome. Male germ cells or sperm undergo meiosis and divide into two separate chromosomes, one X and one Y, so the male may give an X (female) or Y (male) chromosome. This explains why the male partner or sperm determines the sex of the fetus. If an X sperm combines with the ova, the result is XX and the fetus is female. If a Y sperm combines with the ova, the result is XY and the fetus is male. Because each male germ cell division results in one X and one Y, there is a 50/50 chance of the fetus being male or female. These two chromosomes, the sex chromosomes, are in every cell of the body, and are responsible for directing the activity of the cell specifically for a female or for a male.

Chromosomes can be visualized by a process known as **karyotyping** (**CARE**-ee-oh-TYPE-ing). This process involves taking a picture of a cell during mitosis, arranging the chromosome pairs in order of largest to smallest, and numbering them 1 through 23. Sex chromosomes can be evaluated by a simple **buccal smear**. This test is performed by obtaining squamous epithelial cells from the buccal cavity of the mouth, staining the cell, and microscopically observing for X chromosomes called Barr bodies. Barr bodies may be visualized when two X chromosomes are present (female). If there is no Barr body the individual is male. X chromosomes are much larger than Y chromosomes and carry more genetic information. The X chromosome not only carries genes for female characteristics, but also other genes essential to life such as those for blood formation, various activities of metabolism, and immunization. The Y chromosome is smaller in size and only carries the genes related to maleness and masculinity.

Chromosomes are made of ultramicroscopic units of deoxyribonucleic acid (DNA) arranged in a specific order. Each ultramicroscopic unit of DNA is called a **gene**. Each chromosome is composed of

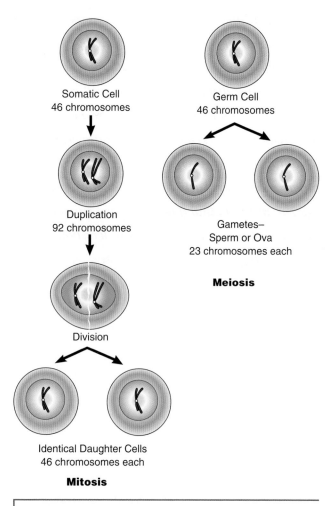

Somatic Cell
46 chromosomes

Duplication
92 chromosomes

Division

Identical Daughter Cells
46 chromosomes each

**Mitosis**

Germ Cell
46 chromosomes

Gametes–
Sperm or Ova
23 chromosomes each

**Meiosis**

**FIGURE 19–1**   Cell division: mitosis and meiosis.

thousands of genes located at specific positions in the chromosome. When the chromosomes (one from each parent) pair up during fertilization of the egg, the genes on the chromosomes align and are called **alleles** (ah-LEELS). This matched gene pair determines heredity, or in other words, expresses those characteristics inherited from parents. When one thinks of genes and heredity, thoughts usually center on facial features such as hair and eye color, but genes also determine the entire physical makeup of the individual from the length of toes to the color and texture of skin. As discussed in previous chapters, heredity is thought to play a part in many other processes such as the development of plaque in arteries and the occurrence of rheumatic fever, obesity, and alcoholism in families, to name only a few.

In order to understand basic heredity, one must look at individual **genotypes**, or the genetic pattern of the individual. Each gene in an allele or matched pair of genes may be **dominant** (in control) or **recessive** (lacking control). Dominant genotypes are expressed with a capital letter (B, for example), whereas recessive genotypes are expressed with a small letter (b, for example). If the alleles or genes in a pair match such as BB or bb, they are said to be **homozygous** (homo = one, zygo = yoked or paired). If the alleles do not match, such as Bb, they are **heterozygous** (hetero = different, zygo = yoked or paired). Expression of a trait such as brown hair or blue eyes is called **phenotype**. Generally speaking, homozygous alleles, whether dominant or recessive, will always express the trait. Heterozygous pairs will express the phenotype of the dominant gene only. Heterozygous pairs are often said to be carriers of recessive disorders as the recessive trait will not be expressed unless paired with another recessive gene (Figure 19-2).

Abnormalities may be due to chromosomal, genetic, or environmental factors, or a combination of these. Chromosomal disorders are usually related to the number or placement of the chromosome. Chromosomes may fail to separate properly during cell division, causing one daughter cell to have an extra chromosome whereas the other daughter cell has no chromosomes. Abnormal number or structure of autosomal (or body) chromosomes is usually incompatible with life as these chromosomes carry

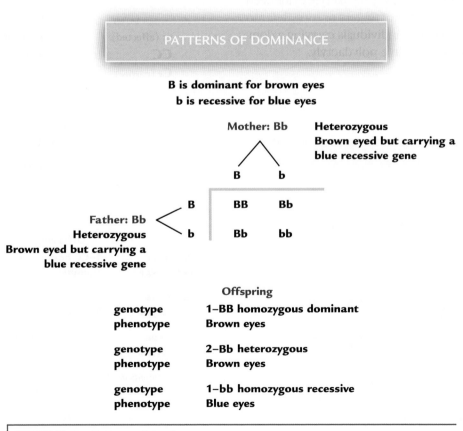

**FIGURE 19-2** Patterns of dominance.

a large number of essential genes. Major chromosomal abnormalities usually lead to spontaneous abortion of the fetus. The most common autosomal chromosomal disorder is Down syndrome. An abnormal number of chromosomes in the sex chromosomes is less serious but does lead to a number of abnormalities. Disorders due to abnormal sex chromosomes are not usually apparent until puberty when sexual characteristics are found to be abnormal.

There are two ways an individual can acquire an abnormal gene: (1) by mutation of the gene during meiosis, affecting the newly formed fetus, or (2) by passage of the abnormal gene from the parents (heredity). Genetic disorders are passed to offspring in four different ways: autosomal dominant, autosomal recessive, sex-linked dominant, and sex-linked recessive.

1. Autosomal dominant—dominant disorders are easily recognized because presence of the disorder identifies those individuals with the dominant gene. The line of inheritance is easily followed from one generation to another. Dominant genes will always be expressed whether homozygous (PP) or heterozygous (Pp). An example of an autosomal dominant disorder is polydactyly, evidenced by an excessive number of fingers or toes. Refer to Figure 19–3 to see how individuals carrying a dominant gene (P) would have polydactyly.

2. Autosomal recessive—recessive disorders are only seen when two recessive genes are paired (cc). Cystic fibrosis is an autosomal recessive disorder. Each parent may be phenotypically normal or without sign of the disorder, but is a heterozygous carrier (Cc) of the disorder. If each parent is heterozygous, the chance of the offspring having the disorder is one in four (Figure 19–4A). If one parent has the disorder (cc), the chances increase to one in two (Figure 19–4B). If one parent is homozygous dominant (CC), none of the offspring will be affected (Figure 19–4C). The occurrence of recessive disorders are often very surprising to a family because this disorder may skip generations and hundreds of years before it is paired with another recessive gene and is expressed.

3. Sex-linked dominant—like autosomal dominant disorders, these are more rare than the recessive disorders and are easily recognized.

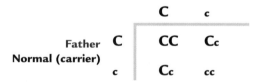

### AUTOSOMAL RECESSIVE PATTERN

| Genotype | Phenotype |
|---|---|
| **cc** (affected) | cystic fibrosis |
| **CC** | normal |
| **Cc** (carrier) | normal |

**Mother**
**Normal (carrier)**

|  |  | **C** | **c** |
|---|---|---|---|
| **Father** **Normal (carrier)** | **C** | **CC** | **Cc** |
|  | **c** | **Cc** | **cc** |

**Offspring**

| genotype | 1–CC homozygous dominant |
|---|---|
| phenotype | **Normal** |

| genotype | 2–Cc heterozygous (carrier) |
|---|---|
| phenotype | **Normal** |

| genotype | 1–cc homozygous recessive |
|---|---|
| phenotype | **Cystic fibrosis** |

*If both parents are heterozygous, there is a 1 in 4 chance of having a child with cystic fibrosis.*

(A)

### AUTOSOMAL DOMINANT PATTERN

**Polydactyly is dominant (P)**
**Normal finger number is recessive (p)**

**Normal mother**

|  |  | **p** | **p** |
|---|---|---|---|
| **Polydactyly father** | **P** | **Pp** | **Pp** |
|  | **P** | **Pp** | **Pp** |

**Offspring**

| genotype (all 4) | heterozygous |
|---|---|
| phenotype | polydactyly |

**FIGURE 19–3** Autosomal dominant pattern.

**FIGURE 19–4** Autosomal recessive pattern.

### AUTOSOMAL RECESSIVE PATTERN

| Genotype | Phenotype |
|---|---|
| **cc** (affected) | cystic fibrosis |
| **CC** | normal |
| **Cc** (carrier) | normal |

**Mother**
**Normal (carrier)**

| | | **C** | **c** |
|---|---|---|---|
| **Father** c | | **Cc** | **cc** |
| **Has** | | | |
| **cystic fibrosis** c | | **Cc** | **cc** |

**Offspring**

| genotype | 2–Cc heterozygous (carrier) |
|---|---|
| phenotype | **Normal** |

| genotype | 2–cc homozygous recessive |
|---|---|
| phenotype | **Cystic fibrosis** |

*If one parent has the disorder, the chances of having a child with cystic fibrosis increase to 1 in 2.*

(B)

### AUTOSOMAL RECESSIVE PATTERN

| Genotype | Phenotype |
|---|---|
| **cc** (affected) | cystic fibrosis |
| **CC** | normal |
| **Cc** (carrier) | normal |

**Mother**
**Normal (carrier)**

| | | **C** | **c** |
|---|---|---|---|
| **Father** | | | |
| **Normal** C | | **CC** | **Cc** |
| **(homozygous** | | | |
| **dominant)** C | | **CC** | **Cc** |

**Offspring**

| genotype | 2–CC homozygous dominant |
|---|---|
| phenotype | **Normal** |

| genotype | 2–Cc heterozygous (carrier) |
|---|---|
| phenotype | **Normal** |

*If one parent is homozygous dominant, none of the offspring will be affected.*

(C)

**FIGURE 19–4**  Autosomal recessive pattern. (continued)

**4.** Sex-linked recessive—these disorders are typically carried by females and passed to males. The reason for this is that recessive gene disorders on the X chromosome of the female are overridden by the dominance of the normal gene on the other X chromosome. In males, the X disorder is expressed because there is no corresponding gene on the Y chromosome. X-linked disorders usually appear every other generation since they are passed from mother to son (Figure 19–5). The affected male (son) will pass this disorder to all of his daughters who then become carriers. The affected male is unable to pass this disorder to his sons because the male gives a Y chromosome to sons, not an X. All the carrier daughters may then pass the disorder to their sons. If the mother is a carrier (XX Hh), there is a possibility that some of her sons will not be affected. If the mother has the disorder (XX hh), which is very rare with X-linked disorders, then all her sons will have the disorder. Hemophilia and muscular dystrophy are both sex-linked recessive disorders.

### SEX-LINKED RECESSIVE PATTERN

Hemophilia is recessive X linked

X and Y are chromosomes

H and h are dominant and recessive genes found only on the X chromosome

**Mother**
**Normal (carrier)**

| | | **XH** | **Xh** |
|---|---|---|---|
| | **Yo** | **XHYo** | **XhYo** |
| | | boy | boy |
| **Father** | | normal | hemophiliac |
| **Normal** | | | |
| | **XH** | **XHXH** | **XHXh** |
| | | girl | girl |
| | | normal | normal (carrier) |

**FIGURE 19–5**  Sex-linked recessive pattern.

Approximately two percent of all newborns have a significant birth defect or **congenital** (kon-JEN-ih-tahl; present at birth) **anomaly** (ah-NOM-ah-lee; abnormality). A high percentage of defects (60%) are due to an unknown cause. Other causes are genetic (20%), chromosomal (10%) and environmental (10%) (Figure 19–6). Chromosomal and genetic causes have been discussed. Environmental causes include maternal radiation, infection, metabolic disorders, drugs, and medications to name only a few.

## COMMON SIGNS AND SYMPTOMS

Signs and symptoms of the various genetic and developmental disorders are varied depending on the disorder, and are discussed individually with each disorder.

## DIAGNOSTIC TESTS

Diagnosis of many of the genetic and developmental disorders begins with a physical examination of the affected individual. Diagnostic tests for these disorders are varied depending on the disorder, and also are discussed individually with each disorder. Prenatal diagnosis of genetic and developmental disorders is beneficial for genetic and family counseling. Tests to diagnose prenatal disorders include:

- ultrasonography of the fetus to detect malformations of the head, internal organs, and extremities

- amniotic fluid analysis to determine genetic and chromosomal disorders

- maternal blood analysis to observe for abnormal fetal substances

## COMMON GENETIC AND DEVELOPMENTAL DISORDERS

There are hundreds of genetic and developmental disorders among populations; however, most of them are very rare in occurrence. Some of the more familiar ones are covered here. Genetic or developmental disorders may affect only one body system or may involve several systems. Muscular dystrophy, for example, which affects the musculoskeletal system, can also be considered a neurological system disease because it affects the neurons, thereby affecting muscle movement.

### Musculoskeletal

Genetic and developmental musculoskeletal disorders are some of the more familiar severe disorders. The severity of the disease varies with the particular disorder and other problems the individual has.

#### ■ Muscular Dystrophy (MD)

**ETIOLOGY** Muscular dystrophy (dys = abnormal, trophic = nourishment, growth) is a group of genetically inherited diseases characterized by degeneration or weakening of the muscles. The affected muscles are unable to store needed protein. Malnourished muscle fibers die, and are replaced with fat and connective tissue. Fat and connective tissue fibers are unable to contract and function like muscle fibers, causing progressive weakness. Over a period of time, the muscle digresses from weak to useless.

The most common type of muscular dystrophy is Duchenne's MD. Duchenne's is also called pseudohypertrophic (pseudo = false, hyper = excessive, trophic = nourishment, growth) MD because the

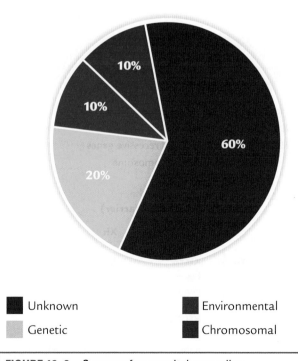

| | |
|---|---|
| ■ Unknown | ■ Environmental |
| ▨ Genetic | ■ Chromosomal |

**FIGURE 19–6**    Causes of congenital anomalies.

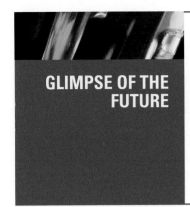

## Looking at the Cause of Muscular Dystrophy

Genetic investigators looking at the cause of muscular dystrophy (MD) found it comes from a warped form of RNA. Normal RNA transmits information from DNA to promote protein production. In MD, the warped RNA prevents the proteins from working correctly. It is not yet clear how this warped mutation occurs but it may be answered in the near future. Researchers act like detectives studying the disease on a cellular level to find the answers. Once the cause is certain, researchers will continue to try to find out how to prevent the disease.

*Source:* The Medical Herald *(2004).*

affected muscle appears healthy and bulging when in reality, the muscle is bulking up in size due to fat deposits. This bulking of muscle mass is especially noticeable in the calf muscle. Duchenne's MD is a sex-linked disorder generally passed from mother to son.

**SYMPTOMS** Onset is usually between the ages of two to five years of age. The pelvic and leg muscles are usually affected first, leading to a characteristic waddling gait, toe walking, lordosis, and Gower's maneuver (a characteristic way of getting up from a squatting position that demonstrates the weakness of the pelvic muscles) (Figure 19-7). Affected children are usually confined to a wheelchair by age nine. Life expectancy is usually in the late teens or early 20s with death due to respiratory or cardiac complications. Diagnosis is made on the basis of physical examination, muscle biopsy, and electromyography.

**TREATMENT** Although there is no cure for MD, physical therapy, orthopedic appliances such as leg braces, and exercise are quite effective in maintaining mobility and quality of life.

## ■ Congenital Hip Dislocation (CHD)

Congenital hip dislocation is an abnormality of the hip joint or acetabulum resulting in the femoral head or ball slipping out of the normal position.

**ETIOLOGY** It is thought that this disorder occurs as a result of (1) improper positioning of the fetus in the uterus prior to or during birth, or (2) the maternal hormones, which relax the mother's pelvic ligaments during labor, also relaxing the joint ligaments in the infant. CHD is more common in girls and is usually obvious during the first few months of life.

**SYMPTOMS** The affected infant may exhibit asymmetrical folds of the affected thigh, a difference in leg length, and limited abduction. This limited

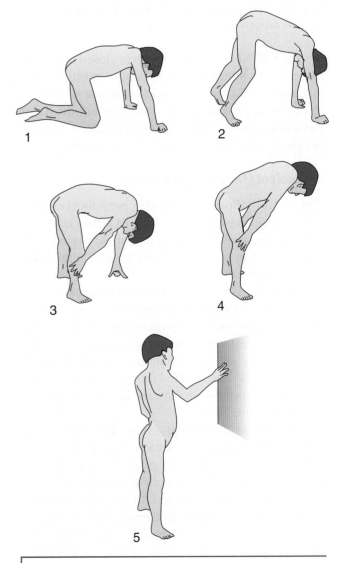

**FIGURE 19–7** Gower's maneuver.

abduction is called a positive Ortolani's sign (Figure 19-8). Diagnosis is confirmed by physical examination and hip joint X-ray studies.

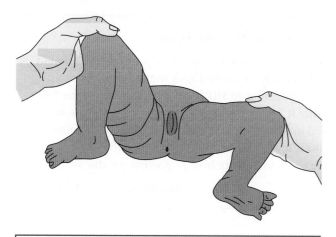

**FIGURE 19–8** Asymmetrical thigh folds and Ortolani's sign in congenital hip dislocation.

**TREATMENT** Treatment involves closed reduction (placing the femoral head in proper position), and maintaining the normal position by use of a splint or cast for approximately two to three months. Treatment may require surgery in older children. The earlier the treatment is begun, the better the prognosis.

### ■ Clubfoot (Talipes Equinovarus)

Clubfoot, or talipes (talus=ankle, pes=foot) equinovarus (TAL-eh-peas ee-KWI-no-**VAY**-rus; equine= horse or toe walking, similar to a horse, varus=bent inward), is a frequently occurring congenital deformity of the foot.

**ETIOLOGY** The cause of clubfoot is unknown, but it is thought to be due to genetic factors or fetal position in the uterus. Some positional deformities may be straightened with manipulation but a true club foot deformity will not straighten with manipulation.

**SYMPTOMS** The affected foot or feet turn inward with the toes pointed downward and the heel drawn upward (Figure 19–9).

**TREATMENT** Treatment is quite successful if begun during infancy. Treatment may involve application of a cast or splints to gradually straighten the foot. The cast or splints are changed frequently until the desired position is achieved. If casting and splinting do not achieve the desired results, surgery may be indicated. Attention must be given to the position of the child's feet throughout childhood to ensure normal position is maintained.

### ■ Osteogenesis Imperfecta

**ETIOLOGY** Osteogenesis (osteo = bone, genesis = beginning) imperfecta (not perfect or normal) is an

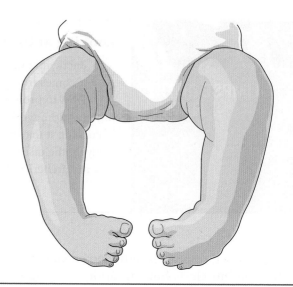

**FIGURE 19–9** Talipes equinovarus (clubfoot).

inherited condition characterized by abnormally brittle bones often leading to frequent fractures.

**SYMPTOMS** Undiagnosed children affected with osteogenesis imperfecta may be suspected as victims of child abuse due to the frequency of bone fractures. Other significant signs are an abnormally blue coloration of the sclera of the eyes, otosclerotic deafness, translucent skin, and thin dental enamel of the teeth.

**TREATMENT** There is no cure for osteogenesis imperfecta, but the tendency of bones to fracture decreases with age and often disappears by adulthood.

## Neurologic

Genetic and developmental neurologic disorders are some of the most severe because of their long-term debilitating effects. Two of the most common disorders in this category are hydrocephalus and cerebral palsy.

### ■ Hydrocephalus

Hydrocephalus (high-droh-SEF-ah-lus; hydro = water, cephal = brain) is an abnormal accumulation of cerebrospinal fluid in the brain.

**ETIOLOGY** Hydrocephalus is generally caused by obstruction of the flow of cerebrospinal fluid out of the brain. This obstruction may be due to a congenital defect, infection, or tumor.

**SYMPTOMS** The head of the affected child may be normal at birth but will rapidly enlarge over the first few months of life as the fluid accumulates. The brain tissue becomes compressed and the skull begins to bulge. Other signs include bulging eyes, a tight scalp, prominent head veins, and a shrill, high-pitched cry. The infant is unable to lift its head, fails to develop normally, and is mentally challenged. Diagnosis is confirmed with skull X-rays and angiography.

**TREATMENT** Treatment of choice is surgical correction by placing a shunt from the brain to the peritoneal cavity or right atrium of the heart to drain the excess fluid (Figure 19–10). Even with early surgical intervention, the prognosis is guarded. Mortality rate is high without surgical correction.

## ■ Cerebral Palsy

Cerebral palsy (SER-eh-bral PAWL-zee) is a congenital bilateral paralysis that results from inadequate blood or oxygen supply to the brain during fetal development, the birthing process, or in infancy.

**ETIOLOGY** Causes of cerebral palsy (CP) include maternal rubella, toxemia, birthing difficulties such as prolonged labor, anoxia, hypoxemia, asphyxia from the umbilical cord being wrapped around the infant's neck, head trauma, and meningitis. Often, the cause

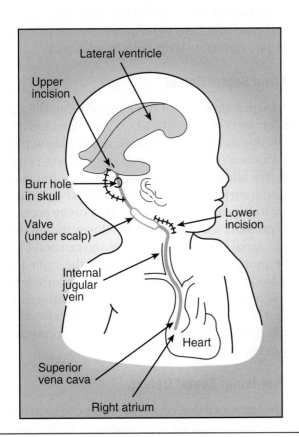

**FIGURE 19–10** A ventricle shunt drains spinal fluid in an infant with hydrocephalus.

of CP is unknown. Cerebral palsy is the most common crippler of children, and more often affects premature infants and males.

**SYMPTOMS** This disorder usually affects motor or muscle performance and may be noticed if the infant has difficulty sucking or swallowing. Other complications include visual and hearing deficits, seizure activity, and mental challenges. Cerebral palsy is characterized by hyperactive reflexes, rapid muscle contraction, and muscle weakness. The affected child commonly has a "scissors gait" exhibited by toe walking and crossing one foot over the other with each step.

**TREATMENT** There is no cure for cerebral palsy. Treatment involves physical therapy, speech therapy, orthopedic cast, braces, and often surgery to help the child reach full potential. Anticonvulsant and muscle relaxant medications also may be of some benefit.

## ■ Spina Bifida

Spina bifida (SPY-nah BIF-ih-dah) is a congenital disorder in which one or more of the vertebrae of the bony spinal column fails to close over the spinal cord, leaving an opening in the column. *Bifid* means split in two parts, which describes the vertebra in this condition. Development of the spinal cord and column occurs during the first trimester of pregnancy.

**ETIOLOGY** The cause of this malformation is unknown, but risk factors include maternal radiation, virus, and genetic factors since children born with spina bifida are more often born to mothers who have other children with this defect. There are several other conditions that tend to accompany spina bifida including hydrocephalus, cleft palate, and clubfoot. Spina bifida can be seen on X-ray examination. There are several forms of spina bifida (Figure 19–11). These forms are described as follows.

1. Spina bifida occulta—**SYMPTOMS** the most common form. There is a spina bifida but it is asymptomatic and hidden (occulta). Signs of the malformation often include a dimpling of the skin, and a tuft of hair or port wine nevus on the skin surface above the defect.

2. Meningocele—**SYMPTOMS** occurs when the meninges of the spinal cord protrude through the opening in the vertebral column, forming a fluid-filled sac on the skin surface. Because nerve tissue is not involved, the infant usually does not have neurologic problems.

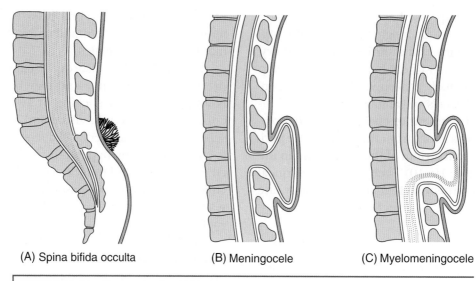

(A) Spina bifida occulta     (B) Meningocele     (C) Myelomeningocele

**FIGURE 19–11**    Types of spina bifida.

**TREATMENT** Surgical intervention to correct the condition is usually performed in the first 24 to 48 hours of life.

3. Myelomeningocele—the most serious spina bifida. **SYMPTOMS** The meninges and a portion of the spinal cord protrude through the opening in the vertebral column, causing neurologic symptoms. Common symptoms include skeletal malformation, deformed joints, paralysis of the legs, and bowel and bladder incontinence.

**TREATMENT** Surgical intervention to correct the condition is usually performed in the first 24 hours of life. Additional procedures may be needed as the child grows. Some of these children are unable to walk, and may die before the age of two or three years.

## Cardiovascular

The heart and its related great vessels are the most common sites of congenital defects. The defects may be small or quite large, and consequences of these deformities may range from asymptomatic to life threatening. Collectively, these malformations of heart structure are called congenital heart defects.

**ETIOLOGY** The cause of these defects is unknown but a genetic tendency is strongly suspected. Certain risk factors include maternal rubella, poor maternal nutrition, and alcoholism. Diagnosis is made by electrocardiogram and physical examination including **auscultation** (listening to the chest with a stethoscope), which usually reveals heart **murmurs** (abnormal heart sounds) if present.

**TREATMENT** Early diagnosis and surgical correction of these defects have improved drastically in recent years and have significantly reduced the mortality rate of infants born with heart defects.

### ■ Atrial Septal Defect

Atrial septal defect is an opening between the right and left atria (Figure 19–12A). This defect is commonly due to the foramen ovale not closing at birth. The foramen ovale is a natural opening between the atria that allows blood to bypass the nonfunctional lungs during fetal life. Once the infant is born, the act of breathing causes a change in chest cavity pressure. This pressure change normally closes the foramen ovale. Atrial septal defects allow oxygenated blood to be pumped from the left atria to the right atria. This blood is again pumped to the right ventricle and to the lungs without ever circulating through the body. This repumping causes an increased workload on the right side of the heart. This defect occurs more commonly in girls than boys.

### ■ Ventricular Septal Defect

Ventricular septal defects are the most common heart defects, accounting for approximately 25 percent of all heart defects. As the name suggests, this defect is a hole between the right and left ventricle (Figure

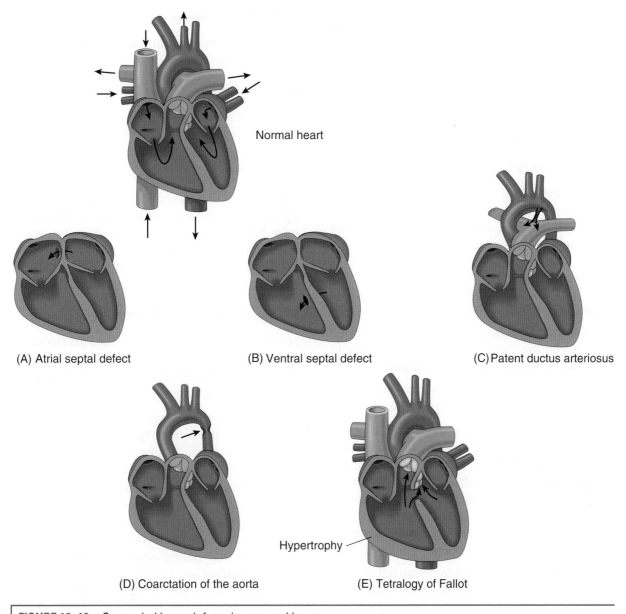

Normal heart

(A) Atrial septal defect

(B) Ventral septal defect

(C) Patent ductus arteriosus

(D) Coarctation of the aorta

Hypertrophy

(E) Tetralogy of Fallot

**FIGURE 19–12** Congenital heart defects in a normal heart.

19-12B) that allows blood from the left ventricle to flow into the right ventricle. Like the atrial septal defect, this oxygenated blood has to be repumped, causing an increase in workload on the right side of the heart.

### ■ Patent Ductus Arteriosus

A ductus arteriosus is a connection between the pulmonary artery and the aorta of the normal fetal heart (Figure 19-12C). This structure allows blood to flow from the pulmonary artery to the aorta, thus bypassing the nonfunctional lungs. The ductus arteriosus, like the foramen ovale, normally closes off shortly after birth. If the structure does not close or remains "patent," the condition is called patent ductus arteriosus. With this condition, oxygenated blood shunts abnormally from the higher pressured aorta back to the pulmonary artery. Once in the pulmonary artery, the blood is recirculated to the lungs. This condition causes an increased workload on the heart and pulmonary system. This condition occurs twice as frequently in girls as in boys.

### ■ Coarctation of the Aorta

Coarctation is a **stricture** or narrowing. A coarctation of the aorta is a narrowing of the descending or thoracic aorta (Figure 19–12D). This condition causes a high blood pressure proximal to the stricture and lower blood pressure distal to the stricture. Infants or children affected with coarctation of the aorta may have a high blood pressure in the arms but a lower blood pressure in the legs. Coarctation increases the workload on the heart as the heart attempts to pump blood through the narrowed vessels.

### ■ Tetralogy of Fallot

Tetralogy of Fallot (TET-traw-lawgee of fall-OH) is a combination of four (tetra) defects (Figure 19–12E) and is one of the most serious of congenital heart defects. The four defects are as follows.

1. Pulmonary valve stenosis—the opening into the pulmonary artery is too small, restricting the amount of blood flow to the lungs

2. Right ventricle hypertrophy—due to the increased workload on the right ventricle as it attempts to pump blood through the stenotic valve

3. Ventricle septal defect—allowing oxygenated blood to flow from the left ventricle to the right

4. Abnormal placement of the aorta—the aorta opens over the ventricle septal defect, allowing blood from both ventricles to be pumped into the aorta. The unoxygenated blood from the right ventricle enters the general circulation without passing through the lungs to become oxygenated. This unoxygenated blood from the right ventricle causes the tissues to become cyanotic or "blue."

**SYMPTOMS** Infants and children with tetralogy of Fallot are truly "blue babies." Cyanosis increases with age, and clubbing of fingers and toes becomes evident. Older children will rest in a squatting position in order to breathe easier. This position also increases venous return. Other symptoms are growth retardation, severe dyspnea with exercise, and frequent respiratory infections.

**TREATMENT** Surgical repair is the treatment of choice.

## Blood

Genetic and developmental disorders of the blood are more common in certain population groups. For example, some anemias are most commonly found in black populations whereas other anemias are more common in European populations. Sickle cell anemia and hemophilia are both discussed in more detail in Chapter 7.

### ■ Sickle Cell Anemia

Sickle cell anemia is a chronic hereditary form of anemia found predominately in black individuals.

### ■ Hemophilia

Hemophilia is an X-linked hereditary bleeding disorder passed from a carrier mother to a son.

## Digestive

Digestive system disorders, both genetic and developmental, range from mild to severe. Many are diagnosed at birth, especially if the disorder interferes with ingestion, digestion, or elimination. Some of them are incompatible with life and must be corrected immediately or the infant would not survive.

### ■ Developmental Malformations

Several developmental malformations occur in the digestive system. Surgical correction is the treatment of choice for these malformations. A few of the more common malformations are briefly discussed here.

■ Meckel's diverticulum—an outpouching or diverticulum of the ileum (Figure 19–13A). During fetal life, the intestine is connected to the yolk sack by a duct. Failure of the duct to disappear leads to formation of this diverticulum. Meckel's diverticulum is the most common malformation of the gastrointestinal system, occurring in approximately two percent of the population. The diverticulum may be asymptomatic the entire life of the individual and found only on autopsy. If symptoms do occur, it is usually during infancy. The most common symptom is painless bloody stools.

■ Esophageal atresia—the absence of part of, or abnormal closure of, the esophagus. An **atresia** (ah-TREE-ze-ah) is the congenital absence or closure of a normal opening or lumen in the body, and may occur in a variety of areas. Esophageal atresia is often accompanied by a fistula connecting the trachea to the esophagus (Figure 19–13B).

■ Congenital diaphragmatic hernia—a congenital hole in the diaphragm. Abdominal organs may herniate through this opening, causing difficulty in breathing and chest pain (Figure 19–13C).

■ Imperforate anus—a failure of the anus to connect to the rectum (Figure 19–13D). Infants with imperforate anus commonly have other developmental anomalies such as those affecting the heart, kidneys, esophagus, and spine.

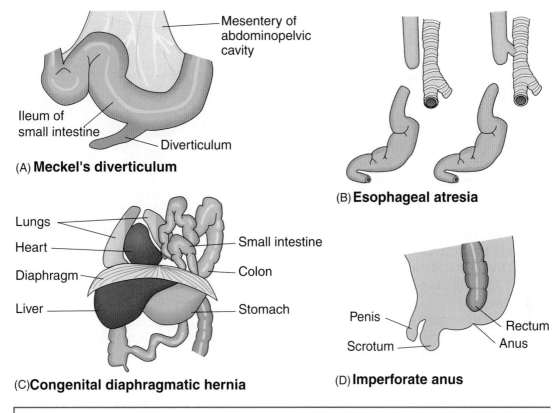

(A) **Meckel's diverticulum**

(B) **Esophageal atresia**

(C) **Congenital diaphragmatic hernia**

(D) **Imperforate anus**

**FIGURE 19–13** Digestive developmental malformations.

## ■ Cleft Lip and Palate

Cleft (a split) lip, formerly commonly called a hare-lip, consists of one or more abnormal splits in the upper lip (Figure 19-14A). This is a common anomaly occurring in approximately one in 1,000 births. The defect occurs more frequently in boys, and may vary from slight to severe.

A cleft palate involves the palate or roof of the mouth (Figure 19-14B). A cleft palate is more serious than a cleft lip as it forms an opening between the nasopharynx and the nose. This anomaly not only leads to difficulty with feeding, but also increases the risk of respiratory and middle ear infections. Cleft palate is more common in girls. Both conditions may occur separately or in combination, and may range from mild to severe.

**ETIOLOGY** The cause of clefts appears to be related to a hereditary factor coupled with an alteration in intrauterine environment.

**TREATMENT** Surgical repair for cleft deformities is usually performed as soon as possible after birth. Several surgeries may be needed to achieve the desired results. Special feeding devices and speech therapy are common needs.

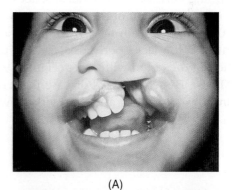

(A)

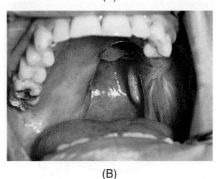

(B)

**FIGURE 19–14** (A) Cleft lip, (B) cleft palate. *(Courtesy of Dr. Joseph Konzelman, School of Dentistry, Medical College of Georgia)*

## ■ Pyloric Stenosis

Pyloric stenosis is a narrowing (stenosis) of the outlet of the lower end of the stomach, the pylorus (Figure 19-15). This condition is one of the most common developmental abnormalities of the digestive tract.

**ETIOLOGY**  It is caused by a hypertrophy or thickening of the pyloric sphincter. This sphincter controls the flow of contents out of the stomach or pyloric area. The hypertrophy of the pyloric sphincter slows the flow of stomach contents, resulting in a backup.

**SYMPTOMS**  The most common symptom of pyloric stenosis is projectile or forceful vomiting. Symptoms of pyloric stenosis usually begin at two to four weeks of age. This condition occurs almost exclusively in boys.

**TREATMENT**  A simple operation called a **pyloromyotomy** (pyloro = pyloric, myo = muscle, otomy = cut into), which involves incising and suturing the pyloric sphincter muscle, can be performed to correct the problem. This surgery is the standard treatment and is usually very effective.

## ■ Hirschsprung's Disease

Hirschsprung's disease is due to an absence of nerves (ganglion) in a segment of the colon, usually the sigmoid colon. Without normal ganglion, the affected segment of colon lacks peristalsis, causing massive distention of the colon with feces (Figure 19-16).

**ETIOLOGY**  Hirschsprung's disease is seen more often in boys and those affected with Down syn-

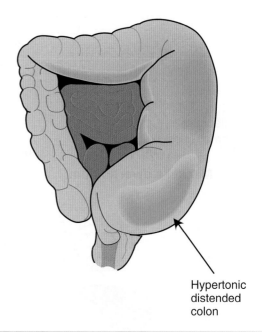

Hypertonic distended colon

**FIGURE 19–16**   Hirschsprung's disease.

drome. It has a familial tendency and occurs in approximately 1 in 5,000 births.

**SYMPTOMS**  Common symptoms include chronic constipation and abdominal distention. Diagnosis is made on the basis of a biopsy to determine the absence of ganglion cells.

**TREATMENT**  Treatment is surgical removal of the affected segment. A temporary colostomy may be necessary to allow adequate healing of the colon.

## ■ Phenylketonuria (PKU)

**ETIOLOGY**  Phenylketonuria (PKU) is a recessive genetic disorder involving faulty metabolism of the protein phenylalanine.

**SYMPTOMS**  Affected individuals do not produce the enzyme necessary to break down the protein phenylalanine. This protein builds up in the blood and becomes present in the urine. Phenylalanine is toxic to brain cells and causes mental retardation if the condition is not corrected. Diagnosis is made by PKU blood testing 72 hours after birth or after the infant has eaten proteins. This testing is mandatory in the United States.

**TREATMENT**  Affected infants are placed on a protein-restrictive diet. If the disease is discovered and treated early, prognosis for normal intelligence is good. If the condition is not discovered until after age two or three years, mental challenges are inevitable and irreversible.

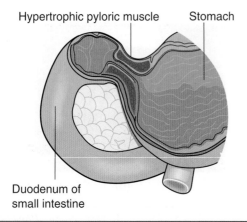

Hypertrophic pyloric muscle          Stomach

Duodenum of small intestine

**FIGURE 19–15**   Pyloric stenosis.

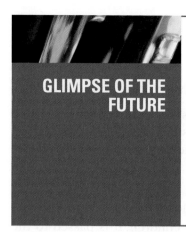

## GLIMPSE OF THE FUTURE

### Potential Changes in PKU Therapy

Phenylketonuria or PKU is a serious genetic disease that is tested for in newborns. If the child is missing the enzyme that breaks down phenylalanine, a complicated diet absent of phenylalanine is prescribed. If an infant is diagnosed with the disease, treatment is life-long. Gene therapy is being studied as a treatment for the disease. In vitro studies and animal studies are being conducted to test the effect of instilling the gene that causes production of the enzyme (phenylalanine hydroxylase) in body organs. If this treatment works, children diagnosed with PKU in the future may not have to be on restricted, complicated, diet therapy.

*Source: Ding, Z., Harding, C. O., & Thony, B. (2004).*

## Urinary

Some genetic and developmental disorders of the urinary system such as hypospadias or epispadias may be obvious at birth. Other disorders such as Wilms' tumor may not present symptoms for many years. If the condition interferes with elimination of urine, it is incompatible with life.

### ■ Hypospadias

Hypospadias is an abnormal congenital opening of the male urinary meatus on the under surface of the penis (Figure 19-17A). This abnormality may be mild, with the opening located just under the tip of the penis, or it may be more severe, with locations midshaft or near the scrotum. Hypospadias is fairly common, occurring in one in 250 boys. Hypospadias may be accompanied by an abnormally downward curvature of the penis called chordee (Figure 19-17B). The cause of chordee is an abnormal fibrous band of tissue. Another similar, but less common, condition is epispadias, characterized by the urinary meatus located on the upper surface of the penis (Figure 19-17C).

**TREATMENT** Mild cases of all these conditions may be left untreated. Surgical repair is the treatment of choice for severe cases.

### ■ Wilms' Tumor

Wilms' tumor is the most common solid tumor affecting children and infants. Most tumors are thought to be present at birth, usually appearing between the ages of two to four years.

**ETIOLOGY** The cause is thought to be genetic. This tumor is highly malignant and usually replaces

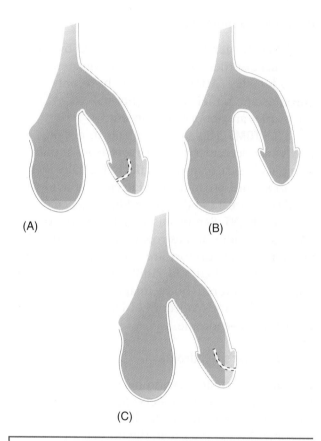

(A)

(B)

(C)

**FIGURE 19–17** (A) Hypospadias, (B) chordee, (C) epispadias.

one entire normal kidney, but rarely affects both kidneys. Most tumors are discovered by palpation of the abdomen during a routine examination by a pediatrician or by a parent.

**TREATMENT** Current treatment involving chemotherapy and surgery has improved a previous dismal prognosis to a survival rate of approximately 85 percent.

# Reproductive

Genetic and developmental disorders of the reproductive system are very rare disorders. Although they are not usually incompatible with life, they can have serious psychological effects on the individual, because of the changes they may cause in the appearance of the person and the gender differences expected in our population.

## ■ Cryptorchidism

This developmental condition of undescended testes (crypt = hidden) is discussed in detail in Chapter 17.

## ■ Turner's Syndrome

**ETIOLOGY** Turner's syndrome is caused by a chromosomal disorder and affects approximately one in 3,000 females. Affected females have only one X chromosome rather than the normal XX. At birth, the ovaries are abnormal or absent.

**SYMPTOMS** This individual fails to develop normal female secondary sex characteristics at puberty. General physical features of affected females include a short stature, broad neck, wide chest, amenorrhea, sterility, dwarfism, and impaired intelligence.

**TREATMENT** Symptoms can be reduced with growth hormone and estrogen therapy. Counseling and emotional support are often needed for the affected individual and family members to help cope with altered body image and self-esteem issues. Turner's syndrome is less common than Klinefelter's syndrome.

## ■ Klinefelter's Syndrome

**ETIOLOGY** Klinefelter's syndrome is caused by a chromosomal disorder and affects approximately one in 1,000 males. Affected males have an extra X chromosome (XXY) rather than the normal XY.

**SYMPTOMS** This disorder is usually not diagnosed until puberty when the affected individual fails to exhibit normal male sexual development. General physical features of affected males include sterility, abnormally small penis and testes, enlarged breasts, absent or scant body hair, decreased muscle development, and impaired intelligence. The affected individual has a general appearance of a eunuch with a tall slender body and long legs.

**TREATMENT** Symptoms can be improved with testosterone therapy. Emotional and psychological counseling are often needed for the affected individual and family members to help cope with altered body image and improve self-esteem.

# Multisystem Diseases and Disorders

Multisystem disorders are complex diseases that affect several body systems. Because of this effect, treatment is complicated and usually long term.

## ■ Cystic Fibrosis

**ETIOLOGY** Cystic fibrosis is a hereditary recessive disorder affecting young children. It is passed to the child by a recessive gene from each parent.

**SYMPTOMS** Cystic fibrosis affects all the **exocrine** glands (glands that excrete through a duct) of the body, causing **viscous** (thick) secretions. These viscous secretions cause obstruction in body passageways. The most serious complication of cystic fibrosis is in the lungs. The thick secretions block bronchi, causing difficulty with breathing. These thick secretions also trap bacteria, and increase the risk of respiratory infections including pneumonia. The most common cause of death with this disease is respiratory failure.

The pancreas is also affected because blockage of these ducts decreases the amount of pancreatic enzymes delivered to the intestine, resulting in poor digestion and weight loss. The sweat glands are also affected. Affected children perspire excessively and lose large amounts of salt or sodium. This loss of sodium causes an increase in the risk for heat exhaustion and electrolyte imbalances. This abnormal excretion of salt is usually the first sign that parents recognize as abnormal. Parents may take the child to the physician and complain that the child, when kissed, tastes salty or has "sweaty baby kisses." This excessive salt excretion is the basis for the "sweat test" that confirms the diagnosis of cystic fibrosis.

**TREATMENT** Major improvements in treatment of cystic fibrosis have been made in the past few decades, but it is still considered a fatal disease. Life expectancy may reach into the late 20s or early 30s. Treatment is directed toward reducing complications and improving quality of life. Aggressive respiratory treatments include postural drainage, chest-clapping, antibiotics, bronchodilators, expectorants, and oxygen therapy. A high-calorie, high-sodium diet is provided with pancreatic enzyme supplementation. Emotional support and extensive education are needed for the affected individual and family members.

## ■ Down Syndrome

Down syndrome was formerly called mongolism because the affected individual has facial features similar to individuals of the Mongolian race. Down syndrome is more correctly called Trisomy 21 because it is a condition resulting in three (tri) chromosomes instead of the normal two in the 21st position of the chromosome chain.

**ETIOLOGY** The cause of Down syndrome is not known, but it is known that during germ cell division (usually affecting the ovum), the 21st chromosome pair fails to separate. This results in a pair of chromosomes in position 21; if fertilized, this ovum—carrying two chromosomes—combines with the sperm—carrying one chromosome—resulting in three chromosomes in position 21. This condition is more common in children born to women 35 years or older, suggesting that chromosomal division is affected by maternal age.

**SYMPTOMS** Signs of Down syndrome include:

- mild to severe mental intelligence.

- facial features that include a flat nasal bridge, low-set ears, slanted eyes with **epicanthus** (a vertical fold of skin across the medial canthus of the eyes, giving them an Oriental appearance), and a thick, protruding tongue (Figure 19–18).

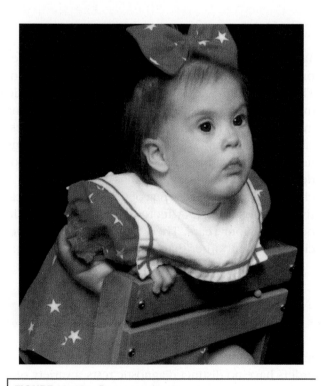

**FIGURE 19–18**　Down syndrome.

- abnormal extremities including short arms and legs. The hands are short and wide with a crease across the entire width of the palm called a "simian" crease. The little finger is short and often crooked. There is an abnormally wide gap between the first (big) and second toes.

- organ defects, especially congenital heart defects. Infertility is common in males but may not affect females.

- other diseases are common including anemia, leukemia, immune deficiencies, and respiratory infections.

Down syndrome occurs in approximately one of every 700 births. It is the most common cause of genetic mental challenges.

**TREATMENT** There is no cure but amniocentesis is an effective tool for discovery. The treatment plan is highly individual, and is directed toward maximizing mental and physical abilities. Improved surgical techniques and antibiotic therapies have increased the life expectancy of affected individuals to an average of 55 years. Individuals affected with Down syndrome are known for their loving, affectionate personalities.

# TRAUMA

## Failure to Thrive

Failure to thrive is a lack of physical growth and development in an infant or child. Usually, this condition may result in individuals with chronic disease processes. For this reason, the condition of failure to thrive is usually reserved for infants and children who are not growing and developing due to emotional or psychological causes. This condition was first noticed by a European psychiatrist who studied the development of infants institutionalized during their early years, and who were deprived of emotional warmth and security.

**ETIOLOGY** The cause of failure to thrive appears to be a disturbance in the mother–child relationship or a failure to bond. This condition tends to be associated with alcohol and drug abuse, economic stress, parental immaturity, and single parenthood. Involved mothers are often found to be victims of maternal deprivation themselves.

**SYMPTOMS** Symptoms of "failure to thrive" include weight loss or failure to gain weight and grow, irritability, anorexia or lack of appetite, vomiting, and diarrhea. Affected infants often are weak and exhibit "rag doll" limpness. They may be unresponsive to affection, wary of parents or caregivers, avoid eye contact, and stiffen when cuddled.

**TREATMENT** Treatment includes the teaching of nurturing and mothering behaviors for the mother, as well as the promotion of her self-esteem, as well as providing for the physical and emotional needs of the child. The prognosis for infants and children with this condition is often unknown. Decreased intelligence, and social and language abilities have been noted in children with failure to thrive. A significant number of these children die early in life.

## Fetal Alcohol Syndrome

**ETIOLOGY** Fetal alcohol syndrome (FAS) is a group of symptoms and birth defects in an infant born to a mother who consumed alcohol during pregnancy. Infants born to mothers who chronically abuse alcohol may go through physical alcohol withdrawal shortly after birth.

**SYMPTOMS** Signs and symptoms of FAS include varying degrees of mental challenges, decreased physical development, irritability in infants and hyperactivity in children, **microcephaly** (micro = small, cephal = brain), and an increased occurrence of ventricular septal heart defects. The exact amount of alcohol consumption needed to cause defects is unknown. For this reason, alcohol consumption during pregnancy should be avoided. The greatest risks for defects occur when alcohol is consumed during and after the third month of pregnancy.

## Congenital Rubella Syndrome

Transmission of the rubella virus across the placenta to the unborn fetus may result in spontaneous abortion or birth of an infant with major birth defects. The most common defects are microcephaly, learning disorders, deafness, growth retardation, heart defects, and ocular lesions such as cataracts, glau-

coma, nystagmus, and strabismus. Prevention includes immunization of all children and women of child-bearing age. Women should avoid becoming pregnant for three months after immunization and should not be immunized during pregnancy.

## RARE DISEASES

## Anencephaly

Anencephaly is a severe congenital malformation resulting in the absence of the brain or cranial vault. This condition is not compatible with life. Infants born with anencephaly are stillborn or die shortly after birth if they are not kept alive by artificial means.

## Achondroplasia

Achondroplasia is a rare genetic disorder characterized by abnormal development of the epiphyseal cartilage, resulting in decreased long bone growth and a type of dwarfism. Interestingly, a similar condition affects basset hounds. Affected individuals may die at birth or shortly thereafter, or may live to a normal life expectancy.

## Tay-Sachs Disease

Tay-Sachs disease is an autosomal recessive disorder primarily affecting families of Eastern Jewish origin. This condition is due to a genetic error in lipid metabolism and results in an accumulation of toxins in the brain. As a result, the brain tissue degenerates, causing mental and physical disabilities. Symptoms usually occur by age six months and include lack of developmental skills, convulsions, and blindness. A cherry red spot on the retina of the eye is one indicative diagnostic test. Affected children usually die before age four years. There is no cure and no specific treatment other than symptomatic treatment.

## SUMMARY

Although there are literally hundreds of genetic and developmental disorders, overall, most are relatively rare. Some are obvious at birth and may be incompatible with life. Others may not be diagnosed

until later in the individual's life. Because some disorders have no distinct diagnostic tests, a variety of testing may have to be completed to obtain a definitive diagnosis. Other disorders can be diagnosed by genetic testing. Many of the genetic and developmental disorders have lifelong effects on the individual, and may be progressively disabling. Because of new research and extended health care services, most individuals with these disorders have longer life expectancy than in past years.

## REVIEW QUESTIONS

### Short Answer

1. How many chromosomes are in the nucleus of each body cell?

2. Which body cells have the ability to reproduce in a process called mitosis?

3. What is a germ cell?

4. Describe the process called meiosis.

5. What is karyotyping?

6. Why is DNA considered to be so important?

7. Name an autosomal dominant disorder.

8. Name an autosomal recessive disorder.

9. Define genotype.

10. Define phenotype.

### Multiple Choice

11. Which of the following statements is the best description of muscular dystrophy?

   a. MD is a degenerative disorder of the nervous system.
   b. MD is a group of genetically inherited diseases characterized by degeneration or weakening of the muscles.
   c. MD is a genetic disorder most common in male children.
   d. MD is a neuromuscular disorder affecting children.

**12.** Which of the following statements is the best description of cerebral palsy?

    **a.** CP is a congenital bilateral paralysis that results from inadequate blood or oxygen supply to the brain during fetal development.

    **b.** CP is a crippling disease caused by a genetic inherited disorder.

    **c.** CP is an abnormal accumulation of cerebrospinal fluid in the brain.

    **d.** CP is a condition of spastic movements and inability to walk, caused by a genetic anomaly.

**13.** Coarctation of the aorta is _____.

    **a.** a combination of four tetra defects of the heart.

    **b.** a constriction or stricture of the major artery of the heart.

    **c.** an abnormal connection of the pulmonary artery and the aorta.

    **d.** a small hole in the artery at birth.

**14.** Some of the problems for the infant with a cleft lip and palate may include _____.

    **a.** a fistula connecting the trachea to the esophagus.

    **b.** increased risk for elimination problems.

    **c.** increased risk for difficulty with feedings, respiratory distress, and middle ear infections.

    **d.** projectile or forceful vomiting.

**15.** Phenylketonuria is best described as _____.

    **a.** an absence of nerves in a particular segment of the colon, causing constipation and distention of the colon.

    **b.** a recessive genetic disorder of metabolism of protein.

    **c.** an autosomal dominant genetic disorder of digestion and absorption.

    **d.** a constriction of the valve in the stomach causing a backup of food and fluid.

**16.** Which of the following is the most common solid tumor affecting children and infants?

    **a.** Osteoma               **c.** Ewings' tumor

    **b.** Sarcoma            **d.** Wilms' tumor

**17.** Which of the following factors are usually present in Down syndrome?

    **a.** dwarf-like body, retardation, spastic movements

    **b.** organ defects, small stature, epicanthal folds, and epispadias

    **c.** retardation, immune deficiencies, and abnormal brain size

    **d.** epicanthal folds, small stature, mild to severe retardation

**18.** When is fetal alcohol syndrome most likely to occur?

    **a.** If the mother drinks alcohol during and after the third month of pregnancy.

    **b.** If the mother drinks more than one glass of alcohol per day during the last trimester.

    **c.** If the mother drinks alcohol during the first two months of pregnancy.

    **d.** Only if the mother drinks more than two glasses of alcohol per day during the pregnancy.

**19.** Tay-Sachs disease is an _____.

    **a.** autosomal dominant disease affecting the brain.

    **b.** autosomal dominant disease affecting metabolism, causing retardation.

    **c.** autosomal recessive disease affecting metabolism, causing retardation.

    **d.** autosomal recessive disease affecting the brain.

**20.** Failure to thrive is defined as which of the following?

    **a.** It is a lack of growth and development due to a genetic disease.

    **b.** It is a lack of physical growth and development in an infant or child.

    **c.** It is an inborn error of metabolism, causing delayed growth and development.

    **d.** It is an inherited disease affecting growth in the infant.

## CASE STUDY

**Heather Lee** is an eight-month-old infant who is brought to the clinic because of chronic respiratory infections. Heather is weak, inactive, underweight, has poor skin turgor, and seems very quiet except for spells of coughing. She is diagnosed with cystic fibrosis. Heather's mother is very upset with this diagnosis, thinking it is her fault the baby is not doing well. Is she correct in thinking this? What can you tell her about this disorder? What is the cause of CF? What is the usual treatment prescribed? What is the prognosis for Heather?

## BIBLIOGRAPHY

Britton, B. (2003). About hemophilia. *Nursing 33*(12), 78.

Capone, G. T. (2004). Down syndrome. *Infants & Young Children: An Interdisciplinary Journal of Special Care Practices 17*(1), 45–58.

Catlin, A. J. (2003). Normalization, chronic sorrow, and murder: Highlighting the case of Carol Carr. *Pediatric Nursing 29*(4), 326–328.

Catlin, A. J. (2003). Thalassemia: The facts and the controversies. *Pediatric Nursing 29*(6), 447–450.

Dave, U. P., Jenkins, N. A., & Copeland, N. C. (2004). Gene therapy insertional mutagenesis insights. *Science 303*(5656), 333.

Ding, Z., Harding, C. O., & Thony, B. (2004). State-of-the-art 2003 on PKU gene therapy. *Molecular Genetics & Metabolism 81*(1), 3–8.

Enderlin, C., Vogel, R., & Conaway, P. (2003). Gaucher disease. *American Journal of Nursing 103*(12), 50–60.

Genetic cops track muscular dystrophy cause. (2004). *The Medical Herald 16*(1), 8.

Gee, L., Abbott, J., Conway, S. P., Etherington, C., & Webb, A. K. (2003). Quality of life in cystic fibrosis: The impact of gender, general health perceptions and disease severity. *Journal of Cystic Fibrosis 2*(4), 206–213.

Gill, D. R., Davies, L. A., Pringle, I. A., & Hyde, S. C. (2004). The development of gene therapy for diseases of the lung. *Cellular & Molecular Life Sciences 61*(3), 355–458.

Hanss, B. (2003). Applications of gene therapy to kidney disease. *Current Opinion in Nephrology & Hypertension 12*(4), 439–445.

McMillan, I. (2003). Parents need support over genetic testing. *Learning Disability Practice 6*(4), 5.

Middleton, L., & Lessick, M. (2003). Inherited urologic malignant disorders: Nursing implications. *Urologic Nursing 23*(1), 15–26.

Mouse research sheds new light on human genetic diseases. (2003, May 23). *Genomics & Genetics Weekly*, 4–5.

Nolan, M. E. (2003). Anticipatory guidance for parents of Prader-Willi children. *Nursing 29*(6), 427–431.

Ratio of reported-to-expected cancer rates in family members approximately 0.7 (2003, July 2). *Biotech Week*, 274–275.

Roizen, N. J., & Patterson, D. (2003). Down's syndrome. *Lancet 361*, 1287–1289.

Scientists discover possible new treatment for genetic diseases. (2003, April 9). *Biotech Week*, 71–72.

Study may help scientists develop safer methods for gene therapy. (2003, July 2). *Biotech Week*, 278–279.

Van Riper, M. (2003). Breast cancer and family genetics—tackling the ethical issues. *Journal of Nutrition 133* (11), 3845S–3846S.

Visual-spatial deficits suitable for neurofibromatosis type-1 diagnosis. (2003, August 3). *Biotech Week*, 284–285

Vitamins reduce risk for congenital anomalies other than neural tube defects. (2004, April 11). *Medical Letter on the CDC and FDA*, 2–3.

Wall, N. R., & Yang, S. (2003, October 25). Small RNA: Can RNA interference be exploited for therapy? *Lancet 362*(9393), 1401–1402.

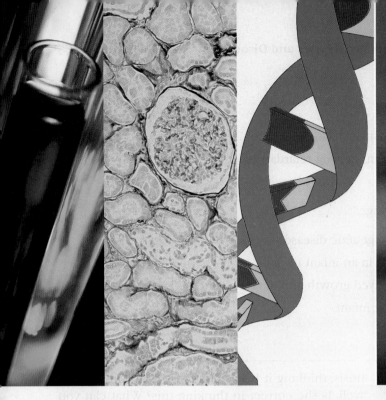
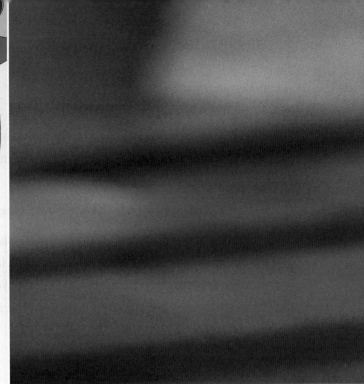

## OUTLINE

## KEY TERMS

# Childhood Diseases and Disorders

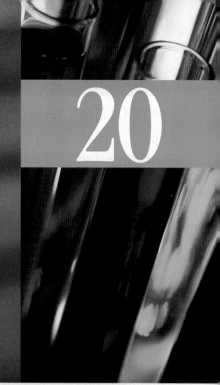

**20**

## LEARNING OBJECTIVES

*Upon completion of the chapter, the learner should be able to:*

1. Define the terminology common to childhood diseases.

2. Identify the important signs and symptoms associated with childhood diseases.

3. Describe the common diagnostics used to determine the type and/or cause of childhood diseases.

4. Describe the typical course and management of the common childhood diseases.

5. State the common drugs abused by children, the effects of the drugs, and the potential health hazards of drug use.

6. List the immunizations available to prevent childhood diseases.

7. Identify the safety precautions for preventing poisonings in children.

## OVERVIEW

*C*hildhood diseases range from common infections such as tonsillitis and colds to more chronic and debilitating diseases such as Ewing's sarcoma and leukemia. In addition, traumatic events such as abuse and poisonings are very common in the young population. Childhood diseases can affect any body system, but the most commonly known ones affect the respiratory system, producing signs and symptoms of a cold or flu. Even though immunizations against many of the common childhood diseases are available, thousands of children in this country have not been immunized at all or do not have adequate immunizations. This increases their likelihood of developing an acute infectious childhood disease. ■

## INFECTIOUS DISEASES

More children are seen yearly by physicians for infectious disease diagnosis and treatment than any other problem. Infectious diseases of childhood fall into four categories: viral, bacterial, fungal, and parasitic diseases. Disorders in these categories include some of the most familiar diseases such as colds, influenza, measles, pertussis, and tonsillitis. Several of the infectious diseases can be prevented by maintenance of a regular immunization schedule (see the Healthy Highlight). Many of these diseases have an **incubation period**, the time between exposure to the disease and the presence of symptoms, which lasts several days. Signs and symptoms, in general, for the common infectious diseases include fever, **malaise** (a feeling of general discomfort), coughing, anorexia, nausea/vomiting, and/or rashes. Treatment varies with the specific disease. In many cases,

treatment consists of symptom relief, good nutrition, and rest. Nonaspirin antipyretics are given to children with fever since aspirin has been linked with Reye's syndrome. Good hand washing is always important to prevent the spread of infectious diseases.

## Viral Diseases

Viral diseases in children are usually treated symptomatically. Most children have mild cases of the disease and recuperate quickly. However, for some children, especially those who have other medical disorders, even a mild viral infection can become a critical health problem. Some viruses invade the host and remain dormant for long periods of time. The viruses activate when triggered by something. Although this concept is not well understood, it is known that stress is a common trigger for initiating the replication of a dormant virus.

 **HEALTHY HIGHLIGHT**

| Schedule for Immunizations | Type of Vaccine | Recommended Age |
|---|---|---|
| | DTP or DTP-Hib (diphtheria/tetanus/ pertussis and *H. influenzae* type b) | Six weeks to two months, four months, six months, 12 to 15 months, four to six years |
| | DTaP (diphtheria/tetanus/acellular pertussis) | Can be given instead of doses four and five above, but should not be given before 15 months of age |
| | TD-adult type (tetanus/diphtheria) | Eleven to 16 years, and every 10 years in adulthood (booster dose) |
| | OPV (oral poliovirus vaccine) | Six weeks to two months, four months, six months, four to six years |
| | MMR (measles, mumps, rubella) | Twelve to 15 months, four to six years |
| | HbOC (*Haemophilus influenzae* type b conjugate vaccine) | Two months, four months, six months, 12 to 15 months |
| | PRP-T (can be given instead of HbOC) | Same as above |
| | PRP-OMP (can be given instead of either of the above) | Two months, four months, 12 to 15 months |
| | Hep B (hepatitis B vaccine) | Birth to two months, two to four months, six to 18 months |
| | Varicella (varicella zoster virus vaccine) | Twelve to 18 months |

## ■ Measles

**ETIOLOGY** Measles, also know as rubeola, is an acute viral disease.

**SYMPTOMS** It is marked by fever, inflammation of the respiratory mucous membranes, runny nose, and a generalized dusky red maculopapular rash over the body trunk and extremities (Figure 20-1). Spots called **Koplik's spots** can be seen in the mouth early in the disease. These spots are rather unique to measles and are often the definitive symptom that confirms the diagnosis (Figure 20-2). Measles is transmitted by contaminated airborne particles. The incubation period is from seven to 14 days.

**TREATMENT** Treatment is usually directed at relief of symptoms and prevention of such complications as dehydration, pneumonia, or high fever. Having had one episode of the disease should provide lifetime immunity, but all children should be immunized to prevent measles (see the Healthy Highlight).

## ■ Rubella

Rubella is a type of measles also known as German measles or three-day measles. It is characterized by a rash similar to measles but lighter in color (Figure 20-3). Rubella is usually a very mild disease in children but can be quite serious in pregnant women. If it occurs during the first three months of pregnancy, there is an increased risk of fetal problems or congenital anomalies occurring. The incubation period is 14 to 21 days. Rubella, like measles, is spread by contaminated airborne droplets.

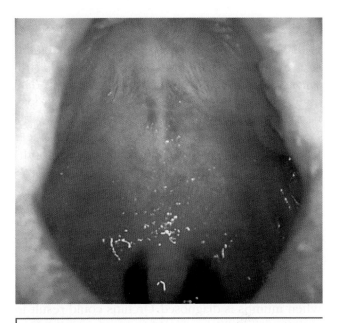

**FIGURE 20–2**  Koplik's spots in the throat of a child with rubeola. *(Courtesy of the Centers for Disease Control and Prevention)*

**SYMPTOMS** Symptoms include lymph node enlargement, rash, nasal discharge, joint pain, chills, and fever.

**TREATMENT** Treatment is usually symptomatic with rest, good nutrition, and prevention of spread of the infection. All children should be immunized to prevent rubella (see the Healthy Highlight).

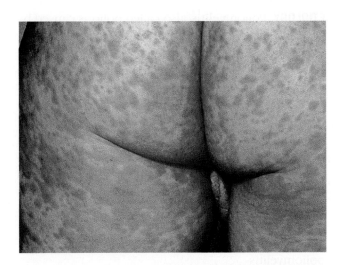

**FIGURE 20–1**  Maculopapular rash in rubeola. *(Courtesy of the Centers for Disease Control and Prevention)*

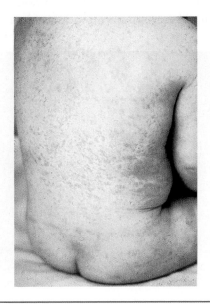

**FIGURE 20–3**  Rubella rash. *(Courtesy of the Centers for Disease Control and Prevention)*

## ■ Mumps

**ETIOLOGY** Mumps is an infectious disease characterized by inflammation of the **parotid glands** (the salivary glands located just in front of the ears). The incubation period is usually 16 to 18 days, but may be as long as 25 days.

**SYMPTOMS** Symptoms include chills, fever, ear pain, and swelling of the parotid glands (one or both) (Figure 20–4). It is transmitted by airborne droplets and secretions of saliva.

**TREATMENT** Treatment varies with the severity of the symptoms but is usually palliative (soothing or relieving symptoms). Complications of mumps includes **orchitis** (or-KYE-tis; inflammation of a testis) in males, and nerve conduction deafness. Although neither is common, they are a concern when mumps is diagnosed. Orchitis could result in sterility. All children should be immunized to prevent mumps (see the Healthy Highlight).

## ■ Varicella

**ETIOLOGY** Varicella, more commonly known as chickenpox, is the result of infection with the varicella-zoster virus. This virus has an incubation period of 10 to 21 days. Varicella can be transmitted by airborne particles or direct contact. It is one of the most common childhood infectious diseases.

**SYMPTOMS** Symptoms of varicella include a macular rash over the face, trunk, and extremities (Figure 20–5). The rash may be quite limited or very widespread. The rash spots develop into **vesicles** (VES-ih-kuls; blister-like eruptions on the skin) in a few days,

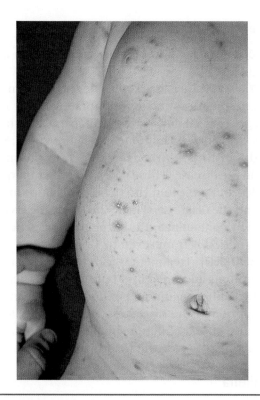

**FIGURE 20–5**    Macular rash in varicella. *(Courtesy of Robert A. Silverman, M.D., Pediatric Dermatology, Georgetown University)*

causing intense itching. The vesicles break, dry, and become crusty.

**TREATMENT** Treatment is usually symptomatic with care taken to prevent a secondary skin infection at the sites of the lesions.

## ■ Poliomyelitis

**ETIOLOGY** Poliomyelitis, also called polio, is caused by the polio virus. It is spread through an oral route or fecal-oral route from an infected individual. Abortive poliomyelitis is a mild form of the disease that does not affect the central nervous system.

**SYMPTOMS** In the more severe form of polio, early symptoms include fever, headache, sore throat, and abdominal pain. This may progress to stiffness of the neck, trunk, and extremities. Although the disease may subside at this point, it can also progress to paralysis. If the respiratory center of the brain is affected, the disease is life threatening. The incubation period is three to six days for abortive poliomyelitis and seven to 21 for the more severe form of poliomyelitis.

**TREATMENT** Treatment of polio is based on the symptoms and severity, but is usually supportive. Phys-

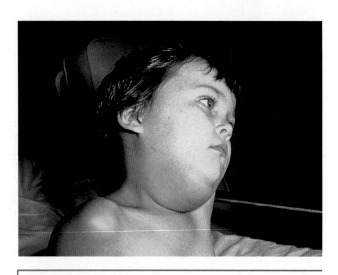

**FIGURE 20–4**    Parotitis (mumps). *(Courtesy of the Centers for Disease Control and Prevention)*

ical therapy is important to prevent wasting of muscles. Ventilator support is needed if the respiratory center is affected. Forty years of an aggressive immunization program in the United States has reduced the threat of polio. However, it could still recur as a major health problem, so all children should be vaccinated against polio (see the Healthy Highlight).

### ■ Influenza

Influenza, or the flu, is an acute infectious respiratory disease.

**ETIOLOGY** It is caused by viruses in the orthomyovirus family.

**SYMPTOMS** Influenza is characterized by chills, fever, headache, joint or muscle aches, runny nose, and a dry cough. It often develops very quickly, and in epidemic proportions in some communities. Very young children or children with other debilitating illnesses are at risk for severe illness.

**TREATMENT** Generally, treatment in children is symptomatic with rest, hydration, and antipyretics if needed. Antiviral drugs can be given for some types of influenza. A newly developed nasal spray flu vaccine is available for children five years of age or older.

### ■ Common Cold

The common cold is appropriately named because it is the most frequently occurring disease.

**ETIOLOGY** There are numerous strains of viruses that can cause the common cold but the rhinoviruses are usually the causative agent. It is transmitted by direct contact and droplet contact. Good hand washing is the best preventive strategy for transmission of the cold virus.

**SYMPTOMS** Symptoms of the common cold include **rhinitis** (RYE-**NIGH**-tis; inflammation of the nasal mucous membrane), nasal discharge, coughing, sneezing, fever, and watery eyes.

**TREATMENT** Treatment is directed at symptom relief, and getting adequate rest, hydration, and good nutrition.

### ■ Mononucleosis

Infectious mononucleosis is a condition where there are abnormally large numbers of mononuclear leukocytes in the circulating blood.

**ETIOLOGY** Most cases of mononucleosis are caused by the Epstein-Barr virus but it can be caused by other viruses. The incubation period may be as long as four to seven weeks.

**SYMPTOMS** Symptoms include sore throat, fever, malaise, fatigue, and enlarged lymph nodes.

**TREATMENT** Treatment is directed at relief of symptoms. Rest and hydration are important.

### ■ Acquired Immunodeficiency Syndrome

Acquired immunodeficiency syndrome, commonly known as AIDS, has now affected thousands of children in the United States.

**ETIOLOGY** It is caused by the human immunodeficiency virus (HIV). This disease is described in detail in Chapter 5 but is addressed here in relation to its effect in children. During the 1980's, most children diagnosed with an HIV infection probably acquired it through a blood transfusion. Most children infected with HIV were hemophiliacs who had received transfusions or other blood products. Today, virtually all HIV infections in children are as a result of maternal-fetal transfer through blood also called perinatal transmission. Children not only suffer the affects of being infected with the disease but also are often orphaned as a result of both parents dying with the disease. By 2010 it is expected that there will be over three million orphans worldwide as a direct result of AIDS. There are also increasing numbers of sexually active teens being diagnosed with HIV/AIDS.

The period of time between the HIV infection and development of AIDS is much shorter in infants and toddlers than in infected older children or adults.

**SYMPTOMS** Many children do not experience symptoms of the disease and live a normal life for years. However, in those with severely compromised immune systems, opportunistic infections can be overwhelming, necessitating repeated hospitalizations to sustain life.

**TREATMENT** Treatment of pediatric HIV infection and AIDS varies with the child and the severity of the symptoms. Therapy focuses on prevention and treatment of opportunistic diseases, good nutrition, antiviral drugs, and other support therapies as needed.

## Bacterial Diseases

Bacterial diseases of childhood are caused by pathogens. There are millions of bacteria in the world, but not all bacteria are pathogenic (see Chapter 4 for more information). Some of the common infection-causing bacteria include *Staphylococcus, Clostridium, Haemophilus, E. coli,* and *Streptococcus*. Symptoms of bacterial infections may include coughing, fever, headache, difficulty breathing, and sore throat. Treatment is based on the causative agent along with relief of symptoms. Some bacterial diseases can be prevented by immunizations.

## ■ Pertussis

**ETIOLOGY** Pertussis, also known as whooping cough, is an acute respiratory infection caused by *Bordetella pertussis*.

**SYMPTOMS** It is characterized by (1) a **catarrhal** (ca-**TAR**-al; inflammation of mucous membranes of the head and mouth with increased mucous flow) stage including cough, runny nose, and low-grade fever; (2) a **paroxysmal** (PAR-ock-**SIZ**-mal; spasm or convulsion) stage including violent "whooping" coughing, cyanosis, distended neck veins, and some vomiting; and (3) a convalescent stage including some periods of the "whooping" coughing but with gradually less frequent episodes. The incubation period is six to 10 days but may be as long as 21 days.

Pertussis is transmitted by direct contact with respiratory droplets.

**TREATMENT** It is treated with antibiotics and supportive therapy. Pneumonia is the most common complication of pertussis and can be life threatening. All children should be immunized to prevent pertussis (see the Healthy Highlight). Infants, prior to receiving vaccinations, are not immune to pertussis so it is a serious threat to them.

## ■ Diphtheria

**ETIOLOGY** Diphtheria is an infectious disease caused by *Corynebacterium diphtheriae* and characterized by severe inflammation of the respiratory system.

**SYMPTOMS** It produces a membranous coating of the pharynx, nose, and sometimes the tracheo-bronchial tree. This membrane becomes a thick fibrinous **exudate** (ECKS-you-dayt; fluid composed of protein and white blood cells that seeps from tissue), causing extreme difficulty breathing. The toxin also can produce degeneration in peripheral nerves, heart muscle, and other tissues. It is transmitted by direct contact with droplets from an infected person. The incubation period is two to five days.

**TREATMENT** Treatment includes antibiotic therapy and diphtheria antitoxin. At one time, diphtheria had a high fatality rate, especially in children, but that is rare now. All children should be immunized to prevent diphtheria (see the Healthy Highlight).

## ■ Tuberculosis

**ETIOLOGY** Tuberculosis (TB) is an infectious disease caused by the tubercle bacillus *Mycobacterium tuberculosis*. For many years, the incidence of tuberculosis was decreasing but in just the last few years, it has been on the rise. Although the disease typically affects the respiratory system, it can also be found in the gastrointestinal system, the bones, brain, and lymph nodes. Tuberculosis is transmitted by contaminated droplets. Once the child is infected with the tubercle bacillus and the incubation period of four to 12 weeks is past, the skin test will be positive. Diagnosis is made by a positive skin test, positive sputum culture, and clinical manifestations, as well as a chest X-ray.

**SYMPTOMS** Signs and symptoms of TB include a persistent cough, bloody sputum, lymph node enlargement, fever, and malaise (see Chapter 9 for more information about tuberculosis).

Most children infected by the bacillus will not develop the symptomatic disease. The greatest percentage of cases of TB infection in children stay

---

## COMPLEMENTARY AND ALTERNATIVE THERAPY

### An Herb for Pertussis

The herb *Gelsemium sempervirens*, yellow jasmine or evening trumpet-flower, is an antispasmotic and a central nervous system depressant. It has been used for neuralgia, migraine headaches, and other health problems including pertussis. Benefits reported include reduction in cough and bronchial spasms, allowing the individual to get needed rest and sleep. Its safety for use in children has not been established, so caution is important for the consumer using the herb to treat pertussis.

*Source:* Mental Health Practice *(2004).*

**dormant** (state of being inactive) and do not develop into the clinical disease.

**TREATMENT** For those children who develop active tuberculosis, treatment consists of drug therapy, rest, good nutrition, and prevention of spread of the disease to other family members. Children at higher risk for developing TB are those who have other chronic diseases, are HIV positive or have AIDS, are malnourished, live in poor hygienic conditions, live with adults with TB, and/or are immunosuppressed.

### ■ Tularemia

**ETIOLOGY** Tularemia, also called rabbit fever or deer fly fever, is caused by *Francisella tularensis*. It is transmitted by the bite of an infected tick, deer fly, or other blood-sucking insect, or by direct contact with an infected animal.

**SYMPTOMS** Symptoms include headache, fever, generalized or localized pain, swelling of lymph nodes, chills, and vomiting.

**TREATMENT** Treatment with antibiotics is usually effective.

### ■ Impetigo

**ETIOLOGY** Impetigo is a contagious superficial **pyoderma** (PYE-oh-**DER**-mah; inflammatory, purulent dermatitis) caused by *Staphylococcus aureus* or group A streptococci. It is commonly found on the face in children (Figure 20–6). It is transmitted by direct contact between contaminated hands and the face.

**TREATMENT** Good hand washing is the best preventive strategy but antibiotics are effective in diagnosed cases of impetigo (see Chapter 18 for more information).

### ■ Acute Tonsillitis

Tonsillitis is an infection of the palatine tonsils, tissue located on the posterior wall of the nasopharynx. The purpose of the tonsils is to help protect the respiratory tract from pathogens; thus, they tend to be a common site for inflammation and infection.

**ETIOLOGY** Most tonsillar infections are caused by group A beta-hemolytic streptococci.

**SYMPTOMS** Symptoms include a sore throat, enlarged tonsils, cough, fever, and pain with swallowing. Diagnosis is made by visual exam and throat culture.

**TREATMENT** Antibiotics are given as supportive treatment. A **tonsillectomy** (TON-sih-**LECT**-toh-me; ectomy = removal; removal of the tonsils) is not rec-

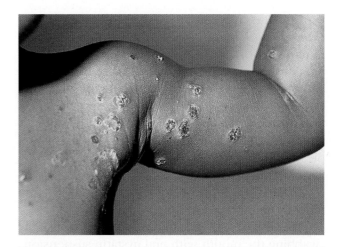

**FIGURE 20–6** Impetigo. *(Courtesy of Robert A. Silverman, M.D., Pediatric Dermatology, Georgetown University)*

ommended for children under three years of age but may be performed on older children with repeated infections.

### ■ Otitis Media

**ETIOLOGY** Otitis media is an acute bacterial infection of the middle ear. It is one of the most common diseases of children. If left untreated, chronic infection may result. It is most often diagnosed in very young children aged six months to three years.

**SYMPTOMS** Signs and symptoms include pain (in the infant this symptom may be indicated by the child pulling on the ear), fever, drainage, and on otoscopic examination, a bulging reddish tympanic membrane.

**TREATMENT** Treatment includes antibiotic therapy and acetaminophen for fever and pain. If the condition persists, a myringotomy with tympanoplasty tubes may be the treatment of choice (see Chapter 16 for more information).

## Fungal Diseases

Fungal diseases are usually seen on the skin or mucous membranes in children. These diseases may be seen in any age, but some, such as candidiasis, are more common in infants than in older children. Most fungal infections are not severe but can be very irritating to the child, and need medical intervention to halt the spread of the infection.

### ■ Candidiasis

Candidiasis, or thrush, is an oral fungal infection common in infants.

**ETIOLOGY** It is caused by an excessive growth of *Candida albicans* on the mucous membranes in the mouth. The organism also can cause a diaper rash if it passes through the intestine because the continually wet diaper area is a good medium for growth of *Candida albicans*. The infant may acquire the infection during delivery, or it may develop later due to antibiotic therapy or from the use of unclean nipples on bottles. Diagnosis is made by visual examination of the mouth.

**SYMPTOMS** White plaques are present on the mucous membranes and the tongue.

**TREATMENT** The treatment of choice is usually swabbing the mouth with oral nystatin suspension.

### ■ Tinea

Tinea infections encompass a group of diseases commonly known as ringworm.

**ETIOLOGY** Tinea capitis (scalp), tinea corporis (face, trunk, and extremities), tinea cruris (groin, buttocks, scrotum, also known as jock itch), and tinea pedis (feet, also known as athlete's foot) are caused by a group of fungi called dermatophytes. These are all common in children, especially tinea capitis. They are transmitted by direct contact, contact with infected articles (such as combs), or contact with infected animals. Tinea infections are usually diagnosed by visual examination.

**TREATMENT** Treatment is usually the application of a topical antifungal agent (see Chapter 18 for more information).

## Parasitic Diseases

Parasitic diseases include all disorders that are caused by an organism that feeds on another organism such as a worm that lives in the intestine of an individual. Parasites are common in areas where poor nutrition, contaminated water, and low socioeconomic conditions are widespread. The parasitic diseases common to children in the United States include giardiasis, pediculosis, and some helminth (worm) infestations.

### ■ Giardiasis

**ETIOLOGY** Giardiasis is an infection by the protozoa *Giardia lamblia*. These protozoa lodge in the small intestines and absorb nutrients from the host.

**SYMPTOMS** Symptoms of giardiasis include diarrhea, nausea, cramping, **flatulence** (excessive gas), fever, and anorexia (loss of appetite). Diagnosis is by laboratory stool examination.

**TREATMENT** Treatment usually includes furazolidone or other similar drugs, and symptom relief as needed. Clear liquids are given to prevent dehydration, a dangerous complication of the disease.

### ■ Pediculosis

**ETIOLOGY** Pediculosis is the condition of being infested with lice. Lice are tiny, wingless, blood-sucking parasites that are transmitted from human to human by direct contact. The type of lice that lives on human hair and feeds on the scalp is *Pediculus humanus capititis*. Lice infestations reach epidemic levels in many school systems throughout the United States. Millions of dollars are spent on lice remedies each year. Lice infestations occur in all socioeconomic populations, and are more commonly found in females because they usually have more hair. An adult parasite produces about six eggs every 24 hours.

The diagnosis is by visual examination of the scalp and hair. The lice eggs (**nits**) can be seen on the hair shafts.

**TREATMENT** The most effective treatment is permethrin 1% crème rinse. In addition, vinegar and water can be used to loosen the nits prior to combing with a delousing comb. This treatment should be performed every day until all nits are removed. Clothes and bedding should be laundered using very hot water and detergent.

### ■ Pinworms

Pinworms are parasitic nematodes (specific type of helminths) that infect the intestines and rectum.

**ETIOLOGY** The causative organism is *Enterobius vermicularis*. Pinworms are transmitted by ingestion or inhalation of the eggs, usually by hand-to-mouth contact.

**SYMPTOM** Usually, the only symptom is anal itching. Diagnosis is by microscopic examination of stool.

**TREATMENT** Treatment includes drug therapy (mebendazole or pyrantel pamoate) and instructions in good hand washing. The child should be discouraged from placing fingers in the mouth or biting the nails. Good toileting habits are also encouraged.

### ■ Roundworms

**ETIOLOGY** Roundworms (*Ascaris lumbricoides*) are parasites that lodge in the intestine, absorbing nutrients from the host. Roundworms, like pinworms, are transmitted by transfer of the eggs to the mouth or nose.

**SYMPTOMS** Symptoms may be more severe than in pinworm infestations, depending on how long they reside in the intestine before treatment. The child may complain of abdominal pain, excessive gas, loss of appetite, or weight loss. Vomiting also may occur. If the helminths are inhaled, symptoms of pneumonia may be present. Diagnosis is usually made by identification of the parasites in a stool specimen.

**TREATMENT** Treatment is the same as for pinworms.

# RESPIRATORY DISEASES

Respiratory illnesses are the most common childhood diseases seen by physicians. Infants are extremely susceptible to upper respiratory problems since their immune systems are not fully developed. Infants also have very small air passages, so even a minor amount of mucus can obstruct a passage and cause respiratory distress. Preschool and school-aged children are very vulnerable to the contagious respiratory diseases since they have a great deal of person-to-person and hand-to-mouth contacts. Several of the viral and bacterial respiratory diseases were covered earlier in this chapter.

## Sudden Infant Death Syndrome (SIDS)

Sudden infant death syndrome, or SIDS, is the abrupt unexplained death of an infant under age one. It is also know as crib death since the infant is found dead after being put in bed to sleep.

**ETIOLOGY** There are several theories about the cause of SIDS but none have been proven at this time. It is now recommended that infants be placed in bed in the **supine** (SUE-pine; on the back) position rather than **prone** (on the stomach side) since more cases of SIDS have occurred in children lying in the prone position. Children at higher risk for SIDS include those with sleep apnea, siblings of SIDS infants, premature infants, and infants with respiratory problems. Diagnosis may be suspected when the child is taken to the emergency department, but SIDS can be confirmed only by autopsy and investigation. A diagnosis of SIDS is very traumatic to parents and families who experience not only loss and grief, but also guilt. Counseling, along with further education, should be available for these families so SIDS might be prevented in future children.

## Croup

**ETIOLOGY** Croup, also known as laryngotracheobronchitis, is caused by parainfluenza viruses 1 and 2.

**SYMPTOMS** It is an upper respiratory infection characterized by a harsh barking cough, fever, **inspiratory stridor** (STRYE-dor; high-pitched sound during inspiration due to blocked airways), laryngeal spasms, and increased difficulty breathing at night. It affects children from three months to three years. Diagnosis is made by physical examination.

**TREATMENT** Treatment usually includes high humidity, fluids, rest, racemic epinephrine, and antipyretics if needed. Complications can be serious if a **patent** (open) airway is not maintained.

## Adenoid Hyperplasia

Adenoid hyperplasia is the enlargement of the pharyngeal tonsils, lymphoid tissues located on the posterior wall of the nasopharynx above the palatine tonsils. Hyperplasia of the adenoids is a very common occurrence in children.

**ETIOLOGY** It can be caused by a congenital defect or from infection.

**SYMPTOMS** The enlarged adenoids can block the eustachian tubes, causing ear problems such as otitis media. Because of the location of the adenoids, enlargement also can cause some obstruction of the airway, resulting in breathing difficulty.

**TREATMENT** Treatment focuses on correcting the cause of the hyperplasia. If repeated infections are the cause, antibiotic therapy is instituted. If the enlargement cannot be corrected, an **adenoidectomy** (AD-eh-noy-**DECK**-toh-me; ectomy = removal; removal of the adenoids) may be necessary.

## Asthma

**ETIOLOGY** Asthma is a serious, chronic, respiratory system disease of unknown cause.

**SYMPTOMS** It is characterized by acute episodes of coughing, wheezing, and shortness of breath. It is one of the leading causes of school absence for illness in children today. Approximately 69 of every 1,000 children are affected by asthma and over 4.8 million children under the age of 18 have been diagnosed with asthma. The cost of asthma in the United States is estimated to be $14 billion a year (Asthma and Allergy Foundation of America, 2004). There are various stimuli (called triggers) of an asthmatic episode. Triggers can include cigarette smoke, dust mites, chemicals, pollen, animal hair and feathers, molds, cold air, and excessive exercise. In spite of the trigger, airway swelling and blockage result, causing the symptoms of respiratory distress.

Diagnosis is made by physical examination, chest X-rays (although they usually show normal results except in severe cases), pulmonary function studies, and allergy tests.

**TREATMENT** Treatment of asthma in the child includes avoidance of the triggers, medications such as bronchodilators and anti-inflammatory agents, and careful monitoring of the disease. A peak flowmeter is used to monitor the breathing capacity of the child. This device measures the flow of air in a forced exhalation and reports it in liters per minute. The value of peak expiratory flow indicates the degree of airway obstruction. The data obtained from the peak flowmeter can help identify the onset of an asthmatic episode. The physician may use the information from the chart of measurements kept by the child to prescribe the appropriate medication regimen.

Education of the child and family is very important in effective asthma management programs. Effective management will allow the child to live a normal life with appropriate activity levels, will prevent acute asthmatic attacks, and will help the child avoid hospitalization for severe episodes (see Chapter 9 for more information on asthma).

## Pneumonia

Pneumonia is an inflammation of the lung parenchyma.

**ETIOLOGY** It may be of viral or bacterial origin. Pneumonia is characterized by the alveolar air spaces in the lungs becoming filled with exudate, inflammatory cells, and fibrin.

**SYMPTOMS** The symptoms include cough, fever, wheezing, and malaise. Diagnosis is made by chest X-ray and auscultation of the chest.

**TREATMENT** Treatment is supportive in viral pneumonia but antibiotics may be used in bacterial pneumonia. Viral pneumonia usually runs its course in children in about five to seven days, but bacterial pneumonia may be more severe (see Chapter 9 for more information).

# DIGESTIVE DISEASES

Ingestion, digestion, absorption, and elimination are essential body functions. Children with digestive diseases may experience serious growth and develop-

ment problems due to a lack of these. Fluid and electrolyte imbalances are frequently more severe in children, especially infants, than in adults. The imbalances may be caused by vomiting or diarrhea, or other digestive diseases that inhibit the child's ability to ingest or digest and absorb food and fluids.

Colic is a common symptom of digestive problems or disease in children. It is particularly common in young infants. Symptoms of colic include paroxysms of gastrointestinal pain with crying and irritability. It may be due to a variety of causes such as the swallowing of air, emotional upset, or overfeeding.

## Fluid Imbalances

**ETIOLOGY** Children have a higher metabolic rate than adults and thus have a higher exchange of fluids. This fact puts them at risk for serious complications if they experience bouts of vomiting or diarrhea. They can become dehydrated and be in severe electrolyte imbalance in a very short period of time. Dehydration is life threatening in very young children and infants.

**SYMPTOMS** Diagnosis is made by reported history of continued vomiting and/or diarrhea, physical examination, and laboratory data.

**TREATMENT** Treatment focuses on replacement of the fluids and electrolytes. If the child cannot retain fluids because of vomiting, intravenous therapy is necessary. If fluids continue to be lost because of diarrhea, treatment focuses on correcting the cause of the diarrhea, administering medications to prevent the hyperactive bowel problems, and giving replacement fluids and electrolytes either orally or intravenously. Nonprescription oral electrolyte solutions are available for infants and young children, and for older children. Children who are active in sports in very warm weather should drink electrolyte replacement fluids frequently to prevent dehydration.

## Food Allergies

**ETIOLOGY** A food allergy is an overreaction of the immune system to a particular food or ingredient in the food. The reaction may occur within seconds after ingestion or several hours after ingestion of the food. Food allergies are more common in children than in adults, but still affect only a small number of children. The greatest incidence occurs in children under age one. The most common allergies are to cow's milk and eggs. Most of these allergies disappear by age three to five. Allergies to peanuts and fish seem to last much longer, but usually disappear by the time the child is in school. If the food allergy develops after age three, it usually continues into adult life. Children at higher risk of developing food allergies are those who have parents with food allergies, or those who were high-risk infants prenatally and at birth. Children with food allergies as infants are at greater risk for developing respiratory allergies as they get older.

**SYMPTOMS** Symptoms of food allergies include nausea, diarrhea, abdominal pain, coughing, wheezing, itching, rash, headache, and swelling of hands, face, and lips.

**TREATMENT** The best method for preventing allergies is to avoid giving children, especially high-risk children, the common allergenic foods. Children can be tested for allergic antibodies if necessary. Medications are not given for food allergies, but some may be necessary to relieve the symptoms of the allergic reaction.

## Eating Disorders

Eating disorders have become a major problem among children, especially adolescent females. The two most common types of eating disorders are anorexia nervosa and bulimia. Anorexia is characterized by the inability to eat over long periods of time, which results in extreme weight loss, fluid and electrolyte imbalances, and a life-threatening state. Bulimia is characterized by binge eating, followed by purging the food.

**ETIOLOGY** Both of the disorders are classified as psychiatric disorders and require a multidisciplinary approach to treatment.

Eating disorders are diagnosed by physical examination, diet history, and reports from the child and close associates. The exact cause is not known but is associated with our societal images of "thin being in," which causes young females to go through cycles of weight gain and dieting to lose weight, decreased self-esteem, physical, sexual, or emotional trauma, and substance abuse.

**SYMPTOMS** The effects of the disorders may range from decreased energy levels, growth retardation, and menstrual dysfunction to more severe effects such as cardiac disturbances, delayed puberty, personality changes, inability to perform activities of daily living, and death.

**TREATMENT** Early intervention for eating disorders is critical to prevent severe complications. Most eating disorders are treated with a combination of medical and psychiatric interventions. The entire

family needs to be involved in the child's recuperation plan. Usually, this can be accomplished on an outpatient basis, but in severe cases, the child may need hospitalization for treatment or forced feedings until stable. There are several clinics in the United States that specialize in treating eating disorders in children. The mental aspects of eating disorders are covered in more detail in Chapter 21.

# CARDIOVASCULAR DISEASES

Most cardiovascular diseases in children are related to genetic or developmental disorders. These are discussed in Chapter 19.

# MUSCULOSKELETAL DISEASES

Musculoskeletal disorders in children are common because of their high activity levels and rapid growth patterns. Musculoskeletal problems range from soft tissue injuries and fractures to joint and bone deformities, and degenerative muscle disorders. Some of these have already been discussed in Chapters 6 and 19.

## Legg-Calvé-Perthes

Legg-Calvé-Perthes (LCP) disease is an avascular necrosis of the upper end of the femur. The blood supply to the femoral head is reduced, causing changes in bone growth. The disease is known as a disorder of growth that is most common in boys age four to eight years.

**ETIOLOGY** The cause is unknown.

**SYMPTOM** In most cases, the only symptom is pain that increases with walking or running. Diagnosis is made by examination and X-ray.

**TREATMENT** The treatment objective is to maintain the correct position of the femoral head in the acetabulum of the hip until healing occurs. This is accomplished by bed rest for a week to 10 days with range-of-motion exercises. Traction, casts, or braces also may be used to maintain the correct position of the femoral head. If this does not correct the condition, surgical intervention may be needed. An osteotomy is performed to place the femoral head in the correct position. If left uncorrected, permanent deformity may result.

# Ewing's Sarcoma

Ewing's sarcoma, also known as Ewing's tumor, is a malignant neoplasm that occurs before age 20. It is more common in males than females. It is usually located in a long bone such as the femur.

**ETIOLOGY** The cause of the tumor is unknown.

**SYMPTOMS** Symptoms include swelling and pain. Diagnosis is made by X-ray, CT or MRI, and bone scan. A biopsy is necessary to differentiate the exact type of tumor from other bone tumors.

**TREATMENT** Treatment usually includes chemotherapy, and in some cases, radiation therapy. Surgery may be performed but is not usually the first choice of treatment, especially if the tumor is in the leg or arm since that would necessitate amputation of the extremity. Ewings sarcoma is quickly metastatic and highly malignant, but if no metastasis has occurred, the prognosis is very good.

# BLOOD DISEASES

One of the most common disorders of the blood and blood-forming organs in children is leukemia, a type of cancer. Many of the other blood disorders diagnosed in children are chronic diseases such as hemophilia and sickle cell disease. These, as well as acute disorders of the blood such as iron deficiency anemia and some cancers such as Hodgkin's disease, were already discussed in Chapter 7, and are not repeated in this chapter.

# Leukemia

Leukemia (leuk = white, emia = blood) is a malignancy of the blood-forming cells located in the bone marrow. It is the most common form of cancer in children. There are approximately 3,400 children diagnosed each year with leukemia (Leukemia and Lymphoma Society, 2004). Leukemia is diagnosed more frequently in boys than in girls.

**ETIOLOGY** The cause of the disease is unknown, but factors that increase the risk for developing leukemia include exposure to radiation and the presence of genetic or immunologic disorders.

The most common type of leukemia in children is acute lymphoblastic leukemia (ALL). It is characterized by a proliferation of white blood cells that are still immature. As the marrow becomes filled with the diseased white cells, platelets, red cells, and

healthy white cell production decrease, causing symptoms to appear.

**SYMPTOMS** Symptoms include pallor (pale skin), easy bleeding or bruising, fatigue, joint, bone, or abdominal pain, and fever. Leukemia is diagnosed by medical history, complete blood count, and bone marrow biopsy.

Childhood leukemias are now among the most curable diseases of all types of childhood cancers.

**TREATMENT** Treatment for ALL in children is directed at killing all cancer cells. Chemotherapy is the treatment of choice. Radiation also may be used in some cases. Three or four chemotherapeutic agents (methotrexate, vincristine, prednisone, L-asparaginase, or others) are used in the first phase of the treatment. **Intrathecal** (IN-trah-**THEE**-kal; intra = within, thecal = spinal cord; injected into the spinal fluid) medications are used to destroy any cancer cells in the central nervous system. Then, other combinations of the chemotherapeutic agents are given to prevent reappearance of the cancer cells. After this initial therapy, the child is placed on a maintenance schedule consisting of daily low-dose chemotherapy medications for two to three years. One of the complications of the therapy is the reduced ability to fight off infections. Children must be carefully monitored and protected during the initial treatment phase. It is important that a team of health professionals—physicians, nurses, social workers, and other pediatric oncology specialists—is involved with the child and family throughout the treatment period.

# NEUROLOGIC DISEASES

There are many neurologic disorders in children. Some of them, such as meningitis and encephalitis, have already been covered in Chapter 15. The genetic and developmental ones, including cerebral palsy, are discussed in Chapter 19.

# Reye's Syndrome

Reye's syndrome is an acute **encephalopathy** (en-SEF-ah-**LOP**-ah-thee; encephalo = brain, opathy = disease; disorder of the brain) seen in children under age 15 who have had a viral infection.

**ETIOLOGY** The cause is unknown, but a relationship has been found between the disease and the use of aspirin for febrile illnesses in children. Thus, it is recommended that aspirin not be given to children, but acetaminophen be used instead.

**SYMPTOMS** It is characterized by nausea, vomiting, liver enlargement, lethargy, seizures, coma, and in many cases, death.

**TREATMENT** Treatment is supportive.

## EYE AND EAR DISEASES

Children are curious, and use their senses even more than adults during the learning and growing process. Problems with the eyes and ears can have profound effects on the child's ability to learn and develop. Some of the common eye and ear problems have been covered in earlier chapters and in other sections of this chapter.

### Strabismus

**ETIOLOGY** Strabismus, also known as lazy eye or crossed eyes, is a condition of lack of parallelism of the eyes. The eyes are not aligned because of muscle imbalance or paralysis of the extraocular muscles.

**SYMPTOMS** This causes one or both eyes to deviate from the normal position. This may be normal in the very young infant, but should not be present after about four months of age.

**TREATMENT** Special glasses, patches, surgery, or medications may correct the problem. The special glasses and patches help the weak eye become stronger. Surgery is done to realign the affected muscle. If left untreated, loss of vision in the affected eye may result.

### Deafness

Hearing losses in children range from mild to complete.

**ETIOLOGY** The cause may be genetic, trauma, infections, exposure to ototoxic drugs, or unknown. Audiometric testing is needed for an accurate diagnosis of the extent of hearing loss.

**TREATMENT** Treatment depends on the cause and severity of the loss. If the hearing loss is the nonconductive type, some medications or surgical interventions may be helpful in restoring all or part of the loss. There are several types of hearing aids designed especially for children: in the ear, over the ear, and attached to the eyepieces of glasses, which can be fitted by professional hearing specialists. Cochlear implants are now being inserted surgically. They stimulate the eighth cranial nerve (vestibulocochlear nerve) and also send out electrical impulses to the inner ear.

## TRAUMA

Trauma in children is a major cause of debility and death. Child abuse is found at all ages, but some types of trauma such as drug abuse and suicide are much more common in adolescents. Poisonings are at peak levels in toddlers.

### Child Abuse

Child abuse is a serious problem in the United States. It is more common than most other pediatric illnesses and is frequently fatal. It has been difficult to define because "limits" of punishment such as spanking are hard to set. However, it is generally defined as purposeful (not accidental), significant, or demonstrable harm to a child. This may be in the form of physical, sexual, or emotional harm. It also may be in the form of neglect, which accounts for a major portion of the child abuse diagnosed. Neglect is defined as failing to provide basic needs such as food, clothes, and schooling for the child.

Physical child abuse, and sometimes neglect, is usually diagnosed by physical examination, review of verbal explanations from the child and parents, and investigation by authorities. It may be difficult to diagnose or prove at times because of conflicting stories reported by those involved. Many children try to cover up the abuse due to fear of retaliation by the abuser or because of shame. The most frequent instrument to inflict physical abuse is the hand. Belts, clubs, and other items are also used. Burns by cigarettes are also common, especially in very young children. Fractures in children under age three are suggestive of physical abuse. One of the most common injuries in infants is the shaken baby syndrome. This is a serious injury to the brain, caused by vigorous shaking of the child. It may result in death.

Sexual abuse has become an epidemic problem. It is defined by specific acts, and may or may not include intercourse. Unfortunately, sexual abuse of children frequently occurs for years before being reported. The emotional effects are often more serious than the physical effects. The easiest way to identify sexual abuse is to listen to the child, ask open-ended questions, and report suspected abuse to appropriate persons.

Emotional abuse is the most difficult form of child abuse to recognize and diagnose. Constant stigmatizing, berating, or ignoring of a child is considered emotional abuse. The effects of this abuse are manifested in symptoms such as failure to thrive, learning disabilities, eating disorders, social isolation, acting out behaviors, depression, and other behavior and personality disorders.

Recognizing child abuse early may save the life of the child. In most states, there are mandatory reporting laws. Usually, these laws protect the person reporting the suspected abuse from any litigation due to the report. Teachers, clergy, health professionals, and law enforcement personnel are usually listed as the persons mandated to report suspected cases, but all individuals should be aware of the problem and report any suspicions of abuse to authorities.

## Suicide

The overall suicide rate among youth has declined in the last decade, but it is still the third leading cause of death among young people. In 2001, over 4,000 suicides occurred in the age group of 15–24 years. Firearms were used in 54 percent of youth suicides (National Center for Injury Prevention and Control, 2004). The incidence is much less for females than males of the same ages but is still significant. The suicide rate for males has increased significantly in the last two decades. It is thought that most teens who commit suicide do so during or immediately after a period of depression. The depression may be due to a variety of factors such as low self-esteem, chemical abuse, sociological makeup, family problems, and/or abuse. Alcohol abuse also has been found to be a contributing factor, as are other risky behaviors such as drug abuse and gang membership. Suicide attempts are highest in incarcerated youths. Females have a higher rate of suicide ideation and attempts than males, but a much lower incidence of death. Sexual abuse also contributes to suicide ideation and suicide attempts. Some children have been involved in suicide "pacts" with others but this is not common. Gay and bisexual youths have a higher suicide rate than heterosexual youths of the same age.

Early intervention is the key to preventing suicides in children. Recognition of problems in ado-lescents and involvement in treatment programs is imperative. Even casual statements about death or killing oneself need to be taken seriously by parents, counselors, teachers, and friends. These youths need to be referred to special counseling programs as soon as possible. In addition, early intervention in dysfunctional families, and prevention of sexual abuse and alcohol and drug abuse is extremely important.

## Drug Abuse

Illicit drug, alcohol and tobacco use among children, especially adolescents, is in epidemic proportions in the United States. The most common drugs used by children and adolescents include marijuana, cocaine, methamphetamine, alcohol, cigarettes, LSD, inhalants, and anabolic steroids. There are also many other drugs and stimulants and/or depressants that children continually use and abuse on a daily basis. Almost any product that gives the individual an altered sense of reality has been used improperly by children and teens. Products such as glue, cough syrup, correction fluid, mouthwash, and a variety of other products have been used to obtain a "high." Unfortunately, many of these can be deadly, especially when mixed with alcohol or other drugs.

Marijuana is a greenish brown mixture of dried flowers and leaves of the hemp plant (*Cannabis sativa*). It is known by a variety of slang terms such as weed, Mary Jane, and pot. All forms of marijuana are mind-altering because they contain THC (delta-9-tetrahydrocannabinol), the active chemical in the plant. Generally, marijuana is smoked like a cigarette but it can also be put in a pipe. THC disrupts the nerve cells in the brain, making it difficult to problem-solve, remember events, and participate in activities with normal skill and coordination. THC is absorbed by fatty tissue in the body and may be detected in urine samples for weeks after use. The short-term effects of marijuana use include memory loss, slowed ability to learn, distorted perception, loss of coordination, and increased heart rate. Long-term effects of use include the short-term effects plus problems in the respiratory, immune, and reproductive systems.

Cocaine is one of the most addictive drugs abused by individuals. The major methods of use are sniffing or snorting, injecting, and smoking. There is a great risk to the user no matter which method is used. "Crack" is a popular type of cocaine that has been processed from cocaine hydrochloride to a freebase for smoking. Cocaine is a very strong central nervous system stimulant. Effects of the drug include increased blood pressure, dilated pupils, increased heart rate, hyperstimulation, reduced fatigue, and a high associated with pleasure. The length of the effect depends on the route of administration and amount used. In some instances, death has occurred with the first dose taken. However, most deaths associated with the drug are related to overdosing, and/or mixing the drug with other drugs or alcohol. When mixed with alcohol, the liver combines the drugs, creating a third substance called cocaethylene, which intensifies the **euphoric** (a sense of well-being) effects of cocaine but increases the risk of sudden death. Treatment for cocaine addiction includes behavior modification along with some pharmacological agents.

Methamphetamine is an addictive, potent stimulant that affects the central nervous system. It was originally a problem drug predominantly in major western cities, but it has now spread across the country and is found in rural sites as much as in urban areas. Methamphetamine has become one of the fastest growing abused drugs today. It is popular among the young because it is relatively cheap. It is also known as meth, crank, and ice. The drug is easily produced in home laboratories using inexpensive ingredients. It can be injected, smoked, or sniffed. The effects of the drug include decreased appetite, decreased fatigue, anxiety, and a general euphoric state. After the initial rush, the effects can last up to eight hours.

LSD (lysergic acid diethylamide) is the most commonly abused drug in the **hallucinogenic** (producing psychedelic or bizarre alterations in mental functioning) class. It is a potent mood-changing drug that became very popular in the 1960s. It is also known as "acid" and using it is called a "trip." The effects of the drug are somewhat unpredictable but generally give the user a mind-altering state of being. The heart rate increases, pupils dilate, blood pressure increases, appetite diminishes, and delusions and hallucinations are experienced. Because LSD does not produce a dependence on the drug, it is not considered to be addictive. However, many individuals have a "bad trip," suffering serious complications or death from its effects.

Inhalants are chemicals that produce a vapor that can be inhaled, and which produce a mind-altering effect. Young people are more likely to abuse inhalants than adults, treating the use of inhalants as a game or as a way to get a "cheap high." This is a very dangerous activity and has caused death in many adolescents. A variety of products are used as inhalants including solvents, gases, nitrites, and some over-the-counter drugs. The effect is similar to alcohol intoxication. Sniffing concentrated amounts can induce sudden heart failure, respiratory failure, and/or death. Irreversible effects from sniffing these products include hearing loss, limb spasms, bone marrow damage, liver and kidney damage, and brain damage.

Anabolic steroids are the synthetic derivatives of testosterone, the male hormone. They are widely abused by athletes and others trying to promote growth of skeletal muscle and increase lean body mass. Because the fitness craze of the 1980s, the use of anabolic steroids has increased significantly in young males, and even females who want to develop athletic, lean bodies. The steroids are taken orally or injected. The drugs do produce increases in muscle strength, lean body mass, and improved performance over periods of time, but the long-term effects are dangerous. The side effects include shrinking of the testes, reduced sperm count, infertility, and baldness in males; and growth of facial hair, changes in menstruation, enlargement of the clitoris, and a deepened voice in females. Adolescents or preteen children may experience accelerated puberty changes and growth cessation due to premature skeletal maturation. Other effects reported include mood swings, depression, and irritability.

Cigarette smoking and alcohol abuse continues to be a major problem among children and adolescents. The short-term and long-term effects of these drugs are well known. Cigarettes are the most widely used drug by adolescents. Alcohol-related accidents are a leading cause of death in several age groups. Regardless of the drug abused, there are significant consequences for the user. Education about the effects of drug uses and abuses has not been entirely successful in stopping or even slowing down the use of drugs by children overall. Drug use is a national problem that needs continued investigation, education, and monitoring.

## Poisoning

Accidental poisoning can occur when a child ingests medications, cleaning products, alcohol, cosmetics, or other toxins. Parents and other adults frequently fail to recognize how toxic certain substances can be or do not even think about the consequences of leaving them in places accessible to children. Accidental poisoning is among the top five causes of death in children under 10 years of age. About three-fourths of all poisonings occur in children under six years of age.

Children are inquisitive and tend to put things in their mouths, with a devastating consequence when the substance is toxic. Most poisonings are due to common substances found in the home such as cleaning products, medicines, and plants. Generally, the poisoning is an acute event, and treatment is provided at a physician's office or emergency room. Symptoms and treatment depend on the substance ingested. Lead poisoning, on the other hand, is a chronic event. Children suffering neurologic symptoms, chronic anemia, or difficulty with coordination should be evaluated for lead poisoning. The diagnosis is made by checking the blood for lead levels. Chelation therapy treatment is instituted to remove the lead from the blood.

There are poison control centers in every state, most with an 800 number to call for emergency information in case of an accidental poisoning. Generally, local hospitals also have an emergency poison control information number. Although over-the-counter medications to induce vomiting are available, it is wise to check with one of the poison control services prior to instituting treatment in the home. Many products should not be vomited up by the child because they are caustic and can do further damage if treated in that manner. All individuals should be aware of the problem of poisoning and prevent poisonings in the home by following a few guidelines as stated in the Healthy Highlight.

 **HEALTHY HIGHLIGHT**

## Preventing Poisonings in Children

### Medication Safety

- Store all medications—prescription and nonprescription—in a locked cabinet, far from children's reach.

- Never leave vitamin bottles, aspirin bottles, or other medications on the kitchen table, countertops, bedside tables, or dresser tops. Small children may decide to emulate adults and help themselves.

- Do not ever tell a child that medicine is "candy."

- Take special precautions when you have houseguests. Be sure their medications are far from reach, preferably locked in one of their bags.

- Do not keep aspirin or other medicines in a pocketbook; children may find them when searching for gum or a toy.

- Child-resistant packaging does not mean childproof packaging. Do not rely on packaging to protect your children.

- Never administer medication to a child in the dark: you may give the wrong dosage or even the wrong medication.

- After taking or administering medication, be sure to reattach the safety cap and store the medication away safely.

### Chemical Safety

- Store household cleaning products and aerosol sprays in a high cabinet far from reach. Do not keep any cleaning supplies under the sink, including dishwasher detergent and dishwashing liquids.

- Never put cleaning products in old soda bottles or containers that were once used for food.

- When cleaning or using household chemicals, never leave the bottles unattended if there is a small child present.

*(continued)*

**HEALTHY HIGHLIGHT (Continued)**

## Preventing Poisonings in Children

### Chemical Safety (Continued)

- Never put roach powders or rat poison on the floors of your home.
- Keep hazardous automotive and gardening products in a securely locked area in your garage.
- Do not leave alcoholic drinks where children can reach them. Take special care during parties; guests may not be conscious of where they have left their drinks. Clean up promptly after the party.
- Keep bottles of alcohol in a locked cabinet far from children's reach.
- Keep mouthwash out of the reach of children. Many brands of mouthwash contain substantial amounts of alcohol.

### Lead Paint

- If you have an older home, have the paint tested for lead.
- Do not use cribs, bassinets, highchairs, painted toys, or toy chests made before 1978. These may have a finish that contains dangerously high levels of lead.

### Other Toxic Items

- Never leave cosmetics and toiletries within easy reach of children. Be especially cautious with perfume, hair dye, hair spray, nail and shoe polish, and nail polish remover.
- Learn the names of all the plants in your house and remove any that could be toxic.
- Discard used button-cell batteries safely and store any unused ones far from children's reach (alkaline substances are poisonous).

## SUMMARY

Childhood is a time for rapid physical, emotional, and intellectual growth and development. Some childhood diseases can interfere with normal growth and development, but most are acute illnesses that are common among young people. The most common diseases in children are infectious respiratory illnesses. Following a regularly scheduled immunization program can prevent many of the infectious diseases of children. Individuals with congenital disorders, premature infants, and children in low socioeconomic households are at highest risk for contracting one of the common childhood diseases. Trauma affects children of all ages, races, and socioeconomic status, and is one of the leading causes of disability and death in children.

## REVIEW QUESTIONS _____

**Short Answer**

1. What are the most common diseases affecting children?

2. What are the common signs and symptoms of these diseases?

3. What immunization is available to prevent the following diseases?

   **a.** Mumps

   **b.** Measles

   **c.** Pertussis

   **d.** Polio

   **e.** Diphtheria

   **f.** Influenzae

   **g.** Rubella

   **h.** Tetanus

   **i.** Hepatitis

4. Tuberculosis is found in which body system?

5. What is the difference between anorexia nervosa and bulimia?

6. What are the four types of child abuse?

7. How do children contract HIV?

8. What is the most common type of cancer diagnosed in children?

9. Why do many adolescents take anabolic steroids?

10. At what age are children at greatest risk for ingesting a poisonous substance?

## Matching

**11.** Match the drugs listed in the left column with the best description in the right column.

| | |
|---|---|
| _____ marijuana | **a.** the most used hallucinogenic drug |
| _____ cocaine | **b.** an addictive stimulant also known as speed and crank |
| _____ methamphetamine | **c.** chemicals with breathable vapors that produce the effect of being intoxicated |
| _____ LSD | |
| _____ anabolic steroids | **d.** the most widely used drug by adolescents |
| _____ alcohol | **e.** contains the active chemical THC |
| _____ nicotine (cigarettes) | **f.** drug taken to enhance muscular development |
| _____ solvents | **g.** an intoxicating drug that is implicated in thousands of motor vehicle accidents |
| | **h.** a strong central nervous system stimulant that produces a euphoric state |

## CASE STUDY

**Jason** is a 13-year-old junior high student. He is on the basketball, soccer, and track teams. Although he is on a rigorous training program, including weightlifting, he is not able to attain the lean body mass and muscular development he would like to have. He confides to you that he has begun taking anabolic steroids purchased at the local athletic club from the trainer. He asks your opinion about this and also asks you not to tell anyone about it. What is your response to Jason? What do you know about the effects of anabolic steroids? Do you have a responsibility to inform someone about this?

## BIBLIOGRAPHY

Bachman, K. H. (2004, February 23). Adverse childhood experiences, obesity and liver disease. *Archives of Internal Medicine 164*(4), 460–461.

Carley, A. (2003). Anemia: When is it not iron deficiency? *Pediatric Nursing 29*(3), 205–211.

Childhood obesity. (2003). *Pediatric Nursing 29*(1), 23–24.

Gelsemium sempervirens (yellow jasmine). (2004). *Mental Health Practice 8*(1), 10.

Hawley, C. A., Ward, A. B., Magnay, A. R., & Mychalki, W. (2004). Return to school after brain injury. *Archives of Disease in Childhood 89*(2), 136–142.

Parmet, S., Lynm, C., & Glass, R. M. (2004, February 18). Chickenpox. *Journal of the American Medical Association 291*(7), 906.

Rassool, G. H. (2003). Current issues and forthcoming events. *Journal of Advanced Nursing 44*(6), 555–557.

Spence, L. J., & Kaiser, L. (2002). Companion animals and adaptation in chronically ill children. *Western Journal of Nursing Research 24*(6), 639–656.

Unusual leukemia caused by rare combination of genes. (2004, February 6). *Drug Week*, 460–461.

Vigneri, S. (2004). Go ask your dad. *Men's Health 19*(2), 129.

Woodgate, R. L., Degner, L. F., & Yanofsky, R. (2003). A different perspective to approaching cancer symptoms in children. *Journal of Pain & Symptom Management 26*(3), 800–817.

Zinkernagel, R. M. (2003). On natural and artificial vaccinations. *Annual Review of Immunology 21*(1), 515–546.

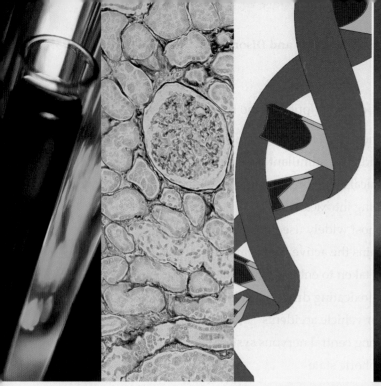
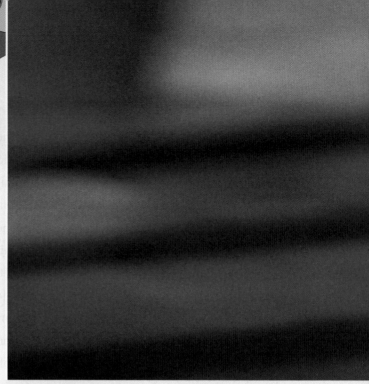

## OUTLINE

## KEY TERMS

# Mental Health Diseases and Disorders

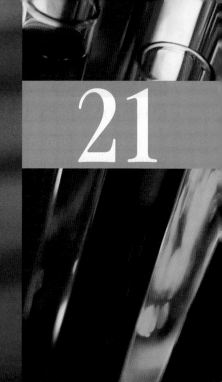

**21**

## LEARNING OBJECTIVES

*Upon completion of the chapter, the learner should be able to:*

1. Define the terminology common to mental health disorders.

2. Identify the important signs and symptoms associated with mental health disorders.

3. Describe the common diagnostic tests used to determine the type and/or cause of mental health disorders.

4. Identify common mental health disorders.

5. Describe the typical course and management of the common mental health disorders.

6. State the mental health disorders found in the older population and the effects of these disorders.

## OVERVIEW

Mental health disorders are some of the most difficult diseases to diagnose and understand. Symptoms may range from mild behavior changes to severe personality disturbances. Because of the variety of symptoms, the difficulty in diagnosing some disorders, and the lack of understanding of the physiologic cause, many mental health disorders are misdiagnosed and can go untreated for years. Although some mental health problems are not yet well understood, many more are relatively easy to diagnose and treat. ■

## COMMON SIGNS AND SYMPTOMS

For mental health disorders, there are only a few common signs and symptoms. Typically, symptoms of mental health problems begin with behavioral changes.

These are often slow developing and very subtle, so symptoms might not be noticed early in the development of a disorder. Many of the symptoms such as forgetfulness, anxiety, or temper tantrums are attributed to age, stress, or other illnesses. Typical symptoms of each mental health problem are discussed with the specific disorder.

## DIAGNOSTIC TESTS

There are a variety of diagnostic tests used to determine the specific mental health problem. When symptoms first appear, the physician usually orders physiologic tests such as laboratory tests, brain scans, EEGs, and MRIs to determine if the cause is an organic problem. Second, an individual may be referred to a psychiatrist for psychological testing to determine a diagnosis. These tests may include an aptitude test, personality test, and several others, depending on the symptoms presented and the severity of the symptoms.

## COMMON MENTAL HEALTH DISORDERS

Mental health disorders range from mild to severe. A few disorders have a genetic base, others are due to behavior choices, and some are of unknown cause. Early diagnosis and treatment are essential to assist the individual to either overcome the disorder or to improve the quality of life.

### Developmental Mental Health Disorders

Developmental mental health disorders are those that are usually discovered during infancy, childhood, or adolescence. These disorders may diminish or worsen as the child matures. Developmental disorders that are carried into adulthood may be mild, allowing the involved individual to function in an adult role, or may be so severe that institutionalization may be needed.

### ■ Mental Retardation

Mental retardation is a condition of decreased intelligence leading to a decrease in the ability to learn, socialize, and mature. Mental retardation varies in degrees from mild and moderate to severe and profound. In the past, these degrees were described as feebleminded, idiot, imbecile, and moron, but these terms are no longer used.

**ETIOLOGY** The cause of mental retardation is often unknown. Known causes of mental retardation fall into two categories: genetic and acquired (Table 21-1). Some types of mental retardation can be avoided by providing prenatal care.

**SYMPTOMS** Affected children may not show signs of mental retardation until entry into school. Difficulty learning and keeping up with other children of the same age may be indicative of mental retardation. Diagnosis is confirmed on the basis of observation and IQ testing.

**TREATMENT** Treatment of mentally retarded individuals varies with the amount of retardation. Many mildly retarded individuals grow up and find employment in a suitable occupation, and lead fairly normal lives. Others may need special dependent living facilities, but very few are retarded to the level of needing institutionalization.

### ■ Autism

Autism, also called autistic disorder, is a severe type of developmental disorder characterized by a preoccupation with inner thoughts, daydreams, fantasies, and **delusions** (a false belief that is firmly adhered to although it is not shared by others).

**TABLE 21–1** Genetic and Acquired Causes of Mental Retardation

| Genetic | Acquired |
|---|---|
| Down Syndrome | Prenatal Maternal Rubella |
| PKU—Phenylketonuria | Prenatal Maternal Syphilis |
| Hypothyroidism—Cretinism | Blood Type Incompatibility |
| | Prematurity |
| | Anoxia |
| | Birth Injury |
| | Poor Nutrition |
| | Head Trauma |

**ETIOLOGY** The cause of autism is unknown although there may be a physical cause.

**SYMPTOMS** Symptoms of autism are usually apparent in infancy when the infant exhibits an eye-to-eye gaze and blank facial expression. Affected children are so involved with themselves that they become inaccessible to others, including parents. These children may play alone happily for hours and become angry if interrupted. Diagnosis is confirmed on the basis of observation of behavior.

**TREATMENT** Behavioral therapy to teach the child how to adapt to situations is beneficial. Prognosis is still relatively poor and affected children rarely recover.

## ■ Attention-Deficit Hyperactivity Disorder

Attention-deficit hyperactivity disorder (ADHD) is a mental health disorder characterized by an inability to concentrate, hyperactivity, and impulsiveness.

**ETIOLOGY** The cause of ADHD is unknown but there does appear to be a familial pattern. This behavior may be apparent at any age, but is usually observed before the age of seven, becoming more obvious in school situations.

**SYMPTOMS** Examples of ADHD behavior include forgetfulness, not appearing to listen, difficulty in remaining seated or waiting one's turn, squirming, excessive running, climbing, talking, inability to complete detailed work, messy work, and an inability to organize. These behaviors tend to become more exaggerated in a group situation. Diagnosis is made on the basis of observation of the age-inappropriate behavior.

**TREATMENT** Treatment of ADHD with amphetamines has shown varying degrees of effectiveness. Behavior modification by rewarding appropriate behavior also has been successful.

## ■ Stuttering

**ETIOLOGY** Stuttering often occurs when children address an impatient or angry parent, or someone who is in authority. The child's anxiety often leads to stuttering. The listener's reaction often enforces the child's anxiety, leading to more difficulties.

**SYMPTOMS** Stuttering, also called stammering, is a speech problem characterized by hesitancy of starting and finishing a sound or word, and prolonged pauses between words or sounds.

**TREATMENT** Treatment is often based on some type of behavior modification and positive reinforcement of proper speech.

## ■ Eating Disorders

Eating disorders currently affect approximately one in 100 females.

**ETIOLOGY** It is thought that a factor in eating disorders centers around the great emphasis Americans place on the thin, perfect, female body. To obtain this ideal figure, many females go to dieting extremes. Two common eating disorders are **anorexia nervosa** and **bulimia**. These are also discussed in Chapter 20 as disorders of adolescents.

Anorexia (AN-oh-**RECK**-see-ah; an = without, orexia = appetite) nervosa is a disorder of self-imposed starvation, resulting from a distorted body image (Figure 21-1). The term anorexia is a misnomer as the appetite is not diminished, but the affected individual simply refuses to eat in fear of becoming fat. The typical characteristics of an individual with anorexia nervosa include:

- adolescent female
- meticulous, high achiever
- body image distortion (feels fat no matter how thin)
- intense fear of becoming fat
- performing excessive exercise

Affected individuals often come from families evidencing "togetherness," characterized by overprotectiveness and conflict avoidance. The mother is often controlling and domineering whereas the father is distant and uninvolved. The family unit often fails to support the idea that the adolescent female is competent and able to function in an independent way.

**SYMPTOMS** The affected female's excessively thin body often appears prepuberty in shape, which can help reduce stress by decreasing the fear of growing up, fear of sexuality, and fear of developing a sexual identity.

**TREATMENT** Treatment is often difficult and lengthy, and involves restoring normal nutrition and resolving psychological problems. Death from starvation is often due to compromised cardiac function.

Bulimia (byou-LIM-ee-ah) is an eating disorder characterized by episodes of binge eating (an intake of approximately 5,000 calories in one to two hours), followed by activities to negate the calorie intake or purging.

**SYMPTOMS** Purging behaviors include self-induced vomiting or excessive laxative use. Excessive vomiting often leads to electrolyte imbalances and erosion of

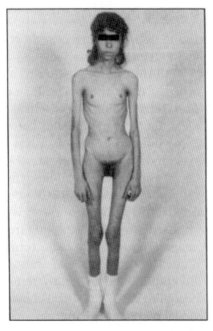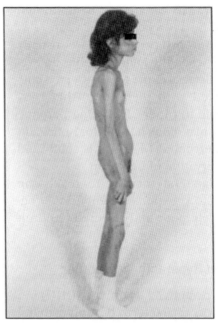

**FIGURE 21–1** Anorexia nervosa: physical manifestations of extreme wasting in an adolescent with anorexia nervosa. *(From R. P. Rawling, S. R. Williams, and C. K. Biel, 1992, Mental Health-Psychiatric Nursing, 3rd ed., St. Louis: Mosby-Yearbook.)*

the teeth. Individuals affected with bulimia are usually older than anorexics, more obese, and experience a wide fluctuation in weight. Bulimic individuals tend to have perfectionist personalities and a dreaded fear of becoming fat, both similar to anorexics.

**TREATMENT** Treatment of bulimia is similar to anorexia including the use of antidepressant drugs and group therapy.

### ■ Tic Disorders

Tic disorders include a variety of conditions characterized by sudden, rapid muscle movement or vocalization.

**ETIOLOGY** The cause of tics is unknown but they tend to develop in children ages five to 10 years. Tics are irresistible but tend to increase with stress and decrease with sleep or preoccupation with another activity.

**SYMPTOMS** Examples of tics include eye blinking, facial grimacing, neck or shoulder jerking, throat clearing, snorting, and grunting to name just a few.

### ■ Enuresis

Enuresis (EN-you-**REE**-sis), commonly called bedwetting, is a condition of urinary incontinence after

the age of bladder training (usually considered as age five years). Enuresis is more common in males than females, and commonly affects firstborn children.

**ETIOLOGY** The cause of enuresis is unknown, but it does have familial tendencies and is thought by some to be due to inadequate or poor attempts at toilet training.

**TREATMENT** Treatment involves encouraging the child to participate in planning and carrying out a program to reduce and finally eliminate the episodes. Planning may include restriction of fluids after the evening meal, bladder training to help enlarge the capacity of the bladder, urinating before bedtime, and awakening the child during the night to void. Reprimanding, ridiculing, and shaming the child should be avoided as these activities tend to make the condition worse.

## Substance-Related Mental Disorders

Substance-related mental disorder is now the diagnosis used in place of the term drug addiction. The cost of substance abuse-related medical care to the health care industry is estimated to be well over $90 billion a year. Common terms used in substance-related mental disorders include addiction, dependency, tolerance, and withdrawal. **Addiction** means a physical and or psychological dependence on a substance. **Dependency** is a psychological craving for a substance that may or may not be accompanied by a physical need. **Tolerance** is the ability to endure a larger amount of a substance without an adverse effect, or the need for a larger amount or dose of the drug to have the same effect. **Withdrawal** is the unpleasant physical and psychological effects that result from stopping the use of the substance after an individual is addicted.

## ■ Alcoholism

Alcoholism is a physical and mental dependence on a regular intake of alcohol. It is a chronic, progressive, and often fatal disease. Onset of alcoholism is often insidious, beginning in the teen years. Excessive use may be related to stress or depression, or some other stressful life event. Alcoholism is a major drug problem adversely affecting the physical, mental, social, and spiritual health of the affected individual. Chronic alcoholism causes physical damage to nearly every organ system. Some of the common problems include heart disease, hypertension, cirrhosis, pancreatitis, peripheral neuropathy, and gastrointestinal problems (including an increased risk of stomach and esophageal cancer). Mental disorders include anxiety, depression, insomnia, impotence, and amnesia. These physical and mental problems, along with the associated accidents, injuries, and violence associated with alcoholism, can be psychologically, socially, and economically devastating to affected individuals and their families.

**ETIOLOGY** The cause of alcoholism is unknown. There is not a universally accepted explanation for alcoholism, although recent research points toward a biologic explanation or at least a genetic predisposition. Other causal factors may include depression, poverty, peer pressure, and condoning of substance abuse by peers and family members. Individuals raised in homes where both parents are alcoholics are at very high risk for also becoming alcoholics.

Alcohol is absorbed in the mouth and small intestine and is broken down by the liver. A normal sized individual can metabolize or break down approximately 10 milliliters of alcohol or one ounce of whiskey every 90 minutes. If taken in higher amounts or consumed more frequently, alcohol causes a sedative effect, and may depress breathing and lead to death. An individual is **intoxicated** when the blood

alcohol level reaches 0.10 percent or more. Four to six hours after intoxication occurs, the individual experiences a hangover with symptoms of nausea, vomiting, fatigue, sweating, and thirst. The primary cause of a hangover is due to the accumulation of alcohol in the blood and hypoglycemia.

**SYMPTOMS** Alcoholics become physically dependent on alcohol, and may experience symptoms of withdrawal if alcohol is withheld for 24 to 48 hours. Symptoms of withdrawal include **hallucinations** (a false sensation of sight, touch, sound, or feel), tremors of the hands, mild seizures, and **delirium tremens (DTs)**. Symptoms of delirium tremens may include agitation, memory loss, anorexia, seizures, and hallucinations. DTs usually last one to five days and may be fatal if not properly treated. Treatment for withdrawal includes tranquilizers, anticonvulsive medication, adequate nutrition, and antiemetic (anti = against, emetic = nausea or vomiting) medications.

**TREATMENT** Treatment of chronic alcoholism includes rehabilitation designed to meet the alcoholic's physical and psychological needs, and supports total abstinence from alcohol. Many alcoholics have found success with self-help groups.

## ■ Marijuana

Marijuana, also called pot, grass, Mary Jane, and weed, is a mixture of dried leaves and flowers of an Indian hemp plant (*Cannabis sativa*). This mixture is crushed and rolled into cigarettes called reefers or joints. *Hashish*, a resin from the flowering top of the hemp plant, is thought to be four to eight times stronger than marijuana. Both marijuana and hashish usually produce a euphoric effect or sense of well-being. This effect is immediate and lasts approximately two to three hours. True tolerance does not develop with marijuana use, but chronic use may lead to a psychological dependence. Marijuana use has not been proven to lead to the use of hard drugs, but users often experiment with other drugs. Beneficial uses of marijuana include a lowering of intraocular pressure in glaucoma patients, and relief of nausea and vomiting in individuals on chemotherapy.

## ■ Cocaine

Cocaine is a powerful stimulant that accelerates the central nervous system and an anesthetic that numbs whatever it touches. Cocaine is obtained from the leaves of the coca plant found in South America or may be produced synthetically. Cocaine is a pure white powder and may be referred to as "coke." This form of cocaine is commonly snorted from a spoon or straw. It also may be mixed with water, heated to help with the dissolving process, and injected. Drug paraphernalia not only includes syringes, spoons, and straws, but also may include a razor blade and mirror, or piece of glass, used to carefully divide the powder dose. Powder cocaine is quite expensive at $100 per gram. Snorting produces a slower response than injecting, with effects lasting approximately 20 minutes. Complications of snorting cocaine include disintegration of the mucous membrane of the nose and ulceration through the nasal septum. Injecting cocaine and sharing needles increases the risk of HIV. The anesthetic properties of powdered cocaine make it an ideal legal medication for patients undergoing nasal surgery.

Another form of cocaine is called "crack" or "freebase." Crack cocaine is currently made by heating a mixture of powder cocaine, water, and ammonia, or baking soda, causing the material to precipitate into a hardened form of small chips or chunks. Historically, this process involved the use of ether and other flammable bases rather than ammonia and baking soda. Processing with the ether method was very dangerous due to the flammability of this product. Crack cocaine is four to five times stronger, and much more addictive, than powder cocaine. Crack is smoked rather than snorted or injected. Manufacturing and smoking crack cocaine is called "freebasing." When smoked, crack reaches the brain within seconds, giving an intense high or rush to the body. The high lasts approximately five minutes, then fades into a restless desire for more of the drug. Crack is sold in small vials (approximately two doses) for $5 to $10. This cost is initially less expensive than powdered cocaine, but the intense addiction this drug causes leads to increased use and cost. Addiction often leads to theft, prostitution, and "dealing" to obtain the money needed to purchase more cocaine. Crack cocaine is usually smoked with marijuana, tobacco cigarettes, or in a glass pipe. Overdosing with crack is more common than with powder cocaine. It is estimated that one in two Americans between the ages of 25 to 35 has tried cocaine, and 1.4 million Americans are regular cocaine users. Infants born to cocaine-using mothers are often addicted and exhibit low birth weight, hyperactivity, tremors, and frantic sucking activities.

## ■ Caffeine and Nicotine

Two of the most common addicting substances in our society are caffeine and nicotine. Caffeine is a stimulant found in coffee, chocolate, tea, cola drinks, and some over-the-counter medications. Caffeine causes vasoconstriction, and over a long period of time, may lead to circulatory problems. Individuals addicted to caffeine often experience severe withdrawal headaches, anxiety, drowsiness, fatigue, and nausea. Caffeine tends to cause breast tenderness in females and intensify the symptoms of premenstrual syndrome (PMS). Caffeine is the cheapest and most abused drug in the United States.

Tobacco use in this country is on the rise, especially among the teen population, despite widespread knowledge of the devastating effects of nicotine on the cardiovascular and respiratory systems. Nicotine is a stimulant that narrows blood vessels, and raises heart rate and blood pressure. It has been theorized that nicotine is as addictive as cocaine. Symptoms of withdrawal include depression, irritability, anger, anxiety, and an increase in appetite and weight gain. Smoking during pregnancy can result in spontaneous abortion and premature birth. Nicotine patches that reduce nicotine intake gradually have been successful in helping millions of affected individuals to quit smoking.

## ■ Sedatives or Depressants

Drugs in this category are commonly antianxiety medications (Librium or Valium), barbiturates (Nembutal and Seconal), and hypnotics (Dalmane and Placidyl). Individuals addicted to these medications may use as much as 65 milligrams of Valium or 600 milligrams of Seconal a day.

The most severely abused group of sedatives or depressants is the barbiturates. Street names for these drugs include downers, barbs, or may be known by the color of the capsules (reds, yellow jackets, or rainbows). These medications are often prescribed to treat insomnia, hypertension, and seizure disorders. Barbiturates distort mood, leading to euphoria, slow down reaction times causing an increase in automobile and home accidents, and in some cases hallucinations. Taking barbiturates with alcohol potentiates or enhances the effect of alcohol. Addiction and tolerance to barbiturates are developed quickly. Tolerance commonly leads to overdosing of barbiturates, causing a slowing of the heart and breathing that often results in death. Barbiturate use is one of the main causes of accidental death and is the most common method of suicide. Sudden withdrawal from barbiturates may be life threatening. It is recommended that withdrawal be under the guidance of a physician. Affected individuals are usually hospitalized and the drug is withdrawn slowly to prevent nausea, delirium, and seizures.

A nonbarbiturate sedative, methaqualone (Quaalude), was introduced in the United States in the mid-1960s, and was marketed as having no effect on sleep patterns and little potential for abuse. Since that time, it has been discovered that Quaalude, commonly called "ludes," does interfere with rapid eye movement (REM) sleep, and does cause psychological and physical dependence. Withdrawal symptoms may last two to three days, and may include insomnia, anxiety, nausea, hallucinations, and nightmares.

## ■ Amphetamines

Amphetamines are stimulant drugs that cause a release of the body's natural epinephrine, leading to an increase in heart rate, respiration, and digestion. Commonly, amphetamines are called "speed," "uppers," "bennies," and "pep pills." These drugs are often used by obese individuals to lose weight, by truck drivers to stay awake, and by college students to stay alert for studying. Amphetamines are addictive and do lead to tolerance. Chronic use often leads to an opposite effect; that is, causing drowsiness. Depression and suicide may occur following sudden withdrawal.

## ■ Hallucinogens

Hallucinogens, also called psychedelic drugs, commonly produce hallucinations. These drugs cause a heightened and distorted response to visual, auditory, and tactile stimuli. This heightened response allows the affected individual to see flat objects take on shape, stationary objects move, and colors that become more vivid. Hallucinogenic drugs include LSD (lysergic acid diethylamide), Mescaline, and PCP. LSD is a colorless, tasteless, and odorless synthetic substance that is primarily produced in illegal laboratories. It may be added to the food or drink of an unsuspecting victim, or may be added to chewing gum, hard candy, postage stamps, or stickers. LSD is a very potent drug. An amount of drug visible to the eye is enough to cause an eight-hour "trip." LSD

causes abnormal thought processes, and may cause temporary or permanent mental changes. Controversy exists over the fact that LSD also may cause chromosomal damage. Suprisingly, LSD is not addictive. It appears that this drug is abused to escape reality rather than make an effort to cope with reality. Abusers of LSD do have a high tendency to abuse marijuana, barbiturates, and amphetamines. The danger of this drug lies in the fact that the activities of an individual under the influence of LSD are totally unpredictable. There may be attempts to "fly," or episodes of violence and self-destruction. Flashbacks (recurrence of a trip) may occur months after the drug was taken because it is stored in fat tissue and may be released at a later time.

Mescaline is similar to LSD but much weaker. Mescaline is an active chemical found in the Mexican peyote cactus that also may be produced synthetically. Native Americans use this cactus as part of their traditional religious ceremonies.

PCP, also known as "angel dust," "peace pill," and "peace weed," is a depressant that was introduced in the 1950s as an animal tranquilizer. Its use has since been abandoned because of unpredictable side effects. PCP is easily produced in illegal laboratories and may be taken as pills, injections, by snorting, or by smoking. Danger lies in the poor and varied quality of the product sold on the street. PCP may cause memory lapses lasting for several days. Other symptoms are coma, convulsions, and respiratory arrest.

## ■ Narcotics

Narcotics are depressants that are primarily prescribed as analgesics or painkillers. Demerol, methadone, morphine, heroin, and opium are classified as narcotics, and are commonly abused. Narcotics slow nerve and muscle action, and slow the rate of the heart and breathing, and lower blood pressure. Physical and psychological dependence and tolerance rapidly develop with the use of narcotics. Overdose symptoms include slurred speech, confusion, staggering, coma, and respiratory arrest.

Opium is an air-dried milky residue obtained from the unripe opium poppy. References to opium smoking are common in Oriental history, and some people in Asian countries still smoke opium. Users in the western countries, including America, prefer opium derivatives like morphine and heroine. Opium contains approximately 10 percent morphine. Heroin is a derivative of morphine but is approximately eight times stronger. Heroin is very addictive, and is commonly called "smack" and "horse." Heroin is the narcotic most widely used by narcotic addicts today. Heroin is a fine white powder that is usually mixed with water and injected intravenously, called "mainlining." It also may be snorted or smoked. Heroin use usually gives a "rush" or intense feeling of well-being, followed by a sleepy, drowsy state. Withdrawal from heroin without medical treatment is called "going cold turkey." Withdrawal is often uncomfortable but usually not life threatening. Symptoms of withdrawal include sweating, shaking, diarrhea, vomiting, and sharp pain and cramps in the stomach and legs.

### ■ Inhalants

Inhalants include over 1,000 legal substances including glue, spray paint, hair spray, nail polish, lighter fluid, and gasoline. These substances commonly contain harmful hydrocarbons and an oily base, that when inhaled, coats the inner lining of the lungs. Inhalant abuse refers to intentionally breathing the vapors of a substance in order to get high. This intentional breathing in is commonly called "huffing," "snuffing," or "bagging." Bagging is the most dangerous as it entails placing a plastic bag over the head to get a longer effect. Using inhalants over a period of time may result in permanent brain, heart, kidney, and liver damage. Some products like paint and gasoline contain lead and may lead to death from lead poisoning. Inhalant abuse is the third most common substance abused by individuals age 12 to 14 years, surpassed only by alcohol and tobacco. Symptoms of inhalant abuse include spots or sores around the mouth, a glassy-eyed look, fumes on the breath or clothing, anxiety, and loss of appetite.

## Organic Mental Disorders

**Organic** mental disorders are those associated with some type of known physical cause. These disorders affect the cognitive abilities or the abilities to think, remember, and make judgments of the affected individual. These disorders may be temporary or permanent.

### ■ Dementia

**ETIOLOGY** Dementia is a progressive deterioration of mental abilities due to physical changes in the brain. The cognitive or mental abilities include severe memory loss, disorientation, impaired judgment, and the inability to learn new information. Dementia may or may not be reversible, depending on cause.

**SYMPTOMS** Symptoms of dementia are usually severe enough to interfere with the individual's ability to care for himself or herself. Dementia is not a part of the normal aging process although most individuals with dementia are older. Factors important in determining whether dementia will occur in an individual include nutritional status, family history, chronic diseases, and general state of health. Onset of dementia may be slow or sudden, depending on the cause. Causes of dementia are listed in Table 21–2.

### ■ Delirium

Delirium is an acute condition that develops suddenly, often as a result of medications, alcohol, fever,

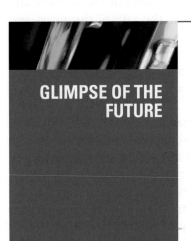

**GLIMPSE OF THE FUTURE**

### Treating Depression in Drug-dependent Individuals

Studies are being conducted on the effects of sertraline for depression in individuals who are on methadone therapy for drug addiction. Sertraline (trade name Zoloft) is a common prescription drug used for depression in adults. In the clinical trials, the researchers are looking at the individual's environment: is it positive or negative? In individuals with positive environments, sertraline has been found to reduce depression and to enhance the effects of the drug withdrawal program. In the future, patients with drug dependencies may be treated with sertraline in combination with some behavioral intervention to reduce their depression and enhance the methadone effects.

*Source: Carpenter, K. M., Brooks, A. C., Vosburg, S. K., & Nunes, E. V. (2004).*

| TABLE 21–2 | Physical Causes of Dementia and Delirium |
| --- | --- |
| **Drugs** | |
| Prescribed medications | |
| Alcohol | |
| Abused substances | |
| **Metabolic Disorders** | |
| Endocrine gland disorders | |
| **Nutritional Disease** | |
| Vitamin deficiencies | |
| Malnutrition | |
| **Infection** | |
| Meningitis | |
| Encephalitis | |
| Brain abscess | |
| AIDS | |
| **Trauma** | |
| Head injury | |
| **Vascular Disorders** | |
| Cerebrovascular accidents (CVA) | |
| Arteriosclerosis | |
| **Neoplastic** | |
| Brain tumors | |
| **Neurologic** | |
| Epilepsy | |

or physical illness. The affected individual is often frightened, disoriented to place and time, has illusions, hallucinations, and incoherent speech. Individuals with delirium expend great amounts of energy, continually wandering and performing aimless activities. Causes of delirium are also listed in Table 21-2.

### ■ Alzheimer's Disease

Alzheimer's disease is a progressive and irreversible form of dementia. Alzheimer's accounts for 50 percent of all dementias and commonly occurs after age 65, but may occur as early as age 40.

**ETIOLOGY** The cause of Alzheimer's is unknown, but some theories include an inherited chromosomal defect, viral infection, a deficiency in neurochemicals in the brain, and an immunologic defect. Interestingly, postmortem studies have revealed a high level of aluminum in the brain and a higher incidence of a serious head injury. Physical changes noted during autopsy include brain plaques and neuronal tangles.

**SYMPTOMS** Symptoms begin with mild memory loss and progress to impaired mental function, personality changes, and speech and language problems. In the final stage, the affected individual is often depressed and paranoid, and may have hallucinations. At this stage, the individual with Alzheimer's is dependent on another individual for total care and may need institutionalization. Death usually occurs in 10 to 15 years from onset and is usually due to complications of immobility.

**TREATMENT** Treatment is aimed at relieving symptoms and managing behavior problems (see Chapter 15 for more information).

## Psychosis

Psychosis is a term describing conditions characterized by a disintegration of one's personality and a loss of contact with reality. Psychotic individuals have impaired communication skills, an inability to deal with life's demands, delusions, and hallucinations. These mental disturbances may or may not have a physical or structural change in the brain. One of the most common psychotic disorders is schizophrenia.

### ■ Schizophrenia

Schizophrenia, meaning "split mind," is a serious type of psychosis. It is not a split personality disorder.

**ETIOLOGY** Various theories exist as to the cause of schizophrenia including genetics, brain biochemical disorders, and structural alterations. It is generally agreed that schizophrenics have a genetic vulnerability, since an individual with a schizophrenic parent, sibling, or other close relative, has an increased possibility of becoming schizophrenic. Another theory suggests that schizophrenic individuals were deprived of meaningful relationships with family members during childhood years. This theory is supported by the fact that most schizophrenics felt that as children, they were unloved, unwanted, and unimportant.

**SYMPTOMS** This disorder often appears in individuals age 16 to 25, and is more common in females than males. Schizophrenics lose touch with reality and act on imagined or fantasized reality.

## ■ Delusional Disorders

Delusional disorders are characterized by a firm belief in a delusion in an otherwise normally adjusted and balanced personality. The delusions often center on feelings of persecution and grandiosity. Areas of delusion often involve romance, religion, and politics. These delusions often develop slowly and involve a false interpretation of an actual occurrence. Delusional individuals become firmly convinced that something is true no matter how convincing evidence is to the contrary. Types of delusional disorders affecting the thinking of an affected individual include:

- Grandiose—an inflated sense of self-worth, power, and knowledge
- Jealous—belief that their sexual partner is unfaithful
- Erotomanic—belief that someone of higher status is in love with them
- Persecutory—suspicious actions and feelings that people are spying on them with harmful intentions
- Somatic—belief that they have a physical disease or disorder

## Mood or Affective Disorders

Mood or affective disorders are those that involve the emotions (**mood**) and the outward expression of those emotions (**affect**). Mood ranges on a spectrum with extreme depression at one end and extreme elation or happiness at the other. Individuals normally experience times of sadness and moments of joy. When these emotions are not appropriate to the events of life, last for an inappropriate length of time, or are extreme in nature, then mood disorders may be suspected. Individuals with mood disorders may have extreme depression, whereas others will exhibit both extreme depression and extreme elation at alternating times (bipolar disorder).

## ■ Depression

**SYMPTOMS** Depression is a prolonged feeling of extreme sadness or unhappiness, despair, and discouragement. Depression is different from grief, which is a realistic sadness related to a personal loss. Pro-

longed grief may become depression because depression is often associated with loss of a loved one, possessions, self-esteem, and youth. A depressed individual often exhibits the following characteristics:

- feels rejected, helpless, and worthless
- is indecisive and disinterested in surroundings
- does not enjoy pleasurable events
- has a low energy level; always feels fatigued
- is unable to sleep or sleeps excessively
- may cry easily and often
- may have thoughts of suicide

Depression more commonly occurs during critical periods along the life cycle including adolescence, menopause, and old age. Depression is often untreated with only one in every three affected individuals seeking assistance.

**TREATMENT** Treatment of depression may include psychotherapy and antidepressant medications. The majority of individuals with serious depression will show improvement in only a few weeks.

## ■ Seasonal Affective Disorder

Seasonal affective disorder (SAD), also called winter depression, is a depressive condition that occurs more commonly during the winter months. Onset of depression typically begins in the fall, becomes progressively worse through the winter months, and clears or improves in the spring. SAD tends to recur each year with the change of seasons.

**SYMPTOMS** Symptoms include chronic fatigue, excessive sleep, and excessive eating with weight gain. SAD occurs more commonly in women and those living at higher latitudes with shorter daylight hours.

**ETIOLOGY** The cause of SAD is thought to be related to an increase in the hormone melatonin. This hormone is released by the pineal gland during dark hours and is suppressed by light. Increased amounts of melatonin cause drowsiness and fatigue. It is thought that individuals with SAD are affected by high levels of melatonin.

**TREATMENT** Medications to reduce melatonin secretion have been of some benefit.

**ETIOLOGY** Another theory suggests that SAD is caused by a delay in the individual's **circadian rhythm** (a normal 24-hour cycle of biological rhythms including sleep, metabolism, and glandular secretions), causing a type of hibernation.

## COMPLEMENTARY AND ALTERNATIVE THERAPY

### Herbs for Mental Health

The herb damiana (*Turnera diffusa*) is a small shrub that grows 1-2 m high and bears aromatic leaves that are the medicinal part of the plant. These leaves are harvested during the flowering season. Damiana is found throughout Mexico, Central America, and the West Indies, as well as in parts of South America. It is reported to be useful in cases of nervous debility and physical and mental exhaustion. It also has been used to reverse depression in adults. There are no known risks associated with using the herb but caution is always important when using herbal preparations with conventional medications.

*Source: Shan, Y. (2004).*

**TREATMENT** This theory is supported by the fact that daily exposure to bright light during the winter months has improved depression in individuals affected by SAD (Figure 21–2).

### ■ Bipolar Disorder (Manic Depressive)

Bipolar disorder is a type of depression in which extreme depression and **mania** (extreme elation or agitation) occur. The mania is not truly a state of happiness but rather a state of elated depression. Affected individuals have a normal state of depression but experience dramatic swings between this state to extreme depression and extreme mania.

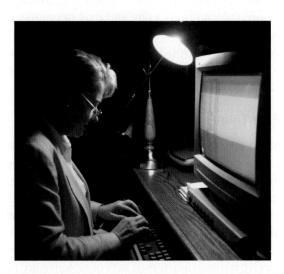

**FIGURE 21–2** Seasonal affective disorder (SAD): many individuals with seasonal affective disorder will experience less depression when using light therapy.

**ETIOLOGY** The cause of bipolar disorder is unknown. Current theories suggest genetics and a deficiency in biochemicals in the brain.

**SYMPTOMS** Symptoms of extreme depression have already been discussed. Symptoms of mania include:

- feelings of euphoria
- increased energy, activity, and restlessness
- rapid thoughts and racing speech
- unrealistic beliefs in one's abilities
- extreme irritability
- unusual behavior and denial that anything is wrong

**TREATMENT** Current treatment includes psychotherapy and lithium medication to control mood swings.

## Dissociative Disorders

Dissociative disorders are characterized by changes in identity or consciousness. These disorders include psychogenic amnesia, psychogenic fugue, depersonalization disorder, and multiple personality.

- Psychogenic amnesia is characterized by a sudden loss of memory that is more than simple forgetfulness. This disorder tends to occur after a major stress event and is considered to be a way of escape.

- Psychogenic fugue is characterized by suddenly leaving home, traveling some distance, forgetting one's identity and past, and often changing one's name. Fugue usually occurs after a major natural disaster such as an earthquake or during wartime. This disorder often lasts only a few days but may last for several months.

- Depersonalization disorders often occur following severe depression, stress, fatigue, or recovery from drug addiction. The affected individuals feel disconnected from mind and body, and may feel like they are viewing life from a distance. Often, individual feel that they are losing their minds.

- Mutiple personality is a rare disorder characterized by an individual exhibiting two or more distinct personalities. The dominant personality determines the actions and activities of the affected individual. The dominant personality is usually not aware of the secondary personality(ies), but the secondary personality(ies) are aware of the dominant personality. Change from one personality to another usually occurs quite suddenly and usually follows a stressful event.

# Anxiety Disorders

Normally, anxiety is a temporary response to stress, but for some individuals, anxiety becomes a chronic problem. Affected individuals often experience anxiety that is exaggerated or of inappropriate proportion to the situation. Anxiety disorders, previously known as neuroses, represent the largest mental health disorder in the United States. The cause of anxiety disorders may be related to genetic factors, severe stress, biochemical alterations, and in some cases, physical causes such as hyperthyroidism. Treatment may include psychotherapy, hypnosis, stress reduction, relaxation therapy including biofeedback, and physical exercise. Types of anxiety disorders include generalized, panic, phobia, obsessive-compulsive, and post-traumatic stress.

## ■ Generalized Anxiety Disorder

Generalized anxiety disorder, also called "excessive worry," is a continuous state of mild to intense anxiety. The anxiety is not related to a specific event, and for this reason, is often called "free-floating anxiety." This state of constant anxiety often leads to physical symptoms including dry mouth, nausea and vomiting, diarrhea, and muscle aches.

## ■ Panic Disorder

Panic disorder is a state of extreme uncontrollable fear. It is commonly called "panic attack." Onset of an attack is usually sudden, and peaks in 10 minutes or less. It may include a feeling of impending doom and a need to escape. Other symptoms include diaphoresis, chest pain, increased pulse, nausea, and dissociation (the feeling that the incident is happening to someone else).

## ■ Phobia Disorder

Phobia disorder is the most common anxiety disorder. A phobia is an intense and irrational fear of an object, situation, or thing, resulting in a strong desire to avoid the feared stimulus. The affected individual usually realizes that the phobia is irrational but is still unable to control the fear. There are over 700 known phobias (see Table 21–3 for a partial listing of these). Fear of spiders, snakes, and enclosed areas are some of the more common phobias.

## ■ Obsessive-Compulsive Disorder

Obsessive-compulsive disorder (OCD), is an anxiety disorder with two distinct parts. **Obsession** is repetition of a thought or emotion. **Compulsion** is a repetitive act the affected individual is unable to resist performing. With OCD, the individual is unable to stop the thought or the action. Behavior becomes ritualistic, and thoughts or attempts to stop the thought or action bring about extreme anxiety. This behavior becomes very time-consuming, usually taking more than an hour a day, and may become so disruptive that the individual is unable to perform daily activities or hold a job. Examples of compulsive activities include hand washing, cleaning objects, checking an object, and locking and unlocking locks.

## ■ Post-Traumatic Stress Disorder

**ETIOLOGY** Post-traumatic stress disorder (PTSD) develops as a response to a psychologically distressing event that could not be controlled and is outside the normal range of human experience. This disorder is a new addition to anxiety disorders and was observed frequently in Vietnam veterans. In addition to war, individuals who are victims of rape, child incest or abuse, or survive natural disasters or acts of violence are often affected. Police and firemen are at great risk for PTSD. The feelings and fears associated with the trauma do

| TABLE 21–3 | Phobias |
| --- | --- |
| **Name of Phobia** | **Fear of** |
| Acrophobia | high places |
| Algophobia | pain |
| Androphobia | men |
| Arachnophobia | spiders |
| Astrophobia | thunder, lightning, storms |
| Avioidphobia | flying |
| Claustrophobia | closed, tight, or narrow spaces |
| Hematophobia | blood |
| Hydrophobia | water |
| Iatrophobia | physicians |
| Kakorrhaphiophobia | failure |
| Lalophobia | public speaking |
| Monophobia | being alone |
| Ochlophobia | crowds |
| Olfactophobia | odor |
| Ophidophobia | snakes |
| Pathophobia | disease |
| Phasmophobia | ghosts |
| Phobophobia | fear |
| Ponophobia | work |
| Pyrophobia | fire |
| Sitophobia | food |
| Thanatophobia | death |
| Toxophobia | being poisoned |
| Traumaphobia | injury |
| Triskaidekaphobia | the number 13 |
| Xenophobia | strangers |
| Zoophobia | animals |

not normally diminish with the passing of time. Affected individuals often experience a reliving of this trauma for weeks, months, or years in painful recollections or dreams. These individuals often go to extremes to avoid any reminder of the trauma.

**SYMPTOMS** Symptoms may occur immediately or may not arise for months after the trauma. Symptoms include:

- flashbacks with the individual reliving the traumatic event
- difficulty developing and maintaining relationships
- irritability and agitation
- depression
- social withdrawal
- drug dependency

## Somatoform Disorders

Somatoform (somato = body) disorders are characterized by physical symptoms that lead one to believe in a physical disease, but no organic or physiologic cause can be found. Additionally, the physical symptoms appear to be associated with unconscious mental factors or conflicts. These symptoms are very real to the affected individual except in the case of factitious disorders (Munchausen and malingering). Individuals with somatoform disorders characteristically are described as frustrated, dependent, emotionally deprived, and resentful of family members and physicians.

### ■ Conversion

Conversion disorder, formerly known as hysterical neurosis, is a very striking disorder characterized by dramatic physical symptoms such as paralysis of an arm or leg, blindness, numbness, and deafness. The affected individual usually exhibits a calm, indifferent attitude about the situation. These physical symptoms enable the individual to avoid a stressful or unacceptable situation, and at the same time, gain attention from others who may not usually give them attention.

### ■ Hypochondriasis

Hypochondriasis is a condition characterized by an abnormal anxiety about one's body and health. Affected individuals are commonly called hypochondriacs. These individuals have an astounding knowledge of medical conditions and are constantly watchful of symptoms. Hypochondriacs have an unrealistic fear that they are ill, despite medical assurance to the contrary. Affected individuals have difficulty establishing and maintaining relationships because so much of their energy and conversation revolve around their perceived illnesses.

## ■ Pain Disorder

Pain disorder may occur at any age, but commonly occurs in adolescent and young females. This disorder is characterized by pain that does not have a physiologic cause; or if a cause is discovered, the pain is greater than normally expected. This pain causes interference with the individual's social, occupational, and basic activities of life. Long-standing pain often leads to depression and suicide. This condition is not fictitious as with malingering.

## ■ Malingering

Malingering is the fictitious display of symptoms in order to gain financial or personal reward. Returning to work after a work-related injury commonly leads to malingering. Symptoms are usually exaggerated and fraudulent. Diagnosis is often difficult because many of the symptoms are subjective and difficult to disprove.

## ■ Munchausen Syndrome and Munchausen by Proxy

Munchausen syndrome is a fictitious disorder. The affected individuals simulate illness for no other apparent reason than to receive treatment. Often, the individuals will go to extremes to present false tests, for example, scratching or cutting themselves in order to add blood to urine specimens. An affected person also may self-inject a variety of substances into the blood or tissues to cause an illness. Generally, this individual has an extensive knowledge of diseases, medical treatments, terminology, and hospital routine. Affected individuals often present to emergency departments with reports of a variety of symptoms. Multiple tests and procedures are undergone willingly. When testing does not support the stated symptoms, the individual often reports different symptoms. There is usually a history of repeated hospitalizations with undetermined diagnosis. When the behavior is discovered, the confronted individual often becomes hostile and seeks attention at a different facility.

Munchausen by proxy is the same disorder except the parent projects the disorder to a child. The parent may inject the child or otherwise cause illness, then presents the child for treatment. Illness tends to commonly be gastrointestinal or genitourinary in nature, and the parent denies any knowledge of the cause of the illness. Munchausen by proxy may be carried to the extreme and actually cause the death of the child.

# Personality Disorders

An individual's basic personality forms during the early years and depends, in large part, on how the individual learns to adapt to situations. This personality remains basically intact throughout life.

**ETIOLOGY** A vast number of people have maladaptive patterns of seeing, relating to, and thinking about their environment. These individuals fit on a mental health spectrum at some point between mentally healthy and mentally ill.

**SYMPTOMS** Most individuals with personality disorders have disturbances in emotional development and are maladjusted socially. Individuals with personality disorders often have incapacitating acute episodes of their mental disorder.

**TREATMENT** Treatment of personality disorders includes psychotherapy and drug therapy. Hospitalization may be needed during acute episodes. Personality disorders include paranoid, schizoid, antisocial, narcissistic, and histrionic.

- Paranoid personalities are characterized by traits of jealousy, suspicion, envy, and hypersensitivity. These individuals exhibit extreme mistrust of others, and suspect the motives and intents as deliberately harmful to them. Paranoid individuals are often angry, hostile, cold, and unemotional.

- Schizoid personalities are loners. They lack warm or tender feelings for others, and have few friends. The opinions of others have little effect on their feelings and they have difficulty expressing anger.

- Antisocial personalities usually are identified in the teen years due to troublesome behavior including fighting, stealing, running away, and cruel behavior. The antisocial individual is selfish, irritable, aggressive, and impulsive. These individuals do not express feelings of guilt and do not learn from mistakes.

- Narcissistic personalities have an exaggerated sense of self-importance and self-love. They need constant attention and admiration. If criticized, they react with rage or humiliation, and lack ability to express empathy.

- Histrionic personalities are overly dramatic with expressions of emotion. They exhibit theatrical mannerisms and overreact to events. This personality is vain and demanding, and needs to be the center of attention while constantly seeking approval and reassurance.

## Gender Identity Disorder

Gender identity disorder is a condition in which the person is uncomfortable or distressed with his or her sexual identity. Affected children may state a preference for being the opposite sex, may cross-dress, choose members of the opposite sex for best friends, play games stereotypic of the opposite sex, show disgust with their genitals, and express a desire for genitals of the opposite sex. In adults, the disorder is characterized by a stated desire to be the opposite sex, a conviction that they have feelings and attitudes of the opposite sex, and that they were born the wrong sex. Adults with gender identity try to rid themselves of secondary sex characteristics, and may seek hormonal and surgical intervention for a sex change.

## Sexual Disorders

Sexual disorders include sexual dysfunction and paraphilias or sexual deviations. Sexual dysfunction has been discussed previously in Chapter 17. Paraphilia is a sexual disorder in which the person experiences repeated and intense sexual arousal from bizarre fantasies, often involving objects or nonconsenting persons. The majority of paraphiliacs are male. Many of these disorders are criminal and considered socially unacceptable. Sexual disorders include exhibitionism, fetishism, transvestic fetishism, frotteurism, pedophilia, sexual sadism, sexual masochism, and voyeurism.

- Exhibitionism is a very common disorder and involves a male exposing his genitals to an unsuspecting female

- Fetishism involves sexual arousal with a nonliving object

- Transvestic fetishism involves arousal by cross-dressing

- Frotteurism involves sexual arousal from touching or rubbing against a nonconsenting person

- Pedophilia is a condition of being sexually aroused by a child. This disorder occurs primarily in impotent men. Pedophiles usually do not

rape the involved child, but more often, they want to fondle the child and request that the child fondle them. This activity is criminally classified as child molestation. Homosexuals are usually not child molesters. The usual case is a teen or adult male with a prepubescent female

- Sexual sadism involves sexual arousal of the sadist when the victim suffers physical or psychological pain

- Sexual masochism involves sexual arousal of the masochist when the masochist is humiliated or made to suffer by being beaten or bound

- Voyeurism is a common disorder, and involves arousal by secretly watching others undress or engage in sexual activity. Voyeurs are commonly called "Peeping Toms"

- Other paraphilia include arousal with animals (zoophilia), corpses (necrophilia), and obscene telephone calls (scatologia)

## Sleep Disorders

Sleep disorders include dyssomnias and parasomnias. Dyssomnias are disorders related to falling asleep and include insomnia, narcolepsy, and sleep apnea. Parasomnias are disorders related to staying asleep and include nightmares, sleep terror, and sleepwalking disorders.

- Insomnia is the inability to fall or stay asleep. The affected individual may awaken early and feel mentally and physically fatigued. Insomnia commonly affects females and tends to increase in incidence with age. Intake of stimulants such as coffee or tea before bedtime often causes the condition, as do other physical disorders including thyroid conditions. Anxiety and stress also may lead to insomnia. Treatment may include treating physical disorders, removing stress and anxiety, psychotherapy, and as a last resort, sleeping medications.

- Narcolepsy is a daily uncontrollable attack of sleep. Affected individuals may fall asleep any time they are sedentary such as driving, studying, reading, or eating. Narcolepsy usually occurs in the late teens or early 20s. Seizure disorder and sleep apnea must be ruled out prior to treatment. Scheduled naps and establishing a sleeping routine will usually resolve the disorder.

- Sleep apnea is a dyssomnia characterized by short periods of breathlessness during sleep. It may be due to respiratory or neurologic problems. This condition was discussed previously in Chapter 15.

- Nightmare disorder is a condition in which the involved individual is awakened by anxiety-provoking dreams. Once awakened, the individual is quickly oriented. Common subjects of nightmares include falling, death, and being attacked. Children usually outgrow this condition, but adults may need treatment with Valium.

- Sleep terror is an awakening due to nightmares, but individuals are so terrified that they do not become quickly oriented. The individual may be confused and cannot be comforted by family members. Night terrors may be reduced by not allowing the child or affected individual to watch disturbing movies or television programs.

- Sleepwalking disorder is a condition characterized by the individual getting up at night and walking without awakening. The individual can be awakened, usually with some difficulty, but does not remember the episode. The primary concern with sleepwalking is the increased potential for injury to the sleeping individual.

# TRAUMA

## Grief

Grief is a natural process of coping with a loss. This loss may involve the loss of a family member, friend, or one's own impending death. The loss may be of lesser weight and include the loss of a body part or body function, a job, or a valued possession. No matter the cause, grief is real and is a natural part of life. Grieving is a healthy process. Those unable to grieve and complete the grieving process often have difficulty coping with life. People grieve differently in different cultures, and individuals in those cultures also may grieve differently. Some individuals are very emotional whereas others remain solemn. The normal grieving process passes through several stages. These stages were developed by Dr. Elisabeth Kübler-Ross in the 1970s and remain true today (Table 21–4). Not everyone is able to move through all the steps. Grieving individuals may stop in one stage and need assistance to move on, or they may retreat back to a lower stage before moving forward again. The speed at which an individual moves through the grieving process is again very different. An important aspect of a funeral ceremony is to allow those who are grieving to say goodbye and to have closure to the situation. Individuals who were never allowed to say goodbye to a deceased or missing loved one such as families of servicemen killed overseas, or missing children or persons, may suffer with extreme depression. Inability to grieve and to complete the grieving process may lead to depression, poor coping skills, and the need for psychological counseling.

## Suicide

Suicide was discussed in Chapter 20 as a major concern for teenagers, but it is also a common problem among those individuals with mental health disorders. Depression is a main cause of suicide. Suicidal individuals have feelings of depression, guilt, hopelessness, and helplessness. As previously stated, changes in the life cycle—including aging—may lead to depres-

**TABLE 21–4** Dr. Elisabeth Kübler-Ross' Five Stages of Grief/Death and Dying

| Stage | Key ideas | Behavior |
|---|---|---|
| Denial | No, not me | Refuses to believe; must be a mistake |
| Anger | Why me? | Envy those not dying or grieving; frustrated |
| Bargaining | If I could have one more chance | Becomes religious and good in an effort to bargain for time |
| Grief/Depression | Realizes bargaining is not working | Depressed, cries, gives up |
| Acceptance | OK, I give up, but I may not like it | Expects death, may call family members near, completes unfinished business, prepares to die |

sion and suicide. It is estimated that over one-third of people over age 65 try to commit suicide. Individuals diagnosed with a terminal illness often consider suicide as a means of living the remainder of life with dignity. Widowed, older white men, minority groups, and the unemployed are also at risk.

## RARE DISEASES

Several of the disorders already discussed in this chapter are considered to be rare, but are included in the chapter to maintain the order of the outline and assist the learner in categorizing mental illnesses. There are, however, many other very rare mental health disorders affecting individuals from children through to the older adult population.

## MENTAL HEALTH DISORDERS IN THE OLDER ADULT

There are many mental health disorders that affect the older adult. Some of these may have begun early in life whereas others occur very late in life. Some dis-

orders of the neurologic system cause symptoms such as memory lapses, behavior changes, and confusion that mimics symptoms of mental health problems, but really are a physiologic or system specific disorder. Others, such as Alzheimer's disease, although a neurologic system problem, are also considered to be a mental health disorder. Many other disorders found in the older adult population are like this. Because of the changes that occur in the aging process, some symptoms seen in the older population may just be normal changes and not related to mental health disorders at all. Unfortunately, older adults are often labeled as having a mental health problem when they are merely dealing with the normal process of aging.

The most common mental health problems in the older population include depression, insomnia, isolation, stress, and disorders related to or caused by other system diseases. In addition, some individual medications or medication interactions may cause symptoms of mental health problems such as confusion, forgetfulness, dizziness, and speech problems.

## SUMMARY

Mental health disorders are some of the most misunderstood health problems. Although some are difficult to diagnose and treat, there are many more that can be either controlled or cured with proper diagnosis and intervention. Some of the symptoms of mental health problems are very slow to appear and are quite subtle, making it difficult to determine if a real problem exists. In the older adult, many neurologic disorders and the normal changes occurring in the aging process are often incorrectly attributed to a mental health disorder. Early diagnosis and treatment of any type of mental health disorder is important to assist the affected individual to live a quality life.

## REVIEW QUESTIONS

### Short Answer

1. What are some of the common signs and symptoms of mental health disorders?

**2.** What are some common tests used to diagnose mental health problems?

**3.** List some of the treatments used to control or cure mental health disorders.

## Matching

**4.** Match the mental health disorder in the left column with the appropriate category in the right column. Items in the right column may be used more than once.

_____ autism

_____ alcoholism

_____ depression

_____ panic disorder

_____ stuttering

_____ dementia

_____ ADHD

_____ PTSD

_____ obsessive-compulsive disorder

_____ drug abuse

_____ mental retardation

_____ Munchausen

_____ schizophrenia

**a.** developmental mental disorders

**b.** substance-related mental disorders

**c.** organic mental disorders

**d.** psychoses

**e.** mood disorders

**f.** anxiety disorders

**g.** somatoform disorders

## CASE STUDY

**Jim Wolf** is a 45-year-old auto parts store owner who constantly washes his hands. He also continually checks and rechecks his employee's schedules, parts lists, and equipment. His wife, Mary, who works in the business with Jim, has convinced him to seek medical intervention for his problem since his anxiety level has been interfering with his work performance and his ability to sleep. After testing and referral to a psychiatrist, he has been diagnosed with an obsessive-compulsive disorder. What can you tell Jim and Mary about this disorder? Jim asks you if you think he is crazy. How would you respond to that question? What type of treatment might he expect?

## BIBLIOGRAPHY

Abayomi, J., & Hackett, A. (2004). Assessment of malnutrition in mental health clients: Nurses' judgment vs. a nutrition risk tool. *Journal of Advanced Nursing 45*(4), 430–437.

Broadbent, M., Jarman, H., & Berk, M. (2004). Emergency department mental health triage scales improve outcomes. *Evaluation in Clinical Practice 10*(1), 57–62.

Carpenter, K. M., Brooks, A. C., Vosburg, S. K., & Nunes, E. V. (2004). The effect of sertraline and environmental context on treating depression and illicit drug substance use among methadone maintained opiate dependent patients: A controlled clinical trial. *Drug & Alcohol Dependence 74*(2), 123–134.

Chan, S., & Yu, I. W. (2004). Quality of life of clients with schizophrenia. *Journal of Advanced Nursing 45*(1), 72–83.

Children and older people with mental illness suffer. (2004). *British Journal of Nursing 13*(1), 8.

Durkin, I., Kearney, M., & O'Siorain, L. (2003). Psychiatric disorder in a palliative care unit. *Palliative Medicine* *17*(2), 212-218.

Elder, J. H., Valcante, G., Won, D., & Zylis, R. (2003). Effects of in-home training for culturally diverse fathers of children with autism. *Issues in Mental Health Nursing* *24*(3), 273-295.

Franks, V. (2004). Evidenced-based uncertainty in mental health nursing. *Journal of Psychiatric & Mental Health Nursing 11*(1), 99-105.

Goss, D., & Grady, J. (2002). Group-based parent training for preventing mental health disorders. *Issues in Mental Health Nursing 23*(4), 367-383.

Jervis, L. L. (2002). An imperfect refuge: Life in an "old-folk's home" for younger residents with psychiatric disorders. *Social Science & Medicine 54*(1), 79-92.

Kübler-Ross, E. (1997). *On Death and Dying.* Simon and Schuster Inc. New York, NY.

Psychiatric disorders rampant among detained youths. (2003). *American Journal of Nursing 103*(3), 22.

Rickelman, B. L. (2004). Anosognosia in individuals with schizophrenia: Toward recovery of insight. *Issues in Mental Health Nursing 25*(3), 227-242.

Shan, Y. (2004). Damiana. *Mental Health Practice 7*(9), 7.

Thomas, S. P. (2004). From the editor—the debate about antipsychotics. *Issues in Mental Health Nursing 25*(2), 113-114.

Whittemore, R., Melkus, G. D., & Grey, M. (2004). Self-report of depressed mood and depression in women with Type 2 diabetes. *Issues in Mental Health Nursing 25*(3), 243-260.

# Common Laboratory Values

| Test | Explanation/Normal Values |
|---|---|
| Complete blood count (CBC) | Indicates oxygen carrying capacity of blood and presence of infection. |
| White blood cells (WBCs) | 5,000–10,000 mm$^3$ |
| Red blood cells (RBCs) | 4.2–5.4/mm$^3$ |
| Hemoglobin (Hg) | |
|    males | 13.5–17.5 g/dl |
|    females | 12–16 g/dl |
| Hematocrit (Hct) | |
|    males | 40–54% |
|    females | 37–47% |
| Electrolytes | Test determines blood electrolyte levels. |
| Sodium (Na) | 136–145 mEq/L |
| Potassium (K) | 3.5–5 mEq/L |
| Chloride (Cl) | 98–106 mEq/L |
| Carbon dioxide ($CO_2$) | 22–30 mEq/L |
| Magnesium (Mg) | 1.5–2.5 mEq/L |
| Arterial blood gases (ABGs) | Indicates respiratory and metabolic functioning. |
| | pH = 7.35–7.45 |
| | $PCO_2$ = 35–45 mm Hg |
| | $HCO_3$ = 21–28 mEq/L |
| | $PO_2$ = 80–100 mm Hg |
| | $O_2$ saturation = 95–100% |
| Culture and sensitivity (C&S) | Culture determines presence of microorganism. Sensitivity determines antibiotic that will kill or inhibit growth of microorganism. Normal value is negative for microorganism growth. |

| Test | Explanation/Normal Values |
| --- | --- |
| Urinalysis | Diagnoses problems in the urinary system |
| Color | Clear to amber |
| Odor | Pleasantly aromatic |
| Albumin (protein) | Negative |
| Acetone | Negative |
| Red blood cells | 2–3/HPF |
| White blood cells | 4–5/HPF |
| Bilirubin | Negative |
| Glucose | Negative |
| Specific gravity | 1.005–1.030 |
| Bacteria | Negative |
| Casts | Rare |
| pH | 4.6–8.0 |

# Metric Conversion Tables

| LENGTH | Centimeters | Inches | Feet |
|---|---|---|---|
| 1 centimeter | 1.00 | 0.394 | 0.0328 |
| 1 inch | 2.54 | 1.00 | 0.0833 |
| 1 foot | 30.48 | 12.00 | 1.00 |
| 1 yard | 91.4 | 36.00 | 3.00 |
| 1 meter | 100.00 | 39.40 | 3.28 |

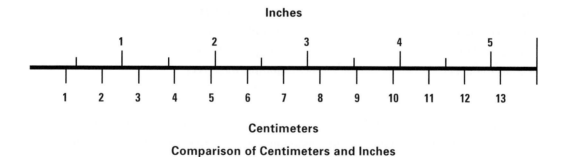

Comparison of Centimeters and Inches

| VOLUMES | Cubic Centimeters | Fluid Drams | Fluid Ounces | Quarts | Liters |
|---|---|---|---|---|---|
| 1 cubic centimeter | 1.00 | 0.270 | 0.033 | 0.0010 | 0.0010 |
| 1 fluid dram | 3.70 | 1.00 | 0.125 | 0.0039 | 0.0037 |
| 1 cubic inch | 16.39 | 4.43 | 0.554 | 0.0173 | 0.0163 |
| 1 fluid ounce | 29.6 | 8.00 | 1.00 | 0.0312 | 0.0296 |
| 1 quart | 946.00 | 255.00 | 32.00 | 1.00 | 0.946 |
| 1 liter | 1000.00 | 270.00 | 33.80 | 1.056 | 1.00 |

| WEIGHTS | Grains | Grams | Apothecary Ounces | Pounds |
|---|---|---|---|---|
| 1 grain (gr) | 1.00 | 0.064 | 0.002 | 0.0001 |
| 1 gram (gm) | 15.43 | 1.00 | 0.032 | 0.0022 |
| 1 apothecary ounce | 480.00 | 31.1 | 1.00 | 0.0685 |
| 1 pound | 7000.00 | 454.00 | 14.58 | 1.00 |
| 1 kilogram | 15432.00 | 1000.00 | 32.15 | 2.205 |

## RULES FOR CONVERTING ONE SYSTEM TO ANOTHER

**Volumes**

| | |
|---|---|
| Grains to grams | divide by 15 |
| Drams to cubic centimeters | multiply by 4 |
| Ounces to cubic centimeters | multiply by 30 |
| Minims to cubic millimeters | multiply by 63 |
| Minims to cubic centimeters | multiply by 0.06 |
| Cubic millimeters to minims | divide by 63 |
| Cubic centimeters to minims | multiply by 16 |
| Cubic centimeters to fluid ounces | divide by 30 |
| Liters to pints | divide by 2.1 |

**Weights**

| | |
|---|---|
| Milligrams to grains | multiply by 0.0154 |
| Grams to grains | multiply by 15 |
| Grams to drams | multiply by 0.257 |
| Grams to ounces | multiply by 0.0311 |

**Temperature**

Multiply centigrade (Celsius) degrees by $\frac{9}{5}$ and add 32 to convert Fahrenheit to Celsius

Subtract 32 from the Fahrenheit degrees and multiply by $\frac{5}{9}$ to convert Celsius to Fahrenheit

## COMMON HOUSEHOLD MEASURES AND WEIGHTS

| | | | |
|---|---|---|---|
| 1 teaspoon | = 4–5 cc or 1 dram | 1 cup | = 8 fluid ounces or ½ pint |
| 3 teaspoons | = 1 tablespoon | 1 tumbler or glass | = 8 fluid ounces or 240 cc |
| 1 dessert spoon | = 8 cc or 2 drams | 1 wine glass | = 2 fluid ounces or 60 cc |
| 1 tablespoon | = 15 cc or 3 drams | 16 fluid ounces | = 1 pound |
| 4 tablespoons | = 1 wine glass or ½ gill | 4 gills | = 1 pound |
| 16 tablespoons (liquid) | = 1 cup | 1 pint | = 1 pound |
| 12 tablespoons (dry) | = 1 cup | | |

# Glossary

**abdominocentesis** (ab-DOM-ih-no-sen-**TEE**-sis)  paracentesis of the abdomen; a procedure in which a puncture is made into the abdominal cavity to withdraw fluid.

**abscess**  a localized collection of pus.

**abrasion**  a scraping away of skin surface.

**achlorhydria** (a-klor-**HIGH**-dree-ah)  absence of hydrochloric acid.

**acromegaly** (ACK-roh-**MEG**-ah-lee; acro=extremity, megaly= enlargement)  a condition of extremity enlargement as a result of excessive growth hormone in the adult.

**acute** (a-**CUTE**)  a disease that is short term.

**addiction**  a physical and/or psychological dependence on a substance.

**Addison's disease**  hypoadrenalism; an uncommon undersecretion of hormones by the adrenal cortex.

**adenoidectomy** (AD-eh-noy-**DECK**-toh-me; ectomy=removal)  surgical removal of the adenoids.

**adenoma** (AD-eh-**NO**-ma; adeno=gland, oma=tumor)  a tumor of glandular tissue.

**adhesions** (ad-HE-zhun)  parts of tissue that cling to the surface of adjoining organs as normal fibrous scar tissue develops in an operative site, resulting in a fibrous band.

**affect**  outward expression of emotions.

**AIDS**  acquired immunodeficiency syndrome.

**albumin** (al-BYOU-men)  a blood protein distributed throughout the body; responsible for osmotic pressure of the blood.

**albuminuria** (al-BYOU-mih-**NEW**-ree-ah; albumin=a blood protein, uria=urine)  albumin in the urine; usually albumin but may also be globulin; usually indicative of a disease process.

**aldosterone** (al-doh-STER-ohn)  a mineralocorticoid; acts on the kidney to assist in maintaining electrolyte balance.

**alleles**  matched pairs of genes; the term used to refer to the product when the chromosomes (one from each parent) pair up during fertilization of the egg, the genes on the chromosomes align.

**allergen**  the environmental substance that causes a reaction.

**allergy**  the state when the immune response is too intense or hypersensitive to an environmental substance.

**alopecia** (AL-oh-**PEE**-shee-ah; in Greek, meaning fox mange, which caused hair loss)  a partial or complete hair loss, usually from the head.

**amblyopia** (AM-blee-**OH**-pee-ah)  a decrease in the vision of the affected eye due to a lack of visual stimuli.

**amenorrhea** (ah-MEN-oh-**REE**-ah; a=without, menorrhea= menses)  the absence or cessation of menses.

**amnesia** (am-NEE-zee-ah)  loss of memory.

**amylase**  an enzyme; often elevated in pancreatic disorders.

**anaerobic** (an=without, aerobic=air)  living without oxygen.

**analgesic** (AN-al-**GEE**-sick)  a medication that relieves pain.

**anaphylaxis** (AN-ah-fih-**LACK**-sis)  an immediate allergic reaction characterized by contraction of smooth muscle and dilation of capillaries, leading to severe respiratory distress or failure.

**anaplastic** (AN-ah-**PLAST**-ic)  abnormal tissue, the more undifferentiated tissue.

**androgens**  hormones secreted by the adrenal cortex and responsible for male characteristics.

**anemia** (ah-NEE-me-ah; an=without, emia=blood)  a condition of low numbers of red blood cells in the blood.

**angiogenesis** (AN-jee-oh-**JEN**-eh-sis; angio=vessel, genesis=formation)  new growth of blood vessels.

**angiography** (AN-jee-**OG**-rah-fee; angio=vessel, graphy=procedure to record)  a radiographic study of blood vessels after injection of fluorescein dye.

**angioplasty** (AN-jee-oh-**PLAS**-tee; angio=vessel, plasty=surgical repair)  a procedure that involves passing a catheter into the artery and inflating a balloon on the catheter to push the plaque against the vessel wall, thus widening the lumen of the vessel.

**anomaly** (ah-NOM-ah-lee)  any abnormality.

**anorexia nervosa** (AN-oh-**RECK**-see-ah; an=without, orexia= appetite)  a disorder of self-imposed starvation, resulting from a distorted body image.

**anoxia** (ah-NOCK-see-ah)  no oxygen.

**antibody(ies)**  immunoglobulins that develop in response to an antigen; also called immune bodies; proteins that the body produces to react to and render the antigen harmless.

**antigen(s)** (AN-tih-jens)   a cell marker that induces a state of sensitivity after coming in contact with an antibody; any substance that causes the body some type of harm, thus setting off this specific reaction.

**antipyretics** (anti=against, pyretic=fever)   a class of medications given to reduce an elevated temperature.

**anuria** (ah-NEW-ree-ah; an=without, uria=urine)   no urine output.

**apnea** (ap-NEE-ah; a=without, pnea=breathing)   the condition of not breathing; a term used to describe the absence of respirations for a period of time.

**arterial blood gases (ABGs)**   the laboratory test that measures the amounts of oxygen and carbon dioxide in blood.

**articular fracture**   one that involves a joint surface.

**articular**   relating to a joint surface.

**ascites** (ah-SIGH-teez)   fluid in the abdomen (peritoneal cavity).

**asymptomatic** (a=without, symptomatic=symptoms)   not displaying symptoms.

**atresia**   the congenital absence or closure of a normal opening or lumen in the body; it may occur in a variety of areas.

**atrophy** (AT-tro-fee)   a decrease in cell size, which leads to a decrease in the size of the tissue and organ.

**audiometry** (AW-dee-OM-eh-tree; audio=sound, metry= measure)   the basic test used to measure hearing.

**aura**   symptoms occurring at the onset of a partial epileptic seizure or migraine headache; it may include tingling of the fingers, ringing in the ears, and visual disturbances.

**auscultation** (AWS-kul-TAY-shun)   using a stethoscope to listen to body cavities and organs.

**autodigestion**   autolysis or digestion of self or one's own cells.

**autoimmunity** or **autoimmune**   the state when the immune response attacks itself.

**autosomes** (auto=self, somes=body)   a chromosome other than a sex chromosome; they determine body function.

**avulsion**   skin pulled or torn away.

**avulsion fracture**   one where there is a separation of a small bone fragment from the bone where a tendon or ligament is attached.

**bacteria**   a one-celled microorganism that may be aerobic or anaerobic and free-living, saprophytic, parasitic, or pathogenic.

**Bence Jones protein**   a special protein found in the blood and urine, indicative of multiple myeloma.

**benign** (beh-NINE)   having limited growth, noncancerous.

**bimanual examination** (bi=two, manual=handed)   an examination in which the physician places one hand on the abdomen and inserts fingers of the other hand into the vagina to feel the female organs between the two hands.

**biopsy** (BYE-op-see)   removing a small piece of tissue for microscopic examination.

**bleeding time**   a test to determine the length of bleeding time or time it takes the blood to clot.

**blood urea nitrogen (BUN)**   a test to determine the level of urea nitrogen or waste in the blood.

**blunt trauma**   a wound or injury (trauma) caused by an object with a flat, dull, or not sharp area (blunt).

**bronchiectasis** (BRONG-key-ECK-ta-sis)   a chronic or long term dilatation of a bronchus or bronchi along with an infection.

**bronchoscopy** (brong-KOS-koh-pee; broncho=bronchus or lung passageways, oscopy=procedure to look into)   a diagnostic or surgical procedure in which a scope is passed through the mouth into the bronchus.

**bronchospasm** (BRONG-ko-SPA-zm)   muscular constriction of the bronchi of the respiratory tract.

**buccal smear**   a test for evaluating chromosomes; this test is performed by obtaining squamous epithelial cells from the buccal cavity, staining the cell, and microscopically observing for X chromosomes called Barr bodies.

**bulimia** (byou-LIM-ee-ah)   an eating disorder, characterized by episodes of binge eating (an intake of approximately 5,000 calories in one to two hours) followed by activities to negate the calorie intake or purging.

**cachexia** (ca-KACK-see-ah)   a term used to describe any individual who has an ill, thin, wasted appearance.

**calcaneal**   the heel area of the foot.

**cancer**   a malignant tumor.

**caput medusae**   tortuous, unsightly varicosities spreading from the umbilicus outward across the front of the abdomen.

**carcinogen** (kar-SIN-oh-jen)   cancer-causing agent or substance.

**carcinogenesis** (KAR-sin-oh-JEN-eh-sis)   cancer development.

**carcinoma** (KAR-sih-NO-mah)   the most common type of malignant neoplasm arising from epithelial tissue.

**carcinoma in situ**   atypical cells residing in the epithelial layer of tissue, not having broken through the basement membrane and invading other local tissues.

**cardiac catheterization** (KATH-eh-ter-eye-ZAY-shun)   an invasive procedure used to sample the blood in the chambers of the heart to determine the amount of oxygen content and blood pressure in the chambers.

**cardiac palpitations**   an unusually strong, rapid, or irregular heart rate that is so abnormal the individual can "feel" it.

**carotid endarterectomy** (END-ar-ter-ECK-toh-me; endo= inside, arter=artery, ectomy=excision of)   surgical intervention to remove plaque in the carotid arteries to improve blood flow and reduce the risk of a thrombus.

**catarrhal** (ka-TAR-all)   inflammation of mucous membranes of the head and mouth with increased mucus flow.

**catheterization** (KATH-er-ter-eye-ZAY-shun)   a sterile procedure consisting of passing a soft catheter through the urethra and into the bladder for the purpose of (1) instilling or pouring fluids or medication into the bladder or (2) removing urine.

**cauterization** (KAW-ter-eye-ZAY-shun)   the electrical burning of tissue to stop bleeding; used most frequently during surgery to stop bleeding from vessels.

**cellulitis** (SELL-you-LYE-tis)   inflammation of connective tissue.

**cephalalgia** (SEF-ah-LAL-jee-ah; cephal=head, algia=pain)   headache.

**cerumen** (se-ROO-men)   ear wax.

**cervicitis** (SER-vih-SIGH-tis)   inflammation of the cervix.

**chancre** (SHANG-ker)   a painless, highly contagious lesion occurring in the primary stage of syphilis.

**chemotaxis**   the movement of cells or organisms in response to chemicals.

**chemotherapy**   utilizing pharmacologic therapy in the treatment of cancer.

**cholecystectomy** (KOH-lee-sis-**TECK**-toh-me; chole=gall or bile, cyst=bladder, ectomy=removal)   surgical removal of the gallbladder.

**chorea** (ko-REE-ah)   a constant, jerky uncontrollable movement.

**chronic**   a disease that persists for a long time.

**circadian rhythm**   a normal 24-hour cycle of biological rhythms including sleep, metabolism, and glandular secretions.

**clean catch**   a term used to describe a clean urine collection method involving cleansing the urethal area prior to urinating and catching the voided urine specimen.

**closed or simple fracture**   a fracture that does not break through the skin.

**clubbing**   a condition affecting the distal portion of the finger; characterized by soft tissue enlargement and an abnormal curvature of the nail.

**Colle's fracture**   a fracture of the lower end of the radius with displacement of the fragment.

**colorectal**   pertaining to both the colon and rectum.

**comedones** (KOM-eh-dohns)   plugged skin pores; the open form is a blackhead; the closed form is a whitehead.

**comminuted fracture**   one in which there are more than two ends or fragments.

**complete blood count (CBC)**   a laboratory test that identifies the number of red blood cells (RBCs), white blood cells (WBCs), and platelets per cubic millimeter.

**complete fracture**   the fracture is completely through the bone.

**complication**   the onset of a second disease or disorder in an individual that is already affected with a disease.

**compound (open) fracture**   a fracture involving the bone puncturing through the skin, or an object puncturing the skin, making an opening through the skin to the fracture site.

**compression fracture**   one in which the bone appears to be mashed down.

**compulsion**   a repetitive act the affected individual is unable to resist performing.

**Computerized Axial Tomography (CAT or CT)**   imaging by a cross-sectional plane of the body; also called computed tomography.

**congenital** (kon-JEN-ih-tahl)   present at birth; usually concerning a congenital anomaly or an abnormality present at birth.

**congenital anomaly** (kon-JEN-ih-tahl ah-NOM-ah-lee; congenital=present at birth, anomaly=abnormality)   a birth defect.

**contusion** (kon-TOO-zhun)   a large bruise.

**convulsion**   an abnormal muscle contraction; a violent spasm or jerking of the face, trunk, or extremities.

**corticosteroids** (KORT-ti-ko-**STEHR**-oyds)   powerful anti-inflammatory hormones.

**cortisol**   hydrocortisone; a steroid hormone secreted by the adrenal cortex.

**cortisone**   a glucocorticoid; it affects carbohydrate metabolism, and influences the nutrition and growth of connective tissues.

**creatinine** (kree-**AT**-in-in)   one of the two most common nitrogenous waste products that are normally filtered from the blood, the final product of creatine catabolism.

**creatinine clearance test**   a diagnostic test for kidney function that measures the rate the kidneys excrete creatinine, a waste product from muscle contraction that is carried in small amounts in the blood, filtered by the kidney and excreted in urine. An increased blood or urine level indicates a disturbance in kidney function.

**cretinism**   congenital hypothyroidism.

**cryptorchidism** (krip-TOR-kih-dizm; crypt=hidden, orchid=testicle, ism=condition)   undescended testicle(s).

**culture and sensitivity**   a test to identify a pathogen and the type of treatment needed.

**curative**   something that corrects or cures the disease or condition.

**cyanosis** (SIGH-ah-**NO**-sis; cyano=blue, osis=condition)   a bluish condition of the skin due to lack of oxygen in the blood.

**cystogram** (cysto=bladder, gram=picture)   an X-ray picture of the bladder that helps determine the shape and function of the bladder.

**cystoscopy** (sis-TOS-koh-pee; cysto=bladder, scopy=procedure to look)   an invasive procedure to look into the urethra and bladder using a lighted scope.

**cytology** (SIGH-**TOL**-oh-jee; cyto=cell, logy= study)   the examination or study of cells.

**cytologic** (SIGH-toe-**LAW**-gic)   pertaining to cytology.

**cytotoxic** (cyto=cell, toxic=killing)   something that kills cells.

**débridement** (day-breed-MON)   a process of washing or cutting away necrotic tissue and foreign material.

**decompression**   a release of pressure.

**defecate**   to have a bowel movement.

**degenerative**   diseases related to aging, or destruction of tissue, functions, and use.

**dehiscence** (dee-HISS-ens)   separation of tissue margins.

**delirium tremens, (DTs)** (dee-LIR-ee-urn TREE-mens)   a serious form of delirium due to alcoholic withdrawal after a period of sustained intoxication.

**delusions**   false beliefs that are firmly adhered to although they are not shared by others.

**dementia** (dee-MEN-she-ah)   a loss of mental ability due to the loss of neurons or brain cells.

**densitometry**   measurement of bone thickness.

**dental plaque**   tough, sticky material that adheres to the tooth enamel; caused by bacteria.

**dependency**   a psychological craving for a substance that may or may not be accompanied by a physical need.

**diabetic retinopathy** (DYE-ah-**BET**-ick RET-ih-**NOP**-ah-thee, retino=retina, opathy=disease)   disease of the retina of the eye, often resulting in blindness; caused by degeneration due to diabetes mellitus.

**diagnosis** (DIE-ag-**KNOW**-sis)   the identification or naming of a disease.

**diapedesis** (DYE-ah-pe-**DEE**-sis)   passage of blood, or its formed elements, through the intact walls of blood vessels.

**diastolic** (dye-as-TOL-ick)   relating to cardiac diastole; the process of the heart resting as the chambers refill with blood.

**differential**   a detailed white blood cell count identifying the number of each type of leukocyte.

**differentiation**   the process of individual specialization of cells.

**digital rectal examination**   a manual examination in which the physician feels the prostate for abnormal enlargement (hypertrophy or hyperplasia) and tumors.

**dilitation and curettage** (**KYOU**-reh-TAHZH)   or D&C a procedure that involves a dilation of the cervix (dilatation) and scraping (curettage) of the uterine endometrial tissue; a D&C is commonly performed for abnormal uterine bleeding and following a spontaneous abortion.

**diplopia** (dih-PLOH-pee-ah)   double vision.

**diskectomy**   surgery to remove a vertebral disk.

**disease**   a change in structure or function within the body that is considered to be abnormal; any change from normal.

**disorder**   a derangement or abnormality of function.

**displaced fracture**   one in which fragments are out of position.

**dominant**   in control.

**Doppler**   a device that may be placed over arteries to magnify the sound of blood flow.

**dormant**   state of being inactive.

**Dowager's hump**   abnormal curvature in the upper thoracic spine.

**dwarfism**   a decrease in growth hormone (GH) that leads to impaired growth of all body tissues.

**dysentery**   an acute inflammation of the colon or colitis.

**dysmenorrhea** (DIS-men-oh-**REE**-ah; dys=painful, menorrhea=menses)   pain with menstrual periods.

**dyspareunia** (DIS-pa-**ROO**-nee-ah)   painful sexual intercourse.

**dysphagia** (dis-FAY-jee-ah; dys=difficulty, phagia=swallowing)   difficulty swallowing.

**dysphasia** (dis-FAY-zee-ah; dys=difficulty, phasia=speaking)   difficulty speaking.

**dysplasia** (dis-PLAY-zee-ah)   an alteration in size, shape, and organization of cells.

**dyspnea** (disp-NEE-ah; dys=difficult, pnea=breathing)   difficulty breathing.

**dysuria** (dis-YOU-ree-ah; dys=difficult or painful, uria=urine)   difficulty or pain with urination.

**ecchymoses** (ECH-ih-**MOH**-ses)   large areas of bruising or hemorrhage.

**eclampsia** (eh-KLAMP-see-ah)   a condition of pregnancy characterized by all the symptoms of toxemia or preeclampsia, plus the symptoms of convulsions.

**ectopic** (eck-TOP-ick)   out of normal place.

**electrocardiogram** (ECG or EKG; ee-LECK-troh-**KAR**-dee-oh-**GRAM**; electro=electrical, cardio=heart, gram=picture)   the graphic drawing produced by an electrocardiograph, a machine that receives electrical information and draws heart action.

**electromyography** (EMG; ee-LECK-troh-my-o-grah-fee)   a diagnostic test in which a small needle is inserted into muscle tissue and the electrical activity is recorded.

**embolus** (EM-boh-lus)   material floating in the blood that may stick in a vessel, and occlude or stop blood flow, leading to ischemia or death of the organs supplied by that vessel.

**empyema** (EM-pye-**EE**-mah)   an accumulation of pus in a body cavity.

**encapsulated**   enclosed in a capsule.

**encephalopathy** (en-SEF-ah-**LOP**-ah-thee; encephalo=brain, opathy=disease)   any disease or disorder of the brain.

**endarterectomy** (END-ar-ter-**ECK**-toh-me; endo=inside, arter=artery, ectomy=excision)   a surgical procedure involving opening an artery and cleaning out the plaque.

**endometritis** (EN-doh-me-**TRY**-tis)   inflammation of the uterus lining.

**enteral**   relating to the small intestine.

**enterotoxin**   intestinal poison.

**enucleation**   removal of the eyeball.

**epicanthus**   a vertical fold of skin across the medial canthus of the eye, giving the eyes an Oriental appearance.

**epidural (hematoma)** (EP-ih-**DOO**-ral; epi=above, dural= dura, outer meninges)   blood collecting between the skull and the dura mater.

**epistaxis** (EP-i-**STACK**-sis)   hemorrhage or bleeding from the nose; nosebleed.

**erythema** (ER-ih-**THEE**-mah)   skin redness.

**erythrocytopenia** (erythrocyte=red cell, penia=decrease)   a deficiency of red blood cells.

**erythrocytosis** (erythrocyte=red cell, osis=condition)   a condition of increased red blood cells.

**esophageal varices** (eh-**SOF**-ah-JEE-al **VAYR**-ih-seez)   varicosities (varicose veins) of the esophagus.

**estrogen**   a term used to describe the hormones responsible for female characteristics.

**etiology** (ET-tee-**OL**-oh-jee)   the study of cause or the cause of a disease.

**euphoric**   a sense of well-being.

**exacerbation** (x-AS-er-**BAY**-shun)   a time when symptoms flare up or become worse.

**exocrine (glands)**   glands that excrete through a duct.

**exophthalmos** (ECK-sof-**THAL**-mos)   abnormal protrusion of the eyeballs.

**exsanguination**   loss of circulating blood volume.

**extracapsular fracture**   a fracture outside or not involving the joint capsule.

**exudate** (ECKS-you-dayt)   fluid that has seeped out of tissue or capillaries because of injury or inflammation.

**familial**   runs in or common to a family; for example, a disease that tends to occur in several members of the same family.

**fascia** (FASH-ee-ah)   a thick fibrous connective tissue.

**fatal**   inevitable or causing death.

**feces** evacuated bowel contents; commonly called bowel movement or BM.

**femoral neck fracture** a fracture involving the neck of the femur.

**fibrillation** (FIH-brih-**LAY**-shun) a heart rhythm that is wild and uncoordinated; a cardiac arrhythmia.

**fissure** a crack, split, or ulcer-like sore; a groove or slit.

**fistula** (FIS-tyou-lah) a tract that connects two organs or cavities to each other or to the surface of the skin.

**flatulence** excessive gas in the stomach or intestine.

**frequency** how often the individual urinates.

**frostbite** the freezing of tissue, usually on the face, fingers, toes, and ears.

**frozen section** a technique that enables a pathologist to make a rapid determination of a tumor condition, either malignant or benign.

**fulminant** (FULL-ma-nant) occurring suddenly, rapidly, and intensely.

**fungi** forms of yeast and molds; microscopic plant-like organisms.

**gangrene** (GANG-green) a condition occurring when saprophytic (dead tissue-loving) bacteria become involved in necrotic tissue.

**gene** the unit on the chromosome that carries DNA information.

**genotypes** the genetic pattern of the individual.

**germ cells** sex cells.

**giantism** a condition of overgrowth due to hyperpituitarism occurring before puberty and during the growing years.

**gingivitis** inflammation of the gums.

**glucagon** a hormone secreted by the alpha cells in the islets of Langerhans in the pancreas; responsible for elevating blood glucose concentration.

**glucocorticoids** a group of steroids of the adrenal cortex that affects metabolism such as causing glycogen storage and causing an anti-inflammatory effect.

**glycogen** (GLYE-ko-jen) the form that extra sugar is stored in, primarily in the liver.

**glycosuria** (GLYE-koh-**SOO**-ree-ah; glyco=glycogen or sugar, uria=urine) the "spilling" of sugar in the urine; a common symptom of diabetes mellitus.

**goiter** (GOI-ter) noticeable protrusion of the thyroid gland.

**goitrogenic** goiter producing, as in foods or drugs such as turnips, cabbage, and lithium.

**gonad** a sex organ; a testis or an ovary.

**grading** determining the degree of differentiation of cells through microscopic examination.

**grand mal** a term applied to seizures that are the type most often thought of as epilepsy; these seizures are characterized by convulsions, loss of consciousness, urinary and fecal incontinence, and tongue biting.

**greenstick fracture** A common incomplete fracture that occurs in children; it appears to have broken partially like a sap-filled green stick.

**gumma** (GUM-mah) a characteristic soft, gummy lesion caused by bacteria that invade organs throughout the body; found in the tertiary stage of syphilis.

**gynecomastia** (GUY-ne-koh-**MAS**-tee-ah) abnormal breast enlargement.

**hallucinations** (hah-LOO-sih-**NAY**-shun) false sensations of sight, touch, sound, or feel.

**hallucinogenic** (hah-LOO-sih-no-**JEN**-ick) producing psychedelic or bizarre alterations in mental functioning.

**heat exhaustion** a reaction to heat, marked by prostration, weakness, and collapse; caused by severe dehydration.

**heat stroke** a serious and possibly fatal illness caused by exposure to excessively high temperatures.

**helminths** intestinal parasites; also called worms; nematodes, cestodes, and trematodes.

**hemarthrosis** (hem=blood, arthro=joint, osis=condition) bleeding into joints.

**hematemesis** (HEM-ah-**TEM**-eh-sis; hema=blood, emesis= vomiting) vomiting blood.

**hematochezia** (HEM-at-toe-**KEE**-zee-ah) bright red blood in the feces.

**hematocrit** (he-MAT-oh-krit) a measurement of the amount of red cell mass as a proportion of whole blood.

**hematoma** (HEM-ah-**TOH**-mah) a large tumor or swelling filled with blood; also called a bruise or contusion.

**hematuria** (HEM-ah-**TOO**-ree-ah; hema=blood, uria=urine) blood in the urine.

**hemiparesis** (HEM-ee-**PAR**-ee-sis; hemi=one half, paresis=paralysis) weakness or paralysis affecting one side of the body.

**hemoglobin (Hgb)** a measurement of the amount of hemoglobin or oxygen carrying potential available in the blood.

**hemolytic** (HE-moh-**LIT**-ick) destruction of red blood cells.

**hemolyzed** broken down cells.

**hemoptysis** (he-MOP-tih-sis; hemo=blood, ptysis=saliva) coughing up blood.

**hemothorax** (hemo=blood, thorax=chest) blood in the chest cavity.

**hepatomegaly** (HEP-ah-toh-**MEG**-ah-lee) enlarged liver.

**heterozygous** (hetero=different, zygo=yoked or paired) having different paired genes.

**hirsutism** (HER-soot-izm) abnormal hair on the face and body of the female.

**histamine** a substance that causes local arterioles, venules, and capillaries to dilate, resulting in an increase in blood flow to the area; it is released in response to injury or irritation.

**holistic medicine** the concept considering the whole person rather than just the physical being.

**homeostasis** (HOME-ee-oh-**STAY**-sis) the state of sameness or normalcy that the body strives to maintain.

**homozygous** (homo=one, zygo=yoked or paired) having identical genes.

**hydrocortisone** a steroid hormone secreted by the adrenal cortex.

**hydrophobia** (hydro=water, phobia=fear) fear of the water.

**hyperemia** (HIGH-per-**EE**-me-ah; hyper=increased, emia= blood) an increased blood flow in response to a release of histamine.

**hyperglycemia** (HIGH-per-glye-**SEE**-me-ah; hyper=excessive, glyc=glycogen or glucose, emia=blood) high blood sugar level.

**hyperplasia** (HIGH-per-**PLAY**-zee-ah)  an increase in cell number; overgrowth in response to some type of stimulus.

**hypersensitivity**  a condition in which there is an excessive response by the body to the stimulus of a foreign body.

**hypertrophy** (HIGH-**PER**-tro-fee)  an increase in the size of the cell, leading to an increase in tissue and organ size.

**hypoglycemia** (HIGH-poh-gly-**SEE**-me-ah; hypo=decreased, glyc=glucose, emia=blood)  a low blood sugar level.

**hypothermia** (hypo=low, thermia=heat or temperature)  a significantly low body temperature.

**hypovolemia** (HIGH-poh-voh-**LEE**-me-ah)  low or decreased blood volume.

**hypoxemia** (high-**POX**-SEE-me-ah; hypo=not enough, ox= oxygen, emia=blood)  not enough oxygen in the circulating blood.

**hypoxia** (HIGH-**POX**-see-ah)  not enough oxygen in tissues.

**hysterosalpingogram** (hystero=uterus, salpingo=fallopian tubes, gram=picture)  an X-ray picture of the uterus and fallopian tubes.

**iatrogenic** (eye-AT-roh-**JEN**-ick; iatro=medicine, physician, genic=rising from)  a problem arising due to or related to a prescribed treatment.

**idiopathic** (ID-ee-oh-**PATH**-ick)  an unknown cause of disease.

**ileus** (ILL-ee-us)  absence of peristalsis.

**immunodeficiency**  the state when the immune response is unable to defend the body due to a decrease or absence of leukocytes, primarily lymphocytes.

**impacted fracture**  one that has a bone end forced over the other end.

**impotent** (IM-poh-tent)  inability in the male to achieve or maintain a penile erection.

**in and out catheterization**  a catheterization procedure where the catheter is removed as soon as the urine is drained; the catheterization is temporary.

**incision**  a laceration or cut with smooth, even edges.

**incomplete fracture**  the bone is fractured but not in two.

**incubation period**  the time between exposure to the disease and the presence of symptoms, which may last several days.

**induration** (IN-dur-**RAY**-shun)  hardened tissue.

**indwelling catheter**  a catheter that is placed for a longer period of time than an in and out catheter as commonly occurs for urinary incontinence; a balloon on the end of the catheter is inflated to hold the catheter in the bladder.

**infarct** (in-FARKT)  necrosis of cells or tissues due to ischemia.

**infection** (in-FECT-shun)  invasion of microorganisms into the tissue, causing cell or tissue injury, thus leading to the inflammatory response.

**inflammation** (IN-flah-**MAY**-shun)  a basic pathologic process of cytologic and chemical reactions that occur in the blood vessels and tissues in response to an injury or irritation; a protective immune response that is triggered by any type of injury or irritant.

**inspiratory stridor** (STRYE-dor)  high-pitched sound during inspiration due to blocked airways.

**insulin**  a hormone secreted by the beta cells in the islets of Langerhans in the pancreas; responsible for glucose utilization.

**intermittent claudication** (KLAW-dih-**KAY**-shun)  the condition of developing muscle cramps that are relieved with rest and increased with activity.

**interphalangeal** (inter=between, phalangeal=finger bones)  usually referring to joints between the finger bones.

**intertrochanteric fracture**  one that is in the trochanteric area of the femur.

**intoxicated**  when the blood alcohol level reaches 0.10 percent or more.

**intracapsular fractures**  a fracture inside the joint capsule.

**intractable**  difficult to stop or control.

**intrathecal** (IN-trah-**THEE**-kal; intra=within, thecal=spinal cord)  injected into the spinal fluid.

**intravenous pyelogram (IVP)** (IN-trah-**VEE**-nus **PYE**-eh-loh-GRAM)  an X-ray picture taken after injecting dye into the individual's bloodstream; the dye accumulates in the urinary tract and improves the ability to identify obstructions, tumors, and deformities.

**intrinsic factor**  a substance secreted by the stomach lining necessary for absorption of vitamin $B_{12}$.

**intussusception** (IN-tus-sus-**SEP**-shun)  the telescoping of one part of the intestine over the adjoining section.

**invasion**  spreading into surrounding or local tissue.

**ischemia** (iss-KEE-me-ah)  hypoxia of cells or tissues caused by decreased blood flow.

**islets of Langerhans**  specialized cells in the pancreas that act as an endocrine gland secreting hormones, primarily insulin.

**isoimmune**  a high level of a specific antibody as a result of antigen stimulation from the red blood cells of another individual; isoimmunization may occur when an Rh negative person is treated with a transfusion of Rh positive blood.

**jaundice** (JAWN-dis)  a yellowish color in the skin and sclera due to increased bile pigments in the blood.

**Kaposi's sarcoma** (KAP-oh-seez sar-KOH-ma)  blood vessel cancer that causes reddish-purple skin lesions.

**karyotyping**  a method of identifying chromosomes; this process involves taking a picture of a cell during mitosis, arranging the chromosome pairs in order from largest to smallest, and numbering them one to twenty-three.

**keloid** (KEE-loid)  excessive collagen formation, often resulting in a hard, raised scar.

**keratin**  a tough protein substance in nails, hair, and body tissues.

**ketoacidosis**  acidosis seen in diabetes mellitus caused by overproduction of ketone bodies.

**ketones**  waste products produced when tissue cells burn fats and proteins.

**kidneys-ureter-bladder (KUB)**  a common X-ray of the structures of the urinary tract to determine abnormalities.

**Koplik's spots**  spots seen in the mouth in the early stage of measles; these spots are rather unique to measles and are often the definitive symptom that confirms the diagnosis.

**laceration**  a cut in the skin.

**laminectomy**  surgery to cut away part of the vertebra to open the area around the spinal nerve.

**laparoscopy** (LAP-ah-**ROS**-ko-pee; laparo=abdomen, scopy= scope procedure)   looking inside the abdominal cavity with a lighted scope; commonly used to view the female organs for abnormalities, diagnose endometriosis, and to perform a tubal ligation.

**lesion** (LEE-zhun)   any discontinuity of tissue.

**lethal**   something that kills.

**leukemia** (loo-KEE-me-ah; leuk=white, emia=blood)   a progressive overgrowth of abnormal leukocytes; a malignant disease of the bone marrow.

**leukocytopenia** (leukocyte=white cell, penia=decrease)   a decrease in white cell count.

**leukocytosis** (leuko=white, cyto=cell, osis=condition)   an increase in white cell count.

**leukorrhea** (LOO-koh-**REE**-ah; leuk=white, orrhea=flow or discharge)   a white, usually foul smelling, vaginal discharge.

**lipids**   fats or fat-like substances.

**lithotripsy** (litho=stone, tripsy=breaking)   a procedure for breaking kidney or gallbladder stones.

**longitudinal fracture**   one that runs the length of the bone.

**lumen** (LOO-men)   the inner open space or width of a tubular structure or anatomical part.

**lymph**   a clear liquid similar to plasma containing many white cells.

**lymphadenopathy** (lim-FAD-eh-**NOP**-ah-thee; lymph=lymph, adeno=gland, opathy=disease)   any disease of the lymph glands.

**lymphangiography** (lim-FAN-jee-**OG**-rah-fee; lymph=lymph, angio=vessel, ography=procedure)   a radiographic procedure consisting of injecting a contrast dye and taking X-rays of lymphatic vessels.

**lymphangiopathy** (lim-FAN-jee-**OP**-ah-thee; lymph=lymph, angio=vessel, opathy=disease)   a general term to describe any disease of the lymph vessels.

**lymphedema** (lymph=lymph, edema=swelling)   an abnormal collection of lymph fluid, usually observed in the extremities.

**lymphocytes**   white blood cells formed in lymphatic tissue.

**lymphocytopenia** or **lymphopenia**   a decrease in lymphocytes.

**lymphocytosis**   increase in number of lymphocytes.

**lymphoma** (lim-FOH-ma)   malignant neoplasms of blood-forming organs.

**macrophage** (macro=large, phage=eat)   a monocyte that leaves the bloodstream and moves into the tissue and becomes phagocytic.

**Magnetic Resonance Imaging (MRI)**   a diagnostic radiological test using nuclear magnetic resonance technology.

**malaise**   general ill feeling.

**malignant** (mah-LIG-nant)   deadly or progressing to death; cancerous.

**mammography** (mam-OG-rah-fee; mammo=breast, ography= procedure to take a picture)   a procedure of taking an X-ray picture of breast tissue.

**mammoplasty** (**MAM**-oh-PLAS-tee; mammo=breast, plasty= surgical repair or restructuring)   a surgical procedure that involves reconstruction of the breast with plastic surgery and prosthetic breast implants.

**mania**   extreme elation or agitation.

**mast cells**   also called tissue histocytes; found in all tissues of the body; play a major role in the inflammatory process.

**mastectomy** (mas-TECK-toh-me; mast=breast, ectomy=excision)   surgical removal of the breast.

**mastoidectomy** (MAS-toy-**DECK**-toh-me; ectomy=removal or excision)   a procedure used to prevent complications and preserve hearing by removing the bony partitions forming the mastoid cells.

**medical ethics**   values and decisions in medical practice including relationships to patient, patient family, peer physicians, and society.

**meiosis**   the process of reproduction of germ cells in which they divide before duplication.

**melena** (meh-LEE-nah)   dark tarry stool due to blood in feces.

**metacarpophalangeal** (meta=beyond, carpo=wrist, phalangeal=finger bones)   referring to the metacarpus and the phalanges; specifically, the articulations between them.

**metaplasia** (MET-ah-**PLAY**-zee-ah)   a cellular adaptation in which the cell changes to another type of cell.

**metastasis** (meh-TAS-tah-sis)   spreading to distant sites.

**metastasize** (meh-TAS-tah-sighz)   move or spread.

**metastatic** (MET-ah-**STAT**-ic)   moves from a site of origin to another secondary site in the body.

**metatarsophalangeal** (meta=between, tarso=foot, phalangeal=toe bones)   referring to the metatarsus and the phalanges; specifically, the articulations between them.

**microcephaly** (micro=small, cephal=brain)   having an abnormally small head; usually associated with mental retardation.

**mineralization**   a process that causes the characteristic hardness of bones.

**mineralocorticoids**   one group of steroids of the adrenal cortex that influences sodium and potassium metabolism.

**mitosis**   the process of reproduction of cells in which the 46 chromosomes duplicate and divide into two identical daughter cells, each containing 46 chromosomes.

**mood**   emotion.

**morbidity**   the state of being diseased.

**mortality**   the quality of being mortal or destined to die.

**motility**   ability to move.

**multiparity** (mul-TIP-ah-rah-tee)   multiple births.

**murmur**   an abnormal sound in the heart or vascular system.

**MVAs**   motor vehicle accidents.

**myelogram**   an X-ray picture taken after injecting dye into the spinal canal to reveal compression on the spinal cord or spinal nerves.

**myringotomy** (MIR-in-**GOT**-oh-me; myringo=eardrum, tomy= incision into)   incision into the eardrum to remove fluid.

**myxedema** (MECK-seh-**DEE**-mah)   advanced hypothyroidism in an adult.

**necrosis** (nee-CROW-sis)   cellular death.

**neoplasia** (nee-oh-PLAY-zee-ah)   the development of a new type of cell with an uncontrolled growth pattern.

**neoplasms** (new growths)   an increase in cell number, leading to an increase in tissue size; commonly called tumors.

**nephrectomy** (neh-FREC-toh-me; nephr=kidney, ectomy=excision or removal)   the surgical removal of the kidney.

**neutropenia**   a decrease in neutrophils.

**nits**   lice eggs.

**nocturia** (nock-TOO-ree-ah; noc=night, uria=urine)   excessive voiding at night.

**nondisplaced fracture**   one in which the fragments are still in correct position.

**nosocomial** (NOS-oh-**KOH**-me-al)   a disease acquired from the hospital environment.

**nuchal rigidity**   a stiffness in the neck that resists bending the neck forward or sideways.

**oblique fracture**   a fracture that runs in a transverse pattern.

**obsession**   repetition of a thought or emotion.

**occult blood**   hidden blood; unable to see except under microscopic examination.

**oliguria** (OL-ih-**GOO**-ree-ah; olig=scanty or few, uria=urine)   a decrease in urine output.

**oncology** (ong-KOL-oh-jee)   the study of tumors.

**oophoritis** (OH-of-oh-**RYE**-tis)   inflammation of the ovary.

**open (compound) fracture**   a fracture involving the bone puncturing through the skin, or an object puncturing the skin, making an opening through the skin to the fracture site.

**ophthalmoscope** (aft-THAL-moh-skope; ophthalm=eye, scope=instrument used to look)   the instrument used for a basic examination of the eye.

**opportunistic**   normal flora bacteria that take the "opportunity" to cause infection in the host.

**orchiectomy** (OR-kee-**ECK**-toh-me; orchi=testicle, ectomy= removal)   removal of the testicle(s).

**orchitis** (or-KYE-tis)   inflammation of a testis.

**organ rejection**   when the body recognizes an organ (after a transplant) as foreign and attacks it, leading to organ death.

**organic**   related to an organ or physical component.

**ORIF (Open-Reduction Internal Fixation)**   surgical opening over a fracture site, and internally fixing the fracture with plates, screws, or pins.

**orthopnea** (or-THOP-nee-ah; ortho=straight, pnea=breathing)   the condition in which an individual has difficulty breathing in a lying position, or is able to breathe with less difficulty when standing or sitting straight up.

**otalgia** (oh-TAL-gee-ah; oto=ear, algia=pain)   ear pain.

**otoscope** (OH-toh-skope; oto=ear, scope=instrument to look)   the instrument used to examine the ear.

**ova and parasite (O&P)**   an examination of a stool specimen for the presence of adult parasites or their eggs (ova).

**palliative** (PAL-ee-ay-tiv)   something that is directed toward relief of symptoms but does not cure.

**pallor** (PAL-or)   lack of color; paleness.

**palmar erythema** (ER-ih-**THEE**-mah)   unusual redness of the palms of the hands.

**palpation**   feeling lightly or by pressing firmly on internal organs or structures.

**pancytopenia** (pan=all, cyto=cell, penia=decrease)   severe decrease or total absence of erythrocytes, leukocytes, and thrombocytes.

**panhypopituitarism** (pan=all, hypo=decreased)   the condition in which the secretion of all anterior pituitary hormones is inadequate or absent; caused by a variety of disorders.

**panhysterectomy** (pan=all, hyster=uterus, ectomy=excision)   the surgical removal of the ovaries, fallopian tubes, and uterus.

**Pap test**   also called Papanicolaou test; a screening for cancer utilizing and examining the cells scraped from the cervical area.

**paralytic obstruction**   a decrease or absence of peristalsis that causes intestinal blockage.

**paraplegia** (PAR-ah-**PLEE**-jee-ah; para=beyond or two like parts, plegia=paralysis)   a loss of movement and feeling in the trunk and both legs.

**parenteral** (pah-REN-ter-al)   a delivery route for fluid or medications that may include subcutaneous, intramuscular, or intravenous administration.

**paresthesia** (PAR-es-**THEE**-see-ah)   abnormal sensation, burning, tingling, or numbness.

**paronychia** (PAR-oh-**NICK**-ee-ah)   an infection of the skin around the nail.

**parotid glands**   the salivary glands located just in front of the ears.

**paroxysmal** (PAR-ock-**SIZ**-mal)   spasm or convulsion.

**patency**   openness.

**patent**   open.

**pathogenesis** (PATH-oh-**JEN**-ah-sis; patho=disease, genesis= arising)   a description of how a particular disease progresses.

**pathogens** (PATH-oh-jens)   microorganisms or agents that cause disease.

**pathologic** (path-oh-LODGE-ick)   caused by a pathogen or a disease.

**pathologic fracture** (path-oh-LODGE-ick)   a fracture caused by weakness from another disease.

**pathologist** (pah-THOL-oh-jist; patho=disease, logist=one who studies)   one who studies disease.

**pathology** (pah-THOL-oh-jee; patho=disease, ology=study)   the study of disease.

**percussion** (per-KUSH-un)   tapping over various body areas to produce a vibrating sound.

**perforation**   an abnormal opening in an organ or tissue.

**perfusion** (per-FYOU-zuhn)   to pour through or supply with blood.

**peristalsis**   the contraction of muscles along the gastrointestinal tract to move food and fluid.

**peritonitis** (PER-ih-toe-**NIGH**-tis)   an inflammation of the peritoneum.

**petechiae** (pee-TEE-kee-ee)   small hemorrhages in the skin.

**petit mal**   a term applied to a type of seizure; these seizures consist of a brief change in the level of consciousness without convulsions; the involved individual may show symptoms of blank staring, blinking, and/or twitching of the eyes or mouth.

**phenotype**   the physical expression of a genetic trait such as eye, hair, and skin color.

**phimosis** (figh-MOH-sis)   abnormally tight foreskin of the penis.

**photophobia** (photo=light, phobia=fear)   an abnormal fear of light.

**pilonidal cyst** (PYE-loh-**NIGH**-dal)   a particular type of sebaceous cyst found in the midline of the sacral area.

**plaque** (PLACK)   a patch; dental plaque is a sticky mass of microorganisms growing on teeth.

**pneumocystis carinii** (NEW-moh-**SIS**-tis kah-RYE-nee-eye) **pneumonia**   a protozoan infection of the lungs, commonly occurring in immunodeficient individuals.

**polydipsia** (POL-ee-**DIP**-see-ah; poly=many, dipsia=thirst or drinking)   excessive thirst.

**polyp** (POL-ip)   an inward projection of the mucosal lining of the colon.

**polyuria** (POL-ee-**YOU**-ree-ah; poly=many, uria=urine)   excessive urination.

**portal hypertension**   increased pressure in the portal system frequently seen in cirrhosis.

**Pott's fracture**   fracture of the lower part of the fibula and tibia, with outward displacement of the foot.

**precocious (puberty)**   premature (early) sexual development.

**predisposing factors**   also known as risk factors; make a person more susceptible to disease.

**preeclampsia** (PREE-ee-**KLAMP**-see-ah)   the development of hypertension with proteinuria and/or edema due to pregnancy; also called toxemia.

**prevalent**   occurring more often.

**preventive**   something that reduces risk.

**primary union**   also called healing by first intention; involves approximating the edges of the wound.

**primigravid** (PRE-mih-**GRAV**-id; primi=first, gravid=pregnancy)   the term used to describe a female who is pregnant with her first child.

**productive cough**   coughing up sputum or excessive mucus.

**progesterone** (pro-**JESS**-ter-ohn)   a female sex hormone produced by the ovary.

**prognosis** (prawg-KNOW-sis)   the predicted or expected outcome of the disease.

**prone**   positioned face down on the stomach.

**prophylactic** (pro-fil-LACK-tic)   something that works to prevent.

**prosthesis** (pros-THEE-sis)   an artificial part.

**proteinuria**   protein in the urine; specific protein or albumin, may be identified, resulting in albuminuria.

**protozoa**   a parasite of the phylum Protozoa; a single-celled microscopic member of the animal kingdom.

**pruritus** (proo-RYE-tus)   itching.

**puerperal** (pyou-ER-pier-al)   relating to childbirth.

**purpura** (PER-pew-rah)   a bleeding disorder characterized by bleeding into the skin and mucus membranes initially turning the affected areas purplish in color.

**purulent** (PURR-you-lent)   loaded with dead and dying neutrophils, tissue debris, and pyogenic (pus-forming) bacteria.

**pus**   white or yellow exudate due to death of numerous neutrophils mixed with exudate or blood fluid.

**pustules** (PUS-tyoul)   small, pus filled lesions.

**pyloromyotomy** (pyloro=pyloric, myo=muscle, otomy=cut into)   a surgical procedure that involves incising and suturing the pyloric sphincter muscle.

**pyoderma** (PYE-oh-**DER**-mah)   inflammatory, purulent dermatitis.

**pyogenic** (PIE-oh-**JEN**-ick; pyo=pus, genic=arising)   pus forming.

**pyuria** (pye-YOU-ree-ah; py=pus, uria=urine)   pus in the urine.

**quadriplegia** (KWAD-rih-**PLEE**-jee-ah; quadri=four, plegia=paralysis)   the loss of movement and feeling in the trunk and all four extremities with the accompanying loss of bowel, bladder, and sexual function.

**radial keratotomy** (KER-ah-**TOT**-oh-me; kerato=cornea, otomy=incision)   a surgical procedure to correct myopia; incisions are made in a radial fashion in the cornea to flatten the cornea, thus shortening the length of the eyeball and correcting the refractive error.

**radiation**   the process of using light, short-waves, ultraviolet or X-rays, or any other rays.

**radical cystectomy** (radical=a treatment that seeks to cure, aggressive, not paliative or conservative, sis-TECT-toh-me, cyst=bladder, ectomy=excision or removal)   the removal of the entire bladder, usually done as treatment for cancer of the bladder.

**radiologic**   relating to medical imaging using X-rays, ionizing radiation, nuclear magnetic resonance, or ultrasound.

**rales** (RALZ)   an abnormal discontinuous breath sound caused by narrowed bronchi and heard primarily on inspiration during auscultation of the chest.

**recessive**   lacking control; weak.

**Reed-Sternberg cell**   a large connective tissue cell found in lymphatic tissue indicative of Hodgkin's disease.

**remission**   a time when symptoms are diminished or temporarily resolved.

**rhinitis** (RYE-**NIGH**-tis)   inflammation of the nasal mucous membrane.

**rhinorrhea** (rhino=nose, orrhea=run through)   a runny nose.

**rhonchi** (RONG-kigh)   abnormal wheezing breath sounds caused by partial airway blockage and heard during inspiration, expiration or both during auscultation of the chest.

**RICE**   acronym for Rest, Ice, Compression, and Elevation, the activities to manage soft tissue trauma like those often associated with sports injuries.

**rickettsiae** (ric-KET-see-ah)   microscopic organisms that are intermediate between bacteria and viruses. They live in the host and are spread by lice, fleas, ticks, and mites.

**RPR (Rapid Plasma Reagin)**   a blood test for syphilis.

**salmonella** (SAL-moh-**NEL**-ah)   a group of gram-negative bacteria often responsible for intestinal infections.

**salpingitis** (SAL-pin-**JIGH**-tis; salping=fallopian tube, itis=inflammation)   inflammation of the fallopian tube.

**sarcoma** (sar–KO–mah)   a malignant neoplasm arising from connective tissue.

**scar**   skin lesion resulting from fibrous connective tissue repair.

**sciatica**   pain along the sciatic nerve, often radiating down the leg and caused by pressure on the spinal nerve.

**sebum**   oil produced by the sebaceous glands.

**secondary union**   also called healing by secondary intention; the same process as primary union, but involves a larger degree of tissue damage and more inflammation to resolve.

**seizure**   a sudden onset or attack, but it is commonly used to indicate a convulsive seizure as occurs in epilespy.

**self-antigen**   the body's own antigen.

**septicemia** (SEP-tih-**SEE**-me-ah; septic=dirty, contaminated, emia=blood)   a systemic disease caused by the spread of microorganisms in the blood; also called "blood poisoning."

**signs**   observable or measurable factors used to determine a diagnosis.

**simple (closed) fracture**   a fracture that does not break through the skin.

**sinus**   a tract or opening to the surface of the body formed by a large ruptured abscess.

**somatic**   related to the body.

**spasms**   uncontrolled muscle contractions.

**spider angiomas**   telangiectasis or small dilated vessels in the skin; commonly seen on the face and chest of individuals with cirrhosis of the liver.

**spinal stenosis** (stenosis=narrowing)   the condition of narrowing of nerve root openings in the spinal column.

**spiral fracture**   a fracture that twists around the bone.

**splenomegaly** (SPLEE-no-**MEG**-ah-lee)   enlargement of the spleen.

**sputum** (SPYOU-tum)   fluid or secretions coughed up from the lungs.

**staging**   determining the degree of spread of a malignant tumor.

**stapedectomy** (STAY-peh-**DECK**-toh-me; stape=stapes, ectomy =removal or excision)   a procedure that removes the stapes bone in the middle ear and replaces it with a prosthesis.

**status asthmaticus** (AZTH-**MAH**-ti-kus)   a severe asthma attack that lasts for several days.

**status epilepticus**   a life-threatening event; a state of continued convulsive seizure with no recovery of consciousness; it is a medical emergency.

**stellate fracture**   a fracture that forms a star-like pattern.

**sterility**   inability to impregnate a female related to sperm quality or quantity.

**stool**   fecal matter; feces; bowel movement (BM).

**strep throat**   an acute form of pharyngitis caused by *Streptococcus*.

**streptococcal** (**STREHP**-toh-KAHK-al)   relating to the organism *Streptococcus*; an anaerobic, gram-positive bacteria.

**stress fracture**   related to too much weight or pressure.

**striae**   stretch marks on the skin.

**stricture**   a narrowing.

**subcapital fracture**   a fracture below (sub) the head (caput) of the femur.

**subdural (hematoma)** (SUB-**DOO**-ral)   blood collecting between the outer (dura mater) layer and the middle (arachnoid) layer of the meninges.

**supine** (SUE-pine)   positioned on the back.

**suppurative** (SUP-you-**RAY**-tive)   formation of pus.

**suprapubic catheter**   a catheter that is inserted surgically through the pelvic wall as is often done after urinary tract surgeries.

**symptoms**   what patients report as their problem or problems.

**syncope** (SIN-koh-pee)   fainting.

**syndrome** (SIN-drome)   a group of symptoms that may be caused by a specific disease but also may be caused by several interrelated problems.

**systemic**   refers to the entire or whole body rather than to a part or region.

**systolic** (sis-TALL-ick)   relating to cardiac systole; the process of cardiac contraction (heartbeat) when blood is ejected into the systemic circulation.

**tachycardia** (TACH-ee-**KAR**-dee-ah; tachy=rapid, cardia=heart rate)   a rapid heart rate; usually a rate over 100 beats per minute.

**tachypnea** (TACK-ihp-**NEE**-ah; tachy=rapid, pnea=breathing) a severely increased respiratory rate.

**tetany** (TET-ah-nee)   hyperirritability of muscles causing a spasm-like condition; usually the result of a lack of calcium.

**thoracentesis** (THOR-rah-sen-**TEE**-sis; thora=chest, centesis= puncture)   a procedure in which a puncture is made into the chest cavity to withdraw air (or fluid); a chest tube also may be inserted to help the lung reexpand.

**thrombocytopenia** (THROM-boh-SIGH-toh-**PEE**-nee-ah; thrombocyte=platelet, penia=decrease)   a decrease in platelets, leading to a coagulation problem.

**thrombocytosis** (THROM-boh-sigh-**TOH**-sis; thrombocyte= platelet, osis=condition of)   an increase in platelets.

**thrombus** (THROM-bus)   a blood clot attached to a vein or artery.

**thyroid storm**   a sudden life-threatening exacerbation of all symptoms of hyperthyroidism.

**tinnitus** (tin-EYE-tus)   ringing in the ears.

**tolerance**   the ability to endure a larger amount of a substance without an adverse effect, or the need for a larger amount or dose of the drug to have the same effect.

**tonometry** (toh-NOM-eh-tree; tono=tone or pressure, metry=measurement)   a procedure to measure the pressure inside the eye.

**tonsillectomy** (TON-sih-**LECT**-toh-me; ectomy=removal)   the surgical removal of the tonsils.

**tophi**   small, whitish nodules of uric acid.

**topical**   placed on the skin.

**TPN**   total parenteral nutrition; intravenously giving a special solution that meets the total nutritional needs of the individual.

**transurethral resection (TUR)** (trans=through, urethral= uretha; resection=partial excision)   a surgical procedure that may be performed to remove a tumor, visualize a structure, or take a piece of tissue for biopsy; a cystoscope is passed through the urinary meatus and the urethra for this procedure.

**transverse fracture**   one that runs across or at a 90-degree angle.

**trauma** (TRAW-mah)   a physical or mental injury.

**triage** (tree-AUZH)   the prioritizing of care.

**trichomonas** (TRICK-oh-**MOH**-nas)   a parasitic protozoan that commonly infects the vagina and causes trichomoniasis.

**tumor**   "swelling" or growth, originally used in the description of the swelling related to inflammation.

**tympanoplasty** (TIM-pah-no-**PLAS**-tee; tympano=eardrum, plasty=surgical correction)   surgery to repair the tympanic membrane.

**tympanostomy** (TIM-pan-**OSS**-toh-me; tympano=eardrum, ostomy=new opening)   a procedure in which tubes, commonly called PE tubes or pediatric ear tubes, are placed through the tympanic membrane to prevent the accumulation of fluid.

**ulcer**   a crater-like lesion in the skin or mucous membranes.

**undifferentiated**   change in a cell that is more general or appears more malignant; not clearly or easily identified.

**urea**   a common nitrogenous waste product that is normally filtered from the blood.

**uremia** (you-REE-me-ah; ur=urine, emia=blood)   a toxic condition of the blood due to high levels of waste products.

**urgency**   the severe need to urinate.

**urinalysis** (YOU-rih-**NAL**-ih-sis; urine analysis)   a laboratory urine tests for pH, specific gravity, protein, glucose or sugar, and blood; it also includes a microscopic examination to determine the presence of bacteria, crystals, and casts.

**urine culture and sensitivity (C&S)**   a laboratory analysis that determines the type of bacteria present and the most effective antibiotic to prescribe for treatment.

**urticaria** (UR-tih-**KAR**-ree-ah)   an allergic reaction resulting in a skin eruption of wheals that causes intense itching.

**vasopressin**   antidiuretic hormone (ADH) secreted by the posterior portion of the pituitary gland.

**VDRL (Venereal Disease Research Laboratory)**   a blood test to screen for syphilis.

**vermiform** (VER-my-form)   worm-like.

**vertigo** (VER-tih-go)   dizziness.

**vesicles** (VES-ih-kuls)   blister-like eruptions on the skin.

**virilism** (VIR-ill-izm)   masculinization; used to describe the occurrence or presence of male characteristics in a female or prepubescent male.

**virulent** (VIR-u-lent; infectious)   difficult to kill; able to produce disease.

**viruses**   a large group of infectious agents; they are much smaller than bacteria and must be viewed with an electron microscope. They can pass through fine filters that would retain most bacteria.

**viscous** (VIS-cuss)   thick.

**volvulus** (VOL-view-lus)   the bowel twisted on itself.

**wheal(s)**   round, slightly reddened, spot(s) on the skin, usually accompanied by intense itching; also called urticarial lesion(s) or hives; caused by an allergic reaction to something such as food or medication.

**wheezing**   a whistling, musical, or raspy sound during breathing, usually indicative of partially blocked respiratory passages.

**withdrawal**   the unpleasant physical and psychological effects resulting from stopping the use of a substance after an individual is addicted.

**xerosis** (zee-ROE-sis)   dry skin.

# The Most Commonly Prescribed Medications*

**Drugs in lowercase italics are generic names.**

| Drug Name | Other Name | Drug Classification | Manufacturer |
|---|---|---|---|
| Accupril | *quinapril* | Antihypertensive | Parke-Davis |
| Accutane | *isotretinoin* | Anti-acne | Roche Labs |
| Aciphex | *rabeprazole* | Anti-ulcer | Eisai |
| Actonel | Risedronate | Used in the treatment of osteoporosis | Aventis Pharmaceuticals |
| Actos | *pioglitazone* | Non-insulin dependent diabetes Tx | Takeda/Eli Lilly |
| Adalat CC | *nifedipine* | Antihypertensive | Bayer Pharmaceuticals |
| Adderall | *dextroamphetamine + racemic amphetamine* | CNS stimulant | Shire Richwood |
| Advair | Fluticasone/ salmeterol | Anti-asthmatic, bronchodilator | GlaxoSmithKline |
| *albuterol* | Ventolin; Proventil | Anti-asthmatic, bronchodilator | Various, e.g., Warrick |
| Alinia | *nitazoxanide* | Used in the treatment of diarrhea | Romark Laboratories |
| Allegra | *fexofenadine* | Antihistamine—non-sedating | Aventis Pharmaceuticals |
| Allegra-D | *fexofenadine + pseudoephidrine* | Antihistamine + decongestant | Aventis Pharmaceuticals |
| *alprazolam* | Xanax | Sedative, hypnotic, benzodiazepine | Various, e.g., Greenstone |

*From Heller, M. E., & Krebs, C. (2004). *Clinical handbook for the medical office* (2nd ed.) (pp. 176–186). Clifton Park, NY: Thomson Delmar Learning.

*(continues)*

| Drug Name | Other Name | Drug Classification | Manufacturer |
|---|---|---|---|
| Amaryl | *glimepiride* | Non-insulin dependent diabetes Tx | Aventis Pharmaceuticals |
| Ambien | *zolpidem* | Sedative, hypnotic | Pharmacia |
| *amitriptyline HCl* | Elavil | antidepressant | Various, e.g., Geneva |
| *amoxicillin* | Amoxil; Polymox; Trimox | Antibiotic | Varous, e.g.,Teva |
| Amoxil | *amoxicillin* | Antibiotic | GlaxoSmithKline |
| *APAP w/ CDN (acetaminophen with codeine)* | Lortab and Vicodin | Narcotic analgesic | Various, e.g.,Teva |
| *atenolol* | Tenormin | Antihypertensive | Various, e.g.,Watson |
| Atrovent | *ipratropium* | Anti-asthmatic, bronchodilator | Boehringer Ingelheim |
| Augmentin | *amoxicillin—clavulanate* | Antibiotic | GlaxoSmithKline |
| Avandamet | *rosiglitazone/ metformin* | Non-insulin dependent diabetes Tx | GlaxoSmithKline |
| Avodart | *dutasteride* | Used in the treatment of BPH | GlaxoSmithKline |
| Avandia | *rosiglitazone* | Non-insulin dependent diabetes Tx | GlaxoSmithKline |
| Azmacort | *triamcinolone acetonide* | Inhaled corticosteroid and anti-asthmatic | Aventis Pharmaceuticals |
| Bactroban | *mupirocin* | Topical antibacterial | GlaxoSmithKline |
| Benicar | *olmesartan medoxomil* | Antihypertensive | Forest Pharmaceuticals |
| Benzamycin | *erythromycin + benzoyl peroxide* | Anti-acne | Dermik |
| Biaxin | *clarithromycin* | Antibiotic | Abbott |
| *bisoprolol + HCTZ (hydrochlorothiazide)* | Ziac | Antihypertensive, diuretic | Various, e.g.,Watson |
| *buspirone* | BuSpar | Anti-anxiety, hypnotic | Various, e.g., PAR |
| Cardura | *doxazosine* | Antihypertensive | Pfizer |
| *carisoprodol* | Soma | Muscle relaxer | Various, e.g.,Watson |
| Cartia XT | *diltiazem* | Antihypertensive | Andrx |
| Ceftin | *cefuroxime* | Antibiotic | GlaxoSmithKline |
| Cefzil | *cefprozil* | Antibiotic | Bristol-Myers Squibb |
| Celebrex | *celecoxib* | NSAID | Pharmacia |
| Celexa | *citalopram* | Antidepressant | Forest Pharmaceuticals |

| Drug Name | Other Name | Drug Classification | Manufacturer |
| --- | --- | --- | --- |
| *cephalexin* | Keflex; Keftab | Antibiotic | Various, e.g., Ranboxy |
| Ciloxan | *ciprofloxacin* | Antibiotic (ophthalmic drops) | Alcon |
| Cipro | *ciprofloxacin* | Antibiotic | Bayer Pharmaceuticals |
| Claritin | *loratidine* | Antihistamine— nonsedating | Schering |
| Claritin-D 12 | *loratidine + pseudoephidrine* | Antihistamine + decongestant | Schering |
| Claritin-D 24 | *loratidine + pseudoephidrine* | Antihistamine + decongestant | Schering |
| Claritin Reditabs | *loratidine* | Antihistamine— nonsedating | Schering |
| Clarinex | *desloratadine* | Antihistamine— nonsedating | Schering |
| *clindamycin* | Cleocin | Antibiotic | Various, e.g., Watson |
| *clonazepam* | Klonopin | Sedative, hypnotic, benzodiazepine | Various, e.g., Purpec |
| *clonidine* | Catapres | Antihypertensive | Various, e.g., Mylan |
| Combivent | *albuterol + ipratropium* | Anti-asthmatic, bronchodilator | Boehringer Ingelheim |
| Coumadin | *warfarin* | Anticoagulant | DuPont |
| Cozaar | *losartan* | Antihypertensive | Merck |
| *cyclobenzaprine* | Flexeril | Muscle relaxer | Various, e.g., Watson |
| Depakote | *valproic acid* | Antiseizure, antimanic | Abbott |
| Detrol | *tolterodine* | Bladder agent; vasopressor | Pharmacia |
| *diazepam* | Valium | Anti-anxiety | Various, e.g., Mylan |
| Diflucan | *fluconazole* | Antifungal | Pfizer |
| Dilantin | *phenytoin* | Anticonvulsant | Parke-Davis |
| Diovan | *valsartan* | Antihypertensive | Novartis |
| *doxycycline* | Vibramycin; Doryx; Doxycin | Antibiotic | Various, e.g., Watson |
| Duragesic | *fentanyl* | Narcotic analgesic | Janssen |
| Effexor XR | *venlafaxine* | Antidepressant, anti-anxiety | Wyeth-Ayerst |
| Elocon | *mometasone furoate* | Topical corticosteroid | Schering |
| *enalapril* | Vasotec | Antihypertensive | Various, e.g., PAR |
| Endocet | *oxycodone + acetaminophen* | Narcotic analgesic | Endo Generics |

*(continues)*

| Drug Name | Other Name | Drug Classification | Manufacturer |
|---|---|---|---|
| Ery-Tab | *erythromycin* | Antibiotic | Abbott |
| Evista | *raloxifene* | Osteoporosis prevention and Tx | Eli Lilly |
| famotidine | Pepcid | Anti-ulcer | Various, e.g., PAR |
| Flomax | *tamsulosin* | Used in the treatment of BPH | Boehringer Ingelheim |
| Flonase | *fluticasone* | Nasal corticosteroid for allergic and nonallergic rhinitis | GlaxoSmithKline |
| Flovent | *fluticasone* | Anti-asthmatic, inhaled corticosteroid | GlaxoSmithKline |
| *fluoxetine* | Prozac | Antidepressant | Various, e.g., PAR |
| Fosamax | *alendronate* | Osteoporosis prevention and Tx | Merck |
| *furosemide* | Lasix | Diuretic | Various, e.g., Mylan |
| Glucophage | *metformin* | Non-insulin dependent diabetes Tx | Bristol-Myers Squibb |
| Glucotrol XL | *glipizide* | Non-insulin dependent diabetes Tx | Pfizer |
| Glucovance | *glyburide/metformin* | Non-insulin dependent diabetes Tx | Bristol-Myers Squibb |
| *glyburide* | Micronase, Diabeta, Glynase | Non-insulin dependent diabetes Tx | Various, e.g., Teva |
| *hydrocodone w/APAP (acetaminophen)* | Lorcet, Lortab | Narcotic analgesic | Various, e.g., Watson |
| *hydrochlorothiazide (HCTZ)* | Oretic, Microzide, Esidrix | Diuretic | Various, e.g., Watson |
| Hyzaar | *losartan + HCTZ* | Antihypertensive and diuretic | Merck |
| *ibuprofen* | Motrin, Advil, Nuprin, Rufen | NSAID | Various, e.g., PAR |
| Imitrex | *sumatriptan* | Migraine Tx | GlaxoSmithKline |
| Inspra | *eplerenone* | Antihypertensive | Pharmacia |
| *isosorbide mononitrate* | Imdur; ISMO | Anti-anginal | Various, e.g., Warrick |
| K-Dur | *potassium chloride* | Potassium supplement | Key Pharmaceuticals |
| Lanoxin | *digoxin* | Anti-arrhythmic | GlaxoSmithKline |
| Levaquin | *levofloxacin* | Antibiotic | McNeil Pharmaceuticals |

| Drug Name | Other Name | Drug Classification | Manufacturer |
|---|---|---|---|
| Levothroid | *levothyroxine* | Thyroid hormone replacement Tx | Forest Pharmaceuticals |
| Levoxyl | *levothyroxine* | Thyroid hormone replacement Tx | Jones Medical Industries |
| Lexapro | *escitalopram oxalate* | Antidepressant | Forest Pharmaceuticals |
| Lipitor | *atorvastatin* | Antihyperlipidemic | Parke-Davis |
| lisinopril | Prinivil and Zestril | Antihypertensive | Various, e.g., Mylan |
| *lorazepam* | Ativan | Sedative, hypnotic, benzodiazepine | Various, e.g., Ranbaxy |
| Lotensin | *benazepril* | Antihypertensive | Novartis |
| Lotrel | *amlodipine + benazepril* | Antihypertensive | Novartis |
| Lotrisone | *clotrimazole + betamethasone* | Topical corticosteroid | Key Pharmaceuticals |
| Macrobid | *nitrofurantoin* | Antibiotic | Procter & Gamble |
| *medroxyprogesterone* | Provera and Cycrin | Hormone replacement Tx | Various, e.g., Greenstone |
| Metaglip | *glipizide/metformin* | Non-insulin dependent diabetes Tx | Bristol-Myers Squibb |
| *methylphenidate* | Ritalin; Ritalin-SR | CNS stimulant | Various, e.g., Geneva |
| *methylprednisolone* | Medrol, Solu-Medrol, Depo-Medrol | Oral corticosteroid | Various, e.g., Barr |
| *metoprolol tartrate* | Lopressor | Antihypertensive | Various, e.g., Mylan |
| Metrogel (vaginal) | *metronidazole* | Antibacterial | Galderma |
| *metronidazole* | Metrogel and MetroLotion | Antibacterial | Galderma |
| Miacalcin | *calcitonin-salmon* | Osteoporosis prevention and Tx | Novartis |
| Monopril | *fosinopril* | Antihypertensive | Bristol-Myers Squibb |
| *nabumetone* | Relafen | NSAID | Various, e.g., PAR |
| *naproxen* | Naprosyn | NSAID | Various, e.g., Watson |
| *naproxen sodium* | Aleve and Anaprox | NSAID | Various, e.g., Teva |
| Nasonex | *mometasone* | Nasal corticosteroid for allergic and nonallergic rhinitis | Schering |
| *neomycin, polymyxin, hydrocortisone* | Cortisporin | Steroidal antibiotic | Various, e.g., Bausch & Lomb |

*(continues)*

| Drug Name | Other Name | Drug Classification | Manufacturer |
|---|---|---|---|
| Neurontin | *gabapentin* | Anticonvulsant, antimanic | Parke-Davis |
| *Nexium* | Esomeprazole | Anti-ulcer | AstraZeneca |
| nifedipine | Procardia XL | Antihypertensive | Various, e.g., Teva |
| Nitroquick | *nitroglycerin sublingual (SL)* | Antianginal | Ethex |
| Norvasc | *amlodipine* | Antihypertensive | Pfizer |
| Ocuflox | *ofloxacin* | Antibiotic (ophthalmic drops) | Allergan |
| *omeprazole* | Prilosec | Antiulcer | Various, e.g., Kremers Urban |
| Ortho Evra | *norelgestromin/ ethinyl estradiol* | Contraceptive patch | Ortho-McNeil Pharmaceuticals |
| Ortho Tri-Cyclen 28 | *norelgestromin/ ethinyl estradiol* | Oral contraceptive | Ortho-McNeil Pharmaceuticals |
| *oxycodone with APAP (acetaminophen)* | Percocet, Roxicet, Tylox | Narcotic analgesic | Various, e.g., Mallinckrodt |
| OxyContin | *oxycodone* | Narcotic analgesic | Purdue Pharmaceuticals |
| Paxil | *paroxetine* | Antidepressant | GlaxoSmithKline |
| Patanol | *olopatadine* | Antihistamine (ophthalmic drops) | Alcon |
| *penicillin VK* | Pen-Vee K; Veetids | Antibiotic | Various, e.g., Teva |
| Pepcid | *famotidine* | Anti-ulcer | Merck |
| Percocet | *oxycodone with APAP (acetaminophen)* | Narcotic analgesic | Endo Labs |
| Phenergan | *promethazine* | Anti-emetic | Wyeth-Ayerst |
| Plavix | *clopidogrel* | Antiplatelet | Bristol-Myers Squibb and Sanofi Pharmaceuticals |
| *potassium chloride* | K-Dur, Klor-Con, Slow-K, Micro-K | Potassium supplement | Various, e.g., Ethex |
| Pravachol | *pravastatin* | Antihyperlipidemic | Bristol-Myers |
| *prednisone* | Deltasone; Pred-Pak | Oral corticosteroid | Various, e.g., Watson |
| Premarin | *estrogens conjugated* | Hormone replacement Tx | Wyeth-Ayerst |
| Prempro | *conjugated estrogens + medroxy- progesterone* | Hormone replacement Tx | Wyeth-Ayerst |
| Prevacid | *lansoprazole* | Anti-ulcer | Tap |

| Drug Name | Other Name | Drug Classification | Manufacturer |
|---|---|---|---|
| Prilosec | *omeprazole* | Anti-ulcer | AstraZeneca |
| Prinivil | *lisinopril* | Antihypertensive | Merck |
| Procardia XL | *nifedipine* | Antihypertensive | Pfizer |
| *promethazine* | Phenergan | Anti-emetic | Various, e.g., Geneva |
| *promethazine with codeine* | Phenergan w/ Codeine | Decongestant, anti-histamine, antitussive | Various, e.g., Alpharma |
| *propoxyphene-N w/ APAP (acetaminophen)* | Darvocet-N | Narcotic analgesic | Various, e.g., Mylan |
| Proventil HFA | *albuterol* | Anti-asthmatic and bronchodilator | Key Pharmaceuticals |
| Prozac | *fluoxetine* | Antidepressant | Lilly Pharmaceuticals |
| *ranitidine* | Zantac | Anti-ulcer | Various, e.g., Apotex |
| Relafen | *nabumetone* | NSAID | GlaxoSmithKline |
| Remeron | *mirtazapine* | Antidepressant | Organon |
| Risperdal | *risperidone* | Antipsychotic | Janssen |
| Ritalin | *methylphenidate* | CNS stimulant | Novartis |
| Roxicet | *oxycodone with APAP* | Narcotic analgesic | Roxane |
| Serevent | *salmeterol* | Anti-asthmatic and bronchodilator | GlaxoSmithKline |
| Serzone | *nefazodone* | Antidepressant | Bristol-Myers Squibb |
| Singulair | *montelukast* | Anti-asthmatic | Merck |
| Skelaxin | *metaxalone* | Muscle relaxer | Carnrick |
| Strattera | atomoxetine HCl | Used in the treatment of ADHD | Eli Lilly |
| *sulfamethoxazole w/ trimethoprim (SMX/TMP)* | Bactrim, Cotrim, Septra, Sulfatrim | Antibiotic | Various, e.g., Teva |
| Synthroid | *levothyroxine* | Thyroid hormone replacement Tx | Knoll Pharmaceuticals |
| *temazepam* | Restoril | Sedative, hypnotic, benzodiazepine | Various, e.g., Mylan |
| Tequin | *gatifloxacin* | Antibiotic | Bristol-Myers |
| Terazol 7 | *terconazole* | Antifungal (vaginal) | Ortho-McNeil Pharmaceuticals |
| *terazosin* | Hytrin | Prostate enlargement Tx | Various, e.g., Geneva |
| TobraDex | *tobramycin + dexamethasone* | Steroidal antibiotic | Alcon |

*(continues)*

| Drug Name | Other Name | Drug Classification | Manufacturer |
|---|---|---|---|
| Toprol-XL | *metoprolol* | Antihypertensive | AstraZeneca |
| *tramadol* | Ultram | Analgesic | Various, e.g., Mylan |
| *triamterene w/ HCTZ* | Dyazide | Antihypertensive, diuretic | Various, e.g., Mylan |
| Trimox | *amoxicillin* | Antibiotic | Apothecon |
| Tussionex | *hydrocodone + chlorpheniramine* | Narcotic antitussive | Medeva |
| Ultram | *tramadol* | Analgesic | Ortho-McNeil Pharmaceuticals |
| Valtrex | *valacyclovir* | Antiviral, antiherpetic | GlaxoSmithKline |
| Vasotec | *enalapril* | Antihypertensive | Merck |
| *verapamil SR* | Calan SR, Isoptin SR, Verelan | Antihypertensive | Various, e.g., Mylan |
| Viagra | *sildenafil* | Erectile dysfunction Tx | Pfizer |
| Vicoprofen | *hydrocodone + ibuprofen* | Narcotic analgesic | Knoll |
| Vioxx | *rofecoxib* | NSAID | Merck |
| *warfarin sodium* | Coumadin | Anticoagulant | Various, e.g., Barr |
| Wellbutrin SR | *bupropion* | Antidepressant | GlaxoSmithKline |
| Xalatan | *latanoprost* | Antiglaucoma | Pharmacia |
| Zelnorm | tegaserod maleate | Used in the treatment of irritable bowel syndrome | Novartis |
| Zestril | *lisinopril* | Antihypertensive | AstraZeneca |
| Zetia | ezetimibe | Used in the treatment of hypercholesterolemia | Merck/Shering-Plough |
| Ziac | *bisoprolol + HCTZ (hydrochlorothiazide)* | Antihypertensive, diuretic | Lederle |
| Zithromax | *azithromycin* | Antibiotic | Pfizer |
| Zocor | *simvastatin* | Antihyperlipidemic | Merck |
| Zoloft | *sertraline* | Antidepressant | Pfizer |
| Zyprexa | *olanzapine* | Antipsychotic | Eli Lilly |
| Zyrtec | *cetirizine* | Antihistamine | Pfizer |

# References

The following references have been used throughout this text and therefore were not listed in the bibliography of any particular chapter:

Austen, K. F., Frank, M. M., Atkinson, J. P., & Canton, H. (2001). *Samter's immunologic diseases, Vol I* (6th ed.). Philadelphia: Williams and Wilkins.

Barry, P. D. (2001). *Mental health and illness* (6th ed.) Philadelphia: Lippincott.

Birrer, R. B., & O'Connor, F. G. (2004) *Sports medicine for the primary care physician* (3rd ed.). Boca Raton, FL: CRC Press.

Braunwald, E., Jameson, J. L., & Kasper, D. L. (2001). *Harrison's principles of internal medicine*. New York: McGraw Hill.

Coggins, C. H. (2001). *Annual review of medicine: Selected topics in the clinical sciences* (vol. 52). Palo Alto, CA: Annual Reviews, Inc.

Daniels, R. (2002). *Delmar's guide to laboratory and diagnostic tests*. Clifton Park, NY: Thomson Delmar Learning.

Ehrlich, A. (2000). *Medical terminology for health professions* (4th ed.). Clifton Park, NY: Thomson Delmar Learning.

Fong, E., & Scott, A. S. (2004). *Body structures and functions* (10th ed.). Clifton Park, NY: Thomson Delmar Learning.

Leifer, G. (2002). *Introduction to maternity and pediatric nursing* (4th ed.). Philadelphia: Saunders.

Lueckenotte, A. G. (2000). *Gerontologic nursing,* (2nd ed.). St. Louis, MO: Mosby.

Mader, S. (2000). *Understanding human anatomy and physiology* (4th ed.). New York: McGraw Hill.

Marieb, E. N. (2002). *Essentials of human anatomy and physiology* (7th ed.). San Francisco: Benjamin/Cummings.

McCance, K. L., & Huether, S. E. (2001). *Pathophysiology: The biological basis for disease in adults and children*. St. Louis, MO: Mosby.

Mulvihill, M. L., Holdaway, P., Tompary, E., & Turchany, T. (2001). *Human diseases: A systemic approach* (5th ed.). East Norwalk, CT: Appleton and Lange.

Neeb, K. (2001). *Fundamentals of mental health nursing*. Philadelphia: F. A. Davis.

Nettina, S. M. (2001). *Lippincott manual of nursing practice* (7th ed.). Philadelphia: Lippincott Williams and Wilkins.

Phipps, W. J., Monahan, F. D., Sands, J. K., Marek, J. F., & Neighbors, M. (2003). *Medical-surgical nursing health and illness perspectives* (7th ed.). St. Louis, MO: Mosby.

Porth, C. M. (2004). *Essentials of pathophysiology concepts of altered states*. Philadelphia: Lippincott Williams & Wilkins.

Price, S. A., & Wilson, L. M. (2002). *Pathophysiology: Clinical concepts of disease processes* (6th ed.). St. Louis, MO: Mosby.

Scherer, J. C., & Timby, B. K. (1998). *Introductory medical-surgical nursing* (7th ed.). Philadelphia: Lippincott.

Shier, D., Butler, J., & Lewis, R. (2002). *Hole's essentials of human anatomy and physiology* (8th ed.) New York: McGraw Hill.

Spratto, G. R., & Woods, A. L. (2004). *PDR nurse's drug handbook* (2004 ed.). Clifton Park, NY: Thomson Delmar Learning.

Thibodeau, G. A. (2003). *Structure and function of the body* (11th ed.). St. Louis, MO: Mosby.

Thibodeau, G. A., & Patton, K. T. (2001). *The human body in health and disease* (3rd ed.). St. Louis, MO: Mosby.

Tierney, L. M., McPhee, S. J., & Papadakis, M. A. (2003). *Current medical diagnosis and treatment*. Stanford, CT: Appleton and Lange.

Venes, D., & Thomas, C. L. (2001). *Taber's cyclopedic medical dictionary* (19th ed.). Philadelphia: F. A. Davis.

Walden-Temparo, C. D., & Lewis, M. A. (2002). *Diseases of the human body* (3rd ed.). Philadelphia: F. A. Davis.

Way, L. W., & Doherty, G. M. (2002). *Current surgical diagnosis and treatment*. Stanford, CT: Appleton and Lange.